Physiotherapy and Rehabilitation in Pelvic and Women's Health-Related Problems

Türkan Akbayrak • Esra Üzelpasaci
Editors

Physiotherapy and Rehabilitation in Pelvic and Women's Health-Related Problems

A Multidisciplinary Approach

Springer

Editors

Türkan Akbayrak
Faculty of Physical Therapy and Rehabilitation
Hacettepe University
Ankara, Türkiye

Esra Üzelpasaci
Gülhane Faculty of Physiotherapy Rehabilitation
University of Health Sciences
Ankara, Türkiye

ISBN 978-3-032-28740-3 ISBN 978-3-032-28741-0 (eBook)
https://doi.org/10.1007/978-3-032-28741-0

This Springer imprint is published by the registered company Springer Nature Switzerland AG
The registered company address is: Gewerbestrasse 11, 6330 Cham, Switzerland

Foreword

The burden of pelvic floor disorders and women-specific health issues is profound, affecting millions of individuals worldwide. Addressing these concerns requires a nuanced understanding of pelvic anatomy, functional systems, and gender-specific pathologies, along with a steadfast commitment to evidence-based, patient-centered care.

This book arrives at a pivotal time, bridging the gap between clinical knowledge and rehabilitative practice. By bringing together a multidisciplinary team—including gynecologists, urologists, gastroenterologists, and physiotherapists—the editors have curated a resource that reflects the collaborative nature of modern pelvic and women's health care.

The breadth of topics and the integration of medical and rehabilitation sciences distinguish this work as a valuable asset for professionals across disciplines. We congratulate the editors and contributors on their commitment to advancing pelvic and women's health through this important academic contribution.

Türkan Akbayrak
Esra Üzelpasacı

Preface

Pelvic and women's health physiotherapy has evolved into a distinct and essential specialty, addressing the unique anatomical, physiological, and psychosocial needs of women across the lifespan. Despite increasing global awareness, interdisciplinary collaboration and evidence-based practice remain critical for advancing care and education in this field.

This book, *Physiotherapy and Rehabilitation in Pelvic and Women's Health-Related Problems*, is designed as a comprehensive reference for clinicians, researchers, and students working in pelvic health, urogynecology, obstetrics, and rehabilitation. The text is organized into four key sections: anatomical and physiological foundations, diagnostic and medical management, physiotherapy and rehabilitation approaches, and special topics. Each chapter provides in-depth, up-to-date, and clinically relevant information, authored by experts in their respective fields.

As editors, our aim was to integrate medical, surgical, and physiotherapy perspectives, ensuring that the content reflects the interdisciplinary nature of pelvic and women's health. We hope this book will serve not only as an educational tool but also as a contribution toward the development of holistic and patient-centered practices in women's health worldwide.

Ankara, Türkiye

Türkan Akbayrak
Esra Üzelpasacı

Acknowledgments

We extend our heartfelt gratitude to all the authors who contributed their experience and time to this book. Their collaborative spirit and academic rigor form the foundation of this work.

We also thank Hacettepe University, Faculty of Physical Therapy and Rehabilitation, and the University of Health Sciences, Gülhane Faculty of Physiotherapy and Rehabilitation, for their continued support of pelvic and women's health research and education. Special thanks go to our contributors from the fields of obstetrics and gynecology, urology, gastroenterology, and physiotherapy and rehabilitation, whose interdisciplinary cooperation made this project possible.

Finally, we are grateful to Springer for providing the opportunity to share this work on a global platform—and to our families for their unwavering support throughout the editing process.

Türkan Akbayrak
Esra Üzelpasacı

Contents

Part I

Anatomy, Physiology and Biomechanics for Pelvic and Women's Health

Anatomy of the Pelvis and Perineum

1

Cem Denk

1.1 Introduction

The pelvis and perineum are regions that are connected to the hip bones and the ends of the spine and are interrelated. The pelvis is divided into two regions:

- The upper part is the false pelvis (greater pelvis) and is generally considered to be part of the abdominal region.
- The true pelvis (lesser pelvis) is related to the hip bones, sacrum, and the lower parts of the coccyx. It has an entrance and an exit.

The bowl-shaped pelvic cavity is surrounded by the true pelvis, which has an entrance (pelvic inlet), walls, and floor. This cavity continues with the abdominal cavity on the upper side and contains structures belonging to the excretory, digestive, and reproductive systems. The perineum is located below the pelvic floor, and its borders form the pelvic outlet.

In the pelvic cavity, the bladder is located in the front in the midline, and the rectum is located behind. As the bladder fills, it rises upward toward the abdominal region. The bladder is supported by the hip bones and the adjacent structures of the pelvic floor. The urethra passes from the pelvic floor to the perineum, opening to the outside in women and to the root of the penis in men.

The rectum, which continues from the sigmoid colon at the S3 vertebra level, continues with the canalis analis while piercing the pelvic floor and opening into the perineum. The canalis analis bends toward the back of the rectum. This bending is created by the pelvic floor muscles and relaxes during defecation. As it passes through the pelvic floor, there is a striated sphincter muscle around the canalis analis and urethra.

The pelvic cavity contains most of the reproductive system in women, while it contains only a portion in men. In women, the vagina pierces the pelvic floor and connects with the uterus in the pelvic cavity. The uterus is located between the rectum and the bladder. The fallopian tubes extend laterally and open into the ovaries in the pelvic wall. In men, the pelvic cavity contains the connection point of the excretory and reproductive systems. It also contains the prostate and two seminal vesicles, which are the largest glands of the reproductive system. In both sexes, the external genitalia, the clitoris and penis, are attached to the bony edge of the anterior half of the pelvic outlet and the thick fibrous membrane perineum that fills the space there. The roots of the external genitalia contain erectile (vascular) tissues and are associated with skeletal muscles.

C. Denk (✉)
Department of Anatomy, Faculty of Medicine, Hacettepe University, Ankara, Türkiye
e-mail: ccdenk@hacettepe.edu.tr

T. Akbayrak, E. Üzelpasaci (eds.), *Physiotherapy and Rehabilitation in Pelvic and Women's Health-Related Problems*, https://doi.org/10.1007/978-3-032-28741-0_1

1.2 Pelvis and Perineum

1.2.1 Pelvis

The term "pelvis" can be broadly defined as the area where the trunk meets the lower extremities. According to the dictionary, the word "pelvis" means "basin" and actually describes the skeleton of this area.

1.2.2 Pelvic Skeleton

The pelvic skeleton consists of four bones: two coxal bones (hip bones), sacrum, and coccyx. Of these, hip bones articulate with each other in the front to form the pubic symphysis and in the back to form the sacroiliac joint by merging with the sacrum.

The pelvis is divided into two parts by the pelvic inlet (or linea terminalis), which is limited by the promontorium at the back, the pecten pubis at the sides, and the pubic symphysis at the front. The part above the pelvic inlet is the greater pelvis (false pelvis) and is the wider part of the pelvis that participates in the structure of the abdominal cavity. The part below the pelvic inlet is called the lesser pelvis (true pelvis).

1.2.2.1 Lesser Pelvis

The lesser pelvis is a cup-shaped structure that contains the lower parts of the intestines and urinary tract and the internal reproductive organs. It has an entrance, an exit opening, and a cavity. The entrance opening, pelvic inlet, is bordered by the promontorium at the back, pecten pubis at the sides, and pubic symphysis at the front. The exit opening, pelvic outlet, is bordered by the coccyx at the back, ischial tuberosities at the sides, and pubic arch at the front. In addition to the ischial tuberosities, there are inflexible ligaments on the sides called sacrotuberous and sacrospinous ligaments. These ligaments divide the sciatic notches into greater and lesser sciatic foramina. The pelvic cavity extends between the pelvic inlet and pelvic outlet. It is a short, oblique canal with a low anterior wall and a posterior wall that is relatively deep compared to the anterior wall.

1.3 Pelvic Bones

The pelvis region consists of four bones: the two coxal bones (hip bones), the sacrum, and the coccyx. The bones in the pelvis region form a solid connection between the trunk and the lower extremities.

1.3.1 Coxal Bone (Hip Bone)

In children, each coxal bone consists of the ilium, ischium, and pubis bones. During puberty, these three bones fuse to form a large and irregular bone. The acetabulum is a deep, rounded depression located on the outer surface of the hip bone and articulates with the head of the femur. The surface of the acetabulum that joins the hip joint, the lunate surface, is horseshoe-shaped and covered with hyaline cartilage. The base of the depression, called the acetabular fossa, does not join the hip joint. There is a wide notch called the acetabular notch on the lower edge of the acetabulum. The ilium forms the upper part of the hip bone. It has two parts, the body and the wing. The body forms the upper part of the acetabulum. The wing is the flat part located on the body and widens upward. The wing has three surfaces: the gluteal surface, the iliac fossa, and the sacropelvic surface. The gluteal surface forms the posterolateral part of the ilium. The wide depression in the middle is called the iliac fossa. The sacropelvic surface is above and behind the arcuate line on the inner surface. Behind this surface, the auricular surface articulates with the auricular surface of the sacrum. The rigid upper edge of the ilium is called the iliac crest. At the anterior end of the iliac crest, there are two protrusions called the anterior superior iliac spine and, below it, the anterior inferior iliac spine. At the posterior end of the crista iliaca, there are two protrusions called the posterior superior iliac spine and, below it, the posterior inferior iliac spine. The ischium consists of the body and the ramus. The most prominent part of the body is called the ischial tuberosity, and the pointed protrusion at the upper back of this is called the ischial spine. There are notches called the greater sciatic notch and the lesser sciatic notch located over and below the ischial spine, respectively. The ramus starts from the ischial tuberosity and extends forward and inward to join the inferior ramus of the pubis. The pubis consists of a body and two rami (superior ramus and inferior ramus). The pubic crest and pubic tubercle are on the body of the pubis. The superior ramus and inferior ramus join at right angles in the front. There is a joint surface called the symphysial surface on the inner surface of the joint. Both pubic bones articulate with each other via the pubic symphysis. The inferior ramus joins with the ischial ramus at the back to form the ischiopubic arm. The hole between the pubis and ischium parts is called the obturator foramen, and this hole is covered by the obturator membrane.

1.3.2 Sacrum–Sacral Vertebrae

The sacrum is a single wedge-shaped bone formed by the union of five immature sacral vertebrae. The promontory is the protrusion extending from the upper and anterior margin of the first sacral vertebra to the pelvic cavity. This protrusion is an important point for birth. The sacral canal is the continuation of the vertebral canal. In this canal, there is a part of the cauda equina, the filum terminale, and the meninges (membranes), extending to the lower border of the second sacral vertebra. The lower part of the canal contains the lower sacral and coccygeal nerve roots up to the filum terminale. The anterior and posterior rami of the first four sacral spinal nerves pass through the anterior and posterior sacral foramina on the anterior and posterior surfaces of the sacrum. The upper edge (or basis) of the sacrum articulates with the fifth lumbar vertebra, and its narrow lower end articulates with the coccyx. The sacrum forms the sacroiliac joint with the hip bones (auricular surface) on the sides.

1.3.3 Coccyx–Coccygeal Vertebrae

The small, triangular-shaped single piece of bone called the coccyx is formed by the fusion of four tail vertebrae.

1.4 Important Ligaments of the Pelvis

The sacrotuberous and sacrospinous ligaments increase the durability of the sacrum and prevent rotation of the sacrum due to the body weight transmitted by the vertebral column.

1.4.1 Sacrotuberal Ligament

This ligament is located between the posterior inferior iliac spine and the lateral parts of the sacrum, coccyx, and ischial tuberosity.

1.4.2 Sacrospinous Ligament

This ligament extends between the lateral parts of the sacrum and coccyx and the ischial spine.

1.5 Important Foramina of the Pelvis

1.5.1 Greater Sciatic Foramen

Via sacrotuberous and sacrospinous ligaments, the greater sciatic notch turns into the greater sciatic foramen.

Structures passing through this hole are:

1. Piriform muscle
2. Sciatic nerve
3. Posterior femoral cutaneous nerve
4. Superior gluteal nerve and inferior gluteal nerve
5. Superior gluteal artery and inferior gluteal artery

6. Nerves to the obturator internus and quadratus femoris muscles
7. Pudendal nerve
8. Internal pudendal artery and vein

1.5.2 Lesser Sciatic Foramen

Via sacrotuberous and sacrospinous ligaments, the lesser sciatic notch turns into the lesser sciatic foramen.

Structures passing through this hole are:

1. The tendon of the obturator internus muscle
2. Nerve to the obturator internus
3. Pudendal nerve
4. Internal pudendal artery and vein

1.6 Joints of the Pelvis

The joints of the pelvis are:

- Sacroiliac joint
- Pubic symphysis
- Sacrococcygeal joint

1.6.1 Sacroiliac Joint

The sacroiliac joints are a very strong pair of synovial joints between the sacrum and the ilium. The very strong *posterior sacroiliac ligament* and *interosseous sacroiliac ligament* nearly suspend the sacrum between the ilium bones. There is limited movement around these joints, and their main function is to transmit body weight from the vertebral column to the pelvic skeleton. Their nerves are branches of the sacral plexus.

1.6.2 Pubic Symphysis

The pubic symphysis is a symphysis-type joint and is located between the pubis bones in the midline. The joint surfaces are covered with hyaline cartilage, and there is a fibrocartilaginous disk in between. The entire joint is surrounded by ligaments. There is almost no movement around this joint.

1.6.3 Sacrococcygeal Joint

The sacrococcygeal joint is a symphysis-type joint located between the sacrum and the coccyx. The sacral cornu and the coccyx are connected by ligaments. A significant amount of movement can be made around this joint.

During pregnancy, the ligaments of the pelvic joints loosen under the influence of the hormones estrogen, progesterone, and relaxin. This allows the pelvic cavity to expand and childbirth to become easier.

1.7 Pelvic Walls

The walls of the pelvis consist of bones and ligaments, partly covered by muscles. The muscles that contribute to the structure of the walls are covered by fascia and parietal peritoneum. The pelvis has anterior, posterior, lateral, and inferior (floor) walls.

1.7.1 Anterior Wall

The anterior wall of the pelvis is the shortest wall and is formed by the body and rami of the pubis and the pubic symphysis.

1.7.2 Posterolateral Wall

The posterolateral wall of the pelvis is broad and is formed by the sacrum, coccyx, piriformis muscle, and the fascia covering them.

1.7.3 Anterolateral Wall

The anterolateral wall of the pelvis is formed by the coxal bone (in the region below the superior pelvic aperture), the obturator membrane, the sacrotuberal ligament, the Sacrospinous ligament, the obturator internus muscle, and its fascia.

1.7.3.1 Obturator Membrane

The obturator membrane is a fibrous membrane that almost completely covers the obturator foramen in the hip bone. The *obturator canal* is a small opening through which the obturator artery, vein, and nerve pass.

1.7.3.2 Sacrotuberal Ligament

The sacrotuberal ligament is a strong ligament that extends from the lateral part of the sacrum and coccyx and from the posterior inferior iliac spine to the ischial tuberosities.

1.7.3.3 Sacrospinous Ligament

The Sacrospinous ligament is a strong, triangular ligament whose base attaches to the lateral part of the sacrum and coccyx and whose apex attaches to the ischial spine.

The sacrospinous and sacrotuberal ligaments prevent the lower end of the sacrum and coccyx from rotating around the sacroiliac joint due to body weight.

1.7.4 Inferior Wall (Pelvic Diaphragm) (Floor of the Pelvis)

The pelvic floor supports the organs in the pelvis and is formed by the pelvic diaphragm. The perineum is located under the pelvic floor.

The pelvic diaphragm is formed by the levator ani muscle and the small coccygeus muscle. The pelvic diaphragm is not complete at the front; there is an opening here that allows the passage of the urethra (and also the vagina in women).

1.7.5 Muscles of the Pelvic Walls

Levator Ani There are two on the right and left. It starts from the pubis, ischial spine, obturator fascia, and the tendinous arch of the levator ani and extends to the perineal body, anococcygeal ligament, and coccyx. This muscle has three parts: pubococcygeus, puborectalis, and iliococcygeus. The fibers extending from the pubococcygeus to the bottom of the prostate are called the levator prostatae muscle, and in women, the fibers extending to the vagina are called the pubovaginalis muscle. Puborectalis extends to the rectum and pulls the rectum forward at a certain angle, thus ensuring that the stool is stored in the rectum for a certain period of time. Its nerves are arising from the pudendal nerve and the S4 spinal nerve.

Coccygeus There are two. It starts from the ischial spine and the Sacrospinous ligament and ends at the coccyx and the fifth sacral vertebra. Its nerves are the S4 and S5 spinal nerves.

Obturator Internus It starts from the inner surface of the obturator foramen (from the obturator membrane). Its fibers unite toward the lesser sciatic foramen and leave the pelvis. It forms the anterolateral wall of the pelvis. Its nerves come from L5 and S1 spinal nerves.

Piriformis It starts from the anterior sacral foramina. It leaves the pelvis through the greater sciatic foramen. It forms the posterolateral wall of the pelvis. Its nerves come from the L5, S1, and S2 spinal nerves.

1.7.6 Pelvic Fascia

Parietal pelvic fascia covers the pelvic walls and is named regionally according to the muscle it covers. It continues with the fascia covering the abdominal walls above the superior pelvic aperture.

Visceral pelvic fascia covers all the organs in the pelvis. In women, this fascia is called the *parametrium* around the cervix uteri.

1.7.7 Peritoneum of the Pelvis

The parietal peritoneum covers the pelvic walls, and from there, it extends over the organs in the pelvis and continues as the visceral peritoneum (peritoneum of organs).

1.8 Nerves of the Pelvis

1.8.1 Sacral Plexus

The sacral plexus is located on the posterior wall of the pelvis, in front of the piriformis muscle. It is formed by the anterior rami of the L4–L5 and S1–S4 spinal nerves. The branch that joins the plexus from the L4 spinal nerve joins the L5 spinal nerve. It descends toward the pelvis, called the *lumbosacral trunk*, and here, it joins the sacral nerves that emerge from the anterior sacral foramina.

1.8.1.1 Branches of the Sacral Plexus

1. The branches that leave the pelvis through the ischial foramina and supply the lower extremity are as follows:
   A. *Sciatic nerve* (L4 and L5 and S1, S2, and S3): This nerve is the largest nerve in the body and is the largest branch of the sacral plexus.
   B. *Superior gluteal nerve:* This nerve innervates the gluteus medius, gluteus minimus, and tensor fasciae latae muscles.
   C. *Inferior gluteal nerve:* This nerve innervates the gluteus maximus muscle.
   D. *The branch to the quadratus femoris:* This branch innervates the quadratus femoris and also the gemellus inferior muscles.
   E. *The branch to the obturator internus:* This branch innervates both the obturator internus and the gemellus superior.
   F. *Posterior femoral cutaneous nerve:* This nerve supplies the buttocks and the back of the thigh.
2. The branches that supply the pelvic muscles, organs in the pelvis, and structures in the perineum are as follows:
   A. *Pudendal nerve (S2, S3, and S4):* This nerve leaves the pelvis through the greater sciatic foramen and enters the perineum through the lesser sciatic foramen.
   B. *The branches to the piriformis muscle.*
   C. *Pelvic splanchnic nerves:* These nerves form the sacral part of the parasympathetic nervous system. These nerves originate from the S2, S3, and S4 sacral nerves and are distributed to the organs in the pelvis.

1.8.2 Lumbar Plexus and Its Branches

1.8.2.1 Lumbosacral Trunk

A portion of the anterior branch of the L4 spinal nerve arises from the medial border of the psoas major muscle and joins the anterior branch of the L5 spinal nerve to form the lumbosacral trunk. This trunk then descends into the pelvis and joins the sacral plexus.

1.8.2.2 Obturator Nerve (L2, L3, and L4)

The obturator nerve originates from the medial border of the psoas major muscle and descends toward the pelvis, together with the lumbosacral trunk. It courses forward on the lateral wall of the pelvis and reaches the obturator foramen. It then passes through the obturator canal and divides into anterior and posterior branches to enter the medial (adductor) region of the thigh.

1.8.2.3 Sensory Branches of the Lumbar Plexus

Sensory branches, namely the iliohypogastric and ilioinguinal nerves, supply the parietal peritoneum covering the lateral wall of the pelvis.

1.8.3 Autonomic Nerves

1.8.3.1 Pelvic Part of the Sympathetic Trunk

The pelvic part of the trunk is continuous with the lumbar part of the trunk above and behind the common iliac a.v. The two parts come together below, in front of the coccyx. Each of the trunks courses downward behind the rectum, in front of the sacrum and the anterior sacral foramina. The trunk has four or five segmental ganglia.

1.8.3.2 Branches

1. Gray ramus communicans, which go to the sacral and coccygeal spinal nerves
2. Branches that join the hypogastric plexuses

1.8.3.3 Pelvic Splanchnic Nerves

The pelvic splanchnic nerves constitute the pelvic portion of the parasympathetic division of the autonomic nervous system. These nerves arise from S2, S3, and S4, as previously described in the sacral plexus. Preganglionic fibers synapse in the ganglia in the hypogastric plexuses.

1.8.3.4 Superior Hypogastric Plexus

The superior hypogastric plexus is located in front of the promontorium belonging to the sacrum. It is divided into the right and left hypogastric nerves below. This plexus is the continuation of the aortic plexus. It consists of branches originating from the L3 and L4 sympathetic ganglia. It contains sympathetic and parasympathetic fibers, as well as visceral afferent fibers.

1.8.3.5 Inferior Hypogastric Plexus

The inferior hypogastric plexus is located on both sides of the rectum, the base of the bladder, and the vagina. It is formed by the union of the hypogastric nerve (a branch of the superior hypogastric plexus) and the pelvic splanchnic nerves. It contains postganglionic sympathetic, preganglionic, and postganglionic parasympathetic fibers and visceral afferent fibers. The branches going to the organs arise from the secondary plexuses formed by the branches coming from this plexus. The parasympathetic fibers coming from the pelvic splanchnic nerve course in the hypogastric nerve and go to the superior hypogastric plexus and the inferior mesenteric plexus and supply the large intestine from the left colic flexure to the upper half of the anal canal.

1.9 Arteries of the Pelvis

1.9.1 Common Iliac Artery

Each of the common iliac arteries ends at the level of the superior pelvic aperture and in front of the sacroiliac joint by dividing into the internal and external iliac arteries.

1.9.2 External Iliac Artery

The external iliac artery extends along the medial border of the psoas major muscle and reaches the superior pelvic aperture. Its branches are the *inferior epigastric artery* and the *deep circumflex iliac artery*. It passes under the inguinal ligament and leaves the greater pelvis, taking the name *femoral artery*.

The arteries in the lesser pelvis are as follows:

1. Internal iliac artery
2. Superior rectal artery
3. Ovarian artery
4. Median sacral artery

1.9.3 Internal Iliac Artery

The internal iliac artery passes toward the pelvis and continues to the greater sciatic foramen, where it divides into two roots, anterior and posterior. The arteries originating from these roots supply the organs in the pelvis, the perineum region, the pelvic walls, and the hip region (buttocks).

1.9.4 Branches Arising from the Anterior Root of the Internal Iliac Artery

1. *Umbilical artery:* The open proximal part of this artery gives off the *superior vesical artery.* The superior vesical artery supplies the upper part of the bladder.
2. *Inferior vesical artery:* This artery supplies the base of the bladder and the prostate gland and seminal vesicles in men. It also gives off the *artery to the ductus deferens.*
3. *Middle rectal artery:* This artery generally originates from the inferior vesical artery. It supplies the muscular layer of the lower rectum and anastomoses with the inferior and superior rectal arteries.
4. *Uterine artery:* This artery courses medially in the pelvic floor and crosses the ureter from above. It passes over the lateral fornices of the vagina and reaches the uterus, where it courses upward between the layers of the broad ligament of the uterus along the lateral edge of the uterus. It continues along the uterine tube to where it anastomoses with the branches of the ovarian artery. The uterine artery also has a branch that supplies the vagina.
5. *Vaginal a.:* This artery supplies the vagina and the base of the bladder.
6. *Inferior gluteal artery:* This artery leaves the pelvis through the greater sciatic foramen. It passes between the S1 and S2 or S2 and S3 spinal nerves.
7. *Obturator artery:* This artery runs on the lateral wall of the pelvis with the obturator nerve and leaves the pelvis through the obturator canal.
8. *Internal pudendal artery:* This artery leaves the pelvis through the greater sciatic foramen and reaches the hip region. It passes through the lesser sciatic foramen and reaches the perineum region, where it enters the pudendal canal; it runs forward with the pudendal nerve. It supplies the muscular layer of the anal canal and the skin and muscles of the perineum region through its branches.

1.9.5 Branches Originating from the Posterior Root of the Internal Iliac Artery

1. *Iliolumbar artery:* This artery courses upward behind the external iliac artery and vein, psoas major, and iliacus muscles.
2. *Lateral sacral arteries:* These arteries descend in front of the sacral plexus and give off branches that feed the neighboring structures.
3. *Superior gluteal artery:* This artery leaves the pelvis by passing through the greater sciatic foramen and supplies the hip region (buttocks).

1.9.6 Superior Rectal Artery

The superior rectal artery is the continuation of the superior mesenteric artery. It supplies the upper half of the rectal mucosa and the anal canal.

1.9.7 Ovarian Artery

The ovarian artery originates from the abdominal aorta at the level of the L1 vertebra. This artery is long and thin and descends behind the peritoneum. At the level of the superior pelvic aperture, it crosses the external iliac artery and enters the suspensory ligament of the ovary. It then passes into the broad ligament of the uterus and courses within the mesovarium to reach the ovary (the testicular artery enters the inguinal canal but does not enter the pelvis).

1.9.8 Median Sacral Artery

The median sacral artery is a small artery that originates at the level of the bifurcation of the abdominal aorta. It descends on the anterior surface of the sacrum and coccyx.

1.10 Veins of the Pelvis

1.10.1 External Iliac Vein

The external iliac vein begins behind the inguinal ligament as a continuation of the femoral vein. It courses medially to its companion artery and joins the internal iliac vein to form the common iliac vein. The inferior epigastric vein and the circumflex iliac vein drain into this vein.

The veins of the pelvis minor are thin-walled and consist of the following veins:

1. Internal iliac v.
2. Superior rectal v.
3. Ovarian v.
4. Median sacral v.

1.10.2 Internal Iliac Vein

The internal iliac vein is formed by the union of the veins that are lateral to the internal iliac artery. It courses upward from the front of the sacroiliac joint and joins the external iliac vein to form the common iliac vein.

1.10.3 Superior Rectal Vein

The superior rectal vein collects the venous blood of the mucosa of the rectum and the upper half of the anal canal. It continues as the inferior mesenteric vein, where it crosses the common iliac artery. *The anastomoses it makes with the middle rectal vein and superior rectal vein are among the important portosystemic (portocaval) anastomoses.*

1.10.4 Ovarian Vein

The right ovarian vein ascends on the posterior abdominal wall and drains into the inferior vena cava, while the left ovarian vein drains into the left renal vein.

1.10.5 Median Sacral Vein

The median sacral vein is a small vein that drains into the inferior vena cava or common iliac vein.

1.11 Lymphatics of the Pelvis

Lymph nodes and lymph vessels are located along the main blood vessels. Lymph nodes are named after the blood vessels they are associated with. Therefore, they are called *internal iliac nodes, external iliac nodes,* and *common iliac nodes.*

1.12 Digestive System Structures in the Pelvis

1.12.1 Sigmoid Colon

The sigmoid colon is approximately 25–38 cm long and begins as a continuation of the descending colon in front of the superior pelvic aperture. It continues as the rectum in front of the S3 vertebra below and makes a curve within the pelvic cavity. The sigmoid colon is attached to the posterior wall of the pelvis by the *sigmoid mesocolon.*

1.12.1.1 Arteries

Sigmoid arteries are the branches of the inferior mesenteric artery.

1.12.1.2 Veins

The sigmoid vein opens into the inferior mesenteric vein. From here, the venous blood is drained into the portal hepatic vein.

1.12.2 Rectum

The rectum is approximately 13 cm long and begins in front of the S3 vertebra as a continuation of the sigmoid colon. It descends by following the curve of the sacrum and coccyx and continues as the anal canal by piercing the pelvic base in front of the tip of the coccyx. The lower part of the rectum is wide and is called the *rectal ampulla*. Only the upper two-thirds of the rectum is covered by the peritoneum. The circular muscle layer and the mucosa layer of the rectum unite to form three semicircular folds (*transverse folds*). The sigmoid veins drain into the inferior mesenteric vein. From here, the venous blood is drained into the portal hepatic vein.

1.12.2.1 Arteries

They are the superior rectal a. (continuation of inferior mesenteric a.), middle rectal a. (branch of internal iliac a.), and inferior rectal a. (branch of internal pudendal a.).

1.12.2.2 Veins

The venous blood of the rectum is drained into the portal vein via the superior rectal vein and into the inferior vena cava via the middle rectal vein and inferior rectal vein. *The anastomoses between the rectal veins are important portocaval anastomoses.*

1.12.2.3 Lymphatics

The lymphatic vessels of the rectum drain into the pararectal nodes and, from there, into the inferior mesenteric nodes, and some lymphatic vessels drain into the internal iliac nodes.

1.12.2.4 Nerves

They are sympathetic and parasympathetic nerves originating from the inferior hypogastric plexus.

1.13 Urinary System Structures in the Pelvis

1.13.1 Ureters

Each of the ureters is a muscular tube extending from the kidney to the back of the bladder.

The ureter enters the pelvis at the point where the common iliac artery divides into two in front of the sacroiliac joint. It then proceeds down the lateral wall of the pelvis to the level of the ischial spine and turns forward in this area to enter the lateral corner of the bladder.

In males, the ureter crosses the ductus deferens in a region close to where it ends. In females, it leaves the region of the ischial spine by turning forward and medially. During this course, it is deep to the base of the broad ligament of the uterus and crosses the uterine artery.

1.13.1.1 Strictures of the Ureter

The ureter has three strictures:

1. Where it joins the renal pelvis
2. Where it crosses the superior pelvic aperture
3. Where it penetrates the bladder wall

1.13.2 Bladder

The bladder is located just behind the pubic bones in the pelvis. The maximum capacity of the bladder is approximately 500 ml.

The empty bladder is pyramidal in shape. The bladder has an apex, a base, an upper surface, two inferolateral surfaces, and a neck. When the bladder is full, it is oval in shape, and its upper surface rises toward the abdomen. In young children, even the empty bladder extends toward the abdomen and becomes a pelvic organ when the pelvis expands at later ages.

The *apex* of the bladder is forward and is connected to the umbilicus by the *median umbilical fold* (the remnant of the urachus). Its *base* is posterior and has a triangular shape. The ureters enter the bladder from the upper-outer corners, and the urethra leaves the organ from the lower corner. The *upper surface* of the bladder is covered by peritoneum, which extends laterally to the lateral wall of the pelvis. As the bladder fills, the upper surface projects into the abdominal cavity, pushing the peritoneum away from the lower part of the anterior abdominal wall. The *neck* of the bladder faces downward.

1.13.2.1 Inner Surface of the Bladder

The inner surface of the bladder's base is called the *trigone of the bladder*. In this region, the mucosa layer is tightly attached to the deep muscle layer, and its surface is always smooth. There are small slits at the outer corners of the trigone, and these areas are the entrance holes of the ureters into the bladder. In the corner below, there is the crescent-shaped hole of the urethra (*internal urethral orifice*). The *interureteric crest* extends between the two ureteral holes. This crest is formed by the deep muscle layer and is the upper limit of the trigone of the bladder. In men, behind the internal urethral orifice, there is a protrusion of the midline lobe of the prostate into the bladder, which is called the *uvula of the bladder*.

1.13.2.2 Muscle Layer of the Bladder Wall

The muscle layer of the bladder (*detrusor*) consists of three interlocking layers of smooth muscle fibers. Circular muscle fibers in the neck of the bladder form the sphincter vesical muscle.

1.13.2.3 Ligaments

The neck of the bladder is held in place by the *puboprostatic ligament* in men and the *pubovesical ligament* in women. These ligaments are formed by the pelvic fascia.

1.13.2.4 Arteries

Superior and inferior vesical arteries (branches of the internal iliac artery).

1.13.2.5 Veins

The veins of the bladder drain into the internal iliac veins.

1.13.2.6 Lymphatics

Drained into the internal and external iliac lymph nodes.

1.13.2.7 Nerves

Sympathetic and parasympathetic fibers from the inferior hypogastric plexus.

1.13.2.7.1 Urination (Bladder Functioning)

When the amount of urine reaches approximately 300 ml in adults, the stretch receptors in the bladder wall transmit the stimulus to the central nervous system. As a result, the person experiences the need to urinate.

Afferent impulses enter the second, third, and fourth sacral segments of the spinal cord. Efferent impulses leave the spinal cord from the same segments and reach the bladder wall via *preganglionic parasympathetic fibers in the hypogastric plexus, where they synapse on postganglionic neurons. After this, the detrusor muscle contracts, and the sphincter vesical muscle relaxes. At the same time, the efferent impulses also travel within the pudendal nerve and reach the external sphincter urethral muscle. Urination is also facilitated by the contraction of the abdominal muscles, increasing intra-abdominal and pelvic pressure and, thus, creating external pressure on the bladder.*

Voluntary control of urination is completed by the contraction of the external urethral sphincter muscle. This event is facilitated by the contraction of the vesical sphincter muscle.

1.14 Reproductive (Genital) Organs in the Pelvis

1.14.1 Male Internal Genital Organs

1.14.1.1 Ductus Deferens

The ductus deferens is a thick-walled, tube-shaped structure approximately 45 cm long. It starts from the tail of the epididymis and enters the abdomen by passing through the inguinal canal. From here, it descends downward, passes into the pelvis, crosses the ureter, and reaches the posterior wall of the bladder. The enlarged part of the posterior wall of the bladder is called the *ampulla*. The ampulla of the ductus deferens unites with the canal of the seminal vesicles, the excretory duct, to form the *ejaculatory duct*.

1.14.1.2 Ejaculatory Duct

There are two ejaculatory ducts. Each of these is formed by the union of the ductus deferens and the excretory ductus, which is the channel of the seminal vesicles. Both ejaculatory ducts open into the prostatic part of the urethra.

1.14.1.3 Seminal Vesicles (Glands)

The seminal vesicles are a pair of organs located on the posterior surface of the bladder and lateral to the last part of the ductus deferens. Each consists of a tube with many folds embedded in connective tissue. The seminal vesicle narrows downward and joins the ductus deferens on the same side, forming the ejaculatory duct. The seminal vesicle produces a fluid that is rich in the fructose, ascorbic acid, and prostaglandin portions of the ejaculate (sperm or semen).

1.14.1.4 Prostate

The prostate is a gland located around the prostatic part of the urethra. It is located below the neck of the bladder and above the urogenital diaphragm. The prostate has an external fibrous capsule and an external fibrous sheath belonging to the visceral layer of the pelvic fascia. The prostate has a base located above the neck of the bladder and an apex facing downward toward the urogenital diaphragm. Both ejaculatory ducts pierce the upper part of the posterior surface of the prostate and open into the prostatic part of the urethra from the lateral edges of the opening of the prostatic utricle. The numerous glands found in the structure of the prostate are embedded in smooth muscle and connective tissue, and the ducts of these glands open into the prostatic part of the urethra. The prostate is divided into a certain number of lobes. The anterior lobe is located in front of the urethra. The middle lobe is behind the urethra and above the ejaculatory duct. The right and left lobes are on both sides of the urethra.

1.14.1.5 Arteries

The branches of the inferior vesical artery and the middle rectal artery.

1.14.1.6 Veins

All veins drain into the prostatic venous plexus and then into the internal iliac vein.

1.14.1.7 Lymphatics

Drain to the internal iliac lymph nodes.

1.14.1.8 Nerves

The nerves originate from the inferior hypogastric plexus.

1.14.2 Female Internal Reproductive (Genital) Organs

1.14.2.1 Ovaries

Each of the ovaries is connected to the back of the broad ligament of the uterus by means of the *mesovarium*. The vessels and nerves of the ovary enter the organ from the *hilum* of the ovary. The ovary is covered by a modified peritoneal section called the germinal epithelium. Deep under this epithelium is a thin fibrous capsule called the tunica albuginea. The ovary has external parts called the *cortex* and internal parts called the *medulla*. There are follicles in the connective tissue of the cortex. The ovary is usually located in the ovarian fossa on the lateral wall of the pelvis. The ovarian fossa is limited by the external and internal iliac arteries.

1.14.2.2 Ligaments of the Ovary

1.14.2.2.1 Suspensory Ligament

The suspensory ligament is the lateral part of the broad ligament of the uterus, which connects the mesovarium to the lateral wall of the pelvis. This ligament contains the vessels and nerves belonging to the ovary.

1.14.2.2.2 Ligamentum of the Ovary

The ligament of the ovary is the remnant of the upper part of the gubernaculum and extends from the medial edge of the ovary to the lateral wall of the uterus. The round ligament of the uterus is also the remnant of the gubernaculum.

1.14.2.3 Arteries

Ovarian arteries, branches of the abdominal aorta.

1.14.2.4 Veins

The ovarian veins drain into the inferior vena cava on the right and into the left renal vein on the left.

1.14.2.5 Lymphatics
Drain into the para-aortic nodes at the level of the L1 vertebra.

1.14.2.6 Nerves
Aortic plexus (branches of this plexus accompany the ovarian artery).

1.14.3 Uterine Tubes

There are two uterine tubes. Each of the tubes is located in the upper part of the broad ligament of the uterus and connects the peritoneal cavity around the ovary to the uterine cavity. The uterine tube is divided into four parts:

1. The most lateral part of the tube with finger-like projections (ovarian fimbriae) toward the top of the ovary, namely the *infundibulum*.
2. The widest part, *ampulla*.
3. The narrowest part, which is immediately lateral to the uterus, is the *isthmus*.
4. Uterine (intramural) part that penetrates the uterine wall.

Sperm pass through the tube and reach the ovum. The uterine tube is where the ovum is fertilized (usually in the ampulla). The tubes are also the places where the fertilized egg is fed, and from there, it is carried to the uterus.

1.14.3.1 Arteries
Ovarian and uterine arteries.

1.14.3.2 Veins
Ovarian and uterine veins.

1.14.3.3 Lymphatics
Lymphatics run with arteries and drain into the internal iliac and preaortic lymph nodes.

1.14.3.4 Nerves
The sympathetic and parasympathetic nerves from the superior and inferior hypogastric plexuses.

1.14.4 Uterus

The uterus consists of the fundus, body, and cervix. The fundus is the region above the entrances of the uterine tubes to the uterus. The body is the biggest part below the entrances of the uterine tubes and continues as the cervix by narrowing below. The cervical canal is continued by the uterine cavity, which is in the body. The cervix pierces the anterior wall of the vagina. The cervical canal is connected to the vagina by the internal os.

1.14.4.1 Positions of the Uterus

Anteversion is the forward bending of the uterus relative to the long axis of the vagina. *Anteflexion* is the name given to the forward inclination of the body of the uterus relative to the cervix. The uterus is normally in an anteflexed and anteverted position.

1.14.4.1.1 Structures That Support the Uterus
The main structures that support the uterus are:

1. *Pelvic diaphragm* (levator ani and coccygeus muscles and their fasciae)
2. *Perineal body* (a fibromuscular structure located in the perineum and supported by the levator ani muscles)
3. *Transverse cervical ligament (cardinal ligament)*, which connects the upper part of the cervix and vagina to the lateral wall of the pelvis
4. *Pubocervical ligament*, which connects the cervix to the pubic bone
5. *Sacrocervical ligament (rectouterine ligament)* connecting the upper part of the cervix and vagina to the lower end of the sacrum

1.14.4.1.2 Broad Ligament of the Uterus
The two peritoneal layers, the broad ligaments of the uterus, extend from the sides of the uterus to the lateral walls of the pelvis. Each broad ligament contains the following structures:

1. At the upper free end, the uterine tubes.
2. Ligament of the ovary.
3. Vessels, nerves, and lymphatic vessels belonging to the uterus and ovary.

The broad ligament provides little support to the uterus.

1.14.4.1.3 Round Ligament of the Uterus

The round ligament starts from the upper and lateral ends of the uterus and extends through the inguinal canal to the subcutaneous tissue of the labium majus. This ligament allows the uterus to remain in anteversion and anteflexion positions.

Arteries

The uterine artery, a branch of the internal iliac artery, and the ovarian arteries supply the uterus.

Veins

The accompanying veins of the ovarian and uterine arteries.

Lymphatics

The lymphatic vessels in the fundus of the uterus course with the ovarian artery and drain into the para-aortic nodes at the level of the L1 vertebra. The lymphatic vessels of the body and cervix drain into the internal and external iliac nodes. In addition, several lymphatic vessels pass through the inguinal canal and drain into the superficial inguinal nodes.

Nerves

The sympathetic and parasympathetic nerves from the inferior hypogastric plexus.

1.14.5 Vagina

The vagina is a flexible sheath belonging to the female reproductive system that receives the male penis during sexual intercourse between a male and a female. The male releases his sperm into the female vagina during sexual intercourse. Menstruation (menstrual bleeding) from the uterus is expelled through this canal. This canal also forms part of the birth canal.

The vagina is a muscular tube that extends between the vulva and the uterus. The cervix pierces this canal from its anterior wall. In people who have never had sexual intercourse, there is a thin mucosal fold with a hole in the middle at the vaginal orifice (*hymen*). The part of the vagina surrounding the cervix is divided into four regions, or fornices (covered chambers): the anterior, posterior, right lateral, and left lateral fornices. The upper half of the vagina is located in the pelvis, between the bladder in front and the rectum behind; the lower half is in the perineum, between the urethra in front and the anal canal behind.

1.14.5.1 Structures that Support the Vagina

Upper one-third: Levator ani muscles, transverse cervical ligaments (cardinal lig.), pubocervical ligament, and sacrocervical ligament (rectouterine lig.)
Middle one-third: Urogenital diaphragm
Lower one-third: Perineal body

1.14.5.2 Arteries

Vaginal artery (a branch of the internal iliac artery) and the vaginal branch of the uterine artery.

1.14.5.3 Veins

Vaginal veins that drain into the internal iliac veins.

1.14.5.4 Lymphatics

The upper third of the vagina drains into the internal and external iliac nodes, the middle third into the internal iliac nodes, and the lower third into the superficial inguinal nodes.

1.14.5.5 Nerves

Inferior hypogastric plexus.

1.15 Visceral Pelvic Fascia in the Female Pelvis

As in men, the visceral pelvic fascia in women also surrounds and supports the organs in the pelvis. This fascia thickens to form the pubocervical, transverse cervical, and sacrocervical (rectouterine) ligaments of the uterus. Clinically, the pelvic fascia around the cervix region is usually called the *parametrium*.

1.16 Peritoneum of the Female Pelvis

The peritoneum continues from the anterior abdominal wall to the upper surface of the bladder. It then reflects to the anterior surface of the uterus and ascends, enveloping the fundus of the uterus. The peritoneal dead end formed here is called the *vesicouterine pouch*. From here, it continues down to the posterior surface of the uterus and covers the posterior surface of the upper part of the vagina. From here, the peritoneum passes to the anterior surface of the rectum and forms the *rectouterine pouch* (Douglas') between the rectum and the uterus. The deepest region of the peritoneal cavity is the rectouterine pouch.

1.17 Perineum

The perineum is located under the pelvic diaphragm. It is rhombic in shape and is bounded by the *pubic symphysis* in front, the tip of the *coccyx* in the back, and the *ischial tuberosities* on the sides. The perineum is divided into two triangles by an imaginary line connecting the ischial tuberosities. The anterior triangle containing the urogenital openings is called the *urogenital triangle*, and the posterior triangle containing the anus is called the *anal triangle*.

1.18 Urogenital Triangle

1.18.1 Urogenital Diaphragm

The urogenital diaphragm is a structure consisting of muscle and fascia that closes the gap between the pubic arches. This structure is formed by the external urethral sphincter and deep transverse perineal muscle located between the upper and lower fasciae. The lower fascia is called the perineal membrane.

1.19 Perineal Body

The perineal body is a small fibrous tissue mass attached to the center of the posterior edge of the urogenital diaphragm. It is larger in women than in men. It supports the posterior wall of the vagina in women and is the attachment point of the muscles in the perineum in both sexes.

1.20 Perineal Spaces

1.20.1 Superficial Perineal Space

The superficial perineal space is a potential space under the skin in the perineum. It is bordered below by the membranous layer of the superficial fascia (Colles' fascia) and above by the urogenital diaphragm. At the back, the membranous layer merges with the posterior edge of the urogenital diaphragm, thus forming the posterior border of the superficial perineal space. At the sides, the membranous layer of the superficial layer and the urogenital diaphragm are attached to the pubic arches. At the front, it is in relation to the potential space between the superficial fascia of the anterior abdominal wall (Scarpa's fascia) and the muscles of the anterior abdominal wall.

1.20.1.1 Structures in the Superficial Perineal Space

In men, the root of the penis and related structures are found in the superficial perineal space. *In women,* there is the root of the clitoris and its related structures.

1.20.2 Deep Perineal Space (= Urogenital Diaphragm)

The deep perineal space is a potential space in which the urogenital diaphragm is located and formed.

1.20.2.1 Structures in the Deep Perineal Space

In men, the following structures are present:

1. Bulbourethral glands
2. Membranous part of the urethra
3. External urethral sphincter
4. Deep transverse perineal muscles
5. Internal pudendal artery and vein
6. Dorsal nerves of the penis

In women, the following structures are present:

1. Some part of the urethra
2. Some part of the vagina
3. External urethral sphincter
4. Deep transverse perineal muscles
5. Internal pudendal artery and vein
6. Dorsal nerves of the clitoris

1.21 Muscles in the Urogenital Triangle

1.21.1 Muscles Found in the Superficial Perineal Space

Superficial transverse perineal muscle: It extends between the ischial tuberosities and the perineal body. It is thought to stabilize the perineal body.

Ischiocavernosus: It originates from the ischial tuberosity and the ischial ramus and surrounds the crus penis/clitoridis. It provides erection of the penis/clitoris.

Bulbospongiosus: It originates from the perineal body and the midline perineal membrane and surrounds the bulb of the penis. In women, it surrounds the vaginal orifice. In men, it ensures the discharge of the urethra during urination. In women, it narrows the entrance to the vagina. It helps with erection in both sexes.

1.21.2 Muscles Found in the Deep Perineal Space

Deep transverse perineal muscle: It originates from the ramus of the ischium and ends in the perineal body. Its fibers mix with the external urethral sphincter muscle. It is thought to fix the perineal body.

External urethral sphincter muscle: It surrounds the membranous part of the urethra. It contracts this part. It ensures retention of urine and relaxes during urination.

The nerve of all muscles in the urogenital triangle is the pudendal nerve.

1.22 Male External Genitalia

1.22.1 Penis

The penis is a male reproductive organ with a mobile cylindrical *body* and a fixed *root.* The expanded distal end of the body is called the *glans penis*. The preputium (foreskin) is the skinfold covering the glans penis. The internal structure of the body is formed by three erectile tissues located in a tube-shaped fascia.

This erectile tissue consists of two *corpora cavernosa* of the *penis,* located on the dorsal side of the penis, and a single *corpus spongiosum* of the *penis* on the ventral side. The corpus spongiosum of the penis expands distally to form the glans penis. The glans penis surrounds the distal ends of the corpora cavernosa. The portion of the urethra within the penis passes through the center of the corpus spongiosum and opens at the *external urethral orifice* on the surface of the glans penis.

The radix penis is located in the superficial perineal space and consists of three erectile tissues: the *bulbus penis* and the *right* and *left crus penis*. The bulbus penis is positioned in the midline, with the urethra passing through it, and its outer surface is covered by the *bulbospongiosus muscle*. Each crus attaches to the margin of the pubic arch, and its outer surface is covered by the *ischiocavernosus muscle*.

The bulbus penis continues anteriorly as the corpus spongiosum penis. The crura penis extend forward to form the corpora cavernosa penis.

1.22.1.1 Arteries

Branches of the deep artery and dorsal artery of the penis.

1.22.1.2 Veins

Deep dorsal vein of the penis.

1.22.1.3 Lymphatics

The lymph from the glans penis drains into the deep inguinal lymph nodes and the external iliac lymph nodes.

Most of the lymph from the penile skin drains into the superficial inguinal lymph nodes.

The lymph from the erectile tissues drains into the internal iliac lymph nodes.

1.22.1.4 Nerves

Pudendal nerve.

1.22.2 Scrotum

The scrotum is a pouch-like extension of the lower part of the anterior abdominal wall. It contains the testes, epididymis, and the lower part of the spermatic cord. The left testis is positioned lower than the right due to the greater length of the spermatic cord.

The wall of the scrotum consists of the following layers:

1. Skin
2. Superficial fascia, in which the fat layer is replaced by the tunica dartos, composed of smooth muscle fibers
3. External spermatic fascia, a continuation of the fascia covering the external oblique abdominal muscle
4. Cremasteric muscle, derived from the fascia of the internal oblique abdominal muscle, along with the cremaster muscle, innervated by the genital branch of the genitofemoral nerve
5. Internal spermatic fascia, derived from the fascia of the transverse abdominal muscle
6. Tunica vaginalis, a closed sac covering the anterior, medial, and lateral surfaces of each testis

1.22.2.1 Vasculature of the Scrotum

Internal pudendal a.v., external pudendal a.v., and cremasteric a.

1.22.2.2 Lymphatics of the Scrotum

The lymph from the scrotum drains into the superficial inguinal lymph nodes.

1.22.2.3 Nerves of the Scrotum

Genital branch of the genitofemoral nerve, ilioinguinal nerve, pudendal nerve, and posterior cutaneous nerve of the thigh.

1.22.3 Testis

The testes are a pair of egg-shaped organs responsible for the production of spermatozoa and testosterone. Normal spermatogenesis (sperm production) occurs at lower temperatures than in the abdominal cavity. Therefore, the testes descend into the scrotum. The opening where the structures entering and exiting the testes are located is called the *mediastinum of the testis*. The fibrous capsule that surrounds the testes externally is called the *tunica albuginea*. The tunica albuginea extends inward, forming septa (*septula testis*). These septa divide the testes into lobules. Within the lobules are the tubules where spermatozoa are produced (convoluted seminiferous tubes and straight tubules). The spermatozoa in these tubules progress to the *rete testis* in the center of the testis. From there, they are transported to the efferent ductules, which exit the mediastinum testis and connect to the epididymis.

1.22.4 Epididymis

The epididymis is a coiled tube, approximately 6–7 m long, that extends downward along the posterior edge of the testis. In this tube, spermatozoa are stored and mature. It consists of three parts: the *head, body,* and *tail* of the epididymis. The cauda epididymis continues as the ductus deferens.

1.22.4.1 Vessels of the Testis and Epididymis

The *testicular artery* is a branch of the abdominal aorta. Small veins emerging from the posterior of the testis and epididymis merge to form a venous network called the *pampiniform plexus*. From this network, the testicular vein originates. Both veins pass through the inguinal canals, with the right testicular vein draining into the inferior vena cava, while the left testicular vein drains into the left renal vein.

1.22.4.2 Lymphatics of the Testis and Epididymis

Drain into the lateral aortic and preaortic lymph nodes.

1.23 Bulbourethral Glands (Cowper Glands)

The bulbourethral glands are a pair of small glands located in the deep perineal space within the fibers of the external sphincter urethrae muscle. The ducts of these glands open into the spongy part of the urethra.

1.24 Male Urethra

The male urethra is divided into three parts: prostatic, membranous, and spongy.

1.24.1 Prostatic Part

The prostatic part of the urethra is located within the prostate, extending from the base to the apex. This segment is the widest and most distensible part of the male urethra. On the posterior wall, the longitudinal ridge in the center is called the *urethral crest*, while the groove-like areas on either side of this ridge are known as the *prostatic sinuses*. The ducts of the prostate gland open into the sinus prostaticus. The depressed area at the most prominent part of the urethral crest is called the *prostatic utricle*, which is considered the homolog of the uterus and vagina in females. The ejaculatory ducts open at the margins of the orifice of the prostatic utricle.

1.24.2 Membranous Part

The membranous part of the urethra passes through the urogenital diaphragm and is surrounded by the external sphincter urethrae muscle. This segment is the shortest and narrowest part of the urethra.

1.24.3 Spongy Part

The spongy part of the urethra passes through the bulb and corpus spongiosum of the penis. The narrowest point of the entire urethra is the *external urethral orifice*. The portion of the urethra within the glans penis expands to form the *navicular fossa*. The bulbourethral glands open into the spongy part of the urethra below the urogenital diaphragm.

1.25 Vulva (Female External Genitalia)

The vulva consists of the mons pubis (the hair-covered skin over the pubic area), the labia majora pudendi, the labia minora pudendi, the clitoris, the greater vestibular glands, and the lesser vestibular glands.

1.25.1 Labium Majus

The labia majora are skinfolds that extend from the mons pubis to meet in the midline. The outer surface of these structures, which contain fatty tissue, is covered with hair (the male equivalent of the labia majora is the scrotum).

1.25.2 Labium Minus

The labia minora are two smaller skinfolds. The outer surface of these structures is not covered with hair and is located between the labia majora. Their posterior ends meet to form a sharp fold. The labia minora separate from each other to cover the clitoris anteriorly and form the *preputium* (foreskin) anteriorly and the *frenulum* posteriorly.

1.25.3 Vestibule of the Vagina

The vestibule of the vagina is the opening between the labia minora. At its top, there is the clitoris, and at its base, there are holes through which the urethra, vagina, greater vestibular glands, and lesser vestibular glands open to the outside.

1.25.4 Clitoris

The clitoris is the equivalent of the penis in males. It has the *glans, body,* and *crura.* The glans part is partially covered by the *preputium*. There are three erectile tissues in the root of the clitoris; these are the bulb of the vestibule and two crura. The two crura unite in front to form the body and then the glans. The crura are covered by the ischiocavernosus muscles. The *bulb of the vestibule* is the equivalent of the bulb of the penis in the male but is divided into two halves by the intervening vagina. It is attached to the lower surface of the urogenital diaphragm and is covered by the bulbospongiosus muscles.

1.25.5 Greater Vestibular Glands

The greater vestibular glands, or the glandulae vestibularis majors, are a pair of glands with a mucous secretion and are covered by the posterior part of the bulb of the vestibule and the labium majus. The duct of each gland opens into the groove between the hymen and the posterior part of the labium minus. These glands secrete a small amount of mucous fluid to provide vaginal lubrication.

1.25.6 Lesser Vestibular Glands

These glands are located in the vestibule of the vagina, below the external urethral orifice, and secrete a few milliliters of a milky fluid.

1.26 Female Urethra

The female urethra is a 3.8-cm-long canal extending from the neck of the bladder to the external urethral orifice. This canal passes through the urogenital diaphragm and external urethral sphincter along its course and reaches the external urethral orifice located under the clitoris and in front of the vagina.

1.27 Anal Triangle

1.27.1 Ischiorectal (Ischioanal) Fossa

The ischiorectal fossa is a triangular prism–shaped space located on both sides of the anal canal. The base of the prism is toward the surface and is covered with skin. Its apex is the junction of the medial and lateral edges. The medial wall is formed by the levator ani and the anal canal. The lateral wall contains the lower part of the obturator internus muscle, which is covered by the pelvic fascia. The urogenital diaphragm is on the anterior wall, and the gluteus maximus is on the posterior wall.

The ischiorectal fossa is filled with fatty tissue that supports the anal canal. Thus, the fossa allows the anal canal to expand easily during defecation. The pudendal nerve and the internal pudendal artery and vein are located in the fascial canal (pudendal canal) located medial to the ischial tuberosity.

1.27.2 Anal Canal

The anal canal, which is approximately 4 cm long, is located under the pelvic diaphragm. This structure, which extends downward and backward from the rectal ampulla, opens to the outside with the *anus*. Its lateral walls are in contact with each other under the influence of the levator ani and the anal sphincters (except during defecation).

The mucosa of the upper half of the anal canal has vertically extending mucosal folds called *anal columns*. These folds meet at their lower ends and form crescent-shaped folds called *anal valves*. The mucosa of the lower half of the anal canal is smooth and meets the skin of the anus.

The muscle layer of the anal canal consists of smooth muscle fibers that run longitudinally on the outside and circularly on the inside. The circular layer thickens at the upper end of the anal canal and forms the involuntary internal anal sphincter. This muscle is surrounded externally by the external anal sphincter. The external anal sphincter is a voluntary muscle and consists of three parts: subcutaneous, superficial, and deep. The deep part is at the top and blends with the puborectal muscle. Its anterior part crosses with the superficial transverse perineal muscle in women, and its posterior part attaches to the anococcygeal ligament. The superficial part is in the middle and extends between the perineal body in front and the coccyx in the back. The subcutaneous part is at the bottom and attaches to the perineal body and the superficial transverse perineal muscle in front and the anococcygeal ligament in the back. Its nerve is the pudendal nerve, and it works voluntarily.

The puborectal fibers of both levator ani form a sling by attaching to the pubic bone anteriorly. This sling surrounds the junction of the rectum and the anal canal and pulls these structures forward, causing a narrow angle between the rectum and the anal canal.

At the junction of the anus and the rectum, the internal anal sphincter, the deep part of the external anal sphincter, and the puborectalis form a separate ring called the *anorectal ring*.

1.27.2.1 Arteries

The upper half of the anal canal is supplied by the superior rectal artery and the lower half by the inferior rectal artery.

1.27.2.2 Veins

The venous blood of the upper half of the anal canal is drained into the superior rectal vein, which is drained into the inferior mesenteric vein, while the venous blood of the lower half is drained into the inferior rectal vein, which is drained into the internal pudendal vein. Anastomoses between rectal veins are important portosystemic anastomoses.

1.27.2.3 Lymphatics

The lymphatic vessels of the upper half of the anal canal drain into the pararectal nodes and, from there, into the inferior mesenteric nodes, while the lymphatic vessels of the lower half drain into the medial group of the superficial inguinal nodes.

1.27.2.4 Nerves

The mucosa of the upper half of the anal canal is sensitive to stretching and is supplied with sensory fibers from the hypogastric plexuses. The lower half is sensitive to pain, temperature, touch, and pressure and is supplied by the inferior rectal nerve (branch of the pudendal nerve). The internal anal sphincter is supplied by sympathetic fibers from the hypogastric plexuses. The voluntary external anal sphincter is supplied by the inferior rectal nerve.

1.28 Sex Differences in the Pelvis

The differences in the pelvis, depending on gender, are as follows:

1. The depth of the greater pelvis is less in women and more in men.
2. When the superior pelvic aperture is examined in the transverse plane, it is oval in women and heart-shaped in men (this is because the promontory is inclined forward in men).
3. The pelvic cavity is more chamber-like in women, and the distance between the superior and inferior pelvic apertures is shorter in women.
4. The inferior pelvic aperture is larger in women than in men. In addition, the ischial tuberosities are outward-facing in women while inward-facing in men.
5. The sacrum is shorter, wider, and flatter in women than in men.
6. The subpubic angle is rounder and wider in women than in men.

References

1. Peter WL. Gray's anatomy. Baskı: Churchill Livingstone; 1995. p. 38.
2. Moore LK, Dalley AF, Agur AMR. Clinically oriented anatomy. Baskı: Lippincott Williams &Wilkins/ Wolters Kluwer Health; 2010. p. 6.
3. Drake RL, Vogl W, Mitchell AWM. Gray's anatomy for students. Churchill Livingstone; 2005.

2 Physiology for Pelvic and Women's Health

Bilge Pehlivanoglu

2.1 Urinary System

The excretory system consists of two kidneys, located retroperitoneally on each side of the spinal cord at the flank region, which produce urine by filtering the blood to ensure the excretion of waste materials that the body does not need and/or are formed as a result of metabolism, and two ureters that transfer the urine from the renal pelvis to the urinary bladder, which stores the urine and allows its excretion in a controlled fashion [19, 21].

Sustaining life and proper functioning depends on the homeostatic balance of the body's internal environment. Like all organs and tissues in our body, the functions of the urinary system are associated with maintaining homeostasis. The main executive organs of this system are the kidneys. The urine formed by the kidneys is transmitted through the ureters to the urinary bladder, a hollow, sac-shaped organ composed of smooth muscle (detrusor muscle). It is controlled mainly through the autonomic nervous system (ANS); however, voluntary control through the cortex is possible as well [5, 6].

B. Pehlivanoglu (✉)
Department of Physiology, Faculty of Medicine, Hacettepe University, Ankara, Türkiye
e-mail: pbilge@hacettepe.edu.tr

2.1.1 Urine Formation

Nephrons, the smallest structural and functional units of the kidney, produce urine. Kidneys contain approximately two million nephrons capable of producing urine, located in the cortical (85%) and juxtamedullary (15%) regions of the parenchyma. The number of nephrons decreases as a result of kidney damage, disease, or degeneration due to aging since they cannot regenerate. After the age of 40, the number of functioning nephrons decreases by about 10% every 10 years. This gradual decline is not a life-threatening condition due to adaptive changes in the remaining nephrons. However, in cases where circulation is disrupted, such as in shock, or when there is an acute reduction in kidney mass and, thus, the number of nephrons due to trauma or surgical interventions, kidney failure may occur before adaptation can take place [5, 6, 19, 21].

Each nephron is composed of two parts:

1. The glomerulus consists of a network of glomerular capillaries between the afferent and efferent arterioles, surrounded by Bowman's capsule. Due to the characteristics of renal blood circulation, glomerular capillaries have a higher hydrostatic (filtration) pressure compared to other capillary systems in the body. The fluid filtered here (ultrafiltrate or urine precursor) passes into the Bowman's space between the two layers of Bowman's capsule and, from there, into the tubules.

T. Akbayrak, E. Üzelpasaci (eds.), *Physiotherapy and Rehabilitation in Pelvic and Women's Health-Related Problems*, https://doi.org/10.1007/978-3-032-28741-0_2

2. The long tubular system starts from Bowman's space and consists of successive segments: the proximal tubule, the loop of Henle, the distal tubule, and the collecting ducts. Through its passage in the tubular system, the composition of the ultrafiltrate changes to the final urine by tubular reabsorption and secretion mechanisms.

Both cortical and juxtamedullary nephrons have all the parts listed above; however, there are some morphological and functional differences. The glomeruli of cortical nephrons are situated in the outer part of the cortex, and since their loops of Henle are short, they traverse only a short distance in the medulla. The peritubular capillaries of cortical nephrons form a network, and there is a difference in diameter between the afferent and efferent arterioles. The glomeruli of juxtamedullary nephrons, on the other hand, are located deeper in the cortex, near the medulla. They have long loops of Henle that extend deep into the medulla, and the peritubular capillaries are in the form of a straight structure known as vasa recta. The vasa recta is situated parallel to the loop of Henle; however, the blood flow is in the opposite direction to ultrafiltrate. This arrangement in the medulla plays an important role in the concentration of urine. In these juxtamedullary nephrons, there is no difference in the diameters of the afferent and efferent arterioles [28].

Urine formation involves three physiological mechanisms:

- Glomerular filtration
- Tubular reabsorption
- Tubular secretion

The amount of any molecule excreted with urine can be formulated as

$$\text{Excreted amount} = \text{Filtered amount} - \text{Reabsorbed amount} + \text{Secreted amount}$$

2.1.1.1 Glomerular Functions

The first step in urine formation is glomerular filtration (GF) or ultrafiltration. Ultrafiltrate contains all the liquid and solid components of blood, except for the formed elements (erythrocytes, leukocytes, and platelets) and proteins. In terms of content, ultrafiltrate is similar to the extracellular fluid. The concentration of all substances in the ultrafiltrate, including organic molecules such as glucose, amino acids, and electrolytes that are not bound to plasma proteins, is the same as in plasma. However, calcium and some small molecular weight fatty acids are not freely filtered, as they are partially bound to plasma proteins. Only the portion of these substances that is not bound to plasma proteins is filtered by the glomeruli. The selective nature of filtration from the glomeruli depends on the filtration membrane formed by the cells of the capillary wall and Bowman's capsule, as well as the properties of the molecules.

The filtration membrane has three layers: glomerular capillary endothelium, which is more porous than any other capillaries to facilitate filtration; basal membrane; and podocytes, forming slits for filtration. The pressures in the nephron determine the forces involved in GF, which are:

- Hydrostatic pressure in the glomerular capillaries (P_G)
- Plasma colloid osmotic pressure (oncotic pressure) in the glomerular capillaries ($\prod_G$)
- Hydrostatic pressure in the Bowman's capsule (P_B)
- Oncotic pressure in the Bowman's capsule ($\prod_B$)

Since $\prod_B$ is zero under physiological conditions, GF pressure can be formulized as

$$\text{Net glomerular filtration pressure}(\text{NFP}) = P_G - \prod\nolimits_G - P_B$$

Under physiological conditions, NFP is 10 mmHg.

The filtration coefficient (K_f), which is the product of the permeability and the surface area of the filtration membrane, is involved in the control of GF. Its normal value is 12.5 mL/min/mmHg.

The amount of filtered plasma in unit time is defined as the glomerular filtration rate (GFR).

$$\mathrm{GFR} = \mathrm{NFP} \times Kf$$

$$\begin{aligned}\mathrm{GFR} &= 10\,\mathrm{mmHg} \times 12.5\,\mathrm{mL/min/mmHg} \\ &= 125\,\mathrm{mL/min}\end{aligned}$$

The properties of the molecules, i.e., the size and electrical charge, are among the determinants of GF as well. The smaller molecules (molecular weight less than 7000 D) filter freely, and GF becomes less and less as the size of the molecule increases. The filtration rate of the negatively charged anionic molecules is lower compared to the neutral and cationic molecules [30].

2.1.1.2 Tubular Functions

Approximately 180 liters of ultrafiltrate is produced daily in the glomeruli in both kidneys. However, the daily urine output is about 1.5 liters. During glomerular filtration, along with the waste molecules and the end products of metabolism, substances necessary for the body are also filtered, except for proteins and protein-bound substances present in the plasma. The processes of reabsorption and secretion, which occur in the tubules following filtration, are selective. Different substances are reabsorbed or secreted through different mechanisms. As a result, the amount of water and solutes excreted with urine is determined. The transportation of water and solutes through different sections of the tubules also varies. For instance, about 99% of the water filtered in the glomeruli is reabsorbed throughout the tubules. Approximately 65% of this occurs in the proximal tubules, 20% in the loop of Henle, and about 12–14% in the distal tubules and collecting ducts.

2.1.1.2.1 Tubular Reabsorption

Remembering that the total volume of plasma is only 3 L, tubular reabsorption becomes a very important function for life. The tubular ultrafiltrate is reabsorbed during its passage through the tubules. Different parts of the tubular system differ in permeability for solutes and water; accordingly, the substances reabsorbed from different tubular sections are different.

Tubular reabsorption is also directed by various pressures; similar to NFP, we can define a net reabsorption pressure (NRP). The forces involved are:

- Hydrostatic pressure in the tubular lumen (P_T)
- Oncotic pressure in the tubular lumen ($\prod_T$)
- Hydrostatic pressure in the interstitial fluid (P_I)
- Oncotic pressure in the interstitial fluid ($\prod_I$)

$$\mathrm{NRP} = \left(P_T - P_I\right) + \left(\prod\nolimits_T - \prod\nolimits_I\right)$$

Under physiological conditions, NRP is 10 mmHg.

Tubular reabsorption in unit time is defined as the tubular reabsorption rate (TRR) and is determined by NRP and the reabsorption coefficient (K_r). The normal value of Kr is 12.4 mL/min/mmHg, and it is affected by the permeability and the reabsorption surface area.

$$\mathrm{TRR} = \mathrm{NRP} \times K_r$$

$$\begin{aligned}\mathrm{TRR} &= 10\,\mathrm{mmHg} \times 12.4\,\mathrm{mL/min/mmHg} \\ &= 124\,\mathrm{mL/min}\end{aligned}$$

Keeping these equations in mind, one can easily figure out that the urine formation rate is 1 mL/min, i.e., approximately 1.5 L/day.

2.1.1.2.2 Tubular Secretion

Various molecules, metabolic end products such as creatinine, urea, organic anions, and organic cations, that need to be removed from the body are secreted along the tubular sections. Moreover, some molecules like urea, sodium, and water shuttle between the tubular lumen and the interstitial fluid to maintain the required osmolarity.

The roles of the tubular sections in urine formation are summarized below.

Proximal Tubule The metabolic activity of proximal tubule cells is quite high. The luminal part of the proximal tubule cells, adjacent to the tubule lumen, has a well-developed brush border structure. This increased surface area in the proximal tubules and the presence of numerous active/passive transport molecules on this surface provide significantly high reabsorption and secretion capacity. Approximately 65% of the water, sodium, chloride, and potassium; all of the glucose and amino acids; and 85% of the bicarbonate in the glomerular ultrafiltrate are reabsorbed in the proximal tubules [8].

The activity of the sodium-potassium ATPase pump on the basolateral membrane of the tubular epithelial cells is crucial to maintain a low intracellular sodium concentration, which facilitates both the passive movement of sodium from the lumen into the cell and the secondary active transport of glucose, amino acids, and many other substances that are sodium-dependent. Glucose, amino acids, and other substances that enter the cell with sodium are passively transferred through the basolateral membrane into the interstitial fluid and, eventually, into the peritubular capillaries. The main mechanism for water transport in the proximal tubule is osmosis; i.e., water can move both transcellularly (through the tubular cells) and paracellularly (through the spaces between cells), following the movement of osmotically active particles.

The glomerular ultrafiltrate is isosmotic because, apart from cells and proteins, its composition is the same as plasma. Since water and solutes are reabsorbed in equal proportions in the proximal tubule, the osmolarity of the fluid in the lumen remains isosmotic.

In addition to its reabsorption function, the proximal tubule cells secrete hydrogen and many drugs into the lumen [19].

The Loop of Henle Three distinct sections of the loop of Henle have different structural and functional characteristics: the descending thin limb, the ascending thin limb, and the thick ascending limb.

The descending and ascending thin limbs have low metabolic activity, contain few mitochondria, and lack a brush border, which is functionally coupled to minimal water or solute transport, generally occurring through passive mechanisms.

In the loop of Henle, approximately 20% of the water, sodium, chloride, and potassium filtered by the glomeruli are reabsorbed. Calcium, magnesium, and bicarbonate are also reabsorbed. The descending limb of the loop of Henle is permeable only to water. Since solutes are not reabsorbed, the tubular fluid becomes hyperosmotic as it moves down the descending limb through the medulla. The thin and thick portions of the ascending limb, however, are impermeable to water. In the thin ascending limb, the reabsorption capacity is very low, but in the thick ascending limb, solutes are reabsorbed through active transport mechanisms. In this section, the Na^+-K^+-$2Cl^-$ transporter facilitates ion transport, driven by the sodium concentration gradient created by the Na^+-K^+ ATPase pump. In contrast to hyperosmolarity in the descending limb, the tubular fluid becomes hyposmolar by the end of the thick ascending limb [8, 19].

Distal Tubule and Collecting Ducts The initial part of the distal tubule is structurally and functionally similar to the thick ascending limb of the loop of Henle, so the osmolarity decreases further. As the hypoosmotic fluid progresses through the distal tubule and collecting ducts, water and solute reabsorption and secretion occur. The osmolarity of the fluid in the later part of the distal tubule and the collecting ducts is regulated by antidiuretic hormone (ADH). ADH increases water reabsorption in these segments, thereby reducing diuresis, or urine output. The second half of the distal tubule shares characteristics with the following segment, the collecting ducts. In these sections, the principal cells are responsible for reabsorbing sodium and water from the tubule lumen and secreting potassium into the lumen via an aldosterone-controlled mechanism. The second cell type, intercalated cells, take part in acid-base balance by secreting hydrogen and reabsorbing bicarbonate and potassium [28].

The unique anatomical location of the distal tubule, passing between the afferent and efferent arterioles, forms a complex known as the juxtaglomerular apparatus (JGA), which plays a crucial role in blood pressure regulation. Specialized macula densa cells of the distal tubule are sensitive to the levels of Na^+ and Cl^- in the tubular fluid, and the juxtaglomerular (granular) cells in the wall of the afferent arteriole secrete renin. When blood pressure decreases or the electrolyte levels in the tubule are low, renin is released, activating the renin-angiotensin-aldosterone (RAA) system, which helps maintain blood pressure and extracellular fluid volume [14].

After all the processes within the nephron are completed, the final urine is collected in the renal pelvis and transported via the ureters to the bladder, where it is stored until excretion. In a person with normal hydration, the rate of urine formation is about 1 mL per minute. Depending on factors such as fluid intake, body fluid osmolarity, blood pressure, and blood volume, the rate of urine formation may increase or decrease. Throughout the later stages of the excretory system, there is no further change in the composition or volume of urine [19].

2.1.2 Ureters

The ureters are a pair of about 30-cm-long muscular tubes that carry urine from the renal pelvis to the bladder. The transmission of urine from the kidneys to the bladder occurs with the effect of gravity and the propulsive peristaltic activity of the smooth muscle. The pacemaker cells stimulated with the tension of the accumulated urine in the renal pelvis initiate peristaltic contractions. The peristaltic waves are under the control of the ANS and are suppressed under the control of the sympathetic nervous system and increase when parasympathetic activity becomes dominant.

Any condition that obstructs urine flow, such as a kidney stone in the ureter, causes excessive accumulation of urine proximal to the blockage. After a certain period, the increase in pressure in the renal pelvis may hinder or even stop glomerular filtration. The tension caused by this pressure increase due to excessive fluid accumulation also leads to continuous peristaltic activity and severe pain experienced by the patient (renal colic).

The ureters enter the bladder after advancing a few centimeters within the smooth muscle of the bladder, also known as the detrusor, from the trigone region. During urination, the contraction of the bladder muscles compresses the part of the ureters that runs within the bladder wall, preventing the backflow of urine into the ureters. However, in some individuals, the portion of the ureter located within the bladder wall is too short or is positioned more steeply. In such cases, some of the urine in the bladder flows backward during urination. This clinical condition, called vesicoureteral reflux, can lead to recurrent kidney infections with serious consequences if the reflux grade is high [5, 6].

2.1.3 Urinary Bladder

The bladder is a hollow, sac-like organ made of smooth muscle that stores urine for a certain period and periodically empties it through the urethra. The bladder consists of the body, where urine collects, and the funnel-shaped neck, which extends toward the urethra. Above the neck, on the back wall of the bladder, there is a triangular area called the trigone. The ureteral openings into the bladder are located at the two corners of the trigone's base, and its lower end continues with the posterior urethra. At this point, there is an internal sphincter composed of the detrusor muscle, which contains a large amount of elastic tissue. The internal sphincter is controlled by the ANS. The tone of the smooth muscles forming the internal sphincter prevents the passage of urine into the urethra until the pressure in the bladder reaches a critical level. The posterior urethra continues with the urethra and passes through the urogenital diaphragm. Here lies the external sphincter, made up of striated muscle tissue, which is under voluntary control. Even when there is an involuntary effort to empty the bladder in response to increased bladder pressure, the external sphincter contracts voluntarily, preventing urine flow [5, 6].

The urethra, transporting urine to the outside, is shorter in women and longer in men. In women, the urethra's sole function is to expel urine, whereas in men, it also serves as the passage for semen during ejaculation.

Bladder functions are under cortical voluntary and autonomic involuntary control. The pelvic nerves that mediate bladder functions contain both sensory and motor fibers. Afferent sensory fibers relay information about bladder tension to the central nervous system. Increased tension triggers a reflex response that stimulates bladder emptying. The motor component of the pelvic nerves consists of parasympathetic nervous system fibers originating from the S2 to segments of the spinal cord. As with all parasympathetic fibers, there is a ganglion located near the organ, and short postganglionic fibers originating from this ganglion innervate the detrusor muscles. Parasympathetic nerve fibers facilitate the contraction of detrusor muscles and the relaxation of internal sphincter muscles, allowing urine to be expelled. In addition to the pelvic nerves, the pudendal nerve and the hypogastric nerve also play a role in bladder innervation. The pudendal nerve contains somatic motor fibers and controls the external sphincter. When the external sphincter is stimulated by the pudendal nerve, it contracts, preventing urine flow. The hypogastric nerve, which arises from the T11 to region of the spinal cord, carries sympathetic nerve fibers, but these fibers are responsible for innervating blood vessels, not the bladder or sphincter muscles. Sympathetic stimulation transmitted through this nerve causes vasoconstriction [32].

All sympathetic and parasympathetic preganglionic fibers that innervate the bladder release acetylcholine (ACh). ACh binds to nicotinic acetylcholine receptors (N_2) located on postganglionic nerve fibers. Norepinephrine released from sympathetic postganglionic fibers causes relaxation of the detrusor muscle via β-adrenergic receptors in the bladder body and contraction of the internal sphincter via the α1 receptor. In this way, the flow of urine (micturition) is prevented. ACh released from parasympathetic postganglionic fibers increases intracellular calcium release through muscarinic M_3 acetylcholine receptors, causing contraction of the detrusor muscles and facilitating micturition [18].

2.2 Gastrointestinal System

The gastrointestinal system (GIS) is the tract between the oral cavity and the anus and associated organs such as the salivary glands, liver, and pancreas. The main functions of the GIS are associated with the processing of ingested food and can be listed as ingestion and digestion of food, macro- and micronutrient absorption, secretion of enzymes and hormones, and excretion of waste products. In addition, the well-documented interaction between microbiota and almost every body system associates GIS with other functions and the well-being of the individual [12, 16].

The long anatomical path and the functions in detail are beyond the scope of this book; that is why they will be summarized briefly; however, the last sections of the GI tract (GIT) responsible for defecation and continence are located in the pelvis and will be discussed in detail.

The GI functions are regulated by the presence of food in the tract, which involves a complex set of hormonal and neural interactions. The food, with its chemical and physical properties, modulates the response of GIS during the cephalic, gastric, and intestinal phases of digestion. The cephalic phase is initiated by the thought, sight, smell, etc. of the food and controls the secretion of digestive juices and contraction pattern. If the overall effect during the cephalic phase is favorable, then the gastrointestinal organs are prepared to digest the foods to be consumed; otherwise, the digestive function is inhibited. The gastric and intestinal phases function when food or its components come in contact directly with the stomach or intestines, respectively. During both of these phases, the mechanical distension of the GI tract, together with the specific composition of the food, stimulates the digestion processes. The GIS is unique with its extensive neural innervation, namely the enteric nervous system (ENS). ENS is located at the wall of the GI tract and is estimated to have as many neurons as the central nervous system. The ENS is capable of controlling all of the digestive functions; however, it is facilitated or inhibited by the ANS. GIS is also considered the richest endocrine organ in the body; among various paracrine hormones, five GI peptides—gastrin, cholecystokinin (CCK), secretin, glucose-dependent insulinotropic polypeptide (GIP), and motilin—control the digestive process. All of them, except motilin, are secreted from discrete enteroendocrine cells following food ingestion and help the food to be digested and absorbed. On the other hand, motilin is secreted between meals and controls GIS activity during fasting periods [10].

The ingested food is broken down into absorbable molecules by mechanical and biochemical processes. Starting with the mouth, both processes go hand in hand down to the large intestines, where mechanical processing and storage functions are the main physiological processes. The different sections and their functions are given in Table 2.1. Each and every one of the constituents of the diet is processed and absorbed, except the ones that are ready to be absorbed (e.g., monosaccharides, amino acids, minerals, water, etc.) or cannot be digested and utilized by the human GIT (e.g., cellulose). Those and secreted substances, together with tissue debris, move to the large intestines through the ileocecal valve. Anatomically, the last sections of the descending colon, sigmoid colon, rectum, and anus are located in the pelvis. These sections function as storage for the feces until it is expelled by defecation [33].

2.2.1 Defecation

Defecation involves integrated and coordinated sensorimotor functions, controlled by central, peripheral, and enteric nervous systems, and requires a morphologically intact GIS, focusing on the pelvic floor and anal sphincters.

Defecation takes place in intervals in a toilet-educated individual; the frequency changes according to habits, diet, etc. It is generally accepted that the "normal" frequency of defecation in adults is between a maximum of three times a day and a minimum of three times a week. But it should be kept in mind that the "normal" changes between the individuals as well as the health professionals, and if someone does not experience discomfort, less than three motions per week can be considered normal [13, 20, 29, 33].

2.2.1.1 Phases of Defecation

There are four physiologically distinct phases: basal, pre-defecatory, expulsive, and termination (Fig. 2.1).

2.2.1.1.1 The Basal Phase

During its stay in the colon, intraluminal contents lose water by absorption and transform from semiliquid to semisolid and eventually solid

Table 2.1 The sections of the gastrointestinal system and their functions

Section	Function

Mouth	Saliva production
	Chewing
	Swallowing
	Initiation of carbohydrate and lipid digestion
	    Amylase
	    Lipase

Esophagus	Passage of swallowed food morsels to the stomach Peristalsis

Stomach	Reservoir function and controlled transmission of contents through the pyloric sphincter
	Mixing and breaking down of the swallowed food
	Endocrine and exocrine secretions required for digestive functions
	    Hydrochloric acid
	    Gastrin
	    Pepsinogen
	    Gastric lipase
	    Histamine
	    Somatostatin
	    Mucus
	Initiation of protein digestion
	    Pepsin
	Absorption of some lipid-soluble molecules

Pancreas	Endocrine and exocrine secretions required for digestive functions
	    Lipolytic enzymes
	    Pancreatic amylase
	    Bicarbonate
	    Secretin

(continued)

Table 2.1 (continued)

Section	Function
Liver	Enterohepatic circulation and first-pass effect on absorbed molecules Detoxification Bile production
Small intestines	Mixing, approaching the absorptive surface, and propulsion of the chyme Peristalsis Segmentation Migrating myoelectric complex Digesting and absorbing micro- and macronutrients in the chyme Pancreatic enzymes Bile Brush border enzymes Gastrin Motilin Cholecystokinin Glucose-dependent insulinotropic polypeptide Controlled transmission of chyme through the ileocecal valve
Large intestines	Reservoir function and controlled defecation Absorption of water and electrolytes Location for microbiota

state. The main motility pattern of the GIS, peristalsis, occurs in the colon as well. The distension-initiated neural and hormonal mechanisms result in the net anterograde propulsion of colonic contents at an adequate rate and temporary storage of feces until it is expelled. After the chyme passes from the terminal ileum into the cecum via controlled opening of the ileocecal valve, luminal contents move distally, while gradual desiccation and mixing occur, and they become progressively more solid.

The transport in the colon has a circadian pattern, increasing after awakening, higher during the day compared to the night, and, specifically, increasing after meals. Actually, this pattern is subject to change if the individual is active during the night, and it is reported that patients suffering from constipation may lack the nocturnal suppression, exhibit reduced response to meals, and lose the spatiotemporal organization of colonic motions. The motor functions in the colon can simply be categorized as transit, i.e., intraluminal movement, and contractile activities. The former can be measured by radiopaque marker studies, colonic scintigraphy, or wireless telemetric capsule methods, and the latter is best measured by intraluminal manometry, but its use is limited to highly selected pediatric cases. These studies indicate that the colonic transit time is around 72 h in adults and 57 h in children.

Colonic motor activity occurs in two forms: phasic, brief contractions and tonic, sustained contractions. Phasic contractions are either propagating or non-propagating sequences. Briefly non-propagated contractions are common and take place as isolated, random bursts, with a frequency of 2–4 Hz. This form of colonic motor activity helps in the mixing of intraluminal contents and the retropulsion of the fecal bolus. Propagated colonic activity can be in both directions in the oral-anal axis: retrograde or anterograde. Retrograde colonic activity is mainly at the proximal colon and is rarer than anterograde activity. However, its frequency increases in constipated individuals.

In addition to propagated contractions, high-amplitude (~100 mmHg) sets of pressure, known as high-amplitude propagated sequences or contractions (HAPSs or HAPCs), have been defined. These sequences occur five or six times a day in adults and significantly more in children below the age of 4, likely to correlate with the increased number of bowel movements. HAPCs can originate anywhere in the colon and migrate distally. Most of the HAPSs terminate at the rectosigmoid segment before reaching the anus. HAPSs are often associated with defecation or passing flatus and are actually equivalent to the mass movements.

The sigmoid colon primarily exhibits motor complexes or periodic colonic motor activity, too. These activities serve to modulate the delivery of fecal material into the rectum. When the sigmoid is distended with the reception of colonic content, contraction at the proximal part and concomitant relaxation of the distal part, i.e., at the rectosigmoid junction, facilitate progression of feces into the rectum. Although there is no solid evidence for an anatomical sphincter between the sigmoid and rectum, the high-pressure zone in the distal sigmoid suggests the presence of a physiological sphincter.

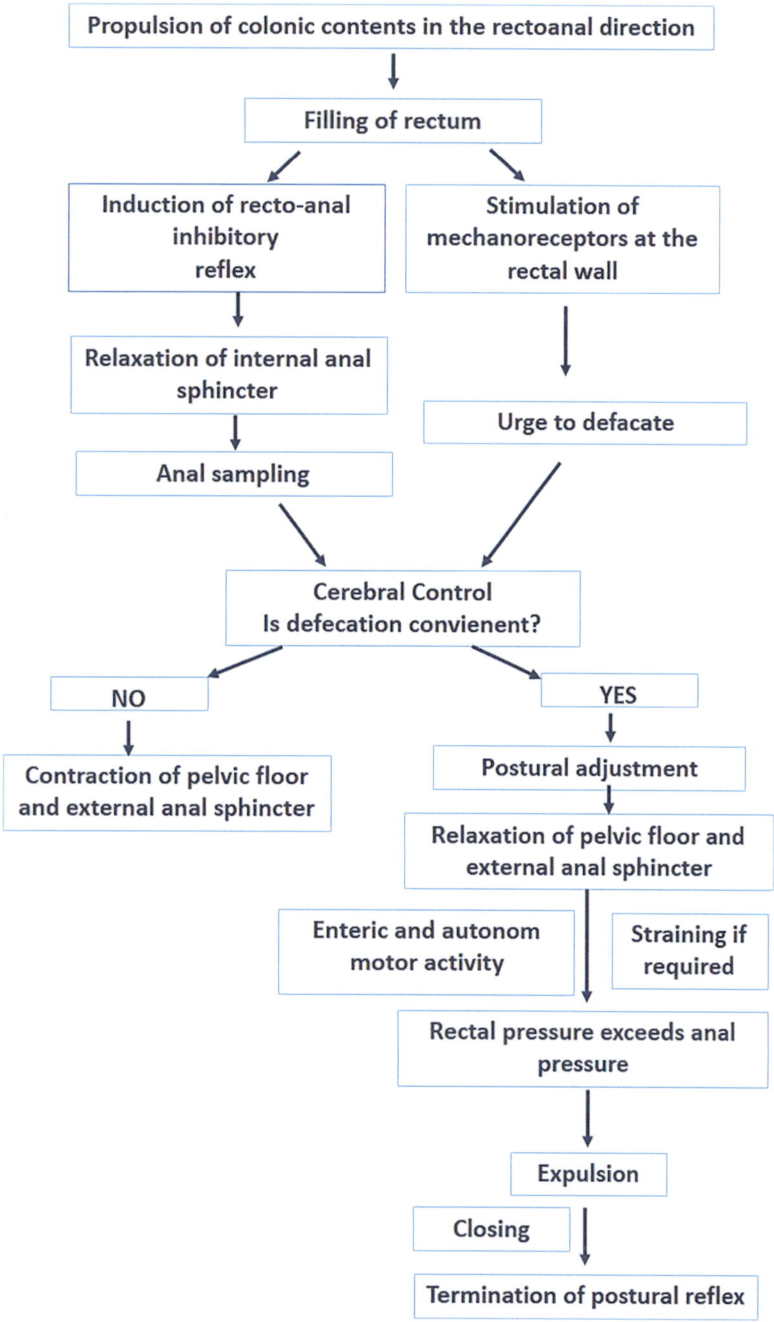

Fig. 2.1 Physiological cascade of defecation

When the feces proceed into the rectum, recurrent motor complexes are activated. However, rectal motor activity propagates in the retrograde direction to keep the rectum empty. It is said to act as a "brake mechanism" to prevent untimely evacuation of the colonic contents. So the rectum remains mostly empty during the basal phase in healthy individuals.

Similar to the rectum, the anal canal is empty at rest. This is achieved by the closed anal sphincter to preserve continence. The anal sphincter complex is controlled by several reflexes and modulated by higher centers, which results in an active seal rather than a passive barrier, except when the individual allows the passage of flatus or feces.

The anal canal is closed by the tonic contraction of the internal anal sphincter (IAS) and the external anal sphincter (EAS). The IAS is composed of slow-twitch, fatigue-resistant smooth muscles and is mainly responsible for continence at rest. The electromyographic studies exhibit a constant IAS activity at rest, interestingly unaffected by respiration and maintained under general anesthesia. Although the contribution of the IAS to the anal canal tone is reported differently under different conditions of rest, active or passive distension, the fact is that it puts the major share at rest. The EAS has a constant tonic activity at rest as well and generates about 30% of the basal resting anal tone. In addition to IAS and EAS, the anal vascular cushions contribute to approximately 15% of the resting tone of the anal canal and add to the sphincteric muscle tone but, more importantly, provide the "hermetic seal."

The anal canal activity is dynamic, and it intermittently and transiently relaxes to allow the passage of rectal contents into the upper anal canal. This is called the sampling reflex, or recto-anal inhibitory reflex, which is also associated with the perception of the physical form of the contents and takes place approximately seven times per hour in healthy individuals but less frequently in patients with incontinence. During this reflex, upper anal canal pressure decreases; lower anal canal pressure, however, remains unchanged. EAS is contracted so that the continence is preserved.

The tonic contraction of the levator ani, puborectalis muscles, and the EAS are helpful to support the weight of the pelvic viscera in the resting state. This is achieved by the postural reflex maintained through the lower lumbar and sacral spinal cord. Among the pelvic floor structures, the puborectalis muscle is probably involved in the defecation process. It maintains the anorectal angle between the long axis of the rectum and the long axis of the anal canal at approximately 90° at rest. This angulation functions in continence; however, it is worth mentioning that increased acuity is related to obstructed defecation. During defecation, the relaxed muscles and the straightened angle facilitate the process.

2.2.1.1.2 The Pre-expulsive Phase

The motor events during this phase end up in the awareness of the person for an urge to defecate. In order to achieve normal defecation, the sensation of "call to stool" is important, and it is likely that the colon, rectum, anus, and pelvic floor structures all contribute to varying degrees.

Defecatory Urge In healthy subjects, HAPSs and the urge to evacuate are closely related. During this phase, the HAPSs start in the proximal colon as unperceived colonic contractions and increase in amplitude to be a full sequence, associated with an urge to defecate as it moves distally. The colonic activity during the pre-expulsive phase moves the colonic contents distally, which stimulates distal afferents in the colon and the rectum. Distension of the distal bowel is associated with an urge to defecate.

The rectum is the primary site of origin of the defecatory urge. The sensation starts with the filling sense and increases gradually with the gradual distension of the rectum. The individual eventually feels a sustained urge to defecate, a sense of discomfort, and an intense urge to defecate when the maximal tolerable volume/pressure is reached. In addition to rectal mechanisms, it has been shown that the need for defecation can be provoked by stimulating nerve endings and stretch receptors in pelvic floor muscles and in the structures adjacent to the rectum.

As explained above, anal canal sensation is essential for the sampling reflex; its role in defecatory urge is unclear, and experimental studies reported a sensation of stool escaping rather than a typical defecatory urge by balloon distension of the anus.

Colonic Motor Activity During the pre-expulsive phase, colonic motor activity exhibits a progressive, time-dependent increase in the frequency and amplitude of the propagated sequences (PSs) up to 1 h before defecation. The origin of PS shifts distally toward the descending colon in the past hour preceding defecation. This pattern reverses in the last 15 min before defecation, when a retrograde shift is seen. PSs are likely to be a part of long colono-colonic reflex pathways.

Rectal Sensorimotor Activity During this phase, rectal filling occurs; physiologically functioning afferent nerves and biomechanical properties of the rectal wall are important for the perception of rectal fullness and the defecatory urge. The fecal bolus, transported by PS activity, deforms the rectal wall and activates mechanoreceptors, inducing reflex rectal contractions in accordance with the volume of the bolus; moreover, the duration of rectal contractile activity correlates with the duration of sensation. Rectal sensation also determines reflex EAS contraction and continence.

In addition to intact receptors and neural connections, the biomechanical properties of the rectum are also important. The rectum is compliant; i.e., it adapts to increasing volume with a slight change in pressure. This is the physiological basis of adaptive relaxation, which enables the rectum to be a temporary storage area, i.e., a reservoir for feces. Rectal distensibility depends on passive mechanical distension or stress relaxation determined by the viscoelastic properties of the rectal wall and active distension as a result of adaptive relaxation, affected mainly by nervous system-mediated smooth muscle tonus.

Pelvic Floor Activity It is contracted to maintain continence, similar to the basal phase. In case a defecatory urge occurs and the timing is inconvenient for defecation, the EAS and pelvic floor muscles contract further voluntarily. The anorectal angle is preserved, elevating the pelvic floor and elongating the high-pressure zone.

Anal Canal Activity Any change in sampling reflex is not documented during the pre-expulsive phase. However, it should be kept in mind that increasing rectal filling during this phase increases the importance of the role of the voluntary contraction in continence.

2.2.1.1.3 The Expulsive Phase

In this phase, evacuation of colonic contents occurs if a conscious decision for defecation is made in the presence of a defecatory urge. The expulsion becomes more effective with straining and with an appropriate posture.

The physiological end point at this phase is elevated intra-abdominal pressure, relaxed pelvic floor, and a relaxed anal canal. The defecation requires voluntary contribution; however, even under physiological conditions, the physical properties and volume of the feces may overcome the voluntary control.

Colonic Activity During defecation, some part of the right as well as the left colon and the rectum empties. Normally, 35–40% of the HAPSs occur during or just before defecation, and all of the defecations are associated with a HAPS. The principle of peristalsis is valid for this phase, too; i.e., the contraction in the colon results in the relaxation of the anal sphincter.

Rectal Activity For defecation, the rectal pressure should exceed the pressure of the anal canal; i.e., increased intrarectal pressure and associated relaxation of the anal canal are essential for evacuation of feces. As straining raises intrapelvic and, hence, intrarectal pressure, it is likely that voluntary straining and cooperative contractions of the bowel affect defecation. However, the modulation of the defecation process by volume and consistency of the stool, as well as the habitual and cultural influences, should always be considered.

Pelvic Floor Activity During this phase, the tonic activity of the pelvic floor is inhibited. Although the exact physiological mechanism of this reflex control is not clear, it is suggested to be via stretch due to increased abdominal pressure. The muscle spindles activated by stretch initially contract pelvic floor muscles, which become inhibitory beyond a critical level. Furthermore, higher centers facilitate or inhibit various stimuli, such as intra-abdominal pressure and pelvic organ distension, to modulate pelvic floor tonus. When the pelvic floor relaxes, it descends and takes the shape of a funnel that tips at the anorectal junction. The angle flattens further when posture is assumed during defecation, which requires a degree of hip flexion.

Anal Canal Activity During the expulsive phase, the anal canal relaxes. Inadequate relaxation of the anal sphincter, as well as the failure of pelvic floor relaxation, is called pelvic floor dyssynergia. IAS relaxes involuntarily in proportion to rectal pressure, which is mediated by the reflex response to rectal distension. The Valsalva maneuver, i.e., contracting the abdominal muscles and diaphragm against a closed glottis and the adequate posture for defecation, results in relaxation of the EAS. The muscles of the anus contract during evacuation, the anorectal angle opens, and further contribution from the contracted pubococcygeus muscle tensing the anterior wall of the anal canal allows only the posterior wall to move backward; the flattening of the anal vascular cushions and shortening of the anal canal help lower the pressure in the anal canal. Evacuation starts and continues with high rectal pressure, augmented by straining. Once an individual starts defecation, propulsive activity continues until the rectum is emptied totally, with the sensory impulses originating from the anus.

2.2.1.1.4 Termination of Defecation

This phase is initiated semi-voluntarily when the individual senses the completion of rectal emptying as a consequence of the ending of the maneuvers to achieve increased intrapelvic pressure. The EAS and pelvic floor are contracted to reverse the pressure gradient. This phase is associated with the "closing reflex," which is important for the recovery of the IAS tonus at the end of defecation. Once the intra-abdominal pressure falls, the postural reflex of the pelvic floor is reactivated. The contraction of the puborectalis tracks the anorectal junction so that the angle regains its basal state. The longitudinal muscles relax, simultaneously elongating the anal canal and letting the anal cushions distend. Collectively, all of the above changes result in the closure of the anal canal [2].

2.3 Reproductive System

The reproductive function is essential for the continuation of the species, is under the delicate control of a complex network of regulatory signals, and is modulated by various endogenous and external conditions. The reproductive system differs from the other body systems so that the differentiation and maturation of the system is a delicately timed phenomenon, a continuous process of events that spans from early fetal life to puberty in both genders and to menopause in women. Not only morphological but also functional changes of the reproductive system are dramatic throughout life, from the neonatal period to puberty, adulthood, and senescence, and, moreover, between genders [17, 37].

In summary, reproductive function involves gametogenesis and steroid hormone production, which are essential both for the facilitation of gametogenesis and gender-specific phenotype. Both of these functions in men and women are activated with pubertal transition and regulated by the hypothalamic-pituitary axis (HPA). The neurons in the arcuate nucleus of the hypothalamus release gonadotropin-releasing hormone (GnRH) in response to various external and internal stimuli (Table 2.2). GnRH is conveyed to the anterior pituitary gland via portal circulation and stimulates gonadotropic cells to synthesize and release luteinizing hormone (LH) and follicle-stimulating hormone (FSH). LH and FSH reach the gonads by circulation and act on correspond-

Table 2.2 The molecules that control the gonadotropin-releasing hormone (GnRH) release

Effecting molecules/conditions	Dominant effect
Glutamate	Stimulator
Noradrenalin	Stimulator
γ-Aminobutyric acid (GABA)	Inhibitor
Serotonin	Inhibitor
Dopamine	Stimulator
Endorphin	Inhibitor
Dark/light input from retina	Inhibitor
Leptin	Stimulator
Stress	Inhibitor
Pheromones	Stimulator/inhibitor

ing cells to stimulate sex steroid hormone synthesis and gametogenesis, respectively [39].

2.3.1 Male Reproductive Function

In men, most of the reproductive organs are located outside of the body, and the genital system functions with the urinary system. The last steps of male reproductive function, erection and ejaculation, involve pelvic structures and the urethra, which proceeds in the penis.

Following pubertal maturation, spermatogenesis is stimulated, and spermatocytes are freed toward the seminiferous tube lumen and travel down the male genital system until they are ejaculated. Through its voyage, the spermatocytes continue to differentiate and mature so that they gain properties required for fertilization, i.e., motility and metabolism shift, and the surrounding medium changes with continuous reabsorption and secretion from the accessory glands, namely the epididymis, seminal vesicles, prostate, and bulbourethral glands.

All the functional aspects and anatomical structures are controlled and maintained by androgens. Testosterone produced by the Leydig cells in the testis acts in paracrine and endocrine fashion to maintain a functional reproductive system lifelong after puberty. The main functions of androgens are listed in Table 2.5 [23–26].

The male reproductive function terminates with two consecutive reflexes: erection and ejaculation.

2.3.1.1 Physiology of Erection

The penile erection is a result of complex neural and vascular mechanisms. The main physiological mechanism to stimulate an erection is mechanical stimulation; however, cortex-induced erection by thoughts, visual stimuli, etc. is possible as well. The hypothalamic medial preoptic area (MPOA), paraventricular nucleus (PVN), and dopamine, as it stimulates oxytocin release, are involved in the central control of erection. Norepinephrine is another erectogenic neurotransmitter acting via α-$_2$ adrenergic receptors; in addition, neurotransmitters such as nitric oxide (NO), α-melanocyte-stimulating hormone (α-MSH), and opioid peptides are involved in the erection process to varying degrees.

For the erection, i.e., penile tumescence, parasympathetic stimulation and sympathetic suppression are both required. Parasympathetic innervation of the penis is derived from the S2 to S4 sacral segments. Patients with spinal cord injury at the sacral level can still experience erections through psychogenic stimulation; if the lesion is above T9, even psychogenic erections do not occur; however, reflexogenic erections may still be maintained. These imply that sympathetic suppression and preservation of the sacral reflex arc may mediate psychogenic and reflexogenic penile erection.

The penis is flaccid when the corporal smooth muscles and cavernous and helicine arteries are constricted. When stimulated, neuronal NO synthase (NOS) is stimulated, and released NO leads to the relaxation of smooth muscles and vasodilation. The initiation of tumescence is via neuronal NO synthase; however, it is maintained through endothelial NOS. The erection starts with the vasodilation of arteries, which eventually results in increased intracorporal pressure and compression of veins, markedly reducing the venous outflow and full erection [22].

2.3.1.2 Physiology of Ejaculation

The stimulation of the penile mechanoreceptors initiates the ejaculation reflex. Ejaculation consists of emission and expulsion phases and is controlled by the ANS [4].

2.3.1.2.1 Emission

The closure of the bladder neck to prevent retrograde spread of the seminal fluid toward the bladder is followed by the ejection of prostatic secretions, mixed with spermatozoa from the vas deferens, into the prostatic urethra. Subsequently, seminal vesicle fluid, constituting 75–80% of the final seminal fluid, is secreted.

The autonomic fibers, predominantly the sympathetic neurons, in the pelvic plexus control organs that are involved in ejaculation. Clinically, the loss of emission after non-nerve-sparing paraaortic lymph node dissection for testicular cancer and induction of emission in paraplegic men through electrical stimulation of the superior hypogastric plexus confirms the role of the pelvic plexus. Similar to the erection reflex, cortical inputs may induce ejaculation.

2.3.1.2.2 Expulsion

Expulsion refers to the ejection of semen through the urethral meatus following emission. The semen is propelled by peristaltic waves as well as the rhythmic contractions of the pelvic skeletal muscles. During expulsion, the bladder neck remains closed, and the external urethral sphincter opens. Even though the external urethral sphincter and the pelvic muscles are innervated by the somatic nervous system, the role of voluntary control in the expulsion process is debatable.

Neuronal Control of Ejaculation The main afferents conveying sensory input from the glans, prepuce, and penile shaft transmit signals to the sacral spinal cord. A secondary afferent route is via the hypogastric nerve, which enters the spinal cord through the thoracolumbar dorsal roots. The efferents consist of sympathetic (T12-L1), parasympathetic (sacral), and motor (sacral Onuf's nucleus) nervous components.

Besides the peripheral nervous system sensory and motor areas, the brain is important for ejaculation. Holstege et al. [15] showed the areas in the brain that are activated during ejaculation by positron emission tomography (Table 2.3).

Neurotransmitter- and Hormone-Mediated Regulation of Ejaculation Many neurotransmitters and hormones are involved in the ejaculation process. The exact role of these molecules varies, as several parameters and different spinal and supraspinal sites and multiple receptor types are affected (Table 2.4).

Ejaculation is a complex process involving several structures and is regulated by extensive neural and hormonal control. However, further research is needed to identify the unknown aspects of these physiological processes [1].

Table 2.3 Central nervous system areas involved in ejaculation

Cerebral cortex
Thalamus   Parvicellular part of the subparafascicular thalamus
Posteromedial bed nucleus of stria terminalis
Posterodorsal medial amygdaloid nucleus
Posterodorsal preoptic nucleus

Hypothalamus
  Medial preoptic area
  Paraventricular nucleus

Mesencephalon   Periaqueductal gray matter
Pons   Paragigantocellular nucleus

2.3.2 Female Reproductive Function

The female reproductive system, although similar to the male reproductive system in fundamental aspects, has anatomical and functional differences. Besides primary functions of gametogenesis and hormone production, in the case of fertilization and pregnancy, it is responsible for the intrauterine development of the offspring during pregnancy and the successful completion of childbirth [11, 23–26].

The primary effector organ of the female reproductive system is the ovary, where gametogenesis and hormone production occur. The fallopian tubes, uterus, cervix, vagina, and breasts are other organs of the reproductive system.

In women who have completed puberty and gained reproductive capability, there is a significant increase in GnRH secretion during different phases of the menstrual cycle. The frequency of GnRH secretion determines whether LH or FSH secretion is predominantly stimulated. When the secretion frequency is higher, LH secretion is dominant and vice versa. LH stimulates the production of steroid hormones in the ovaries. FSH, on the other hand, promotes follicular development in the ovaries and plays a role in the steps of steroid hormone synthesis [7].

This cyclic pattern, repeating approximately every 28 days under the HPA, leads to changes both in the blood levels and the effects of steroid

Table 2.4 The hormones and neurotransmitters, their effects, and the receptors involved in the regulation of ejaculation

Neurotransmitter/ hormone	Dominant effect	Receptor subtype
Dopamine	Stimulates ejaculation	D2, D3, and D4
Serotonin	Inhibits ejaculation (brain) Stimulates ejaculation (medulla spinalis)	1A, 1B, and 2C
Nitric oxide	Inhibits ejaculation (reduction of seminal vesicle contraction and seminal emission)	
Oxytocin	Facilitates ejaculation (epididymal contractions and sperm motility) Stimulates ejaculation (brain)	
Prolactin	Inhibitor (through inhibition of GnRH and dopamine production)	
Thyroid hormones	Delayed ejaculation (hypothyroidism) Premature ejaculation (hyperthyroidism)	
Glucocorticoids	No known effect under physiological conditions Improves disturbed function	
Estrogens	Facilitates ejaculation (epididymal contractions)	
Androgens	Delayed ejaculation (hypoandrogenism) Premature ejaculation (hyperthyroidism) Facilitates the ejaculatory reflex (brain) Stimulates pelvic floor muscles involved in ejaculation	

and protein hormones synthesized by the ovaries. Under the control of cellular programs and hormonal milieu, follicle development results in ovulation approximately on the 14th day of each menstrual cycle. The interactions between germ cells and somatic cells, involving gap junctions, cytokines, and growth factors are crucial for the control of gametogenesis. Under normal physiological conditions, this process prepares a single follicle for ovulation.

The ovulated ovum freed into the pelvic cavity is captured by the fimbriae of the fallopian tubes and begins its journey toward the uterus. The remaining cells of the follicle luteinize, forming the corpus luteum (CL), the endocrine structure responsible for hormone production during the second (luteal) phase of the menstrual cycle.

If the ovum is not fertilized, the lifespan of the CL is fixed at 10 days. Afterward, CL begins to degenerate, and within approximately 4 days, it loses its function entirely, transforming into fibrous tissue. This grayish-white structure, called the corpus albicans, remains on the ovary surface as a lifelong scar, representing each ovulation event.

The ovaries, through the formation of follicles and CL and their control of hormone secretion, regulate the monthly rhythm of the female reproductive system from puberty until menopause. The first day of menstrual bleeding is considered the first day of the cycle. The period up to ovulation, around day 14, is called the follicular phase. The 14 days following ovulation are referred to as the luteal phase, and the 28-day cycle concludes with the onset of a new menstrual period.

The two steroid hormones, estrogen and progesterone, are produced in the ovaries in monthly cycles. In the female reproductive system, cholesterol-initiated hormone biosynthesis requires both LH and FSH, as well as both thecal and granulosa cells. The main hormone in the first 14 days of a monthly cycle is estrogen, produced by the follicles, whereas estrogen and progesterone are produced by CL in the second half of the cycle.

The effects of sex steroid hormones are given in Table 2.5.

The cyclic hormonal changes affect other reproductive organs, too. All the organs serve for a possible fertilization in the first 14 days, for implantation of the zygote in the last 14 days, and to prevent polyspermy.

The uterus is composed of a thick muscular layer (myometrium) and the endometrium, which lines it internally. The cyclical changes observed in the uterus primarily occur in the innermost

Table 2.5 The physiological effects of sex steroid hormones

Testosterone	Estrogen	Progesterone
Negative feedback to the hypothalamus and hypophysis	Negative feedback to the hypothalamus and hypophysis	Negative feedback to the hypothalamus and hypophysis
Stimulation of spermatogenesis	Stimulation of growth Internal and external genital organs (prenatal, postnatal) Breasts (duct formation, fat deposition) Follicle (paracrine and autocrine) Linear growth	Prepares the endometrium for the implantation of the embryo
Development, maintenance, and function of male accessory glands Penis Scrotum Urethra Epididymis Prostate Bulbourethral glands	Proliferation and increased function of smooth muscles and epithelial surfaces Contraction of fallopian tubes, ciliary activity Uterine contraction and response to oxytocin Vaginal epithelial cornification Mucus secretion Coagulation factors in liver	Decreases contraction of fallopian tubes and myometrium
Anabolic effects	Bone deposition	Decreases vaginal cornification
Libido and aggressive behavior	Stimulation of neurogenesis and dendrite proliferation	Increases the tendency to sleep
Prenatal development of male phenotype and postnatal maintenance	Stimulation of prolactin (PRL) release	Inhibits the milk-producing effect of PRL
Body hair distribution	Decrease the fat content of skin secretions	Stimulate the growth of breasts (glands)
Unfavorable lipid profile	Favorable lipid profile	Increases body temperature
Abdominal fat accumulation	Female body contours	Anesthetic effect

layer, the endometrium. This layer undergoes renewal (proliferative phase), differentiation (secretory phase), and shedding (menstrual phase) in cycles of approximately 28 days if pregnancy does not occur.

The functional layer of the endometrium is 1–2 mm thick at the end of menstruation, and it thickens throughout the follicular phase under the proliferative effects of estrogen. Endometrial proliferation is accompanied by elongation and thickening of the spiral arteries, which defines this phase as the "proliferative" phase.

In the postovulatory phase, proliferation and thickening of the endometrium continue under the combined effects of progesterone and estrogen secreted by CL. Progesterone induces a secretory appearance in the endometrium, which begins producing significant amounts of secretions. Therefore, the second half of the cycle is referred to as the "secretory" phase. The fluid secreted into the uterine lumen is rich in nutrients to support the zygote before implantation. As long as the trophic effects of steroid hormones persist, the endometrium continues to thicken, and the spiral arteries elongate, thicken, and become coiled.

In the cycles where the ovum is not fertilized, CL begins to degenerate on the 24th day, and it loses its function completely within 4 days, so hormone levels decrease to their lowest value. The loss of trophic support causes the upper layers of the endometrium to shed. Reduced blood flow due to compression of the arteries in the thinning endometrium initially leads to spot-like bleeding, which culminates in menstrual bleeding on day 28. From day 25 onward, the decline in estrogen and progesterone from CL degeneration triggers the release of proteolytic enzymes, which digest tissues. Constriction and compression of endometrial vessels induce ischemia, initiating bleeding. Moreover, increased prostaglandin F2α during the secretory phase facilitates the release of acid hydrolases from lysosomes and stimulates myometrial contractions that help in the expulsion of the degenerated endometrial tissue. Menstrual bleeding lasts an average of 4 days, with an estimated 30 ml of arterial blood loss. Including the fluid and tissue debris from the uterine lumen, the total volume expelled is higher.

The cervix and vagina under estrogenic effect secrete more alkaline and less cellular mucus to ease the passage of spermatocytes. On the other hand, when progesterone is the dominating hormone, mucus gains the characteristics of a mechanical and chemical barrier as its acidity increases, and it becomes a thick cellular medium.

2.3.2.1 Physiology of Pregnancy

All the functions summarized above aim to ensure the fertilization of a single ovum by a single sperm, which is vital for the continuation of the species. Pregnancy, the period between fertilization and delivery of the baby, lasts an average of 280 days (9 months and 10 days) and occurs within the female reproductive system [36].

2.3.2.1.1 Fertilization

Approximately 300 million sperm released into the female reproductive system during ejaculation progress through the vagina, cervix, and uterus toward the fallopian tubes. During this process, prostaglandins in the semen and oxytocin released by sexual arousal stimulate smooth muscle contractions, facilitating the movement of sperm. Capacitation, which occurs in the female reproductive system, enhances the effectiveness of this progression. However, only about 100 sperm complete this journey, as most perish due to the conditions of the female reproductive system, such as acidic pH and a lack of nutrients and oxygen. If the spermatocytes that are fastest and those with metabolic adaptations meet the ovum during the fertilization window, i.e., 3 days before and 1 day after ovulation, the likelihood of pregnancy is very high.

2.3.2.1.2 Physiological Changes During Pregnancy

The pregnancy period involves both fetal growth and maternal adaptations. For the point of pelvic health, the growing uterus, initially in the pelvis and then eventually growing toward the abdominal cavity, is a big challenge for abdominal and pelvic floor structures.

The detailed physiological changes during pregnancy are beyond the scope of this chapter; that is why we will focus mainly on pelvis-associated changes and adaptations.

The physiological events observed during pregnancy result from both changes caused by the growing fetus and the body's adaptive mechanisms. Throughout pregnancy, the fetus continues to grow and differentiate, acquiring the characteristics necessary for adaptation to extrauterine life. On the other hand, all of the changes in the maternal physiology serve to meet the needs of the fetus, ensure the silence of the uterus until term, prepare the uterus for labor, and support lactation after birth [27].

When considering the whole body, the most significant change in the mother during pregnancy is weight gain. The average physiological weight gain during gestation ranges between 10.5 and kg, attributed to the growth of the fetus and increases in maternal body fluids and fat stores. However, it is more appropriate to evaluate weight gain during pregnancy based on the prepregnancy body mass index (BMI). It is important to note that weight gain during pregnancy outside the physiological limits—either below or above—may pose risks to the health of the baby and/or the mother. Regarding the major share of the weight gain, it is in the pelvis: the fetus (2.6–3.2 kg), amniotic fluid and fetal membranes (1 kg), placenta (0.7 kg), and uterus (1 kg). The load on the pelvic floor increases gradually and affects the urinary and gastrointestinal systems.

During pregnancy, the kidneys shift upward due to the pressure exerted by the growing uterus. Additionally, increased vascularization, interstitial volume, and dead space enlarge the kidneys by approximately 1 cm [9]. The anatomical and functional changes can be summarized as:

- Increased glomerular filtration rate (GFR) of approximately 60% as a result of increased blood volume, enhanced renal blood flow, and compression of the abdominal aorta by the growing uterus. Increased GFR leads to decreased levels of serum creatinine (Cr) and blood urea nitrogen (BUN), as well as glycosuria and aminoaciduria due to a high filtration load.
- Increased deoxycorticosterone (DOC) produced by conversion from progesterone promotes water and salt retention in the kidneys.
- Dilation of the collecting systems is observed from the first trimester onward, which can lead to hydronephrosis. The main reasons for this dilation are the effects of progesterone and the increased pressure on the ureters.
- Increased ureteral pressure is associated with increased risk of urinary retention, nephrolithiasis, urinary tract infections (UTIs), and pyelonephritis.
- Reduced bladder tone resulting in frequent urination, urgency, and urinary incontinence [3].

These complaints intensify in the third trimester as the baby's head descends into the pelvis.

From the early stages of pregnancy to delivery, although manifesting with varying symptoms, GIS is affected. In the early period, nausea and vomiting associated with hCG may occur, while as pregnancy progresses, increased intra-abdominal and intragastric pressure can lead to reflux and heartburn in the esophagus. Additionally, gastrin produced from the placenta increases gastric acid production, contributing to GIS symptoms in 50–80% of pregnant individuals.

The relaxation of the lower esophageal sphincter due to progesterone further raises the likelihood of reflux. This relaxing effect also prolongs stomach emptying and gastrointestinal transit time, which explains why a significant number of pregnant women experience bloating and constipation.

During delivery, the mother's anxiety, pain, and, sometimes, the anticholinergic and/or opioid drugs used, which reduce smooth muscle tone, can increase the risk of aspiration, particularly in cases requiring general anesthesia.

Throughout the pregnancy, alkaline phosphatase levels increase due to placental production, while transaminase and bilirubin levels decrease slightly as the volume of extracellular fluid increases.

The adjustments in the cardiovascular system (CVS) are crucial for both the mother and the baby. The cardiac output (CO) is maintained to meet the body's demands. CO is determined by stroke volume (SV), the amount of blood pumped per cardiac cycle, and heart rate (HR). During pregnancy, total peripheral resistance (TPR) decreases, and total blood and plasma volumes expand, resulting in increased SV and, consequently, CO by up to 40% compared to prepregnancy levels. Increased sympathetic tone and altered sensitivity to catecholamines, leading to positive chronotropic (increased HR) and inotropic (enhanced myocardial contractility) effects, have a role in increased CO.

The decreased TPR can be explained by the transformation of the uterine spiral arteries into low-resistance, high-compliance vessels to support increased uteroplacental blood flow. This contributes to reduced TPR as well as the estrogen-stimulated nitric oxide production that facilitates vasodilation.

Mean arterial pressure (MAP), which drives tissue perfusion, depends on CO and TPR. Until late pregnancy, BP generally remains normal. Total body volume increases by up to 8 liters due to the expansion of body fluids. This volume includes maternal and fetal circulatory systems, the uteroplacental circulation, and the growing amniotic sac. To accommodate the increasing demands of the growing fetus, uteroplacental blood flow increases, and blood volume rises by up to 50%. Approximately 25% of the total blood flow is directed to the uteroplacental unit during pregnancy, with additional increases in blood flow to the skin, breasts, and kidneys. However, low CO or hypoxic conditions in the mother can lead to growth restriction, miscarriage, or preterm birth due to compromised fetal blood flow.

During labor, uterine contractions inject 200–500 mL of blood into systemic circulation with each contraction, increasing SV and CO by 15% at the early stages of labor and up to 50% at the later stage. Contractions and stressors such as pain and anxiety via sympathetic activation lead to further increases in BP and HR. Epidural anesthesia is often recommended for pregnant women with underlying cardiovascular diseases (CVDs) to manage pain and stress, except in conditions like aortic stenosis, where it is contraindicated.

After the delivery of the baby, the contracting uterus relieves pressure on the inferior vena cava, and increased venous return leads to a 60% rise in CO. In women with CVD, this surge can elevate the risk of pulmonary edema from the second stage of labor onward. CO begins to decline within the first hour after birth and normalizes to prepregnancy levels within about 2 weeks postpartum.

The hemodynamic system is affected significantly by the postural changes. After the second trimester, the vena cava is compressed in the supine position, reducing venous return and CO. This can decrease uterine and fetal blood flow. Hence, during prolonged labor, women should avoid being in the supine position for extended periods.

Significant adaptations occur in the respiratory system from the beginning to the end of pregnancy. Increasing progesterone and relaxin hormones loosen the costo-sternal ligaments; the anterior-posterior and lateral thoracic diameters increase due to the upward displacement of the diaphragm. As a result, compliance decreases, respiratory rate increases, vital capacity remains unchanged, total lung capacity decreases, functional residual capacity (FRC) and residual volume decrease, and tidal volume and minute ventilation increase, leading to a reduction in partial carbon dioxide pressure (Pco_2). Moreover, the mechanical compression of the diaphragm by the expanding uterus and fetus, the elevated metabolic rate associated increase in oxygen consumption and carbon dioxide production as well as lowered central threshold for carbon dioxide regulation by the elevated progesterone levels ultimately leads to a state of highly enhanced ventilation. Spirometry parameters do not change during pregnancy [35].

Approximately 15% acceleration in metabolism and around 30% increase in oxygen consumption, alongside a decreased FRC, compromise maternal oxygen reserves and increase the vulnerability to hypoxia during pregnancy. Although minute ventilation increases oxygenation, the amount of carbon dioxide decreases, resulting in respiratory alkalosis. However, this alkaline state is fully compensated by the kidneys through bicarbonate excretion. Bicarbonate levels are about 25% lower during pregnancy, reducing the buffering capacity for potential acidosis. In healthy pregnant women, plasma ketone levels are higher, leading to earlier ketoacidosis during fasting periods. Insulin resistance and low serum bicarbonate concentration are the reasons for fasting ketoacidosis, even in nondiabetic pregnant women.

During labor, pain, anxiety, and breath control lead to hyperventilation, which is prominent, especially during the second stage of labor. Narcotic analgesics used during this period may suppress respiration. Within 48 h after delivery, all respiratory parameters return to normal values.

Blood volume expands for adequate blood flow from the 7th week onward and peaks between the 30th and 34th weeks. During pregnancy, erythropoietin production in the kidneys rises, stimulating erythrocyte production. However, *dilutional anemia* is inevitable, as the plasma volume increases more than the red blood cell mass. Hemoglobin and hematocrit (Htc) levels decrease. Reduced blood viscosity associated with the lower Htc significantly facilitates blood flow. The maternal iron requirement increases (5–6 mg/day), and iron deficiency anemia can lead to obstetric complications.

In a normal pregnancy, the leukocyte counts average around 14,000/mm^3 and may increase to 30,000/mm^3 during labor and the postpartum period. It is mediated by the adrenocortical hormones observed during pregnancy. Platelet counts are generally within normal range; however, increased aggregation may result in lower counts. Pregnancy is considered a *prothrombotic state*, with a four times higher risk of venous thromboembolism (VTE). This elevated risk primarily results from increased production of procoagulant clotting factors such as fibrinogen and factors VII, VIII, IX, X, and XII. Additionally, a decrease in protein S activity, increased resistance to protein C, and elevated levels of plasminogen activator inhibitors reduce fibrinolysis, further contributing to the risk of VTE. Furthermore, factors like *venous stasis* and impaired venous return due to uterine compression make venous thromboembolism one of the leading causes of maternal mortality during pregnancy [34, 35].

The hormonal milieu changes very significantly during pregnancy. First of all, a new endocrine organ, the placenta, is functional during pregnancy. Following implantation, various hormones are initially produced by trophoblasts, and as the placenta develops, it takes over and plays a crucial endocrine role in maintaining hormonal balance throughout pregnancy and initiating labor when the time comes, including maintaining the state of pregnancy, growth, and development of the mammary gland; adapting maternal metabolism to support the growing fetus; regulating fetal development and timing; and managing the progression of labor. Some of the hormones secreted from the placenta are listed in Table 2.6.

Besides placental hormones, all of the maternal endocrine organs adapt to pregnancy; some of them are listed in Table 2.7 [38].

The delivery of the baby is the termination of the pregnancy, and labor has four stages (Table 2.8).

The pregnancy period and obstetric trauma challenge the pelvic structures. Perineal trauma, especially, is a very common complication of vaginal delivery. On the other hand, the increasing load on the pelvic floor throughout the pregnancy increases complications like pelvic prolapses, urinary dipping, and/or incontinence even after cesarean section.

Table 2.6 Hormones produced and released from the placenta [34]

Human chorionic gonadotropin (hCG)
Human placental lactogen (hPL)
Progesterone
Estrogens
Corticotropin-releasing hormone (CRH)
Somatostatin
Thyrotropin-releasing hormone (TRH)
Oxytocin
Insulin-like growth factors (IGF)
Adrenocorticotropic hormone (ACTH)
Placental growth hormone (PGH)
Transforming growth factor-β (TGF-β)
Activin
Follistatin
Inhibin A/B
Leptin
Ghrelin

Table 2.7 The main endocrine organs and the increased hormones during pregnancy

Endocrine organ	Hormones
Hypophysis	Prolactin Growth hormone Adrenocorticotropic hormone
Thyroid gland	Total thyroxine Total triiodothyronine
Adrenal cortex	Cortisol Aldosterone
Ovaries	Relaxin Inhibin Activin

Table 2.8 The stages observed in the uterus during pregnancy and active labor

Stage	Duration	Observation	Dominant hormones
0 Quiescence	Throughout pregnancy	Myometrium is silent	Progesterone Prostacyclin Relaxin Nitric oxide Parathormone-related peptide hPL
I Cervical	Primigravid ~12 h Multigravid ~6 h	From not effaced/not dilated To fully dilated	Estrogen Prostaglandins CRH
II Expulsion	Primigravid ~2 h Multigravid ~30 min	From full cervical dilatation To the expulsion of the fetus	Prostaglandins Oxytocin
III Expulsion of placenta	~15 min	From the expulsion of the fetus To the expulsion of the placenta	Prostaglandins Oxytocin
IV. Involution	1 h to a few weeks	From the expulsion of the placenta To the stabilization of the mother and fetus	Oxytocin Prostaglandins Thrombin

2.4 Pelvic Floor

The pelvic floor is made up of muscles, and their functions are crucial for all the above-summarized systems. Pelvic floor muscles support the pelvic organs by coordinated contraction and relaxation. The active support by muscular contraction, together with the passive support provided by the surrounding connective tissue and fascia, is important. Briefly, when intra-abdominal pressure increases, the pelvic floor muscles contract reflexively with upward movement and close the vagina and urethral and anal sphincters. The normally functioning pelvic floor is critical in maintaining continence. Pelvic floor relaxation occurs transiently for brief periods during micturition and defecation. The involvement of the pelvic floor for urinary and fecal continence and expulsion is explained above.

The pelvic floor muscles, genitalia, and ANS are coordinated for normal sexual function. As the reproductive system is anatomically and functionally different between men and women, the contribution of the pelvic floor is different accordingly. However, the sexual response in both genders is under the control of the parasympathetic system during the excitement phase and the sympathetic system during the orgasm phase. In women, the arousal stage of sexual intercourse involves both psychological and physical factors, with generalized congestion and lubrication. Then, if sexual orgasm is achieved, a spinal reflex mediated by the pudendal nerve coordinates the repeated contractions of 0.8-s intervals in the pelvic floor muscles, anal sphincter, and uterus. The erection and ejaculation reflexes in male sexual function, initiated by the mechanical stimulation and/or cortical input via parasympathetic nerves, relax the corpus cavernosa so that they are filled with blood; at the same time, the pelvic floor muscles contract to promote rigidity.

In women, pelvic floor functions are especially important and change during the period of pregnancy. Various musculoskeletal adaptations take place during this period for the well-being of the growing fetus and mother and to prepare the mother's body for delivery. These are increased maternal weight, elongated abdominal muscles, increased lumbar lordosis, anterior pelvic tilt and pelvic width, and an anteriorly shifted center of gravity as the fetus grows and hormones, namely progesterone and relaxin, mediate joint laxity.

When taken together, advancing pregnancy increases the load on hip extensors, hip abductors, ankle plantar flexors, and the pelvic floor muscles. It is recommended that women who plan pregnancy start exercises to strengthen the pelvic floor and continue during pregnancy.

The pelvic floor muscles work with coordinated contraction and relaxation as a unit, voluntarily or involuntarily. Voluntary control is on demand; on the other hand, involuntary contraction is a reflex response to an increased intra-abdominal pressure to prevent incontinence, e.g., during a cough. Involuntary relaxation allows normal micturition or defecation, e.g., during straining or the Valsalva maneuver [31].

References

1. Alwaal A, Breyer BN, Lue TF. Normal male sexual function: emphasis on orgasm and ejaculation. Fertil Steril. 2015;104(5):1051–60. https://doi.org/10.1016/j.fertnstert.2015.08.033.
2. Bajwa A, Emmanuel A. The physiology of continence and evacuation. Best Pract Res Clin Gastroenterol. 2009;23:477–85. https://doi.org/10.1016/j.bpg.2009.06.002.
3. Beers K, Patel N. Kidney physiology in pregnancy. Adv Chronic Kidney Dis. 2020;27(6):449–54. https://doi.org/10.1053/j.ackd.2020.07.006.
4. Clement P, Giuliano F. Physiology and pharmacology of ejaculation. Basic Clin Pharmacol Toxicol. 2016;119(Suppl 3):18–25. https://doi.org/10.1111/bcpt.12546.
5. de Groat WC, Yoshimura N. Anatomy and physiology of the lower urinary tract. Handb Clin Neurol. 2015a;130:61–108. https://doi.org/10.1016/B978-0-444-63247-0.00005-5.
6. de Groat WC, Yoshimura N. Neural control of the lower urinary tract. Handb Compr Physiol. 2015b;5(1):327–96. https://doi.org/10.1002/cphy.c130056.
7. D'Souza AC, Wageh M, Williams JS, Colenso-Semple LM, McCarthy DG, McKay AKA, Elliott-Sale KJ, Burke LM, Parise G, MacDonald MJ, Tarnopolsky MA, Phillips SM. Menstrual cycle hormones and oral contraceptives: a multimethod systems physiology-based review of their impact on key aspects of female physiology. J Appl Physiol (1985). 2023;135(6):1284–99. https://doi.org/10.1152/japplphysiol.00346.2023.
8. Fogo AB, Harris RC. Crosstalk between glomeruli and tubules. Nat Rev Nephrol. 2024; https://doi.org/10.1038/s41581-024-00907-0.
9. Gabbe SG, Niebyl JR, Simpson JL. Obstetrics: normal and problem pregnancies. 5th ed. Philadelphia: Churchill Livingston; 2007. p. 70.
10. Greenwood-Van Meerveld B, Johnson AC, Grundy D. Gastrointestinal pharmacology. In: Handbook of experimental pharmacology, vol. 239. Cham: Springer; 2017. p. 1–16. https://doi.org/10.1007/164_2016_118.
11. Hall JE. Female physiology before pregnancy and female hormones. In: Guyton and Hall textbook of medical physiology. 14th ed. Philadelphia: Elsevier; 2020.
12. Hamid MS. Physiology of the gastrointestinal tract. 6th ed. London: Academic; 2018.
13. Heitmann PT, Vollebregt PF, Knowles CH, Lunniss PJ, Dinning PG, Scott SM. Understanding the physiology of human defaecation and disorders of continence and evacuation. Nat Rev Gastroenterol Hepatol. 2021;18(11):751–69. https://doi.org/10.1038/s41575-021-00487-5.
14. Higashihara E, Harada T, Fukuhara H. Juxtaglomerular apparatus-mediated homeostatic mechanisms: therapeutic implication for chronic kidney disease. Expert Opin Pharmacother. 2024;25(7):819–32. https://doi.org/10.1080/14656566.2024.2357188.
15. Holstege G, Georgiadis JR, Paans AM, Meiners LC, van der Graaf FH, Reinders AA. Brain activation during human male ejaculation. J Neurosci. 2003;23(27):9185–93. https://doi.org/10.1523/JNEUROSCI.23-27-09185.2003.
16. Johnson LR. Gastrointestinal physiology: Mosby physiology series. 9th ed. Philadelphia: Elsevier; 2018.
17. Jones EE. Fertilization, pregnancy, and lactation. In: Boron W, Boulpaep EL, editors. Textbook of medical physiology. 3rd ed. Philadelphia: Elsevier; 2021.
18. Jung J, Ahn HK, Huh Y. Clinical and functional anatomy of the urethral sphincter. Int Neurourol J. 2012;16(3):102–6. https://doi.org/10.5213/inj.2012.16.3.102.
19. Koeppen BM, Stanton BA. Renal physiology. 6th ed. Philadelphia: Elsevier; 2018.
20. Kola JB, Docsa T, Uray K. Mechanosensing in the physiology and pathology of the gastrointestinal tract. Int J Mol Sci. 2022;24(1):177. https://doi.org/10.3390/ijms24010177. PMID: 36613619; PMCID: PMC9820522.
21. Lote CJ. Principles of renal physiology. 5th ed. New York: Springer; 2012.
22. MacDonald SM, Burnett AL. Physiology of erection and pathophysiology of erectile dysfunction. Urol Clin North Am. 2021;48(4):513–25. https://doi.org/10.1016/j.ucl.2021.06.009.
23. Mesano S, Jones EE. Female reproductive system. In: Boron W, Boulpaep EL, editors. Textbook of medical physiology. 3rd ed. Philadelphia: Elsevier; 2016a.
24. Mesano S, Jones EE. Male reproductive system. In: Boron W, Boulpaep EL, editors. Textbook of medical physiology. 3rd ed. Philadelphia: Elsevier; 2016b.
25. Molina PE. Female reproductive systems. In: Endocrine physiology. 5th ed. New York: Mc Graw Hill; 2018a.
26. Molina PE. Male reproductive systems. In: Endocrine physiology. 5th ed. New York: Mc Graw Hill; 2018b.
27. Morton A, Teasdale S. Physiological changes in pregnancy and their influence on the endocrine investigation. Clin Endocrinol. 2022;96(1):3–11.

28. Nawata CM, Pannabecker TL. Mammalian urine concentration: a review of renal medullary architecture and membrane transporters. J Comp Physiol B. 2018;188(6):899–918. https://doi.org/10.1007/s00360-018-1164-3.
29. Palit S, Lunniss PJ, Scott SM. The physiology of human defecation. Dig Dis Sci. 2012;57(6):1445–64. https://doi.org/10.1007/s10620-012-2071-1.
30. Pollak MR, Quaggin SE, Hoenig MP, Dworkin LD. The glomerulus: the sphere of influence. Clin J Am Soc Nephrol. 2014;9(8):1461–9. https://doi.org/10.2215/CJN.09400913.
31. de Tayrac R, Jundt K, Letouzey V, Cayrac M, Masia F, Mousty E, Marès P. Anatomy and physiology of the pelvic floor. In: Ismail KMK, editor. Perineal trauma at childbirth. 1st ed. Birmingham; 2016. https://doi.org/10.1016/j.gtc.2008.06.003.
32. Roy HA, Green AL. The central autonomic network and regulation of bladder function. Front Neurosci. 2019;13:535. https://doi.org/10.3389/fnins.2019.00535.
33. Santucci NR, Velez A. Physiology of lower gastrointestinal tract. Aliment Pharmacol Ther. 2024;60(Suppl 1):S1–S19. https://doi.org/10.1111/apt.17900.
34. Smith R. The placenta as an endocrine organ/placental endocrinology. In: Petraglia F, Di Tommaso M, Mecacci F, editors. Hormones and pregnancy: basic science and clinical implications. Cambridge: Cambridge University Press; 2022.
35. Tan EK, Tan EL. Alterations in physiology and anatomy during pregnancy. Best Pract Res Clin Obstet Gynaecol. 2013;27(6):791–802. https://doi.org/10.1016/j.bpobgyn.2013.08.001.
36. Vannuccini S, Paternò I, Challis JRG, Petraglia F. The neuroendocrinology of pregnancy. In: Petraglia F, Di Tommaso M, Mecacci F, editors. Hormones and pregnancy: basic science and clinical implications. Cambridge: Cambridge University Press; 2022.
37. White BA. Male and female reproductive system. In: Koeppen BM, Stanton BA, Hall JM, Swiatecka-Urban A, editors. Berne and Levy physiology. 8th ed. Philadelphia: Elsevier; 2023.
38. White BA, Harrison JR, Mehlmann LM. Fertilization, pregnancy, and lactation. In: Endocrine and reproductive physiology. 5th ed. Amsterdam: Elsevier; 2019.
39. Xie Q, Kang Y, Zhang C, Xie Y, Wang C, Liu J, Yu C, Zhao H, Huang D. The role of kisspeptin in the control of the hypothalamic-pituitary-gonadal axis and reproduction. Front Endocrinol (Lausanne). 2022;28(13):925206. https://doi.org/10.3389/fendo.2022.925206.

3 Biomechanics for Pelvic and Women's Health

Senem Demirdel and Tezel Yıldırım Şahan

3.1 Introduction

The pelvic system is drastically understudied from a biomechanical perspective. In order to comprehend how a structure changes shape in response to an applied force, biomechanics applies mechanical engineering concepts to biological systems [36]. The complex and interrelated supportive tissues and muscles that make up the pelvic floor are intended to counteract the effects of intra-abdominal pressure and gravity while simultaneously giving the pelvic organs the necessary support [179]. Biomechanical investigations of the pelvic region and women's health represent a complex and dynamic field that requires a multidisciplinary approach. Understanding the relationships between female physiology, anatomy, and biomechanics is of great importance for both clinical practice and academic research. Issues such as pelvic floor muscle function; biomechanical changes during and/or after pregnancy, childbirth, and menopause; the effects of menopause; and pelvic dysfunction are important components of women's health [50].

This chapter emphasizes the role of pelvic floor biomechanics in women's health and includes the latest scientific data and clinical applications in this field. Increasing biomechanical knowledge in women's health aims to improve the quality of life of women by contributing to the development of more effective treatment and rehabilitation approaches. Preventive and therapeutic strategies can be developed by examining and comprehending these systems from a biomechanical standpoint [50].

The goal of this chapter is to describe the pelvic region's biomechanical makeup, physiological alterations, and clinical implications in depth. Clinical evaluation techniques and rehabilitation strategies will also be covered concurrently, offering a thorough viewpoint for academic researchers and health professionals. This chapter presents the mechanical properties of the female and male pelvic systems, the biomechanics of the joints associated with the pelvis, the biomechanical properties of the pelvic organs, and pelvic biomechanics in different conditions such as pregnancy or menopause and addresses the main challenges and issues in research and treatments. Its primary aim is to analyze the relevant literature, aiming to improve our understanding of the mechanisms that influence pelvic biomechanics or predispose to pathomechanics.

S. Demirdel (✉) · T. Y. Şahan
Department of Orthopedic Physiotherapy and Rehabilitation, Gülhane Faculty of Physiotherapy and Rehabilitation, University of Health Science, Ankara, Türkiye
e-mail: senem.demirdel@sbu.edu.tr; tezelyildirim.sahan@sbu.edu.tr

T. Akbayrak, E. Üzelpasaci (eds.), *Physiotherapy and Rehabilitation in Pelvic and Women's Health-Related Problems*, https://doi.org/10.1007/978-3-032-28741-0_3

3.1.1 Biomechanics of the Pelvic Ring

The ischium, pubis, ilium, sacrum, and coccyx make up the pelvis [9]. The os coxae is made up of the pubis, ischium, and ilium bones. Each os coxa connects to the sacrum posteriorly via the sacroiliac joint and anteriorly via the symphysis pubis. At these joints, there is a slight amount of rotation and translation. In the os coxae, the acetabulum and the femoral head articulate to form the hip joint [89].

The pelvic girdle transmits and supports the weight of the upper body to the lower extremities when standing or moving and when sitting. It also provides attachment points for many lower extremity and trunk muscles [95]. The pelvis is crucial to a woman's ability to give birth and support her pelvic organs [43].

Fetal pelvic development begins in the fifth week of pregnancy and ossifies from the third month [180]. After birth, the growth of the pelvis progresses rapidly until the age of 3; then, the growth rate slows down [163, 180]. Fusion of the three bony centers in the acetabulum is completed between the ages of 11 and 14 [65, 180]. Around the age of 30, the female pelvis's size and form stabilize [66]. The bony pelvis expands by more than 20 mm between the ages of 20 and 80 [11].

The bony structure that forms the pelvis consists of trabecular bone surrounded by thin cortical bone. In the pelvic girdle, forces are transferred mainly through the cortical bone [39]. The area around the acetabulum is the most important weight-bearing area in the bony pelvis. The pubic region, ischium, and iliac crest play a lesser role in weight-bearing [107]. The stresses acting on the pelvis are compression, tension, bending, and shear forces. The maximum stress is compression in the upper part of S1, the sacroiliac joint, and the acetabular roof [60]. Compared to other sacral levels (S2–S5), the S1 body is exposed to greater compression forces [166]. In the acetabulum, most of the loads are transmitted through the acetabular roof, i.e., the upper and lateral part of the acetabulum. The posterior part of the acetabulum plays a minor role in load transmission. Muscle and joint reaction forces create compression and tensile stress in the acetabulum. Compression forces are more common on the lateral side. Tensile stresses are lower than compression forces; they are more common in the infero-posterior and supero-anterior quadrants of the acetabulum [39, 60, 166]. The pressures on the pubis and iliac wings are mostly complex stresses that arise from several muscle connections during walking, as these stresses do not play a significant role in the weight-bearing function [60, 166].

The pelvic floor is at the bottom of the pelvic cavity, and the abdominal cavity is above the pelvic cavity. There are two parts of the pelvic cavity: the true pelvis and the false pelvis [32]. The area between the pelvic inlet and the pelvic outlet is called the true pelvis. The true pelvis is the birth canal and an attachment site for muscles, fascia, and ligaments. The tension of this elastic tissue system affects the size and form of the true pelvis [66].

3.1.1.1 Sagittal Pelvic Parameters

Maintaining postural and spinal balance is significantly influenced by the pelvic sagittal alignment. Sagittal pelvic parameters can be assessed with lateral radiography during standing. Positional and anatomical pelvic parameters can be determined from two-dimensional sagittal radiography. Positional pelvic parameters are determined by measuring the angles between the individual's position and horizontal or vertical reference lines. To compare these parameters between subjects, they must be measured in a standard position. Sacral slope and pelvic tilt are examples of positional pelvic parameters. Anatomical pelvic parameters are determined by reference lines related to the individual's anatomy. Since these parameters remain constant in different positions of the individual, they can be compared between subjects regardless of their positions. Pelvic incidence angle is the most frequently evaluated anatomical parameter [167].

Pelvic tilt is the angle formed by the reference vertical line and the line that connects the femoral head axis and the sacral plate center [148, 167]. The average pelvic tilt angle in the standing position was found to be 13° ± 6° [164]. The greater the pelvic tilt angle, the more posterior the center of gravity is relative to the femoral head [85]. When lumbar degeneration begins and lumbar lordosis decreases, pelvic tilt increases and sacral slope decreases [18]. Pelvic tilt depends on position. Standing causes lumbar lordosis to increase and sacral slope and pelvic tilt to decrease. Pelvic tilt increases, sacral slope decreases, and lumbar lordosis reduces while one is seated [117]. It has been reported that pelvic tilt increases by 20° in the sitting position [73]. A less popular method of measuring pelvic tilt is to use the anterior pelvic plane tilt in the sagittal plane. This angle is formed by the vertical line that joins the symphysis pubis to the middle of the superior iliac spines [128].

The angle formed by the horizontal reference line and the sacral plate is known as the sacral slope [167]. Sacral slope change is an important parameter, as it affects the overall biomechanics of the spine [77].

The angle formed by the line drawn perpendicular to the sacral plate center and the line connecting the femoral head axis and the sacral plate center is known as the pelvic incidence angle [167]. The average value is stated to be 55° ± 10° [164]. Pelvic incidence increases slightly until skeletal maturation is complete and then remains constant [93]. This angle is an anatomical feature specific to the individual. This angle has a direct effect on the balance of the spine standing on the sacral plateau [87, 164].

The equation "Pelvic incidence = Pelvic tilt + Sacral slope" is used to calculate pelvic incidence [148, 167]. As the pelvic tilt increases, the sacral plateau becomes more horizontal, and the sacral body assumes a more vertical position. Thus, the pelvic incidence value is a fixed angle independent of position. In non-pathological cases, the pelvic tilt should be less than 50% of the pelvic incidence. The sacral slope should be more than 50% of the pelvic incidence [86].

Individuals with a very low pelvic incidence have a vertical pelvis with a narrow anteroposterior diameter, a horizontally narrow pelvis, and femoral heads just below the sacral plate. Individuals with a very high pelvic incidence have a wide anteroposterior diameter of the pelvis and a horizontal pelvis. The femoral heads are anterior to the sacral plate [86].

3.1.2 Pelvic Movements

When standing with equal weight on both lower limbs, the pelvis is in its neutral posture if the anterior superior iliac spines (ASISs) are at the same height, the anterior superior iliac spine (ASIS) and the posterior superior iliac spine are in the same transverse plane, and the symphysis pubis and the ASIS are located in the same frontal plane [89].

Pelvic movements are very important in terms of regulating sagittal balance. Since the pelvic ring is a closed chain, the translation and rotation movements that occur in the symphysis pubis require the opposite movement in the sacroiliac joint [89]. The rotations in the pubic symphysis in the frontal and sagittal planes are less than 1.5°. An average translational movement of 1 mm occurs in the transverse and sagittal directions and approximately 2 mm in the vertical direction. These values are greater in multiparous individuals than in nulliparous individuals [169].

The movements of the pelvis around the mediolateral axis are called anterior and posterior tilt, or anteversion and retroversion. In anterior pelvic tilt movement, each ASIS moves in an anterior and inferior direction. In posterior pelvic tilt movement, each ASIS moves in a superior and posterior direction [89, 111]. When the pelvis is in the posterior pelvic tilt position, the pelvic tilt angle increases. The anterior pelvic tilt position causes the pelvic tilt angle to decrease [86].

Movements of the pelvis around the anteroposterior axis, which cause one side of the pelvis to point downward and the other side upward in the frontal plane, are often referred to as a pelvic drop or hike. Pelvic movement in the frontal plane is most common in the single support phase of walking and is managed by the hip abductor muscles [89, 111].

The movement of the pelvis on the vertical axis causes the pelvis to rotate forward or backward in the transverse plane. The transverse plane movement of the pelvis is based on the movement of the opposite side of the leg in the stance phase. In other words, when standing on one lower limb, the opposite side moves forward, causing forward rotation. When the opposite side of the pelvis moves backward, backward rotation occurs. In addition, the movements of the pelvis in the transverse plane are also called internal or external rotation [89, 111].

During walking, the pelvis moves in the transverse, sagittal, and frontal planes. As walking speed increases, the magnitude of pelvic movements increases. Pelvic movements during walking cause the center of mass to move less vertically and horizontally [89]. Throughout the gait cycle, the pelvis is held in a more anterior tilt in the sagittal plane. The movement in the sagittal plane is 2–5° [22, 89, 151]. The pelvis is neutral during the initial contact phase of walking, then drops, and then rises again in the frontal plane. At the preferred walking speed, total frontal plane pelvic motion is 6–11° [22, 89, 151]. In the transverse plane, the pelvis is in a backward rotation, with the right ASIS more posterior during the initial contact phase of the left lower extremity in walking. Forward rotation then occurs. At the preferred walking pace, total transverse plane pelvic motion is 3–14° [22, 38, 89, 151].

Pelvic movements during walking differ in women and men. Anterior pelvic tilt is greater in women during walking. It has been found that pelvic movement in the transverse plane and frontal plane is greater in women than in men when walking at a similar pace [22, 35, 89].

The range of motion of the hip is determined by pelvic morphology. Vertically oriented pelvises with low pelvic incidence and low sacral slope have less pelvic retroversion capability. Therefore, the hips have a very broad range of motion in these individuals. These individuals are called “hip users.” Pelvic incidence and sacral slope are higher in pelvises with a more horizontal orientation. Hip range of motion is more limited in these individuals. These individuals are called “spine users” [128].

3.1.3 Sexual Dimorphism in the Pelvis

Sexual dimorphism in the pelvis is often contrasted with body size dimorphism due to differing evolutionary pressures and developmental factors. Body size is larger in men; pelvic size is larger in women. The main reason for this is that women give birth [43]. Sexual dimorphism in the pelvis has led to its frequent use in determining biological sex in adult individuals [23, 144]. One reason for the differences in pelvic morphology may be the effect of sex-specific hormones on bone growth. Female hormones, especially during puberty, have been reported to affect the pelvic obstetric dimensions [72]. In addition to hormonal factors, biomechanical stresses also play a role in differences in pelvic morphology. The male pelvis offers mechanical advantages because it must adapt to the higher biomechanical stresses created by larger body size [15].

In females, the ischial spines are less noticeable, and the pelvis is broader [83]. The bispinous width is greater in the female pelvis, but the biacetabular width is not very different between the sexes. The less noticeable ischial spines, broader sacrum, and wider subpubic angle of the female pelvis all contribute to the birth canal’s enlargement [83, 157].

3.1.4 Pelvic Diameters and Energy Expenditure

The female pelvis must be wide enough to birth babies yet narrow enough to be suitable for walking on two legs [173]. As a result of simple biomechanical analyses, it has been assumed that having wider hips increases the energy cost of walking. In fact, the term “obstetrical dilemma” refers to the challenges associated with women having wider hips than men, particularly concerning childbirth and bipedal locomotion. Accordingly, the distance between the two acetabula must be narrow for an efficient bipedal gait, but the birth canal must be wide for the birth of large-brained offspring [140, 174]. However, recent studies have shown that hip width does not predict the energy expenditure of the abductor muscles, suggesting that the muscle energy requirements for maintaining pelvic stability in the frontal plane during walking are not very different between men and women [82]. It has even been reported that a wide pelvis, which allows for a wider birth canal, does not increase the energy cost of walking [173] and that a greater bitrochanteric width saves energy costs while carrying loads [170, 172]. This may be attributed to the fact that a wider pelvis is associated with reduced hip adductor and hamstring muscle activity during walking [171]. By extending stride length through pelvic rotation, individuals with a wider pelvis can also lower energy costs by lowering the number of steps taken over a given distance [134, 172, 175]. When taking longer steps, individuals with wider hips move less in the sagittal plane, and in this case, they expend less energy because the vertical displacement of the center of mass is less [43].

3.1.5 Joints Associated with the Pelvis and Their Relationship with Pelvic Biomechanics

3.1.5.1 Lumbopelvic Joint Biomechanics

Pelvic tilt and pelvic position are associated with lumbar lordosis at the lumbopelvic junction. The sacrum moves anteroinferiorly, and the pubis moves posterosuperiorly when the pelvis is inclined posteriorly in the hypolordotic posture. Therefore, a hypolordotic departure from a person's normal standing posture might shorten the pelvic floor muscles by altering the direction of their attachments at the sacrum, coccyx, and pubis. This brings the pubis and coccyx attachments of the pubococcygeus muscle closer together during hypolordotic standing posture. The process ultimately shortens the pubococcygeus muscle, the key pelvic floor muscle where electromyography (EMG) activity is recorded [21, 52].

It has been demonstrated that a muscle can receive more excitatory input from the central nervous system when it is kept in a shortened condition [41, 120]. When people stand with less lumbar lordosis, their resting activity increases, a phenomenon that can be explained by the role of the pelvic floor muscles. The position of the ligaments in the lumbopelvic area determines the degree of neuromodulation and muscle shortening, which may vary in wedded or older women [27].

By activating the pelvic floor muscles, lumbopelvic posture impacts coordination through the trunk muscles. Thus, when treating women who have lumbopelvic pain or stress incontinence, lumbopelvic posture is a crucial factor. During static postures and dynamic tasks, the contractility of the pelvic floor muscles and the quantity of vaginal pressure generated are both influenced by changes in lumbopelvic posture [27]. Studies in the literature have examined the effects of changing body position (i.e., from supine to standing) on the activation of pelvic floor muscles [6, 16, 80]. Sapsford et al. [146] conducted a comparison of voluntary pelvic floor muscle contractions in a seated, erect, and unsupported posture. Their findings indicated that a collapsed posture yielded a higher level of pelvic floor muscle activity than a supported posture. Furthermore, the activation of the pelvic floor muscle is enhanced when standing compared to supine, regardless of whether the individual is standing at a hypo-, hyper-, or normal lordotic angle. Hypolordotic posture exhibits higher resting pelvic floor muscle activation compared to normal and hyperlordotic postures. It has been demonstrated that when people are in their normal posture, rather than in hyper- or hypolordotic postures, their pelvic floor muscles activate considerably more during maximal voluntary contraction, coughing, Valsalva, and load-lifting exercises [27]. In conclusion, changes in lumbopelvic posture affect both the contractility of the pelvic floor muscles and the amount of intravaginal pressure generated during both static and dynamic tasks but do not have a significant effect on the timing of pelvic floor muscles (PFM) activation during lumbopelvic posture, coughing, or load-catching tasks. This supports the results reported by Shafik et al., who found higher electromyography

(EMG) activity in the M. levator ani in the standing position compared to the lying position [149]. Given the role that the pelvic floor muscles play in supporting the pelvic contents, it is anticipated that their activity would be higher in the gravity-dependent (standing) position, where the weight of the viscera is directly applied to the pelvic floor muscles (PFM), as opposed to the gravity-independent (supine) position, where the viscera rests on the posterior abdominal wall.

Urinary incontinence in women is epidemiologically associated with lumbopelvic postural problems [29, 152]. In women with stress urinary incontinence (SUI), the dual tasks placed on the pelvic floor muscles (postural control and continence maintenance) increase the risk of episodes of urinary incontinence, especially during tasks where postural stability is challenged. For example, delayed or inadequate pelvic floor muscle activation during postural perturbations leads to ineffective urethral closure during tasks that challenge spinal stability [79, 152].

The rectus abdominis, gluteus maximus, and adductor magnus muscles are recognized as the synergist muscles of the pelvic floor. The abdominal muscles are important because they provide support to the internal organs with breathing mechanics and reduce the pressure on the pelvic floor. When the effect of lumbopelvic posture on the activation of these muscles was examined, the highest activation was seen in posterior pelvic tilt compared to normal lumbopelvic posture [27, 132]. Capson et al. [41] and Sapsford et al. reported that the highest activation of the internal and external oblique abdominal muscles was observed in the relaxed standing position compared to the standing position in which the lordosis angles increased or decreased. Sapsford et al. [146] found that abdominal and pelvic floor muscles (PFM) activity was lower in the loosely supported sitting position with trunk flexion compared to the upright sitting position, which may prove synergistic co-activation of these muscles. While Bo and Stien [17] found that contraction of the hip adductors, gluteus medius (GMed), and abdominal muscles led to the contraction of the pelvic floor muscles in accordance with the principles of muscular synergy, Soljanik et al. [153] demonstrated a correlation between levator ani and gluteus medius.

According to research by Hodges et al. [69], women with urinary incontinence have delayed pelvic floor muscle activation, whereas in healthy women, these muscles are recruited slightly before the prime mover as part of anticipatory postural regulation. Since the pelvic floor muscles work synergistically with the abdominal muscles [17, 94, 112], physiotherapists include postural correction training in programs aimed at improving both continence function and postural control [110, 145].

Pelvic floor muscles, abdominal muscles, and bladder neck elevation have been shown to functionally interact. Proper functioning of the abdominal muscles can lower intravaginal pressure during contractions of the pelvic floor muscles. This effect is due to their additional function of supporting the internal organs and regulating intra-abdominal pressure [78]. Devreese et al. [44] suggested that an imbalance between the pelvic floor muscles (PFM) and the lower abdominal muscles may be the cause of stress urinary incontinence.

3.1.5.2 Sacroiliac Joint Biomechanics

The sacroiliac joints (SIJs), the largest axial joints in the body, are located on either side of the sacrum and pelvic bones. Until the early eighteenth century, it was thought that the SIJs could only move during pregnancy and birthing [78]. According to recent research, the sacroiliac structure provides upper trunk stability and flexibility. Its kinematics also influence the lumbosacral intervertebral discs, particularly L5–S1, and result in kyphosis and lordosis [28]. They preserve a degree of mobility that does not limit activities of daily living by connecting the spine to the pelvis, allowing load transmission from the lumbar spine to the lower extremities [156].

The SIJ is subjected to a shear force of up to 4800 N, slides 1.6 mm in the anteroposterior plane, and can rotate up to 4° in motion. When lying supine and performing straight leg raises, the ilium of the resting leg rotates 0.8° backward and 0.3° inward. Biomechanical studies have shown that small differences in the length of the legs during load transfer can increase the load on the SIJ by up to five times [81]. The load transmitted to the extremities during normal walking can reach 300% of body weight, suggesting an adverse stress condition that is potentially associated with joint degeneration in the sacroiliac joint [127].

The stabilization of the joint was defined by the principles of form and force closure, according to Vleeming et al. [165]. The stability provided by the complementary convex and concave surfaces of the iliac and sacral articular surfaces is known as the form closure concept. The force closure theory explains how muscles and ligaments work across a joint to provide support and motion. The link made by the thoracolumbar fascia between the gluteus maximus and the contralateral latissimus dorsi is a crucial part of the force closure concept. According to Barker et al. [10], the gluteus maximus can exert 70% of its muscular force perpendicular to the SIJ plane, with 14% of that power being transmitted through the thoracolumbar fascia. Carvalhais et al. [47] provided in vivo evidence of force transfer through the thoracolumbar fascia between the latissimus dorsi and contralateral gluteus maximus. Furthermore, van Wingerden et al. [161] demonstrated that by compressing the sacroiliac joint (SIJ) and avoiding excessive shear forces, gluteus maximus muscle movements significantly contribute to the force closure principle. This implies that having a muscle synergy between these muscles could benefit the SIJ by providing more stability [56]. With an unbalanced SIJ affecting form closure or force closure principles, muscle synergy can be impaired, and load transfer across the pelvis can create excessive loads on the surrounding tissues, causing pain [129].

The sacroiliac joint (SIJ) lacks inherent stability under shear loads, relying on the surrounding ligaments, such as the sacroiliac ligaments, and the tight interlocking of the sacrum between the hip bones to resist shear forces and maintain joint integrity. In particular, the sacrospinous ligament unites the fibers of the sacrotuberous ligament, which connects the sacrum to the posterior superior iliac spine and the ischial spine to the lateral portion of the sacrum and coccyx. These two ligaments stabilize the sacrum by limiting its movement relative to the ischium. The degree of stiffness of these ligaments has been demonstrated by research. Muscles also provide support to this self-support mechanism. Because they increase the compressive stress across the SIJ, the transversus abdominis and pelvic floor muscles (levator ani and coccygeus muscles) have been demonstrated to be crucial for SIJ stability [46, 121].

The auricular surface of the SIJ is covered in a coarse layer of hyaline cartilage that is about 4 mm thick on the sacral surface and 1–2 mm thick on the iliac surface. Furthermore, pathological situations such as surgical fixation of the thoracolumbar spine can intensify the loads transmitted by the SIJ. In these cases, applying large flexion moments due to high spinal stiffness might further raise the likelihood of developing joint arthrosis [28].

The sacrum can move in 6° of freedom relative to the ilium, but this movement is minimal, and hyper- or hypomobility of the joint can cause pain in the joint area. In comparison to the male SIJ, the female SIJ is more mobile and experiences greater stress, pressure, and strain on the pelvic ligaments. The majority of cases of lower back pain (LBP) are believed to come from the lumbar spine, although the sacroiliac joint is another potential cause of LBP that is frequently disregarded [109, 162]. Recent studies have found that the sacroiliac joint (SIJ) is the primary source of pain in 15%–30% of low back pain cases [91].

Sacroiliac joint pain can be caused by pathological alterations and injuries unique to various SIJ structures. Capsular and ligamentous stress, hypo- or hypermobility, compression or shear forces, micro- or macrofractures, soft tissue damage, and inflammation are some of the alterations or disorders. Sacroiliitis, rheumatism, infectious diseases, and cancer are pathological disorders associated with SIJ. In many cases, SIJ pathologies are difficult to diagnose because the symptoms can be confused with nonspecific low back pain, but there are differences in kinesiological movements between patients with low back pain and SIJ disorders [2]. SIJ pain leads to ineffective muscle contraction, preventing the joint from closing with the force necessary to maintain stability [1]. These alterations impact limb coordination and muscle force control, while aberrant joint loading, in particular, results in joint deterioration [33]. In addition to SIJ pain, lower back and hip pain are common signs of sacroiliac joint dysfunction, which is known to decrease muscular strength and endurance and affect gait and muscle coordination [55]. Research has shown that individuals with SIJ dysfunction preferentially load on their unaffected legs when rising from a chair and exhibit lower maximum hip moments and joint angles on the affected side [26, 55]. These altered movement patterns result from reducing the amplitude and speed of a painful movement or avoiding it altogether. According to research, people with SIJ dysfunction have lower maximum hip moments and joint angles on the affected side. They preferentially load their unaffected legs when getting out of a chair. Reducing the amplitude and speed of an action that causes pain or avoiding it completely results in changes in movement patterns. It has been demonstrated that, in comparison to age-matched controls, people with SIJ dysfunction walk with greater leg asymmetry and less activation of the gluteus maximus.

In women with sacroiliac joint dysfunction, the synergy between the painful side's gluteus maximus and contralateral latissimus dorsi is impaired during gait, and there are differences in hip extension angle and ground reaction force. By restricting the joint's force closure principle, decreased muscle strength in the synergy of the injured side's gluteus maximus and the contralateral latissimus dorsi may jeopardize pelvic stability and change kinematics [56, 105].

3.1.6 Hip Joint Biomechanics

The most crucial muscles for maintaining and regulating the pelvis during movement are the hip abductor muscles [176]. It is well-recognized that the gluteus medius (GMed) muscle is essential for regulating coronal pelvic movement [57]. Additionally, people with a variety of knee issues, such as patellofemoral discomfort and knee osteoarthritis (OA), exhibit excessive trunk lateral flexion when this muscle is dysfunctional [30]. It has been proposed that ipsilateral trunk flexion and contralateral pelvic drop during stance, a mechanism that increases the load on the knee's medial compartment, are involved in coronal plane motion impairment in individuals with GMed weakness. This has been found to be a significant contributing factor to the development of genu varum [30].

Normally, anterior pelvic tilt is maintained by a pair of forces between the hip flexors and lumbar extensor muscles (Fig. 3.1). Contraction of the hip flexor muscles on a fixed femur causes rotation of the pelvis around the mediolateral axis. If the hip flexors, such as the iliopsoas and sartorius, are able to flex the pelvis on the femur, they also cause anterior pelvic tilt. Clinically, the most important symptom of anterior pelvic tilt is increased lumbar lordosis.

Functional tasks like stair climbing are commonly employed in clinical assessment to identify aberrant motions and examine movement symmetry. While ipsilateral pelvic fall is noted during stair descent, the pelvis falls to the opposite side during the first 50% of the stance phase of walking.

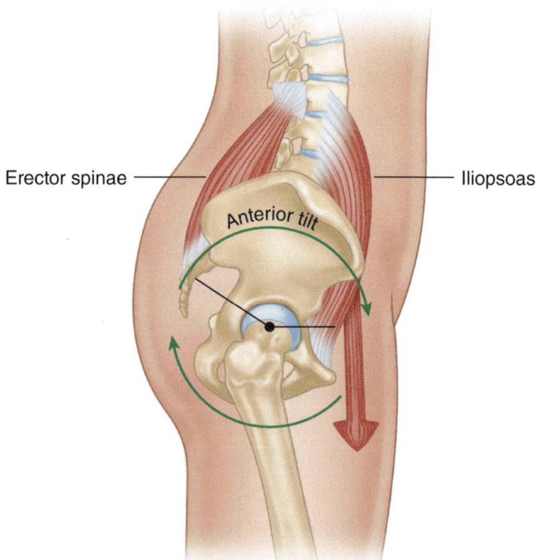

Fig. 3.1 Pairs of forces that cause the pelvis to tilt anteriorly

Despite stair climbing and gait being both closed-chain kinetic activities, this example illustrates how the control techniques of pelvic movement vary depending on the activity. When walking and climbing stairs, a contralateral pelvic drop of about 3–4° was noted. Walking causes noticeably more lateral trunk flexion excursions and pelvic oblique excursions than stair descent [150]. Walking on a treadmill was associated with less pelvic tilt than walking on the ground. According to findings, the average pelvic drop for men and women when walking on the ground was 4.93° and 6.04°, respectively [34]. When descending stairs, the gluteus medius muscle is used more than it is when walking. This highlights how crucial GMed strength is for hip and pelvic control during stair descent, where the latter should exhibit less pelvic excursion than walking normally [150].

The development of knee issues such as patellofemoral pain (PFP), noncontact anterior cruciate ligament (ACL) injuries, and knee osteoarthritis has been linked to coronal plane movements of the trunk, pelvis, and lower leg joints [30, 68, 130]. As a risk factor for the development of injuries, larger motions with asymmetries are frequently observed and linked to clinical conditions such as knee valgus, pelvic drop, and trunk lateral flexion [181].

Even for the purpose of increasing shooting speed, research on upper-limb athletes highlights the significance of the pelvic–trunk interactions. Pelvic movement starts the power generation process, after which energy is progressively transported to the trunk, upper arm, forearm, hand, and ball [118]. Additionally, Stodden et al. [155] discovered a relationship between ball speed and the rotational velocities of the pelvis and trunk.

3.1.6.1 Pelvic Biomechanics in Different Pathomechanical States

3.1.6.1.1 Femoroacetabular Impingement

About 37% of young adults have femoroacetabular impingement (FAI), a hip structural condition that is known to increase the incidence of hip osteoarthritis [58]. The most noticeable aspect of FAI is pain. Hip adduction and internal rotation are both involved, and pain intensifies with repeated hip flexion movements. It has been demonstrated that these segments are also impacted by individual variations in movement style and the interactions between neighboring body segments (such as the pelvis and trunk). Treatment insufficiency may be explained by a failure to consider such factors. Few studies have examined pelvic and trunk control in the frontal plane, although some biomechanical changes have been found in the sagittal plane during squatting and in the trunk during stair climbing in FAI syndrome. This is despite the fact that it may be significant, given its potential effects on hip joint loading [13].

Hip impingement can be prevented by proper pelvic posture in the frontal plane while on one leg. Pain and weakening of the hip abductor muscles, which are typical in FAI syndrome, might impair pelvic postural control. People with painful hip osteoarthritis have been shown to have altered anterior plane control of the trunk, which can lessen provocative hip joint contact forces (i.e., the demand for hip abductor muscles) [159]. Step climbing puts more strain on the hip joint than straight-line walking because it necessitates compressive hip action [108]. Studies have shown that people with FAI have altered pelvic and/or trunk control. During locomotion, people with FAI syndrome exhibited ipsilateral trunk tilt and pelvic elevation toward the affected side when on one leg, indicating stress on the hip joint. Additionally, it was discovered that people with FAI experienced pain when they performed pelvic elevation. Pelvic elevation on the symptomatic side may increase the severity of pathology by shifting the affected hip into adduction, especially when combined with hip flexion, when increased load is placed on one leg during activities such as stepping. However, studies have shown that individuals with FAI who have good pelvic postural control experience neither pelvic elevation nor pain [45].

The decrease in posterior pelvic tilt may bring the femoral head–neck junction closer to the acetabulum, potentially aiding in the development of

FAI. Furthermore, lower hip extensor movements imply that a reduction in hip extensor muscle activity could be a factor in a reduction in posterior pelvic tilt [8].

3.1.6.1.2 Pelvic Biomechanics in Dynamic Valgus Pathomechanics

Dynamic valgus, also known as frontal plane knee projection angle (FPKPA), is a movement disorder that is typified by medial knee displacement during dynamic tasks. It is typically brought on by combinations of excessive contralateral pelvic drop, hip adduction, and internal rotation [178]. Dynamic valgus in female recreational runners has been associated in recent research with patellofemoral pain, plantar fasciitis, and medial tibial stress syndrome [54]. Dynamic valgus was biomechanically linked to a number of factors, including insufficient ankle dorsiflexion range of motion, excessive passive internal hip rotation range of motion, posterolateral hip muscle weakness, and dynamic ankle eversion. Additionally, in runners with dynamic valgus, ankle eversion and stride cadence were positively connected with contralateral pelvic drop and hip adduction [114].

3.2 Biomechanical Properties of the Pelvic Floor and Organs

3.2.1 Biomechanical Properties of the Pelvic Floor

The pelvic floor is a structure made up of connective tissue and striated muscles that maintains the pelvic organs' position by resisting the force of gravity and intra-abdominal pressure [49]. The female pelvic floor must prevent incontinence and pelvic organ prolapse (POP) and facilitate the excretion of urine and feces. It must also allow for childbirth [5].

To provide continence and support to the pelvic organs, the soft tissues supporting the pelvic floor, such as ligaments, muscles, and fasciae, work together to form a hammock-like support system. Their biomechanical characteristics are examined to understand how these tissues work to resist deformation and provide support. The pelvic floor tissues are loaded and deformed by physiological conditions such as age, breathing, parity, jumping, and walking or pathological conditions such as coughing, obesity, and vomiting [142]. Obesity, coughing, vomiting, constipation, and pregnancy increase intra-abdominal pressure, causing more pressure to be applied to the pelvic floor muscles [4, 40, 74]. Knowing the biomechanical properties of these tissues is important for understanding pelvic floor diseases. While individuals with weak tissues develop pelvic floor diseases under high loads applied to the pelvic floor tissues, individuals with strong tissues can resist these loads [142].

Pelvic floor muscles consist of approximately 66% type I and 34% type II fibers. Slow-twitch fibers are responsible for maintaining resting tone and providing support to the pelvic organs at rest. Fast-twitch fibers (type II) are activated in situations that cause a sudden increase in intra-abdominal pressure, such as sneezing and coughing [133]. The superficial layer of the pelvic floor muscles includes the ischiocavernosus, bulbospongiosus, and superficial transverse perineal muscles, as well as the deep transverse perineal muscles. The deep layer includes the coccygeus and levator ani muscles [51]. The pelvic floor muscles, especially the levator ani, support the pelvic organs and also play an important role in defecation, sexual, and urinary functions [9]. The puborectalis, pubococcygeus, and iliococcygeus are the three separate components that make up the levator ani muscle. The main component of the levator ani muscle is the pubococcygeus, which extends from the pubis to the coccyx [97]. The pubococcygeus and puborectalis muscles, which form the anterior part of the levator ani muscle complex, undertake the task of closing the urethral hiatus and pulling the urethra, vagina, perineum, and anorectum toward the pubis. The iliococcygeus muscle, which forms the more horizontal posterior part, serves to support the pelvic organs. The stable resting tone of the pelvic floor muscles serves to close the urethra and anal sphincter and support the pelvic organs. The levator ani and sphincter muscles have the ability to contract rapidly during coughing or sneezing to maintain continence [9]. The levator ani muscle expands excessively during birth and contracts after birth. Since the upright position in humans requires very strong pelvic floor support, muscular support alone is not sufficient; the endopelvic fascia plays an important role in pelvic support. If there is an unstable pelvic floor, the pressure from the abdomen and diaphragm cannot be adequately counteracted, causing the intestines and pelvic organs to be pressed downward by the forces coming from above. The lengthening of the pelvic floor muscles prevents optimum force production. As a result, the risk of incontinence, POP, and chronic pelvic pain increases [63].

The connective tissue that surrounds the pelvic organs and joins them to the supporting muscles and bones is called endopelvic fascia. The uterosacral ligament (USL), mesovarium, mesosalpinx, cardinal ligament, and broad ligament are not true ligaments but are condensed portions of the endopelvic fascia. The pelvic floor muscles' optimal tone reduces the stress on the connective tissue [9].

Although the USL, which has a significant impact in supporting the uterus and vagina, is called a "ligament," it has a very different structure from joint ligaments. They consist of collagen, blood vessels, nerves, lymph, and smooth muscles. The distal region of the USL is connected to the cervix. The proximal region is connected to the sacral spine via the endopelvic fascia. While the distal region contains more smooth muscle, the smooth muscle content in the proximal region is much reduced, and loose connective tissue is more abundant. When the pelvic floor muscle support decreases, more load is placed on the USLs to support the pelvic organs; long-term tension causes damage, and the risk of POP increases [48].

The biomechanical properties of tissues include active and passive components. The ability of the tissue to produce force through muscle contractions is related to its active properties. The ability to transmit forces and resist deformation is an inherent passive property of tissue. Passive properties can be classified as either mechanical or structural. Structural properties express loads and elongation; mechanical properties express stress and strain. The uniaxial tensile test is often used to evaluate passive biomechanical properties. In this test, the tissue is stretched until failure/rupture occurs. During this time, the load–displacement curve is obtained from the measurements made, and the stiffness of the structure is assessed. At the same time, the mechanical properties of the tissue can be understood by obtaining the stress–strain curve. Stress is the force per unit of the tissue's cross-sectional area. Strain is the alteration in the tissue's length divided by its initial length. A tissue is linearly elastic if its stress–strain curve is linear, and the Young modulus, which is an indicator of tissue stiffness, is the slope of the curve. Nonetheless, because of their viscoelastic characteristics, the majority of biological tissues exhibit stress–strain curves with time-dependent behavior [142].

Different pelvic tissues have different stiffness properties. In the uniaxial tensile test, the vagina showed strain up to 20%, the rectum up to 30%, and the bladder up to 80% [141]. The uterosacral ligament (USL) complex is an important connective tissue supporting the upper vagina and cervix. Connective tissues supporting the vagina show viscoelastic properties. Therefore, their mechanical properties vary according to the duration of exposure to loading [49]. When the uterosacral ligament, round ligament, and broad ligament were analyzed, it was found that the USL was the most rigid ligament and the round ligament was more rigid than the broad ligament [139]. The cervical portion of the USL can support a weight of up to 17 kg [24]. It has been shown that the stiffness of the ligaments and vaginal wall is greater than that of the rectum and bladder. It has been reported that the mechanical behavior of vaginal tissues and pelvic floor ligaments differs with aging [31].

Biomechanical properties of tissues may vary according to anatomical position. For example, in women under 50 years of age, the posterior vaginal wall was found to be stiffer than the anterior wall [99]. The anterior vaginal wall was shown to be stiffer than the posterior vaginal wall in women over 50 [99, 141]. In women with POP, anterior vaginal wall stiffness was found to be higher than posterior wall stiffness [99].

3.2.2 Biomechanical Properties of Pelvic Organs

The vagina, bladder, and rectum—three organs that are essential for preserving pelvic support—have different biomechanical characteristics. Differences in tissue stiffness between the anterior and posterior vaginal wall tissues were found, in addition to the anisotropic mechanical behavior of the bladder tissue at high strain levels. It is evident that using the same prosthetic material or surgical technique for diverse anatomical sites is inappropriate, given the reported variations in stiffness and anisotropism under substantial deformations [141].

From the data on tissue stiffness, it is thought that vaginal tissue is a key structure in terms of pelvic support. Because of the alignment of its tissue fibers, human bladder tissue is known to display mechanical anisotropy. However, these distinctions between the front and posterior bladder walls, as well as between the longitudinal and circumferential orientations, were found only at high strain levels. The same is true for the anterior and posterior walls of the vagina. This is especially important in the selection of tissue to be used as a surgical mesh for POP. The anterior and posterior wall biomechanical characteristics of rectal tissue do not differ significantly from those of vaginal and bladder tissue. This could be because of variations in the organ's physiological function, histomorphology, and form [124]. Their moderate flexibility allows the bladder and rectum to undergo large deformations without rupturing, aligning with their filling role and organ mobility. Consequently, the bladder and rectum can carry out their role of storing urine and feces [177].

The rectum can be thought of as a tube, in contrast to the bladder, which can be characterized and represented as a sphere. Bladder smooth muscle cells respond to temporary strain by releasing enhanced tensile stresses that allow for incredibly quick actin filament separation and activate signaling pathways. Smooth muscle, collagen, and elastin make up the bladder wall, which remodels in response to mechanical stress from a variety of pathological diseases. The bladder uses newly produced elastin fibers to increase its compliance in response to extended periods of severe stress [177]. Consequently, depending on the various matrix layers, distinct mechanical behaviors can be seen in the same bladder [61].

Pelvic floor biomechanics depend on active and passive structures. Passive structures are provided by bone and connective tissues, i.e., ligaments and fascia, while active structures are provided by the pelvic floor muscles, which can actively contract to elevate the pelvic floor and, thus, compensate for increased intra-abdominal pressure and maintain the normal position of the pelvic organs [122].

More modern hypotheses of pelvic floor disorders have been put forth after the establishment of the two most recognized ideas [14, 70, 126, 158], DeLancey's Hammock Theory [42] and Petros and Ulmsten's Integral Theory [126]. Despite the fact that these ideas differ somewhat in how each pelvic floor component contributes to particular illnesses [84], to a certain degree, everyone agrees that the many supporting systems in the pelvis, including muscles, ligaments, tendons, and fascia, work in unison to sustain appropriate pelvic floor activities; if this coordination is disrupted, functional deficits will result [122].

3.2.2.1 DeLancey's Hammock Theory

This theory was developed in 1992, and the understanding of pelvic– pathophysiology was derived from anatomical dissection and, later, from MRI and biomechanical modeling [4]. The theory is based on the "paravaginal support" in the pelvic wall, which consists of fasciae and ligaments that support the middle region of the vaginal wall [100]. Muscular attachments link the periurethral tissue to the pubovaginal muscle, whereas fascial attachments link the anterior vaginal wall and periurethral tissue to the pelvic fascial tendon arch (arcus tendineus fasciae pelvis (ATFP)). The vaginal wall and endopelvic fascia (EF) connected to the ATFP form a hammock with this musculofascial support in the region where the urethra expands and is crushed by abdominopelvic pressure. DeLancey's theory states that urine continence is facilitated by the suburethral support system [42].

3.2.2.2 Tansatit's Theory

The two mechanical structures that form the basis of the third and most recent theory are the arcus tendineus fasciae pelvis (ATFP) and the levator ani muscle, an adipose cushion that fills the ischioanal fossa and guarantees pelvic organ functional interdependence and pelvic stability, and an Endopelvic fascia (EF) suspension system on the ATFP that is crucial for support. These pelvic chambers, which are filled with connective tissue, have an unclear anatomophysiological function [158].

3.2.2.3 Urethral Sling Theory (UST)

In the urethral sling theory, the urethral funneling feature, which is an unexplained structure, is emphasized. This anatomical characteristic of the proximal urethra emphasizes the association between female stress and urinary incontinence. According to UAT, stress urinary incontinence occurs when the proximal urethra moves lower than the bladder neck, causing a funnel effect due to tensile forces. This downward movement is typically countered by suburethral support that compresses the urethra and prevents leakage during increased intra-abdominal pressure, such as coughing. UAT suggests that inadequate support of the urethra can lead to its downward movement, which, in turn, affects its ability to maintain closure, resulting in urine leakage. Overall, UAT provides a framework for understanding the relationships of biomechanics and functionality that contribute to stress urinary incontinence in women [14].

3.2.2.4 Integral Theory

According to Petros et al.'s Integral Theory, the foundation of stress urinary incontinence and the reason behind the creation of suburethral slings is a fixed suburethral point [126].

Integral theories primarily use the flexibility of the ligamentous–fascial structures and connective tissue of the vaginal wall to explain pelvic problems. According to the hypothesis, a sagittal ligamentous–fascial support—which includes the pubourethral ligaments and the pubocervical fascia—extends from the posterior pubis to the S3/4 sacral concavity, and it enters the cervical ring. The urethra, bladder, uterus, and upper rectum extend via this wide sagittal hammock that is formed by the two uterosacral ligaments from front to back. The pelvic muscle complex, a dynamic pelvic organ support that creates the hammock's "wings," is added to this [125]. The system's integrity determines how well the pelvic–perineal muscles work. According to Petros, ligamentous–fascia insufficiency has two effects: It weakens the support of the pelvic organs and destabilizes the pelvic–perineal muscles, which together cause organ prolapse and dysfunction. Petros demonstrated that the muscular force acting on the vagina plays a major role in the initiation of cystocele, and he explained pelvic organ function by the combination of organ displacement brought on by muscle group contraction. He identified two vaginal areas, nine essential anatomical features, and three muscular forces that underlie the suspension of the pelvic organs. This idea states that anatomical abnormalities are the cause of all pelvic complaints. Consequently, laxity of the uterosacral ligament destabilizes the pubourethral ligaments and pubocervical fascia, increasing the likelihood of cystocele. Urinary incontinence and cystocele are, thus, at risk due to the destabilization of the pubourethral ligaments and pubocervical fascia caused by uterosacral ligament hyperlaxity; a ligamentous–fascial condition far from the afflicted organ may be the cause of a visceral complaint [125].

The interosseous sacroiliac ligaments serve as suspension rods, the sacrum serves as the central bridge, and the posterior superior iliac processes serve as pillars in the suspension bridge concept. To improve stability and stop lateral spreading, the anterior pelvic ring serves as a strut [122].

At the intersection of the three stress zones (iliac–femoral, iliac–pubic, and iliac–ischial strains), the posterior pelvic ring serves as the primary structure responsible for bearing the majority of the body weight. To maintain general

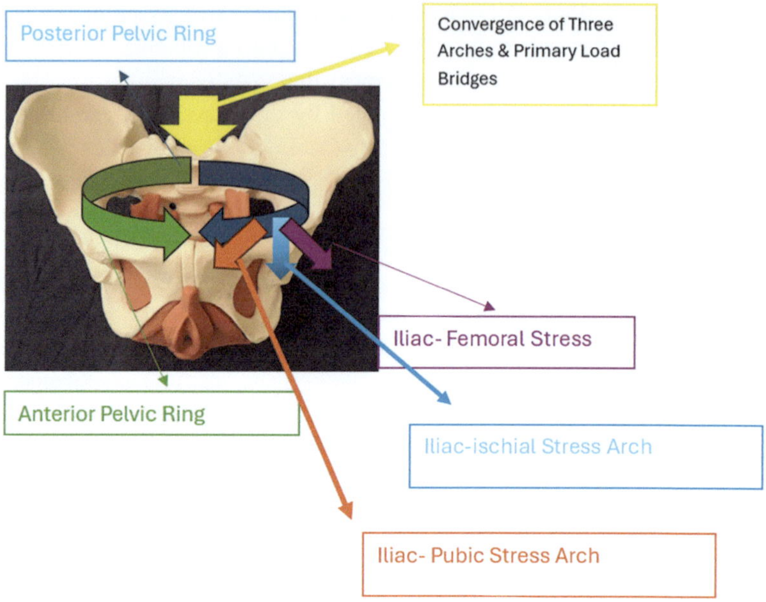

Fig. 3.2 Posterior–anterior pelvic ring and loads

stability and balance the stress distribution in the posterior ring, the anterior pelvic ring takes on a secondary load-bearing role. For long-term stability, the anterior and posterior pelvic rings must be harmoniously integrated (Fig. 3.2) [71, 122].

3.3 Changes in Pelvic Biomechanics in Women in Different Situations

3.3.1 Pelvis During Pregnancy

Physiological, anatomical, and hormonal changes that occur during pregnancy, postpartum, or postmenopausal conditions affect the musculoskeletal system as well as the cardiovascular and urinary systems. All these changes result in changes that affect gait and posture [137].

When abdominal muscles, especially the transversus abdominis, are weakened, e.g., during pregnancy or in the postmenopausal period due to inactivity, contraction of the hip flexor muscles causes anterior pelvic tilt. The increase in lumbar lordosis leads to anterior pelvic tilt. As this condition becomes chronic, compression forces increase in the apophyseal joints in the spine, and consequently, low back pain may develop [111].

With the progression of pregnancy, the displacement of the center of gravity of the trunk and weight gain affect the lumbar lordosis and, thus, the position of the pelvis. In the second and third trimesters, the condition gradually increases. In a healthy individual, lumbar lordosis and pelvic positioning are achieved by balancing the forces between the hip flexors and lumbar extensor muscles, abdominal muscles, and gluteus maximus muscles. As seen in Fig. 3.4, the deterioration of this balance during pregnancy, postpartum, and postmenopausal periods affects pelvic positioning and lumbar lordosis. Factors such as the increase in fetal, the lengthening of sarcomere length in the abdominal muscles, loss of flexibility due to excessive tension, the relaxing effect of hormones, and postural adaptation to changes in the body's center of gravity contribute to increased lumbar lordosis and anterior pelvic tilt (Fig. 3.3) [111].

Biomechanical changes, especially during pregnancy, are seen in pregnant individuals exhibiting gait types such as waddling gait [103, 147]. In the postpartum period, these changes do not return to normal quickly and continue for some time. During pregnancy, there is a decrease in pelvic elevation changes in the frontal plane. This condition returns to normal immediately

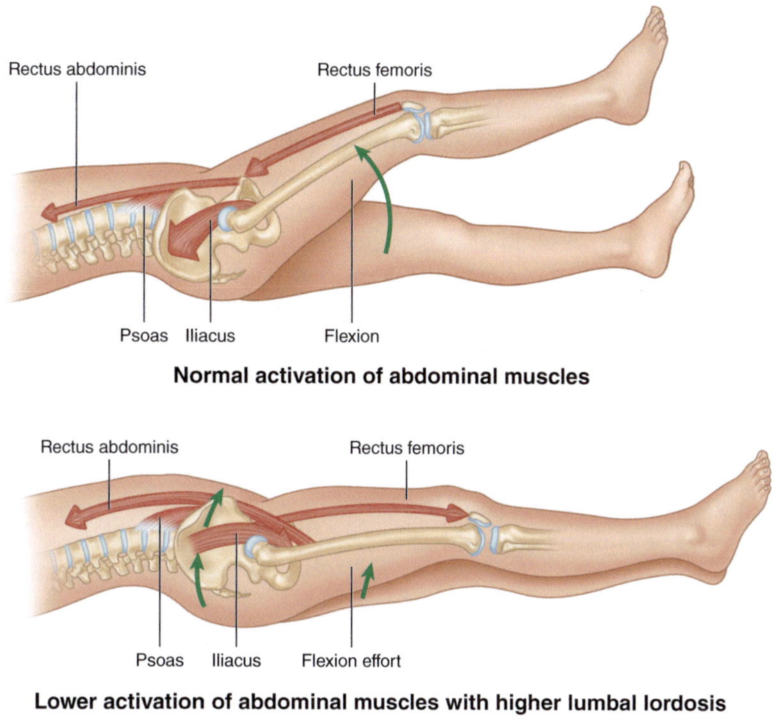

Fig. 3.3 Effects of abdominal muscle activation on lumbar lordosis and pelvis

after delivery. This pelvic mobility is necessary to achieve balance in the trunk during this period [98]. In both pregnant and nonpregnant women, a significant increase in bispinous diameter, bituberous diameter, mid-pelvic plane, and pelvic outlet was found in the kneeling squat position compared to the supine position. This suggests that pelvic diameters change in different positions, and this information should be taken into consideration for delivery [136].

A complex structure, the human pelvic floor is made up of muscles and other connective tissues that are connected to the organs it supports. The levator ani muscle and its fascial sheath make up the pelvic diaphragm. The striated muscle of the anterior abdominal wall works in tandem with the levator ani muscle, which is primarily in charge of supporting the pelvic and abdominal organs, to produce intra-abdominal pressure. Any rise in intra-abdominal pressure brought on by sneezing or coughing is distributed equally across the abdominal and pelvic walls. One side of the pelvic organ may experience more pressure than the other, allowing the organ to descend (genital prolapse) if the levator ani is pathologically compromised or momentarily ineffective [76].

Although the etiology of prolapse is multifactorial, pregnancy and childbirth are known to be risk factors [7, 64]. Mazza et al. [102] demonstrated by aspiration the in vivo evolution of the biomechanical properties of the uterine cervix at different stages of pregnancy. A significant reduction in cervical stiffness was observed. The cervical rigidity of a nonpregnant woman is six times higher than during pregnancy. This change is due to hormonal changes in all pelvic tissues and organs, such as muscles and ligaments [88].

When examining the biomechanical effects of pelvic organ prolapse (POP) in premenopausal or postmenopausal women, the influence of the pelvic support structures becomes evident. These pelvic support tissues contain blood vessels, nerves, and fibrous connective tissue and, therefore, function as a combined neurovascular and supportive structure. One of the causes of POP in both premenopausal and postmenopausal women is related to connective tissue, including collagen abnormalities and joint hypermobility. Collagen has been found to be the most important biomechanical factor. Collagen, the main component of pelvic support tissue, is responsible for resistance to tensile force. Previous biomechanical studies on premenopausal women have shown that the collagen content in the upper vaginal epithelium of women with POP is lower than that of those without POP [62, 139]. In a study conducted on 1961 nonpregnant women in the USA in 2008, it was reported that the prevalence of at least one pelvic floor disorder was 23.7%; 15.7% of women had urinary incontinence (UI), 9.0% had fecal incontinence (FI), and 2.9% had POP [116].

3.3.2 Female Pelvis During the Aging Process

Aging plays a significant role in the development of both POP and urinary incontinence (UI). The decrease in estrogen in the postmenopausal period also increases the risk of these dysfunctions [160]. Additionally, with advancing age, the number and diameter of periurethral muscle fibers decline, leading to changes in muscle function [123].

It has been found that fibrotic degeneration occurs in the pelvic floor muscles with aging and that intramuscular lipid accumulation increases. Interestingly, age-related degeneration has been found to affect the pelvic floor muscles more than the appendicular muscles [138]. It has been found that with aging, the physiological cross-sectional area and muscle mass of all pelvic floor muscles decrease, and the collagen content in the muscle increases [3]. However, it has been suggested that in healthy nulliparous women, advanced age causes a decrease in the cross-sectional area and volume of the obturator internus muscle but does not cause atrophy in the levator ani muscle [106]. Pelvic floor muscle stiffness also increases with age [25].

Postmenopausal hypoestrogenism is associated with pelvic floor muscle and connective tissue quality [19]. Since estrogen and estrogen receptors play a role in maintaining pelvic supporting structures by decreasing the degradation or increasing the synthesis of collagen and extracellular matrix proteins, estrogen reduction in the postmenopausal period may lead to weakening of the supporting tissues of the pelvis [37]. It has been shown that pelvic floor muscles in women over the age of 40 are approximately 20% weaker than those in younger women. However, it has been reported that pelvic floor muscle endurance is greater in women over the age of 40, which may be due to the increase in the type I fiber ratio with increasing age [133].

With aging, there is a decrease in lumbar lordosis and sacral slope [104, 131]. Age-related atrophy of the pelvic floor muscles, birth traumas, increased pelvic tilt due to age, and decreased sacral slope cause the pelvic floor to become more horizontal, causing the effect of gravity to increase the pressure on the pelvic floor. In this case, first the pelvic floor, and then the pelvic organs descend, causing the pelvic floor structures to become excessively stretched, and if the pressure becomes too strong, the stretched connective tissue, nerves, muscles, and ligaments can cause pain, thus increasing the risk of chronic pelvic pain [63, 104].

3.3.3 Biomechanical Changes in Dysfunctions Related to the Pelvis

Pelvic diameters may be associated with the risk of pelvic floor disorders (PFD) because they are related to tension in the elastic support system formed by the muscles and connective tissue in the pelvic floor [66]. Pelvic inlet and pelvic outlet diameters of women with UI were found to be significantly larger than those of continent women. In addition, the cross-sectional area of the psoas major, levator ani, and transverse perineal muscles was found to be smaller, and their muscle densities were lower in women with UI than in continent women. This shows that pelvic anatomy and muscle mass are important risk factors for the development of UI [154]. The subpubic angle was found to be wider in women with postpartum stress urinary incontinence (SUI). However, there is no significant difference in pelvic dimensions between middle-aged women with SUI and continent women [12]. This shows how the effect of birth on pelvic biomechanics is important in the development of UI. When the pelvic shape is examined in three dimensions, it is stated that in women with pelvic floor disorders, the bispinous diameter increases with the mediolateral expansion of the pelvic floor at the level of the ischial spines, and the ischium is in more eversion. These factors cause more strain on the pelvic floor connective tissue throughout the individual's life [20]. Increased pelvic anteroposterior diameter increases the risk of pelvic floor dysfunction [119]. A pelvic outlet transverse diameter of greater than 9.5 cm can be used as a threshold value for pelvic floor dysfunction. Women with a large pelvic outlet transverse diameter should begin preventive measures as early as possible, such as treating constipation, avoiding heavy physical exertion, and performing strengthening exercises for the pelvic floor muscles [66].

A reduced lumbar lordosis and pelvic inlet that is less vertically oriented may increase the risk of POP. The pelvic inlet that is less vertically oriented is thought to redirect intra-abdominal forces normally directed anterior to the symphysis pubis toward the pelvic viscera and their muscular and ligamentous supports [101, 113]. A more horizontally oriented pelvic inlet has been shown in women with POP [63, 113]. This means that, as the angle between the pelvic inlet plane and the transverse plane decreases and lumbar lordosis decreases, the pelvic floor becomes horizontal. The distance from the promontorium to the edge of the upper pubic symphysis has decreased from 9–11 to 4–5 cm over the decades (Fig. 3.4). The horizontalization of the pelvic floor with age places the pelvic floor under greater pressure from the abdominal organs above and gravity below (Fig. 3.5). This increases the risk of POP and also causes overstretching of pelvic floor structures, such as the USL, which increases the risk of chronic pelvic pain [63]. Every 10° increase in pelvic incidence value increases the risk of POP by 2.9 times [92]. An increase in the transverse diameter of the pelvic inlet also increases the risk of POP [67]. Another risk factor for POP is the vast anterior pelvic area defined by the inferior pubic point at the lower margin of the symphysis pubis at the anterior, the medial edges of the obturator internus muscles on the sides, and the ischial spines posteriorly [143].

The quality and amount of collagen in pelvic support tissues are lower in women with POP [75, 96]. It has been reported that women with POP

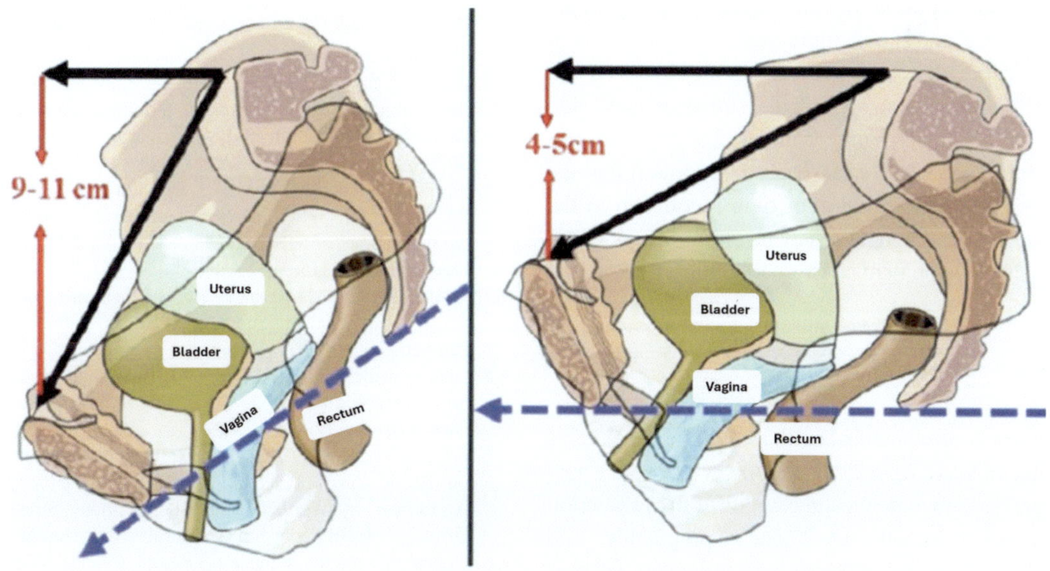

Fig. 3.4 Natural rotation of the female pelvis during aging. Left: In the normal standing female pelvis, the distance from the promontory to the superior pubic symphysis margin varies between 9 and 11 cm. The orientation of the pelvic floor is approximately 45°. Right: Pelvis of an elderly woman standing. Due to the rotation of the pelvis, the promontory descends, and the symphysis pubis rises; the distance between them varies between 4 and 5 cm. The direction of the pelvic floor is horizontal [63]

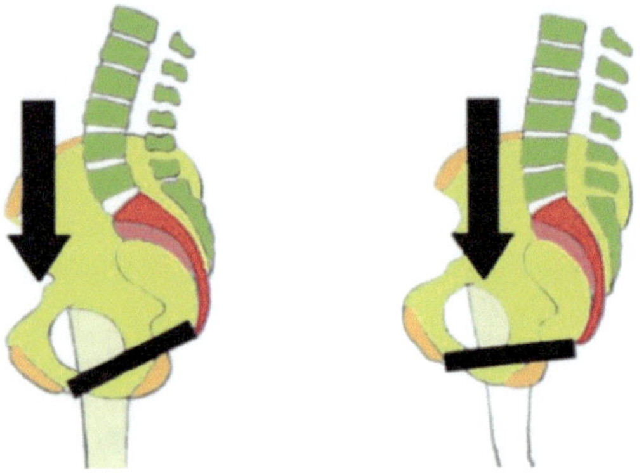

Fig. 3.5 The change in the angle of inclination of the pelvic floor due to pelvic rotation determines the forces acting on it. Left: Normal position. Right: The pelvic floor is under pressure when it becomes horizontal [63]

have less type 1 collagen in their uterosacral ligaments [168]. It has been found that women with POP have a higher proportion of type 3 collagen in their pelvic connective tissue, especially among women without USL. Since type 3 collagen plays an important role in tissue elasticity, the tissue laxity seen in women with POP may be related to the increase in type 3 collagen [59, 115]. Structural abnormalities in the smooth muscles of the USL have been reported in women with POP [135]. It has been reported that the vaginal skin of women with POP can stretch more than the vaginal skin of women with normal pelvic support. However, this difference is not seen in the forearm skin, and therefore, local biomechanical changes (not systemic) cause POP [53]. It has been found that the decrease in the amount of type 3 collagen in the pubocervical ligament may be an important factor in the development of stress incontinence [90].

3.4 Conclusion

In terms of women's health, pelvic biomechanics plays a key role in trunk and lower extremity posture and movements and is vital for the protection of pelvic organs, continence, pregnancy, and labor. However, physiological processes such as pregnancy and menopause significantly alter pelvic biomechanics, potentially leading to dysfunctions. Changes in pelvic alignment, joint mechanics, and soft tissue properties can contribute to musculoskeletal pain and pelvic floor disorders. A comprehensive understanding of these biomechanical variations is crucial for developing preventive and therapeutic strategies to maintain pelvic health. The integration of biomechanical principles into clinical assessments and rehabilitation programs can enhance the management of pelvic floor dysfunctions and musculoskeletal disorders. Health professionals should adopt a comprehensive approach that considers the complex interactions between the pelvis, joints, and surrounding structures. Future research should focus on innovative interventions to optimize pelvic function and improve women's quality of life.

Acknowledgments We would like to thank our fourth-grade physiotherapy student, Özlem Telli, for her support in drawing the pictures.

References

1. Agarwal Y, Doebele S, Windolf M, Shiozawa T, Gueorguiev B, Stuby FM. Two-leg alternate loading model–A different approach to biomechanical investigations of fixation methods of the injured pelvic ring with focus on the pubic symphysis. J Biomech. 2014;47(2):380–6.
2. Akçali Ö, Satoglu IS, Çakiroğlu MA. Kinesiology of the lumbar vertebral column. In: Comparative kinesiology of the human body. Amsterdam: Elsevier; 2020. p. 325–37.
3. Alperin M, Cook M, Tuttle LJ, Esparza MC, Lieber RL. Impact of vaginal parity and aging on the architectural design of pelvic floor muscles. Am J Obstet Gynecol. 2016;215(3):312e1-e9.
4. Ashton-Miller JA, DeLancey JO. On the biomechanics of vaginal birth and common sequelae. Annu Rev Biomed Eng. 2009;11(1):163–76.
5. Ashton-miller JA, DeLancey JO. Functional anatomy of the female pelvic floor. Ann N Y Acad Sci. 2007;1101(1):266–96.
6. Auchincloss, C. C. (2024). The Influence of Posture on Pelvic Floor Muscle Activation and Sensory Awareness in Women With and Without Stress Urinary Incontinence (Doctoral dissertation). Queen's University, Kingston, Ontario, Canada 2023.
7. Badir S, Bajka M, Mazza E. A novel procedure for the mechanical characterization of the uterine cervix during pregnancy. J Mech Behav Biomed Mater. 2013;27:143–53.

8. Bagwell JJ, Snibbe J, Gerhardt M, Powers CM. Hip kinematics and kinetics in persons with and without cam femoroacetabular impingement during a deep squat task. Clin Biomech. 2016;31:87–92.
9. Barber MD. Contemporary views on female pelvic anatomy. Cleve Clin J Med. 2005;72(Suppl 4):S3–11. https://doi.org/10.3949/ccjm.72.suppl_4.s3.
10. Barker PJ, Hapuarachchi K, Ross J, Sambaiew E, Ranger T, Briggs C. Anatomy and biomechanics of gluteus maximus and the thoracolumbar fascia at the sacroiliac joint. Clin Anat. 2014;27(2):234–40.
11. Berger AA, May R, Renner JB, Viradia N, Dahners LE. Surprising evidence of pelvic growth (widening) after skeletal maturity. J Orthop Res. 2011;29(11):1719–23.
12. Berger MB, Doumouchtsis SK, DeLancey JO. Bony pelvis dimensions in women with and without stress urinary incontinence. Neurourol Urodyn. 2013;32(1):37–42.
13. Bergmann G, Deuretzbacher G, Heller M, Graichen F, Rohlmann A, Strauss J, Duda G. Hip contact forces and gait patterns from routine activities. J Biomech. 2001;34(7):859–71.
14. Bergström BS. Urethral hanging theory. Neurourol Urodyn. 2017;36(3):826–7.
15. Best KC, Garvin HM, Cabo LL. An investigation into the relationship between human cranial and pelvic sexual dimorphism. J Forensic Sci. 2018;63(4):990–1000.
16. Bø K, Finckenhagen HB. Is there any difference in measurement of pelvic floor muscle strength in supine and standing position? Acta Obstet Gynecol Scand. 2003;82(12):1120–4.
17. Bø K, Stien R. Needle EMG registration of striated urethral wall and pelvic floor muscle activity patterns during cough, Valsalva, abdominal, hip adductor, and gluteal muscle contractions in nulliparous healthy females. Neurourol Urodyn. 1994;13(1):35–41.
18. Boulay C, Tardieu C, Hecquet J, Benaim C, Mouilleseaux B, Marty C, et al. Sagittal alignment of spine and pelvis regulated by pelvic incidence: standard values and prediction of lordosis. Eur Spine J. 2006;15:415–22.
19. Brito LGO, Pereira GMV, Moalli P, Shynlova O, Manonai J, Weintraub AY, et al. Age and/or postmenopausal status as risk factors for pelvic organ prolapse development: systematic review with meta-analysis. Int Urogynecol J. 2022:1–15.
20. Brown KM, Handa VL, Macura KJ, DeLeon VB. Three-dimensional shape differences in the bony pelvis of women with pelvic floor disorders. Int Urogynecol J. 2013;24:431–9.
21. Brown SH, McGill SM. Co-activation alters the linear versus non-linear impression of the EMG–torque relationship of trunk muscles. J Biomech. 2008;41(3):491–7.
22. Bruening DA, Frimenko RE, Goodyear CD, Bowden DR, Fullenkamp AM. Sex differences in whole body gait kinematics at preferred speeds. Gait Posture. 2015;41(2):540–5.
23. Brůžek J, Santos F, Dutailly B, Murail P, Cunha E. Validation and reliability of the sex estimation of the human os coxae using freely available DSP2 software for bioarchaeology and forensic anthropology. Am J Phys Anthropol. 2017;164(2):440–9.
24. Buller JL, Thompson JR, Cundiff GW, Sullivan LK, Ybarra MAS, Bent AE. Uterosacral ligament: description of anatomic relationships to optimize surgical safety. Obstet Gynecol. 2001;97(6):873–9.
25. Burnett LA, Cook M, Shah S, Wong MM, Kado DM, Alperin M. Age-associated changes in the mechanical properties of human cadaveric pelvic floor muscles. J Biomech. 2020;98:109436.
26. Capobianco RA, Feeney DF, Jeffers JR, Nelson-Wong E, Morreale J, Grabowski AM, Enoka RM. Patients with sacroiliac joint dysfunction exhibit altered movement strategies when performing a sit-to-stand task. Spine J. 2018;18(8):1434–40.
27. Capson AC, Nashed J, Mclean L. The role of lumbopelvic posture in pelvic floor muscle activation in continent women. J Electromyogr Kinesiol. 2011;21(1):166–77.
28. Casaroli G, Bassani T, Brayda-Bruno M, Luca A, Galbusera F. What do we know about the biomechanics of the sacroiliac joint and of sacropelvic fixation? A literature review. Med Eng Phys. 2020;76:1–12.
29. Chaitow L. Chronic pelvic pain: pelvic floor problems, sacro-iliac dysfunction and the trigger point connection. J Bodyw Mov Ther. 2007;11(4):327–39.
30. Chang A, Hayes K, Dunlop D, Song J, Hurwitz D, Cahue S, Sharma L. Hip abduction moment and protection against medial tibiofemoral osteoarthritis progression. Arthritis Rheum. 2005;52(11):3515–9.
31. Chantereau P, Brieu M, Kammal M, Farthmann J, Gabriel B, Cosson M. Mechanical properties of pelvic soft tissue of young women and impact of aging. Int Urogynecol J. 2014;25:1547–53.
32. Chaudhry, S. R., Nahian, A., Chaudhry, K. Anatomy, abdomen and pelvis, pelvis. StatPearls Publishing, Treasure Island; 2023. PMID: 29489173.
33. Cher D, Polly D, Berven S. Sacroiliac joint pain: burden of disease. Medical Devices: Evidence and Research. 2014;7:73–81.
34. Chockalingam N, Chatterley F, Healy AC, Greenhalgh A, Branthwaite HR. Comparison of pelvic complex kinematics during treadmill and overground walking. Arch Phys Med Rehabil. 2012;93(12):2302–8.
35. Chumanov ES, Wall-Scheffler C, Heiderscheit BC. Gender differences in walking and running on level and inclined surfaces. Clin Biomech. 2008;23(10):1260–8.
36. Clark–Patterson G, Domingo M, Miller KS. Biomechanics of pregnancy and vaginal delivery. Current Opinion in Biomedical Engineering. 2022;22:100386.
37. Cox DA, Helvering LM. Extracellular matrix integrity: a possible mechanism for differential

clinical effects among selective estrogen receptor modulators and estrogens? Mol Cell Endocrinol. 2006;247(1–2):53–9.
38. Crosbie J, Vachalathiti R, Smith R. Age, gender and speed effects on spinal kinematics during walking. Gait Posture. 1997;5(1):13–20.
39. Dalstra M, Huiskes R. Load transfer across the pelvic bone. J Biomech. 1995;28(6):715–24.
40. De Keulenaer B, De Waele J, Powell B, Malbrain M. What is normal intra-abdominal pressure and how is it affected by positioning, body mass and positive end-expiratory pressure? Intensive Care Med. 2009;35:969–76.
41. Del Valle A, Thomas CK. Motor unit firing rates during isometric voluntary contractions performed at different muscle lengths. Can J Physiol Pharmacol. 2004;82(8–9):769–76.
42. DeLancey JO. Structural support of the urethra as it relates to stress urinary incontinence: the hammock hypothesis. Am J Obstet Gynecol. 1994;170(5):1713–23.
43. DeSilva JM, Rosenberg KR. Anatomy, development, and function of the human pelvis. Anat Rec. 2017;300(4):628–32.
44. Devreese A, Staes F, De Weerdt W, Feys H, Van Assche A, Penninckx F, Vereecken R. Clinical evaluation of pelvic floor muscle function in continent and incontinent women. Neurourol Urodyn. 2004;23(3):190–7.
45. Diamond LE, Bennell KL, Wrigley TV, Hinman RS, Hall M, O'Donnell J, Hodges PW. Trunk, pelvis and hip biomechanics in individuals with femoroacetabular impingement syndrome: strategies for step ascent. Gait Posture. 2018;61:176–82.
46. Diemerbroeck IV. The anatomy of human bodies: comprehending the most modern discoveries and curiosities in that art to which is added a particular treatise of the small-pox & measles, together with several practical observations and experienced cures. Whitwood, William; 1969.
47. do Carmo Carvalhais VO, de Melo Ocarino J, Araújo VL, Souza TR, Silva PLP, Fonseca ST. Myofascial force transmission between the latissimus dorsi and gluteus maximus muscles: an in vivo experiment. J Biomech. 2013;46(5):1003–7.
48. Donaldson K, Huntington A, De Vita R. Mechanics of uterosacral ligaments: current knowledge, existing gaps, and future directions. Ann Biomed Eng. 2021;49(8):1788–804.
49. Easley DC, Abramowitch SD, Moalli PA. Female pelvic floor biomechanics: bridging the gap. Curr Opin Urol. 2017;27(3):262–7.
50. Egorov V. Biomechanical mapping of the female pelvic floor. Amsterdam: Elsevier; 2023.
51. Eickmeyer SMJPM, Clinics R. Anatomy and physiology of the pelvic floor. Physical Medicine and Rehabilitation Clinics. 2017;28(3):455–60.
52. Enck P, Vodušek DB. Electromyography of pelvic floor muscles. J Electromyogr Kinesiol. 2006;16(6):568–77.
53. Epstein LB, Graham CA, Heit MH. Systemic and vaginal biomechanical properties of women with normal vaginal support and pelvic organ prolapse. Am J Obstet Gynecol. 2007;197(2):165. e1-6.
54. Esculier J-F, Roy J-S, Bouyer LJ. Lower limb control and strength in runners with and without patellofemoral pain syndrome. Gait Posture. 2015;41(3):813–9.
55. Falla D, Hodges PW. Individualized exercise interventions for spinal pain. Exerc Sport Sci Rev. 2017;45(2):105–15.
56. Feeney DF, Capobianco RA, Montgomery JR, Morreale J, Grabowski AM, Enoka RM. Individuals with sacroiliac joint dysfunction display asymmetrical gait and a depressed synergy between muscles providing sacroiliac joint force closure when walking. J Electromyogr Kinesiol. 2018;43:95–103.
57. Flack N, Nicholson H, Woodley S. The anatomy of the hip abductor muscles. Clin Anat. 2014;27(2):241–53.
58. Frank JM, Harris JD, Erickson BJ, Slikker W III, Bush-Joseph CA, Salata MJ, Nho SJ. Prevalence of femoroacetabular impingement imaging findings in asymptomatic volunteers: a systematic review. Arthroscopy: J Arthroscopic & Relat Surg. 2015;31(6):1199–204.
59. Gabriel B, Denschlag D, Göbel H, Fittkow C, Werner M, Gitsch G, Watermann D. Uterosacral ligament in postmenopausal women with or without pelvic organ prolapse. Int Urogynecol J. 2005;16:475–9.
60. Garnon J, Jennings JW, Meylheuc L, Auloge P, Weiss J, Koch G, et al. Biomechanics of the osseous pelvis and its implication for consolidative treatments in interventional oncology. Cardiovasc Intervent Radiol. 2020;43:1589–99.
61. Gilbert TW, Wognum S, Joyce EM, Freytes DO, Sacks MS, Badylak SF. Collagen fiber alignment and biaxial mechanical behavior of porcine urinary bladder derived extracellular matrix. Biomaterials. 2008;29(36):4775–82.
62. Gimenez C, Alperin M, De Vita R. The effect of menopause on vaginal tissue mechanics: A brief review. J Biomech Eng. 2024;146(6):060903.
63. Goeschen K, Liedl B. Chronic pelvic pain and pelvic organ prolapse: a consequence of upright position? Pelviperineology. 2020;39(2):55.
64. Goh JT. Biomechanical and biochemical assessments for pelvic organ prolapse. Curr Opin Obstet Gynecol. 2003;15(5):391–4.
65. Grissom LE, Harty MP, Guo GW, Kecskemethy HH. Maturation of pelvic ossification centers on computed tomography in normal children. Pediatr Radiol. 2018;48:1902–14.
66. Hai-Nan X, Zhi-Jun X, Bao-Xiang L, Yi-Tong Y, Fei W, Qing H, Ying Z. Investigation of correlation between diameters of pelvic inlet and outlet planes and female pelvic floor dysfunction. Eur J Obstet Gynecol Reprod Biol. 2011;159(2):461–4.
67. Handa VL, Pannu HK, Siddique S, Gutman R, VanRooyen J, Cundiff G. Architectural differ-

ences in the bony pelvis of women with and without pelvic floor disorders. Obstet Gynecol. 2003;102(6):1283–90.
68. Hewett TE, Torg JS, Boden BP. Video analysis of trunk and knee motion during non-contact anterior cruciate ligament injury in female athletes: lateral trunk and knee abduction motion are combined components of the injury mechanism. Br J Sports Med. 2009;43(6):417–22.
69. Hodges PW, Sapsford R, Pengel LH. Postural and respiratory functions of the pelvic floor muscles. Neurourol Urodyn. 2007;26(3):362–71.
70. Hoyte L, Damaser M. Biomechanics of the female pelvic floor. Cambridge: Academic Press; 2016. p. 109–26.
71. Hu X, Lu M, Wang Y, Luo Y, Zhou Y, Yang X, et al. 3D-printed custom-made hemipelvic endoprosthetic reconstruction following periacetabular tumor resection: utilizing a novel classification system. BMC Musculoskelet Disord. 2024;25(1):384.
72. Huseynov A, Zollikofer CP, Coudyzer W, Gascho D, Kellenberger C, Hinzpeter R, Ponce de León MS. Developmental evidence for obstetric adaptation of the human female pelvis. Proc Natl Acad Sci. 2016;113(19):5227–32.
73. Ike H, Dorr LD, Trasolini N, Stefl M, McKnight B, Heckmann N. Spine-pelvis-hip relationship in the functioning of a total hip replacement. JBJS. 2018;100(18):1606–15.
74. Iqbal A, Haider M, Stadlhuber RJ, Karu A, Corkill S, Filipi CJ. A study of intragastric and intravesicular pressure changes during rest, coughing, weight lifting, retching, and vomiting. Surg Endosc. 2008;22:2571–5.
75. Jackson S, Eckford S, Abrams P, Avery N, Tarlton J, Bailey A. Changes in metabolism of collagen in genitourinary prolapse. Lancet. 1996;347(9016):1658–61.
76. Janda S. Biomechanics of the pelvic floor musculature, vol. Vol. 55. University Park: Citeseer; 2006.
77. Jiang Y, Sun X, Peng X, Zhao J, Zhang K. Effect of sacral slope on the biomechanical behavior of the low lumbar spine. Exp Ther Med. 2017;13(5):2203–10.
78. Junginger B, Baessler K, Sapsford R, Hodges PW. Effect of abdominal and pelvic floor tasks on muscle activity, abdominal pressure and bladder neck. Int Urogynecol J. 2010;21:69–77.
79. Karaaslan Y, Karaaslan U, Celenay ST. A comparison of lumbopelvic muscle endurance, stability, mobility, and respiratory functions in children and adolescents with and without nocturnal enuresis. Clin Biomech. 2023;101:105829.
80. Kelly M, Tan B, Thompson J, Carroll S, Follington M, Arndt A, Seet M. Healthy adults can more easily elevate the pelvic floor in standing than in crook-lying: an experimental study. Aust. J. Physiother. 2007;53(3):187–91.
81. Kiapour A, Abdelgawad AA, Goel VK, Souccar A, Terai T, Ebraheim NA. Relationship between limb length discrepancy and load distribution across the sacroiliac joint—a finite element study. J Orthop Res. 2012;30(10):1577–80.
82. Kramer PA, Sylvester AD. Hip width and metabolic energy expenditure of abductor muscles. PLoS One. 2023;18(4):e0284450.
83. Kurki HK. Pelvic dimorphism in relation to body size and body size dimorphism in humans. J Hum Evol. 2011;61(6):631–43.
84. Lamblin G, Delorme E, Cosson M, Rubod C. Cystocele and functional anatomy of the pelvic floor: review and update of the various theories. Int Urogynecol J. 2016;27:1297–305.
85. Lazennec J-Y, Riwan A, Gravez F, Rousseau M, Mora N, Gorin M, et al. Hip spine relationships: application to total hip arthroplasty. Hip Int. 2007;17(5_suppl):91–104.
86. Le Huec J-C, Aunoble S, Philippe L, Nicolas P. Pelvic parameters: origin and significance. Eur Spine J. 2011;20:564–71.
87. Legaye J, Duval-Beaupere G, Hecquet J, Marty C. Pelvic incidence: a fundamental pelvic parameter for three-dimensional regulation of spinal sagittal curves. Eur Spine J. 1998;7(2):99–103. https://doi.org/10.1007/s005860050038.
88. Lepage J, Jayyosi C, Lecomte-Grosbras P, Brieu M, Duriez C, Cosson M, Rubod C. Biomechanical pregnant pelvic system model and numerical simulation of childbirth: impact of delivery on the uterosacral ligaments, preliminary results. Int Urogynecol J. 2015;26:497–504.
89. Lewis CL, Laudicina NM, Khuu A, Loverro KL. The human pelvis: variation in structure and function during gait. Anat Rec. 2017;300(4):633–42.
90. Liapis A, Bakas P, Pafiti A, Frangos-Plemenos M, Arnoyannaki N, Creatsas G. Changes of collagen type III in female patients with genuine stress incontinence and pelvic floor prolapse. Eur J Obstet Gynecol Reprod Biol. 2001;97(1):76–9.
91. Lingutla KK, Pollock R, Ahuja S. Sacroiliac joint fusion for low back pain: a systematic review and meta-analysis. Eur Spine J. 2016;25:1924–31.
92. Liu T, Hou X, Xie B, Wu J, Yang X, Sun X, Wang J. Pelvic incidence: A study of a spinopelvic parameter in MRI evaluation of pelvic organ prolapse. Eur J Radiol. 2020;132:109286.
93. Mac-Thiong J-M, Labelle H, Berthonnaud E, Betz RR, Roussouly P. Sagittal spinopelvic balance in normal children and adolescents. Eur Spine J. 2007;16:227–34.
94. Madill SJ, McLean L. Quantification of abdominal and pelvic floor muscle synergies in response to voluntary pelvic floor muscle contractions. J Electromyogr Kinesiol. 2008;18(6):955–64.
95. Mahadevan V. Anatomy of the pelvis. Surgery (Oxford). 2018;36(7):333–8.
96. Mäkinen J, Söderström K-O, Kiilholma P, Hirvonen T. Histological changes in the vaginal connective

tissue of patients with and without uterine prolapse. Arch Gynecol. 1986;239:17–20.
97. Mannella P, Palla G, Bellini M, Simoncini T. The female pelvic floor through midlife and aging. Maturitas. 2013;76(3):230–4.
98. Marshall MR, Montoye AH, Conway MR, Schlaff RA, Pfeiffer KA, Pivarnik JM. Longitudinal changes in walking cadence across pregnancy and postpartum. Gait Posture. 2020;79:234–8.
99. Martins P, Lopes Silva-Filho A, Maciel R, da Fonseca AM, Santos A, Santos L, Mascarenhas T, et al. Biomechanical properties of vaginal tissue in women with pelvic organ prolapse. Gynecol Obstet Investig. 2013;75(2):85–92.
100. Martins PA, Jorge RMN, Ferreia AJ, Saleme CS, Roza T, Parente MM, et al. Vaginal tissue properties versus increased intra-abdominal pressure: a preliminary biomechanical study. Gynecol Obstet Investig. 2011;71(3):145–50.
101. Mattox TF, Lucente V, McIntyre P, Miklos JR, Tomezsko J. Abnormal spinal curvature and its relationship to pelvic organ prolapse. Am J Obstet Gynecol. 2000;183(6):1381–4.
102. Mazza E, Nava A, Bauer M, Winter R, Bajka M, Holzapfel GA. Mechanical properties of the human uterine cervix: an in vivo study. Med Image Anal. 2006;10(2):125–36.
103. McCrory JL, Chambers AJ, Daftary A, Redfern MS. The pregnant "waddle": an evaluation of torso kinematics in pregnancy. J Biomech. 2014;47(12):2964–8.
104. Merrill RK, Kim JS, Leven DM, Kim JH, Meaike JJ, Bronheim RS, et al. Differences in fundamental sagittal pelvic parameters based on age, sex, and race. Clin Spine Surg. 2018;31(2):E109–14.
105. Milosevic M, Yokoyama H, Grangeon M, Masani K, Popovic MR, Nakazawa K, Gagnon DH. Muscle synergies reveal impaired trunk muscle coordination strategies in individuals with thoracic spinal cord injury. J Electromyogr Kinesiol. 2017;36:40–8.
106. Morris VC, Murray MP, DeLancey JO, Ashton-Miller JA. A comparison of the effect of age on levator ani and obturator internus muscle cross-sectional areas and volumes in nulliparous women. Neurourol Urodyn. 2012;31(4):481–6.
107. Müller DA, Capanna R. The surgical treatment of pelvic bone metastases. Advances in orthopedics. 2015;2015(1):525363.
108. Nadeau S, McFadyen BJ, Malouin F. Frontal and sagittal plane analyses of the stair climbing task in healthy adults aged over 40 years: what are the challenges compared to level walking? Clin Biomech. 2003;18(10):950–9.
109. Nakipoglu GF, Karagoz A, Ozgirgin N. The biomechanics of the lumbosacral region in acute and chronic low back pain patients. Pain Physician. 2008;11(4):505–11.
110. Navarro Brazález B, Sánchez Sánchez B, Prieto Gómez V, De La Villa Polo P, McLean L, Torres Lacomba M. Pelvic floor and abdominal muscle responses during hypopressive exercises in women with pelvic floor dysfunction. Neurourol Urodyn. 2020;39(2):793–803.
111. Neumann DA. Kinesiology of the musculoskeletal system-E-book: kinesiology of the musculoskeletal system-E-book. Amsterdam: Elsevier Health Sciences; 2016.
112. Neumann P, Gill V. Pelvic floor and abdominal muscle interaction: EMG activity and intra-abdominal pressure. Int Urogynecol J. 2002;13:125–32.
113. Nguyen JK, Lind LR, Choe JY, McKindsey F, Sinow R, Bhatia NN. Lumbosacral spine and pelvic inlet changes associated with pelvic organ prolapse. Obstet Gynecol. 2000;95(3):332–6.
114. Noehren B, Schmitz A, Hempel R, Westlake C, Black W. Assessment of strength, flexibility, and running mechanics in men with iliotibial band syndrome. J Orthop Sports Phys Ther. 2014;44(3):217–22.
115. Norton P. Abnormal collagen ratios in women with genitourinary prolapse. Neuro Urodyn. 1992;11:2–4.
116. Nygaard I, Barber MD, Burgio KL, Kenton K, Meikle S, Schaffer J, et al. Prevalence of symptomatic pelvic floor disorders in US women. JAMA. 2008;300(11):1311–6.
117. Ochi H, Baba T, Homma Y, Matsumoto M, Nojiri H, Kaneko K. Importance of the spinopelvic factors on the pelvic inclination from standing to sitting before total hip arthroplasty. Eur Spine J. 2016;25:3699–706.
118. Orishimo KF, Kremenic IJ, Mullaney MJ, Fukunaga T, Serio N, McHugh MP. Role of pelvis and trunk biomechanics in generating ball velocity in baseball pitching. J Strength Cond Res. 2023;37(3):623–8.
119. Özgül S, Gürşen C, Toprak Çelenay Ş, Baran E, Üzelpasacı E, Nakip G. Contributory effects of individual characteristics on pelvic floor distress in women with pelvic floor dysfunctions. Physiother Theory Prac. 2024;40(3):625–36.
120. Pasquet B, Carpentier A, Duchateau J. Change in muscle fascicle length influences the recruitment and discharge rate of motor units during isometric contractions. J Neurophysiol. 2005;94(5):3126–33.
121. Pel J, Spoor C, Pool-Goudzwaard A, Hoek van Dijke G, Snijders C. Biomechanical analysis of reducing sacroiliac joint shear load by optimization of pelvic muscle and ligament forces. Ann Biomed Eng. 2008;36:415–24.
122. Peng Y, Miller BD, Boone TB, Zhang Y. Modern theories of pelvic floor support: a topical review of modern studies on structural and functional pelvic floor support from medical imaging, computational modeling, and electromyographic perspectives. Curr Urol Rep. 2018;19:1–10.
123. Perucchini D, DeLancey JO, Ashton-Miller JA, Peschers U, Kataria T. Age effects on urethral striated muscle I. Changes in number and diameter of

striated muscle fibers in the ventral urethra. Am J Obstet Gynecol. 2002;186(3):351–5.
124. Petersen P, Gao C, Rössel P, Qvist P, Arendt-Nielsen L, Gregersen H, Mohr Drewes A. Sensory and biomechanical responses to distension of the normal human rectum and sigmoid colon. Digestion. 2001;64(3):191–9.
125. Petros PE, Woodman PJ. The integral theory of continence. Int Urogynecol J. 2008;19:35–40.
126. Petros PEP, Ulmsten UI. An integral theory of female urinary incontinence: experimental and clinical considerations. Acta Obstet Gynecol Scand. 1990;69(S153):7–31.
127. Phillips A, Pankaj P, Howie C, Usmani AS, Simpson A. Finite element modelling of the pelvis: inclusion of muscular and ligamentous boundary conditions. Med Eng Phys. 2007;29(7):739–48.
128. Pizones J, García-Rey E. Pelvic motion the key to understanding spine–hip interaction. EFORT Open Rev. 2020;5(9):522–33.
129. Pool-Goudzwaard A, Vleeming A, Stoeckart R, Snijders C, Mens JM. Insufficient lumbopelvic stability: a clinical, anatomical and biomechanical approach to 'a-specific'low back pain. Man Ther. 1998;3(1):12–20.
130. Powers CM. The influence of abnormal hip mechanics on knee injury: a biomechanical perspective. J Orthop Sports Phys Ther. 2010;40(2):42–51.
131. Pries E, Dreischarf M, Bashkuev M, Putzier M, Schmidt H. The effects of age and gender on the lumbopelvic rhythm in the sagittal plane in 309 subjects. J Biomech. 2015;48(12):3080–7.
132. Ptaszkowski K, Zdrojowy R, Ptaszkowska L, Bartnicki J, Taradaj J, Paprocka-Borowicz M. Electromyographic evaluation of synergist muscles of the pelvic floor muscle depending on the pelvis setting in menopausal women: A prospective observational study. Gait Posture. 2019;71:170–6.
133. Quartly E, Hallam T, Kilbreath S, Refshauge KJP. Strength and endurance of the pelvic floor muscles in continent women: an observational study. Physiotherapy. 2010;96(4):311–6.
134. Rak Y. Lucy's pelvic anatomy: its role in bipedal gait. J Hum Evol. 1991;20(4):283–90.
135. Reisenauer C, Shiozawa T, Oppitz M, Busch C, Kirschniak A, Fehm T, Drews U. The role of smooth muscle in the pathogenesis of pelvic organ prolapse—an immunohistochemical and morphometric analysis of the cervical third of the uterosacral ligament. Int Urogynecol J. 2008;19:383–9.
136. Reitter A, Daviss B-A, Bisits A, Schollenberger A, Vogl T, Herrmann E, et al. Does pregnancy and/or shifting positions create more room in a woman's pelvis? Am J Obstet Gynecol. 2014;211(6):662.e1–9.
137. Ribeiro AP, João SMA, Sacco ICN. Static and dynamic biomechanical adaptations of the lower limbs and gait pattern changes during pregnancy. Womens Health. 2013;9(1):99–108.
138. Rieger M, Duran P, Cook M, Schenk S, Shah M, Jacobs M, et al. Quantifying the effects of aging on morphological and cellular properties of human female pelvic floor muscles. Ann Biomed Eng. 2021;49:1836–47.
139. Rivaux G, Rubod C, Dedet B, Brieu M, Gabriel B, Cosson M. Comparative analysis of pelvic ligaments: a biomechanics study. Int Urogynecol J. 2013;24:135–9.
140. Rosenberg KR. The evolution of modern human childbirth. Am J Phys Anthropol. 1992;35(S15):89–124.
141. Rubod C, Brieu M, Cosson M, Rivaux G, Clay J-C, de Landsheere L, Gabriel B. Biomechanical properties of human pelvic organs. Urology. 2012;79(4):968.e17–22.
142. Ruiz-Zapata AM, Feola AJ, Heesakkers J, de Graaf P, Blaganje M, Sievert K-D. Biomechanical properties of the pelvic floor and its relation to pelvic floor disorders. Eur Urol Suppl. 2018;17(3):80–90.
143. Sammarco AG, Sheyn DD, Krantz TE, Olivera CK, Rodrigues AA, Kobernik MEK, et al. A novel measurement of pelvic floor cross-sectional area in older and younger women with and without prolapse. Am J Obstet Gynecol. 2019;221(5):521.e1–7.
144. Santos F, Guyomarc'h P, Rmoutilova R, Bruzek J. A method of sexing the human os coxae based on logistic regressions and Bruzek's nonmetric traits. Am J Phys Anthropol. 2019;169(3):435–47.
145. Sapsford R, Hodges P, Richardson C, Cooper D, Markwell S, Jull G. Co-activation of the abdominal and pelvic floor muscles during voluntary exercises. Neurourol. Urodyn. 2001;20(1):31–42.
146. Sapsford RR, Richardson CA, Maher CF, Hodges PW. Pelvic floor muscle activity in different sitting postures in continent and incontinent women. Arch Phys Med Rehabil. 2008;89(9):1741–7.
147. Sawa R, Doi T, Asai T, Watanabe K, Taniguchi T, Ono R. Differences in trunk control between early and late pregnancy during gait. Gait Posture. 2015;42(4):455–9.
148. Schwab F, Lafage V, Patel A, Farcy J-P. Sagittal plane considerations and the pelvis in the adult patient. Spine. 2009;34(17):1828–33.
149. Shafik A, Doss S, Asaad S. Etiology of the resting myoelectric activity of the levator ani muscle: physioanatomic study with a new theory. World J Surg. 2003;27:309–14.
150. Sinsurin K, Valldecabres R, Richards J. An exploration of the differences in hip strength, gluteus medius activity, and trunk, pelvis, and lower-limb biomechanics during different functional tasks. Int Biomech. 2020;7(1):35–43.
151. Smith LK, Lelas JL, Kerrigan DC. Gender differences in pelvic motions and center of mass displacement during walking: stereotypes quantified. J Womens Health Gend Based Med. 2002;11(5):453–8.
152. Smith MD, Coppieters MW, Hodges PW. Postural activity of the pelvic floor muscles is delayed during

rapid arm movements in women with stress urinary incontinence. Int Urogynecol J. 2007;18:901–11.
153. Soljanik I, Janssen U, May F, Fritsch H, Stief CG, Weissenbacher ER, et al. Functional interactions between the fossa ischioanalis, levator ani and gluteus maximus muscles of the female pelvic floor: a prospective study in nulliparous women. Arch Gynecol Obstet. 2012;286:931–8.
154. Stav K, Alcalay M, Peleg S, Lindner A, Gayer G, Hershkovitz I. Pelvis architecture and urinary incontinence in women. Eur Urol. 2007;52(1):239–44.
155. Stodden DF, Fleisig GS, McLean SP, Lyman SL, Andrews JR. Relationship of pelvis and upper torso kinematics to pitched baseball velocity. J Appl Biomech. 2001;17(2):164–72.
156. Sturesson B, Selvik G, UDÉN A. Movements of the sacroiliac joints: a roentgen stereophotogrammetric analysis. Spine. 1989;14(2):162–5.
157. Tague RG. Sexual dimorphism in the human bony pelvis, with a consideration of the Neandertal pelvis from Kebara cave, Israel. Am. J. Phys. Anthropol. 1992;88(1):1–21.
158. Tansatit T, Apinuntrum P, Phetudom T, Phanchart P. New insights into the pelvic organ support framework. Eur J Obstet Gynecol Reprod Biol. 2013;166(2):221–5.
159. Thurston A. Spinal and pelvic kinematics in osteoarthrosis of the hip joint. Spine. 1985;10(5):467–71.
160. Tinelli A, Malvasi A, Rahimi S, Negro R, Vergara D, Martignago R, et al. Age-related pelvic floor modifications and prolapse risk factors in postmenopausal women. Menopause. 2010;17(1):204–12.
161. van Wingerden J-P, Vleeming A, Buyruk H, Raissadat K. Stabilization of the sacroiliac joint in vivo: verification of muscular contribution to force closure of the pelvis. Eur Spine J. 2004;13:199–205.
162. Vaz G, Roussouly P, Berthonnaud E, Dimnet J. Sagittal morphology and equilibrium of pelvis and spine. Eur Spine J. 2002;11:80–7.
163. Verbruggen SW, Nowlan NC. Ontogeny of the human pelvis. Anat Rec. 2017;300(4):643–52.
164. Vialle R, Levassor N, Rillardon L, Templier A, Skalli W, Guigui P. Radiographic analysis of the sagittal alignment and balance of the spine in asymptomatic subjects. J. Bone Joint Surg. 2005;87(2):260–7.
165. Vleeming A, Schuenke M, Masi A, Carreiro J, Danneels L, Willard F. The sacroiliac joint: an overview of its anatomy, function and potential clinical implications. J Anat. 2012;221(6):537–67.
166. Volinski B, Kalra A, Yang K. Evaluation of full pelvic ring stresses using a bilateral static gait-phase finite element modeling method. J Mech Behav Biomed Mater. 2018;78:175–87.
167. Vrtovec T, Janssen MM, Likar B, Castelein RM, Viergever MA, Pernuš F. A review of methods for evaluating the quantitative parameters of sagittal pelvic alignment. Spine J. 2012;12(5):433–46.
168. Vulic M, Strinic T, Tomic S, Capkun V, Jakus IA, Ivica S. Difference in expression of collagen type I and matrix metalloproteinase-1 in uterosacral ligaments of women with and without pelvic organ prolapse. Eur J Obstet Gynecol Reprod Biol. 2011;155(2):225–8.
169. Walheim G, Olerud S, Ribbe TJA o S. Mobility of the pubic symphysis: measurements by an electromechanical method. Acta Orthop Scand. 1984;55(2):203–8.
170. Wall-Scheffler CM. Women carry for less: body size, pelvis width, loading position and energetics. Evol. Hum. Sci. 2022;4:e36.
171. Wall-Scheffler CM, Chumanov E, Steudel-Numbers K, Heiderscheit B. Electromyography activity across gait and incline: the impact of muscular activity on human morphology. Am J Phys Anthropol. 2010;143(4):601–11.
172. Wall-Scheffler CM, Geiger K, Steudel-Numbers KL. Infant carrying: the role of increased locomotory costs in early tool development. Am. J. Phys. Anthropol. 2007;133(2):841–6.
173. Warrener AG, Lewton KL, Pontzer H, Lieberman DE. A wider pelvis does not increase locomotor cost in humans, with implications for the evolution of childbirth. PLoS One. 2015;10(3):e0118903.
174. Washburn SL. Tools and human evolution. Sci Am. 1960;203(3):62–75.
175. Whitcome KK, Lopez J, Miller EE, Burns JL. Revisiting the human obstetrical dilemma: effect of pelvic rotation stride length. Am J Phys Anthropol. 2012;147:302.
176. Widler KS, Glatthorn JF, Bizzini M, Impellizzeri FM, Munzinger U, Leunig M, Maffiuletti NA. Assessment of hip abductor muscle strength. A validity and reliability study. J Bone Joint Surg. 2009;91(11):2666–72.
177. Wognum S, Schmidt DE, Sacks MS. On the mechanical role of de novo synthesized elastin in the urinary bladder wall. J Biomech Eng. 2009;131(10):1–11.
178. Wyndow N, De Jong A, Rial K, Tucker K, Collins N, Vicenzino B, et al. The relationship of foot and ankle mobility to the frontal plane projection angle in asymptomatic adults. J Foot Ankle Res. 2016;9:1–7.
179. Yang M, Chen C, Wang Z, Long J, Huang R, Qi W, Shi R. Finite element analysis of female pelvic organ prolapse mechanism: current landscape and future opportunities. Front Med. 2024;11:1342645.
180. Young M, Selleri L, Capellini TD. Genetics of scapula and pelvis development: an evolutionary perspective. Curr Top Dev Biol. 2019;132:311–49.
181. Zhang S, Derrick TR, Evans W, Yu Y-J. Shock and impact reduction in moderate and strenuous landing activities. Sports Biomech. 2008;7(2):296–309.

Part II

Diagnosis and Treatment for Pelvic and Women's Health

Diagnosis and Treatment of Lower Urinary Tract Disorders

4

Rabia Hizarci Bal and Naşide Mangir

4.1 Introduction

Lower urinary tract disorders (LUTDs) in women include a variety of conditions that affect the bladder, urethra, and the surrounding structures, leading to various symptoms and dysfunctions. These disorders can severely affect a woman's physical, emotional, and social well-being. Issues like incontinence can lead to embarrassment, social withdrawal, and decreased physical activity, which can ultimately impact mental health.

As the population ages, LUTDs become increasingly more common, and the costs associated with the diagnosis, treatment, and management of LUTDs can be substantial, both for individuals and healthcare systems. LUTDs often lead to increased healthcare visits, diagnostic testing, and treatment interventions, placing a burden on healthcare systems.

LUTDs can also indicate or be associated with other more significant health conditions, such as neurological disorders, diabetes, or pelvic floor dysfunction, necessitating comprehensive evaluation and management.

The most common types of LUTDs in women are urinary incontinence, overactive bladder (OAB) syndrome, pelvic organ prolapse (POP), and bladder pain syndrome/interstitial cystitis. In this chapter, we will review the diagnosis and treatment of the two most commonly encountered LUTDs in women: stress urinary incontinence (SUI) and overactive bladder syndrome.

4.2 Terminology Used in the Assessment of LUTD in Women

Understanding and using the correct terminology in the assessment of LUTD in women is essential for effective communication between clinicians by ensuring that the terms and diagnosis are consistent. The most common lower urinary tract symptoms (LUTS) and their standard International Continence Society (ICS) definitions are shown in Table 4.1. Further details related to this standardized terminology can be found at https://www.ics.org/glossary.

The lower urinary tract symptoms consist of storage, voiding, and post-micturition symptoms, according to ICS definitions. Storage symptoms can be categorized as general storage symptoms, sensory symptoms, and urinary incontinence (UI) symptoms. General storage symptoms include increased urinary frequency, increased daytime frequency, nocturia, and polyuria. Sensory symptoms include urgency and increased/reduced/absent and nonspecific (atypical) bladder-filling sensation. Incontinence

R. Hizarci Bal (✉) · N. Mangir
Department of Urology, Faculty of Medicine, Hacettepe University, Ankara, Türkiye
e-mail: rabiahizarci@hacettepe.edu.tr; n.mangir@hacettepe.edu.tr

T. Akbayrak, E. Üzelpasaci (eds.), *Physiotherapy and Rehabilitation in Pelvic and Women's Health-Related Problems*, https://doi.org/10.1007/978-3-032-28741-0_4

Table 4.1 The standard definitions of the most commonly encountered lower urinary tract symptoms. (definitions as reported by the International Continence Society https://www.ics.org/glossary)

Symptom	ICS standard definition
Storage symptoms	Lower urinary tract symptoms occurring during the bladder storage phase
Increased urinary frequency	Complaint that voiding occurs more frequently than deemed normal by the individual (or caregivers)
Nocturia	The number of times urine is passed during the main sleep period. Each urination must be followed by sleep or the intention to sleep
Polyuria	Complaint that the urine excretion volume over 24 h is noticeably higher than the previous experience
Urgency	Complaint of a sudden, compelling desire to pass urine, which is difficult to defer
Urgency urinary incontinence (UUI)	Complaint of involuntary loss of urine associated with urgency
Stress urinary incontinence (SUI)	Complaint of involuntary loss of urine on effort or physical exertion, including sporting activities, or on sneezing or coughing
Mixed urinary incontinence (MUI)	Complaints of both stress and urgency urinary incontinence
Voiding symptoms	Lower urinary tract symptoms during the voiding phase (experienced during micturition)
Hesitancy	Complaint of a delay in initiating voiding (when the individual is ready to pass urine)
Straining to void	Complaint of the need to make an intensive effort to either initiate, maintain, or improve voiding or the urinary stream
Slow (urinary) stream	Complaint of a urinary stream perceived as overall slower than the previous performance or in comparison with others
Intermittency	Complaint of urine flow that stops and starts on one or more occasions during one voiding episode
Dysuria	Complaint of pain, burning, other discomfort, or difficulty during voiding
Post-voiding symptoms	Lower urinary tract symptoms experienced after voiding have ceased
Feeling of incomplete (bladder) emptying	Complaint that the bladder does not feel empty after voiding has ceased

symptoms include urgency UI (UUI), stress UI, mixed UI (MUI), postural UI, continuous UI, overflow UI, sexual arousal UI, and enuresis. Voiding symptoms include hesitancy, straining to void, slow stream, intermittency, and dysuria, whereas post-micturition symptoms include feelings of incomplete emptying and a need to immediately re-void [1].

4.3 Prevalence of LUTS in Women

Lower urinary tract symptoms are highly frequent in women and have a significant impact on health-related quality of life [2]. The prevalence of LUTS differs according to the study design and the population chosen. Yet there is general agreement about the high prevalence and physical, social, and economic burdens in the studies.

Based on the population-based epidemiology of lower urinary tract symptoms, Prevalence of Incontinence and Comorbidities study (EPIC) [3] and Epidemiology of LUTS (EpiLUTS [4] studies, both of which assessed LUTS using the standardized terminology mentioned in the previous section, the overall prevalence of at least one LUTS is 66.6–76.3% in women. Unlike men, voiding symptoms (19.5%) and post-micturition symptoms (14.2%) are less prevalent in women. Terminal dribble is the most common voiding symptom in women (9.9%), whereas incomplete emptying is the most common post-micturition symptom (12.3%).

Storage symptoms (34.2–59.2%) are the most common symptoms among the three symptom groups, and the prevalence increases with age in both sexes. Nocturia, when defined as one or more nocturnal micturitions per night, is the most frequent symptom (54.5–76.3%) in the female population. Urgency, which is the cardinal symptom of overactive bladder syndrome, is reported by 12.8–35.7% of women. UI is reported in nearly half of the women who have OAB symptoms. Among all the subtypes, stress incontinence is the most frequent incontinence in women and has been reported by 6.4% of women aged ≥18 years in the EPIC study. Mixed urinary incontinence and urgency urinary incontinence are the second and third most prevalent subtypes, with a prevalence of 2.4% and 1.5%, respectively. Like the EPIC study, incontinence was highly prevalent in women aged ≥40 years in the EpiLUTS study; SUI was reported by 31.8%, and UUI was reported by 24.4% of women.

4.4 Diagnosis of LUTD in Women

4.4.1 History and Physical Examination

Taking a detailed clinical history should be the first step in the clinical evaluation of a patient with LUTS. A thorough questioning of the LUTS and sexual, neurological, and gastrointestinal symptoms should be included in the history. Storage, voiding, and post-micturition symptoms should be questioned separately. Symptoms of sexual dysfunction, anorectal symptoms, lower urinary tract pain and/or other pelvic pain, and lower urinary tract infection (UTI) history must be included in the history. If a urinary tract infection is present at the time of the assessment, the patient must be reassessed after the treatment. Factors that may affect LUTS, such as previous surgeries, childbearing and menopausal status, comorbidities, smoking status, and current medication, should be questioned. A neurological, obstetric, and gynecological history should be included in the history to figure out the underlying causes and factors that may have an impact on treatment decisions and identify patients who would need referral to other specialties [5].

Physical examination should include abdominal examination for the detection of abdominal mass and palpable urinary bladder and digital examination of both the vagina and the rectum. Physical examination for urinary incontinence should be performed when the bladder is comfortably full [6]. A cough test must be performed to assess SUI, and urethral mobility must be assessed. Extra-urethral incontinence (due to fistula or other issues) should be observed. Examinations for pelvic organ prolapse should be done with the woman's bladder empty [6]. The presence of any prolapse can be staged using POP-Q staging (Table 4.2).

Vulvar examination should be included to check for abnormalities such as cysts and atrophic changes. Urethral palpation should be done to assess mucosal prolapse, urethral caruncle, and diverticulum. Vaginal examination should be included to assess the estrogen status and the presence of pain. The location of any vaginal pain and tenderness over the course of the pudendal nerve should be noted. Pelvic floor muscle function and anal sphincter tone and strength should be examined carefully. Finally, a neuro-urological examination should be undertaken.

4.4.2 Patient-Reported Outcome Measures Used in the Assessment of LUTD

Patient-reported outcome measures (PROMs) are frequently used in the clinical management of

Table 4.2 Simplified POP-Q staging [6]

Stage	Definition
Stage 0	No prolapse is demonstrated
Stage I	The most distal portion of the prolapse is more than 1 cm above the level of the hymen
Stage II	The most distal portion of the prolapse is 1 cm or less proximal to or distal to the plane of the hymen
Stage III	The most distal portion of the prolapse is more than 1 cm below the plane of the hymen
Stage IV	Complete eversion of the total length of the lower genital tract is demonstrated

patients with LUTD. PROMs mainly consist of symptom scores and QoL scores and can complement patient history and help physicians better understand the nature and impact of LUTS in the patient's overall well-being. PROMs are useful and objective tools for the baseline evaluation of lower urinary tract symptoms and the assessment of the severity of the symptoms and their effects on the quality of life; most importantly, PROMs are generally sensitive to change, making them a useful follow-up measure [7]. Symptom scores/questionnaires must be validated for the language being used and must be sensitive to change if they are aimed to be used for treatment evaluation [5]. To date, numerous questionnaires have been developed to assess different aspects of LUTS in women, yet there is no gold standard tool to evaluate all LUTS symptoms in women [8].

There are several questionnaires, such as the International Consultation on Incontinence Questionnaire Female Lower Urinary Tract Symptoms (ICIQ-FLUTS), ICIQ short form (ICIQ-SF), and The Questionnaire for Urinary Incontinence Diagnosis (QUID), that can differentiate UI types and assess the symptoms and effects of UI in women. The short form of ICIQ (ICIQ-SF) is a useful tool to assess symptoms and the impact of urinary incontinence and pelvic floor dysfunction in clinical practice. It has been shown to correlate with 1-h and 24-h pad test assessments of the severity of stress urinary incontinence [9, 10]. International Consultation on Incontinence Questionnaire Female Lower Urinary Tract Symptoms (ICIQ-FLUTS) is one of the most preferred forms to evaluate female LUTS, especially incontinence; measure the impact on QoL; and evaluate the treatment outcome. It is validated in 31 languages and has a grade A level of validation according to ICI grades of recommendation. The questionnaire consists of 12 question items and evaluates filling, voiding, and incontinence symptoms. Bother scales are not incorporated in the overall score but indicate the impact of individual symptoms for the patient [11].

Apart from the symptom scores focusing on UI, there are questionnaires such as The Overactive Bladder Questionnaire Short Form (OABQ-SF), the bladder control self-assessment questionnaire (B-SAQ), and Overactive Bladder Questionnaire-Version 8 (OAB-V8) that are developed to assess symptoms and bother in overactive bladder and other LUT symptoms in women. Among these, OABQ-SF focuses on both continence and incontinence symptoms of overactive bladder and their impact on health-related quality of life. The OAB-V8 form (OAB Awareness Tool) is an eight-item screening tool for use in a primary care setting to identify patients who may have OAB and the need for treatment [12]. The questionnaire has a grade A level of validation according to ICI grades of recommendation and can be used in both men and women.

There are also several forms that are developed to assess other LUTS-related problems, such as POP symptoms and QoL (Pelvic Floor Distress Inventory (PFDI) and Pelvic Floor Impact Questionnaire (PFIQ)), urgency (Indevus Urgency Severity Scale (IUSS)), and sexual matters (ICIQ-FLUTSsex). Due to the variety of symptom scoring tools and QoL scores, clinicians are advised to choose a tool according to the intended purposes.

4.4.3 Bladder Diary, Pad Testing, Uroflowmetry, and PVR

4.4.3.1 Bladder Diary

Bladder diary is a semi-objective tool that can be used to quantify fluid intake and measure the frequency and severity of LUTS. It also provides the patient with insights into their voiding behaviors [5].

The frequency volume chart (FVC) includes the recording of the time of each micturition, together with the voided volume for at least 24 h. A bladder diary contains information about the fluid intake, pad usage, incontinence episodes, the degree of incontinence, and the circumstances at the time of the leakage, in addition to the information in the FVC.

FVCs and bladder diaries are adjuncts to the diagnosis and management of LUTS and can be used as more reliable tools to measure the severity of LUTS than the subjective history that depends on patient recall since patient recalls might not be as accurate as the diaries. In a retrospective study that included 601 patients who underwent a suburethral sling procedure and whose complete medical history and bladder diaries were present, it was found that only 47% of the women were accurate about daytime frequency and that 51% overestimated daytime frequency. Overestimation was distinct, particularly in patients who reported a daytime frequency of greater than ten voids per day [13]. Similarly, in another prospective study that compared the International Prostate Symptom Score (IPSS) scores and 3-day FVC in 164 patients, overestimation of the number of nocturia episodes has been found more common than underestimation in patients older than 60 years old [14]. Therefore, the use of FVC or bladder diary is essential in preventing recall bias in the management of patients with LUTS.

Apart from being semi-objective, FVC and bladder diaries are useful in diagnosing patients with nocturnal polyuria. By the ICS definition, nocturnal (nighttime) polyuria is increased proportional production of urine during the nighttime compared with the 24-h urine volume. Nocturnal polyuria may be an indicator of systemic diseases other than the urinary system, such as diabetes, heart failure, and peripheral edema. FVC and bladder diaries are the most practical way of diagnosing nocturnal polyuria.

In the literature, there are several studies showing the reproducibility, feasibility, reliability, and validity of the bladder diaries. Although diaries should not replace medical history, they are cost-effective and reliable when used in conjunction with history. It should be kept in mind that requesting longer diaries may increase the accuracy while decreasing patient compliance. Although the optimum number of days required varies in different studies, 3–7 days are routinely reported in the literature. In the

DAY 1			DAY 2			DAY 3		
Time	Fluid Intake (Amount/Type)	Voided Volume	Time	Fluid Intake (Amount/Type)	Voided Volume	Time	Fluid Intake (Amount/Type)	Voided Volume
7 am			7 am			7 am		
8 am			8 am			8 am		
9 am			9 am			9 am		
10 am			10 am			10 am		
11 am			11 am			11 am		
12 am			12 am			12 am		
1 pm			1 pm			1 pm		
2 pm			2 pm			2 pm		
3 pm			3 pm			3 pm		
4 pm			4 pm			4 pm		
5 pm			5 pm			5 pm		
6 pm			6 pm			6 pm		
7 pm			7 pm			7 pm		
8 pm			8 pm			8 pm		
9 pm			9 pm			9 pm		
10 pm			10 pm			10 pm		
11 pm			11 pm			11 pm		
12 pm			12 pm			12 pm		
1 am			1 am			1 am		
2 am			2 am			2 am		
3 am			3 am			3 am		
4 am			4 am			4 am		
5 am			5 am			5 am		
6 am			6 am			6 am		

Fig. 4.1 A sample of frequency/volume chart, where patients can note their total fluid consumptions and the time and volume of each void

European Association of Urology (EAU) guidelines, at least 3 days of bladder diaries are recommended.

In Fig. 4.1, a sample of frequency volume chart (FVC) used by the author has been shown. A three-day bladder diary sample can be found on the official website of the International Continence Society: https://www.ics.org/.

4.4.3.2 Pad Testing

Measurement of the amount of urine leakage using an absorbent pad at specific times or during physical exercise can be used to assess the presence and severity of urinary incontinence and the response to treatment. Pad testing is a noninvasive, cheap, and easy method that can diagnose UI accurately. A positive pad test can be defined as an increase in pad weight by 1 g and 4 g in 1 h and 24 h, respectively [15]. The test is sensitive to response to treatment, so the change in urine leakage on pad tests can be used to measure treatment outcome rather than providing an indication of disease severity.

Different durations of pad tests, varying from 1 h to 24–48 h, as well as numerous provocations, varying from everyday activities to provocation regimens, can be chosen by the clinicians. Despite there not being a gold standard for the duration of the pad test, longer-duration tests seem to be more reproducible with lower patient compliance. On the other hand, a systematic review of 18 studies concluded that the 1-h pad test was more accurate but less reproducible when compared to the longer-duration pad tests [16]. In EAU guidelines, it is suggested that 24 h is a sufficient duration for home-based testing, balancing diagnostic accuracy and adherence, and a pad test can be used when quantification of urinary incontinence is required, especially to assess response to treatment.

4.4.3.3 Uroflowmetry and Post-void Residual Urine Volume

Uroflowmetry is a noninvasive test assessing the voiding phase of micturition and is accepted as a simple form of urodynamic evaluation. The maximum flow rate (Q_{max}), voided volume, the pattern of the curve, and the post-void residual (PVR) volume are the most significant parameters to be evaluated.

It is advised that the bladder be sufficiently full, as Q_{max} is dependent on volume, but there is no consensus on the threshold of the minimum volume in women [5]. Provided that the bladder is full, reduced Q_{max} can be an indication of incomplete bladder emptying, resulting from weakness in the contractility of the detrusor muscle, such as an underactive bladder, or increased functional or anatomical outlet resistance, such as a urethral stricture. Voided volumes can show the functional urinary bladder capacity. The voiding pattern is expected to be a bell-shaped pattern. A bell-shaped voiding pattern does not exclude underlying pathologies, but abnormal patterns may provide insights into the underlying pathology. For instance, a staccato pattern may be indicative of dysfunctional voiding, whereas a plateau-shaped pattern may show bladder outlet obstruction (BOO). A tower-shaped pattern may indicate an overactive bladder, while an interrupted pattern may indicate low detrusor contractility with abdominal straining.

The volume of urine left in the bladder at the completion of voiding is referred to as post-void residual (PVR). It can be measured either by catheterization after voiding or by ultrasound. Ultrasound is the recommended choice for measuring PVR in the guidelines, as it is noninvasive.

Although there is no consensus on the significant volume of PVR in women, PVR > 100 cc is routinely accepted as significant in the literature [5]. Significant PVR can potentially indicate bladder outlet obstruction and/or detrusor underactivity, and importance must be attached when significant PVR is detected, as it may cause/worsen symptoms, UTI, upper urinary tract dilatation, and renal insufficiency. Both the EAU 2023 guideline and the American Urological Association/ Society of Urodynamics, Female Pelvic Medicine & Urogenital Reconstruction (AUA/SUFU) guideline (2023) recommend measuring PVR for the initial evaluation of LUTS and before considering invasive treatments in patients with SUI since increased PVRs may elevate the risk of voiding difficulties postoperatively [5, 17]. Patients who are candidates for anti-incontinence surgeries or for medical therapies which aim to decrease bladder contractility in urinary urgency are also recommended to be evaluated with PVR before and after the treatments.

4.4.4 Urodynamics

Urodynamic studies (UDs) can be used where the first-line assessment tools, including history, physical examination, symptom scores, bladder diaries, and simple tests such as urinalysis and PVR measurement, are insufficient for disease management. UDs can be used to provide or confirm a diagnosis, predict treatment outcome, understand the reasons for failure of previous treatments, and facilitate discussion during counseling [18].

Urodynamic studies are essential to objectively show the presence of detrusor overactivity (Fig. 4.2). However, while evaluating patients with OAB, failure to demonstrate Detrusor overactivity (DO) in the UDs does not rule out a diagnosis. In the current clinical practice, the use of UDs in the management of patients with OAB is recommended before invasive treatments such as botulinum toxin injection and sacral neuromodulation (SNM). In a Cochrane review of seven randomized trials, it is shown that UDs change the clinical decisions in the treatment of incontinence in women and increase the likelihood of recommending medical treatment. Yet there was no statistically significant change in the treatment outcome despite the change in clinical decisions [19]. Thus, urodynamic studies are not recommended to be routinely carried out while offering first-line treatment to patients with uncomplicated OAB symptoms.

Urodynamic studies are often performed before surgical treatment of SUI. The main purposes of carrying out UDs before surgery are to find out the best treatment modality, predict the treatment success, and predict the likelihood of voiding dysfunction after the surgery. UDs are shown to increase the likelihood of avoiding surgery, but the change in decision-making could not be shown to change the clinical outcome of the treatment [19]. In the Stress Incontinence Surgical Treatment Efficacy Trial (SISTEr), a multicenter randomized trial that included 655 subjects who had UDs before surgery for SUI, the presence or absence of DO, urodynamic stress incontinence, and Valsalva leak point pressures are not shown to predict treatment success and likelihood of voiding dysfunction after surgery. The National Institute for Health and Care Excellence (NICE) 2019 guidelines and EAU 2023 guidelines do not recommend performing urodynamic studies before primary surgery for SUI or stress-predominant MUI in uncomplicated patients. UDs before surgery are recommended in patients who have urge-predominant MUI, in cases in

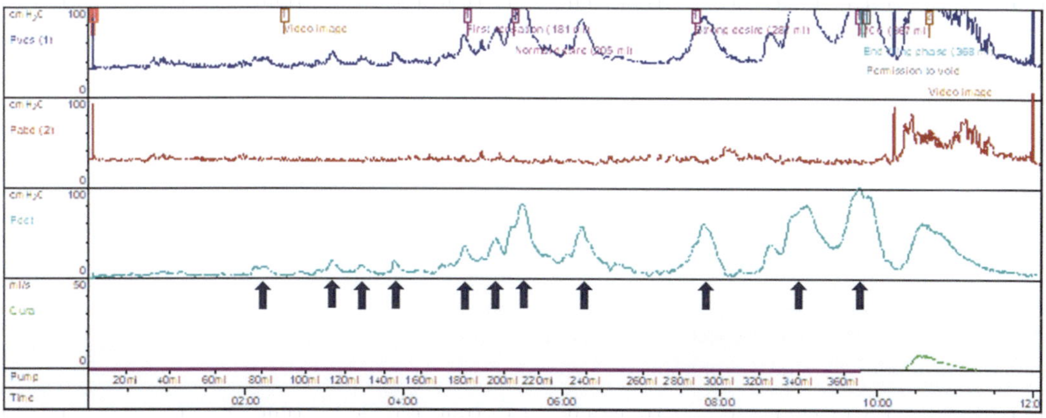

Fig. 4.2 Urodynamic investigation of a patient with overactive bladder syndrome. Detrusor overactivity (blue arrows) associated with a sensation of urgency started from a bladder volume of 80 ml in the filling cystometry, but no incontinence was observed. The voiding phase shows a normal pressure and normal flow pattern

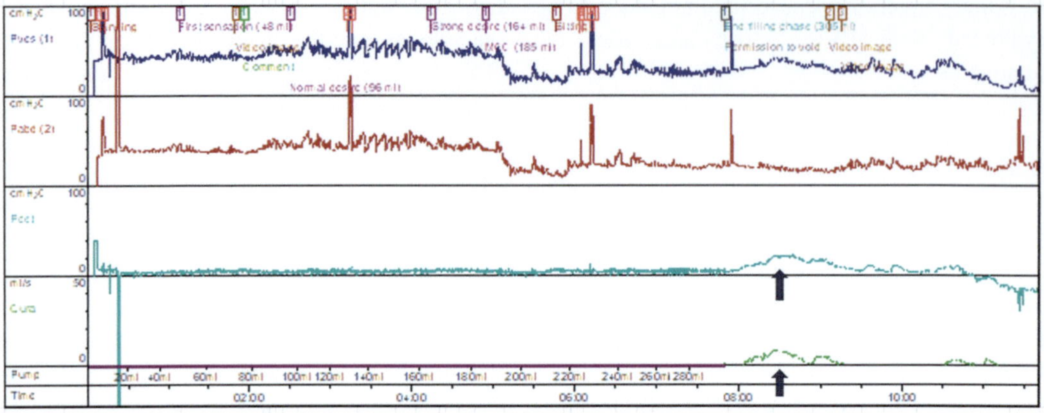

Fig. 4.3 The urodynamic trace of a male patient presenting with frequent voiding and nocturia. A normal detrusor function is observed in the storage phase; however, a low-pressure, low-flow pattern with incomplete emptying is observed in the voiding phase. This patient was diagnosed with detrusor underactivity

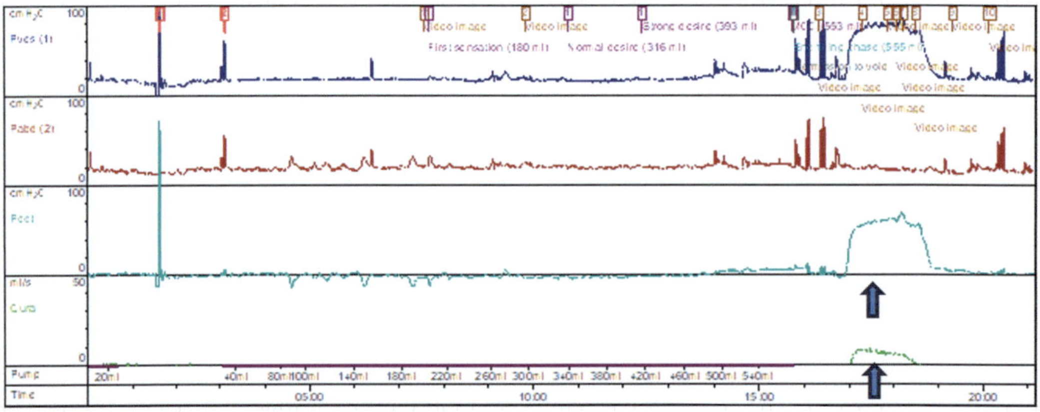

Fig. 4.4 The urodynamic study of a male patient presenting with voiding problems showed normal bladder storage functions, together with a high-pressure, low-flow pattern (blue arrows) in the voiding phase, which indicates bladder outlet obstruction

which the type of UI is unclear, when there is a suspicion of voiding dysfunction, when the case is associated with POP, and when the patient has a history of prior surgery for SUI.

Apart from its use in OAB and SUI, urodynamic studies can be used as a reliable tool to distinguish an underactive bladder from bladder outlet obstruction. Although symptoms and uroflowmetry and PVR findings in both underactive bladder and BOO overlap, invasive UDs can reliably distinguish if the patient has detrusor underactivity (Fig. 4.3) or BOO (Fig. 4.4).

4.5 Treatment of LUTD in Women

In this section, the treatment approach for the most commonly encountered LUTDs in women will be discussed.

4.5.1 Overactive Bladder

By the ICS definition, overactive bladder (OAB) syndrome is urinary urgency, usually accompanied by increased daytime frequency and/or nocturia, with urinary incontinence (OAB-wet) or without it (OAB-dry), in the absence of urinary tract infection or other detectable disease [20]. OAB is a chronic condition that has a significant negative impact on daily life and Health-Related Quality of Life (HRQOL), including work productivity, sleep patterns, social relations, and low self-esteem [21].

In patients with uncomplicated OAB symptoms, detailed history, physical examination, urinalysis, and bladder diaries are generally adequate before offering the first-line treatment. Advanced evaluation, such as urodynamic studies, cystoscopy, and urinary ultrasound, is only needed in complicated patients who do not respond to first-line conservative treatments and medical therapy and before surgical treatments.

Treatment of OAB consists of conservative treatments, medical therapies, and surgical treatments.

4.5.1.1 Conservative Treatments

The first-line treatment of OAB consists of lifestyle interventions and behavioral and physical therapies.

4.5.1.1.1 Lifestyle Interventions

Lifestyle interventions include reduction in caffeine and fluid intake, weight loss, regulation of bowel habits, and smoking cessation. High doses of caffeine have an acute diuretic action, but regular caffeine users become accustomed to the effects of caffeine, and the diuretic effect diminishes [22]. Although caffeine reduction has not been shown to reduce urinary incontinence in a consistent way, it is shown to improve other OAB symptoms, such as urgency and frequency. A scoping review shows that complete caffeine cessation or a reduction under 100 mg of caffeine per day leads to a reduction in urgency and nocturnal enuresis [23].

Modification of the total volume of fluid intake is a common method used by patients with OAB. As a healthcare provider, advice should be given based on the bladder diary of the patient, and the patient should be provided with sufficient fluid intake to avoid thirst, constipation, and underhydration. A randomized controlled trial (RCT) showed that restriction of fluid intake by 25% did not improve UI but resulted in a marked reduction in OAB symptoms, including daytime frequency, urgency, and nocturia [24]. Considering the improvement in OAB symptoms, fluid restrictions should be encouraged when feasible.

In epidemiological studies, there is evidence indicating that both SUI and UUI are more prevalent with increasing body mass index. Weight loss is primarily associated with decreased SUI, yet it also reduces the UUI episodes. In a prospective study evaluating urinary incontinence in overweight and obese individuals after an intensive weight loss program, a mean weight loss of 7.8 kg was shown to be associated with an increased likelihood of decreased UUI episodes when compared to a mean weight loss of 1.5 kg [25]. In EAU guidelines, it is recommended to encourage overweight and obese adults with overactive bladder (OAB)/urinary incontinence to lose weight and maintain weight loss.

Smoking (both former and current smoking) has been shown to be weakly associated with urinary incontinence and other OAB symptoms in several studies [26]. In the EAU guidelines, it is recommended to provide smoking cessation strategies to patients with OAB who smoke.

4.5.1.1.2 Behavioral and Physical Therapies

Behavioral and physical therapies, such as timed voiding, urgency suppression, bladder training, and pelvic floor muscle training (PFMT), are included in the first-line treatment of OAB and are recommended to be offered to all patients with OAB by AUA/SUFU guidelines [27].

Timed voiding is a fixed time interval toileting assistance program that has been promoted for the management of people with urinary incontinence, with or without cognitive impairment [28]. The main goal of timed voiding is emptying the bladder before it reaches full capacity to decrease the urine leakage, which is associated with detrusor contraction with a full bladder, especially in patients with SUI [29]. It is considered a passive program that can be used predominantly with frail older adults suffering from UI. Yet the data on the efficiency of timed voiding is of insufficient quality to provide support for or against the intervention of timed voiding [26].

Bladder training is a gradual voiding program with patient education that includes teaching strategies for suppressing urgency and delaying voiding. The program starts with a scheduled voiding regimen, after which the voiding intervals increase gradually. This program is used for individuals with no cognitive or physical impairments. The main goals of the program include improving the bladder capacity, enhancing the patients' control over urgency, and correcting erroneous patterns of frequent urination [5]. There are several randomized controlled trials reporting statistically significant improvements in urinary incontinence with bladder training when compared to no treatment. Yet it is unclear whether bladder is more effective than drug therapy for women with DO or UUI. Considering the lack of adverse effects of bladder training and its efficacy, it is an appropriate first-line conservative therapy for UI in women [30].

Pelvic floor muscle training consists of repetitive contraction and relaxation of pelvic floor muscles, which provides strength, endurance, and control over the pelvic floor and improves the structural support in pelvic organs. PFMT is aimed at resulting in hypertrophy in striated muscles, which increases the external mechanical pressure on the urethra, yields more effective inhibition of the detrusor, and improves structural support of the bladder neck [5, 31]. In a systematic review of 11 randomized controlled trials, 5 studies have shown that PFMT significantly reduced OAB symptoms such as UUI and frequency when compared to no treatment, a placebo drug, or an inactive control treatment, whereas in the remaining studies, no significant difference could be shown [32]. Although there is no consensus on the optimal duration, it is recommended in the EAU guidelines to ensure that pelvic floor muscle training programs are as intensive as possible.

4.5.1.1.3 Pharmacological Management

Medical treatment is considered the second-line treatment in OAB and predominantly consists of antimuscarinic agents as well as beta-3 (β3) agonists. Oral antimuscarinic agents and β3 agonists are recommended as standard treatment according to the AUA/SUFU AAM 2024 guidelines (strong recommendation; evidence level: Grade A). Similarly, in the EAU 2023 guidelines, antimuscarinics and the β3 agonist mirabegron are recommended with strong evidence in cases where conservative treatments are inadequate.

Antimuscarinic Drugs

Antimuscarinic drugs currently form the basis of OAB treatment. Darifenacin, fesoterodine, oxybutynin, propiverine, solifenacin, tolterodine, and trospium are the main agents that could be chosen for antimuscarinic treatment. In a systematic review of 12 studies, all these antimuscarinic agents were shown to be more effective than placebo in terms of improving the mean symptom score on OAB—reducing frequency, urgency, and UUI episodes and increasing functional bladder capacity in the short term. All the antimuscarinic agents were found to cause significantly higher rates of adverse effects, such as dry mouth, cognitive impairment, UTI, and constipation, than placebo [33]. In terms of cure or improvement, none of the agents was found to be superior, and no single agent improved QoL more than another [5].

According to the AUA/SUFU 2024 guidelines, clinicians should counsel patients on the side effects (dry mouth, constipation, cognitive effects such as dementia and cognitive impairment and visual impairment) of all oral medication options, and treatment should be chosen based on side effect profiles and in the context of shared decision-making. In patients who have narrow-angle glaucoma or impaired gastric emptying, extreme caution should be taken, and the patients should be referred to the relevant departments before initiating treatment. For all patients being assessed for LUTD, it is recommended to measure PVR before the treatment. Antimuscarinics are not advised to be used in elderly patients who have mobility impairment and decreased cognitive functions. Therefore, methods other than pharmacological treatment should be preferred in older-age-group patients.

If an antimuscarinic is to be started, it should be started at a low dose due to the undesirable effects specific to this age group, and the treatment should be continued with slow titration, observing the balance of symptoms and undesirable effects. After the treatment is started, the physician should carefully monitor whether there is a change in mental status throughout the treatment process.

Considering the chronic nature of OAB, adherence to treatment is of great importance. However, a high discontinuation rate is reported (62–77.2% at 12 months and 87–92% at 36 months) in several studies [34]. Factors associated with low adherence are mainly identified as low levels of efficacy, adverse events, and costs. Although immediate-release antimuscarinic preparations provide maximum dosage flexibility, they have a greater risk of adverse effects than extended-release forms. Thus, extended-release formulations should be prescribed where possible to increase adherence to treatment. Alternative formulations, such as transdermal oxybutynin, which is superior to oral formulations in terms of dry mouth, can also be considered.

Clinicians are encouraged to conduct early reviews of patients who have initiated pharmacotherapy for efficacy and side effects by the AUA/SUFU 2024 and EAU 2023 guidelines. If the patient experiences insufficient symptom control and/or unacceptable adverse effects, dose modification, using an alternative antimuscarinic agent, or the use of mirabegron (alone or in combination) can be tried [5, 35].

Beta-3 Agonists

Beta-3 adrenoceptors are the predominant beta receptors expressed on the detrusor smooth muscle, and stimulation of these receptors induces detrusor smooth muscle relaxation [36]. Mirabegron is the first and the most common beta-3 agonist agent used in the treatment of OAB.

In several phase III trials and Systematic Reviews (SRs), 25-mg, 50-mg, and 100-mg doses of mirabegron are shown to be more effective than placebo in terms of reducing micturition frequency, urge incontinence, and urgency episodes and improving the mean voided volume. As for the adverse effects, the incidence of dry mouth, which is the most prevalent and bothersome adverse effect of antimuscarinic agents, is similar to placebo [37, 38]. The most common adverse effects of mirabegron are hypertension (7.3%), nasopharyngitis (3.4%), and UTI (3%); thus, caution should be taken before prescribing mirabegron to patients with uncontrolled hypertension.

In a systematic review including 21 studies, the use of mirabegron for 12 weeks resulted in a reduction in all OAB symptoms, but no significant difference was shown between mirabegron and antimuscarinic agents in terms of efficacy, except that mirabegron has been shown to be more effective than antimuscarinic agents in terms of reducing nocturia episodes [39]. In the AUA/SUFU 2024 and EAU 2023 guidelines, clinicians are advised to offer either antimuscarinic agents or beta-3 agonists to improve OAB symptoms. It is also advised to offer beta-3 agonists as an additional therapy to those who are inadequately treated with antimuscarinic agents. While recommending medical therapies, the clinicians should choose the agent by considering the patient's medical history and comorbidities and individualize the regimen.

4.5.1.1.4 Surgical Management

Onabotulinumtoxin A

Intravesical injection of onabotulinumtoxinA (onabotA; BOTOX (BTX)) 100U is licensed for the treatment of persistent and refractory OAB/UUI in adults of both sexes. In multiple RCTs and SRs, intravesical BTX injection has been shown to be superior in curing and improving all components of OAB and HRQOL when compared to placebo in both short-term and long-term use. When compared to antimuscarinic agents, BTX has been shown to be significantly more effective in curing UUI, but no significant difference was found in the reduction of mean UUI episodes [31, 40, 41].

The most significant adverse effects of BTX injection are a two-to-three times increased risk of UTI and a six-to-eight times increased risk of urinary retention, which may result in the need for clean intermittent self-catheterization (CISC) when compared to placebo. Thus, all patients must be informed about the potential risks and must be taught CISC before the injection.

The effect of each injection diminishes between 5 and 9 months, which causes the need for repeated injections. The median time to request repeat injection is reported as 24 weeks, yet repeated injections generally result in consistent or increasing duration for subsequent injections, with a median of 7.6 months. Despite BOTOX injections being efficient in both short- and long-term use, discontinuation rates are considerably high. In a study in which 268 patients were followed over a period of 7 years, almost two-thirds of patients (61.3%) discontinued the intravesical therapy, mainly due to tolerability issues, including UTI and the need for CISC [42].

In both the EAU 2023 guidelines and the AUA/SUFU 2024 guidelines, intravesical injection of onabotulinumtoxin A is recommended for patients who are refractory to conservative or medical therapies or who are intolerant to the adverse effects of medical treatment. Clinicians are advised to measure PVR before starting the treatment and inform the patients about the limited duration of BTX, the increased risk of UTI, and the possible need for CISC.

Sacral Neuromodulation/Sacral Nerve Stimulation

Sacral neuromodulation (SNM), or sacral nerve stimulation (SNS), involves the implantation of stimulating electrodes adjoining the sacral nerve roots through the sacral foramina of typically S3. The electrodes stimulate the nerve, and the stimulation results in the modulation of neural activity and the stabilization of the bladder's electrical activity. In the first session of this technique (test stimulation), which is applied in two sessions in most centers, a temporary wire electrode is placed percutaneously under fluoroscopic control in the foramen along the sacral nerve. Those who have a ≥50% improvement in OAB symptoms during the test period are considered candidates for a permanent device [43].

SNM is an FDA-approved surgical treatment that is shown to be effective in refractory OAB. In a prospective study that compared SNM vs. medical treatment, therapeutic success (which is defined as an improvement of 50% or above in OAB symptoms in this study) was significantly higher in the SNM group (76%) than the standard medical therapy group (49%). Similarly, improvement in QoL was significantly greater in the SNM group (86%) than in the medical treatment group (44%). Similar rates of adverse effects were reported as 30% and 27% in the SNM and antimuscarinic groups, respectively. SNM was associated with higher rates of UTIs and implant site infection, and lead migration occurred in 3.4% of cases each [44].

In The Refractory Overactive Bladder: Sacral NEuromodulation vs. BoTulinum Toxin Assessment (ROSETTA) trial, which involved 386 female patients who had refractory OAB and were randomized to be treated with either onabotulinumtoxinA (BTX) or SNM, no statistically significant difference was found between the two interventions in terms of improving OAB symptoms, and both interventions were found to be efficient. Higher satisfaction was reported in the BTX group, but recurrent UTIs were also higher in the BTX (24% vs. 10%) group, and clean intermittent catheterization after the second injection was needed in 6% of the patients. On the other hand, for the SNM group, revision and removals were needed in 3% and 9% of the patients, respectively [45].

Both EAU 2023 guidelines and AUA/SUFU 2024 guidelines recommend offering sacral nerve stimulation to patients who have OAB/UUI refractory to anticholinergic therapy and/or who experience intolerable side effects due to pharmacotherapy.

4.5.2 Stress Urinary Incontinence (SUI)

By the ICS definition, stress urinary incontinence is defined as a complaint of involuntary loss of urine on effort or physical exertion, including sporting activities, or on sneezing or coughing [18]. Stress incontinence is the most frequent incontinence in women and has been reported by 6.4% of women aged ≥18 years. The prevalence has a peak between 45 and 59 years of age. Stress incontinence is more common in women and is associated with pregnancy, childbirth, constipation, and obesity.

Diagnostic evaluation of SUI includes a detailed history; physical examination, including a standardized cough stress test; and urinalysis. The use of appropriate questionnaires, bladder diaries, and PVR should be included in the standard evaluation. Pad testing is recommended to evaluate the presence and severity of SUI. Urodynamics and imaging are not included in the routine assessment, but both can be used before any surgical interventions or in patients with complicated SUI [5].

The treatment of SUI mainly consists of conservative and surgical management.

4.5.2.1 Conservative Management of SUI

Weight loss and pelvic floor muscle training form the basis of conservative management of SUI. Being overweight or obese is associated with an increased risk of LUTS and SUI. There are several SRs and RCTs that have concluded that weight loss in the overweight population is beneficial in terms of improving UI [23, 46, 47]. In a prospective study, in which 160 women who underwent bariatric surgery were evaluated, surgically induced weight loss was associated with a significant improvement in pelvic floor disorders, including UI, and pelvic organ prolapse [48].

Since both nonsurgical and surgical weight loss improve SUI in obese women, clinicians are advised to encourage overweight patients with SUI to lose weight to improve SUI symptoms.

As mentioned previously in the conservative management of OAB, pelvic floor muscle training forms an essential part of the management of UI. The exercises briefly improve the function and morphology of the pelvic floor and the urethral stability by increasing the PFM strength and volume, lifting the bladder neck and rectum, and increasing the urethral closure pressure [49, 50]. PFMT is a useful method both in preventing and curing SUI.

In a systematic review of 31 trials, women with SUI who were assessed at the end of active PFMT were eight times more likely to report a cure and six times more likely to report a cure or improvement when compared to no treatment and inactive control treatment groups. The study showed significant improvement in QoL due to incontinence and reduced leakage episodes in pad tests in the active PFMT group [51].

The National Institute for Health and Care Excellence (NICE) 2019 guidelines state that PFMT is just as effective as surgery for about half of the women with SUI [52]. Therefore, considering the noninvasive nature and the efficacy of PFMT, both the NICE and EAU guidelines recommend at least 3 months of supervised PFMT as the first-line treatment for SUI and MUI, and both guidelines recommend ensuring that the PFMT is as intensive as possible [5, 51].

4.5.2.2 Surgical Treatment of SUI

4.5.2.2.1 Burch Colposuspension (Open/Laparoscopic/Robotic-Assisted)

Burch colposuspension was considered to be the gold standard surgical treatment method for SUI for a long time, and it is still of value when compared with newer, less invasive methods [53]. The general principle of this surgery is to suspend the bladder neck and proximal part of the urethra to maintain its high retropubic position. By doing so, pressure around the urethra, as well as the length of the functional urethra, is increased [54]. Therefore, incontinence resulting from the lack of urethral resistance is significantly overcome. Suspension is performed in a retropubic fashion. Sutures that provide tension are put on both sides of the bladder neck and then tied with Cooper ligaments on each side. The method was finalized by John Christopher Burch in 1961 and was defined as an open surgery [55]. Regarding the advancements in minimally invasive surgical techniques, laparoscopic and robotic-assisted methods are getting more popular. Outcomes are slightly in favor of the open technique, in which 70% of the patients are expected to be continent in 5 years after the surgery [56]. Complications, such as bladder or urethral injury, are found to be higher in the laparoscopic approach, but there is no significant difference in the presentation of de

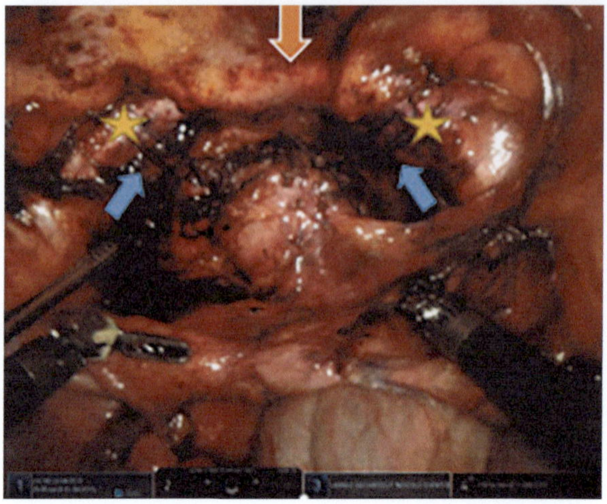

Fig. 4.5 Robotic-assisted Burch colposuspension. Sutures (blue arrows) are placed through the periurethral and paravaginal tissues to elevate and support the bladder neck. These sutures are anchored to the Cooper's ligament (yellow stars) or the pubic periosteum (orange arrow), which is located near the pubic symphysis

novo incontinence compared with other surgical techniques for SUI (Fig. 4.5).

4.5.2.2.2 Mid-urethral Sling

Mid-urethral slings (MUSs) occupy a significant role in the surgical management of SUI. Multiple subtypes of this procedure have been defined throughout the years. However, the main goal is similar: supporting the urethra ventrally in a strap-like fashion to increase resistance, thus improving the continence status of the patient. Surgical methods are divided in terms of approaching routes to the urethra (retropubic/transobturator) and the material that is functioning as the strap *(synthetic/autologous)*. There are various types of synthetic materials that are used (polypropylene, polyester, polyethylene terephthalate (PET), and polyvinylidene fluoride (PVDF)). Polypropylene is the most used type, and its effectiveness is shown to be the highest compared to other types. Erosion and infections are the most common types of complications in synthetic sling procedures, and there is no significant difference between the materials that are used. In recent years, the use of synthetic materials is strongly discouraged in European countries, such as the United Kingdom, which banned their use in 2018. Studies showed that a considerable number of patients are suffering from a variety of postoperative complications, as explained above [57]. This novel insight has increased the use of autologous tissues such as rectus sheath or fascia lata grafts. Effectiveness and patient satisfaction of autologous sling turned out to be better compared to retropubic MUS, Transobturator Tape (TOT), and open colposuspension [58] (Fig. 4.6).

4.5.2.2.3 Urethral Bulking Agents

In terms of surgical complications, urethral bulking agents are considered to be the safest. Therefore, their use in clinical practice is getting more frequent, even though the efficacy of treatment is questionable compared to other surgical methods explained above [59]. This minimally invasive method aims to form artificial cushion-like bulks in submucosal or periurethral tissues, resulting in increased urethral resistance. Various types of biocompatible polymers have been manufactured, one example being a 2.5% cross-linked polyacrylamide and 97.5% non-pyrogenic water combination (*Bulkamid®*).

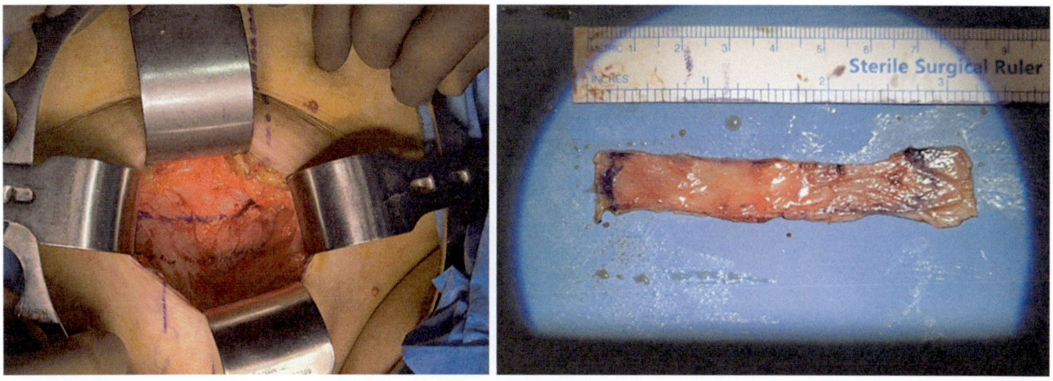

Fig. 4.6 The harvesting of the rectus fascia (in the left photo) by a horizontal incision above the pubic hairline for the autologous sling procedure. The fascia is carefully dissected and harvested, ensuring that the tissue is healthy and strong to provide adequate support. After harvesting, the fascia is processed to remove any excess fat or tissue and create a uniform, flat strip suitable for use as a sling (in the right photo)

Injection is applied at the proximal urethra corresponding to the 1-cm distal part of the bladder neck. Injection sites are 3, 6, and 9 o'clock, and the injection is performed in a submucosal fashion. Each injection consists of 0.5 mL of *Bulkamid®*, resulting in 1–2 mL of material at the urethral wall in total [60]. When compared to other surgical methods, efficacy duration is short-lived in bulk injections, resulting in the need for recurrent applications. In terms of complications, urinary tract infections are observed most frequently (Fig 4.7).

4.5.2.2.4 Artificial Urinary Sphincter

Patients suffering from failed previous surgeries are ideal candidates for external compression devices such as artificial urinary sphincters. The advantageous part of this procedure is that patients are in total control of their voiding routines. An artificial refillable cuff prosthesis is placed around the urethra through a perineal approach. This cuff is connected to a pump that is placed inside the labia and connected to a reservoir that is located in the anterior abdominal wall. The reservoir contains fluid that is required for cuff activation. The

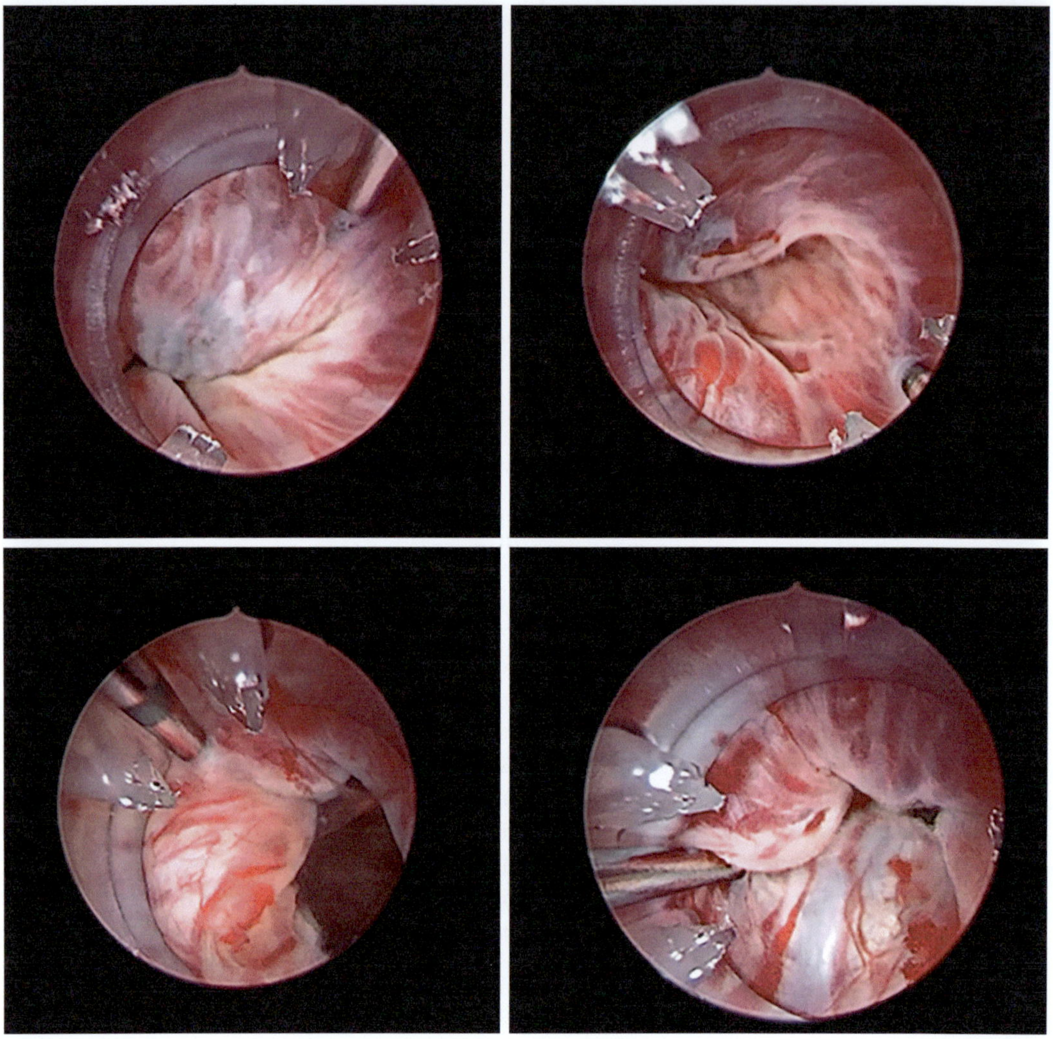

Fig. 4.7 Bulkamid injection. Injection is applied at the proximal urethra corresponding to the 1-cm distal part of the bladder neck at 3,6, and 9 o'clock. Each injection consists of 0.5 mL of *Bulkamid®*, resulting in 1–2 mL of material at the urethral wall in total. Bulking is visible at the urethra at the end of each injection

patient deactivates the cuff via the pump and, after micturition, reactivates the cuff, making it almost identical to normal voiding physiology. Success rates of this procedure are up to 60–100%; however, the complicated nature of its connectable parts makes this system prone to mechanical failures, which can be seen up to 44%, as reported in several systematic reviews [61].

4.6 Conclusion

LUTDs are common in women, and their effective management is crucial for improving their overall health and quality of life. These disorders are significant for several reasons, including their prevalence, impact on quality of life, and potential for underlying health issues. Awareness, appropriate diagnosis, and effective treatment options are essential for managing these conditions. Recognizing the significance of LUTDs can lead to better education, research, and clinical practices, ultimately benefiting women's health.

References

1. D'Ancona C, Haylen B, Oelke M, Abranches-Monteiro L, Arnold E, Goldman H, Hamid R, Homma Y, Marcelissen T, Rademakers K, Schizas A, Singla A, Soto I, Tse V, de Wachter S, Herschorn S. The International Continence Society (ICS) report on the terminology for adult male lower urinary tract and pelvic floor symptoms and dysfunction. Neurourol Urodyn. 2019;38(2):433–77. https://doi.org/10.1002/nau.23897.
2. Coyne KS, Wein AJ, Tubaro A, Sexton CC, Thompson CL, Kopp ZS, Aiyer LP. The burden of lower urinary tract symptoms: evaluating the effect of LUTS on health-related quality of life, anxiety and depression: EpiLUTS. BJU Int. 2009;103(Suppl 3):4–11. https://doi.org/10.1111/j.1464-410X.2009.08371.x.
3. Irwin DE, Milsom I, Hunskaar S, Reilly K, Kopp Z, Herschorn S, Coyne K, Kelleher C, Hampel C, Artibani W, Abrams P. Population-based survey of urinary incontinence, overactive bladder, and other lower urinary tract symptoms in five countries: results of the EPIC study. Eur Urol. 2006;50(6):1306–14. https://doi.org/10.1016/j.eururo.2006.09.019.
4. Coyne KS, Sexton CC, Thompson CL, Milsom I, Irwin D, Kopp ZS, Chapple CR, Kaplan S, Tubaro A, Aiyer LP, Wein AJ. The prevalence of lower urinary tract symptoms (LUTS) in the USA, the UK and Sweden: results from the epidemiology of LUTS (EpiLUTS) study. BJU Int. 2009;104(3):352–60. https://doi.org/10.1111/j.1464-410X.2009.08427.x.
5. EAU Guidelines. Presented at the EAU annual congress, Paris; 2024. ISBN 978-94-92671-23-3.
6. Haylen BT, de Ridder D, Freeman RM, Swift SE, Berghmans B, Lee J, Monga A, Petri E, Rizk DE, Sand PK, Schaer GN. An International Urogynecological Association (IUGA)/International Continence Society (ICS) joint report on the terminology for female pelvic floor dysfunction. Int Urogynecol J. 2010;21(1):5–26. https://doi.org/10.1007/s00192-009-0976-9.
7. Partin AW, editors. Campbell-walsh-wein urology 12th ed. Volume 3, part XIII: urine transport, storage, and emptying, section 112: evaluation and management of women with urinary incontinence and pelvic prolapse; 2024. p. 11551 [E-book].
8. Graham CW, Dmochowski RR. Questionnaires for women with urinary symptoms. Neurourol Urodyn. 2002;21(5):473–81. https://doi.org/10.1002/nau.10015.
9. Franco AV, Lee F, Fynes MM. Is there an alternative to pad tests? Correlation of subjective variables of severity of urinary loss to the 1-h pad test in women with stress urinary incontinence. BJU Int. 2008;102(5):586–90. https://doi.org/10.1111/j.1464-410X.2008.07612.x.
10. Karantanis E, Fynes M, Moore KH, Stanton SL. Comparison of the ICIQ-SF and 24-hour pad test with other measures for evaluating the severity of urodynamic stress incontinence. Int Urogynecol J Pelvic Floor Dysfunct. 2004;15(2):111–6. https://doi.org/10.1007/s00192-004-1123-2.
11. International Continence Society. n.d.. ICIQ-FLUTS. Retrieved 21 Dec 2024, from https://iciq.net/iciq-fluts.
12. Partin AW, editors. Campbell-walsh-wein urology (12th ed.). Volume 3, part xiii: urine transport, storage, and emptying, section 112: evaluation and management of women with urinary incontinence and pelvic prolapse, p. 11553; 2024 [E-book].
13. Stav K, Dwyer PL, Rosamilia A. Women overestimate daytime urinary frequency: the importance of the bladder diary. J Urol. 2009;181(5):2176–80. https://doi.org/10.1016/j.juro.2009.01.042.
14. Ku JH, Hong SK, Kim HH, Paick JS, Lee SE, Oh SJ. Is questionnaire enough to assess number of nocturic episodes? Prospective comparative study between data from questionnaire and frequency-volume charts. Urology. 2004;64(5):966–9. https://doi.org/10.1016/j.urology.2004.06.027.
15. Staskin D, Kelleher C, Bosch R, Coyne K, Cotteril N, Emmanuel A, Yoshida M, Kopp Z. Initial assessment of urinary and faecal incontinence in adult male and female patients. In: Abrams P, Cardozo L, Khoury S, Wein A, editors. Incontinence. 4th ed. Birmingham: Health Publications Ltd.; 2009. p. 333–412.
16. Medeiros Araujo C, de Morais NR, Sacomori C, de Sousa Dantas D. Pad test for urinary incontinence diagnosis in adults: systematic review of diagnostic test accuracy. Neurourol Urodyn. 2022;41(3):696–709. https://doi.org/10.1002/nau.24878.
17. Kobashi KC, Vasavada S, Bloschichak A, et al. Updates to surgical treatment of female stress urinary incontinence (SUI): AUA/SUFU guideline. J Urol. 2023;209(6):1091–8.
18. Partin AW, editor. Campbell-walsh-wein urology (12th ed.), volume 3, part XIII: urine transport, storage, and emptying, section 114: urodynamic and video-urodynamic evaluation of the lower urinary tract, p. 11645; 2024 [E-book].
19. Clement KD, Lapitan MC, Omar MI, Glazener CM. Urodynamic studies for management of urinary incontinence in children and adults. Cochrane Database Syst Rev. 2013;2013(10):CD003195. https://doi.org/10.1002/14651858.CD003195.pub3.
20. The International Continence Society (ICS). The ICS report on the terminology for adult male lower urinary tract and pelvic floor symptoms and dysfunction. Neurourol Urodyn. 2019;38(2):433–77. https://doi.org/10.1002/nau.23897.

21. Milsom I, Kaplan SA, Coyne KS, Sexton CC, Kopp ZS. Effect of bothersome overactive bladder symptoms on health-related quality of life, anxiety, depression, and treatment seeking in the United States: results from EpiLUTS. Urology. 2012;80(1):90–6. https://doi.org/10.1016/j.urology.2012.04.004.
22. Maughan RJ, Griffin J. Caffeine ingestion and fluid balance: a review. J Hum Nutr Diet. 2003;16(6):411–20. https://doi.org/10.1046/j.1365-277x.2003.00477.x.
23. Le Berre M, Presse N, Morin M, Larouche M, Campeau L, Hu YX, Reid I, Dumoulin C. What do we really know about the role of caffeine on urinary tract symptoms? A scoping review on caffeine consumption and lower urinary tract symptoms in adults. Neurourol Urodyn. 2020;39(5):1217–33. https://doi.org/10.1002/nau.24344.
24. Hashim H, Abrams P. How should patients with an overactive bladder manipulate their fluid intake? BJU Int. 2008;102(1):62–6. https://doi.org/10.1111/j.1464-410X.2008.07463.x.
25. Subak LL, Wing R, West DS, Franklin F, Vittinghoff E, Creasman JM, Richter HE, Myers D, Burgio KL, Gorin AA, Macer J, Kusek JW, Grady D, Investigators PRIDE. Weight loss to treat urinary incontinence in overweight and obese women. N Engl J Med. 2009;360(5):481–90. https://doi.org/10.1056/NEJMoa0806375.
26. Hannestad YS, Rortveit G, Daltveit AK, Hunskaar S. Are smoking and other lifestyle factors associated with female urinary incontinence? The Norwegian EPINCONT study. BJOG Int J Obstet Gynaecol. 2003;110(3):247–54.
27. Cameron AP, Chung DE, Dielubanza EJ, et al. The AUA/SUFU guideline on the diagnosis and treatment of idiopathic overactive bladder. J Urol. 2024; https://doi.org/10.1097/JU.0000000000003985.
28. Ostaszkiewicz J, Johnston L, Roe B. Timed voiding for the management of urinary incontinence in adults. Cochrane Database Syst Rev. 2004;2004(1):CD002802. https://doi.org/10.1002/14651858.CD002802.pub2.
29. Partin AW, editor. Campbell-Walsh-Wein urology (12th ed.), volume 3, part XIII: urine transport, storage, and emptying, section 121: conservative management of urinary incontinence, p. 12562; 2024 [E-book].
30. Dumoulin C, Adewuyi T, Booth J, et al. Adult conservative management. In: Abrams P, Cardozo L, Wagg A, et al., editors. Incontinence, 6th International Consultation on Incontinence. Bristol: International Continence Society; 2017. p. 1443–628.
31. Partin AW, editor. Campbell-Walsh-Wein urology (12th ed.), volume 3, part XIII: urine transport, storage, and emptying, section 121: conservative management of urinary incontinence, p. 12531; 2024 [E-book].
32. Bo K, Fernandes ACNL, Duarte TB, Brito LGO, Ferreira CHJ. Is pelvic floor muscle training effective for symptoms of overactive bladder in women? A systematic review. Physiotherapy. 2020;106:65–76. https://doi.org/10.1016/j.physio.2019.08.011.
33. Farag F, Sakalis VI, Arteaga SM, Sihra N, Karavitakis M, Arlandis S, Bø K, Cobussen-Boekhorst H, Costantini E, de Heide M, Groen J, Peyronnet B, Phé V, van Poelgeest-Pomfret ML, van den Bos TWL, van der Vaart H, Harding CK, Lapitan MC, Omar IM, Nambiar AK. What are the short-term benefits and potential harms of therapeutic modalities for the management of overactive bladder syndrome in women? A review of evidence under the auspices of the European Association of Urology, Female Non-neurogenic Lower Urinary Tract Symptoms Guidelines Panel. Eur Urol. 2023;84(3):302–12. https://doi.org/10.1016/j.eururo.2023.05.014.
34. Kalder M, Pantazis K, Dinas K, Albert US, Heilmaier C, Kostev K. Discontinuation of treatment using anticholinergic medications in patients with urinary incontinence. Obstet Gynecol. 2014;124(4):794–800. https://doi.org/10.1097/AOG.0000000000000468.
35. Partin AW, editor. Campbell-walsh-wein urology (12th ed.), volume 3, part XIII: urine transport, storage, and emptying, section 117: overactive bladder, p. 12070; 2024 [E-book].
36. Frazier EP, Peters SL, Braverman AS, Ruggieri MR Sr, Michel MC. Signal transduction underlying the control of urinary bladder smooth muscle tone by muscarinic receptors and beta-adrenoceptors. Naunyn Schmiedeberg's Arch Pharmacol. 2008;377(4-6):449–62. https://doi.org/10.1007/s00210-007-0208-0.
37. Chapple CR, Cardozo L, Nitti VW, Siddiqui E, Michel MC. Mirabegron in overactive bladder: a review of efficacy, safety, and tolerability. Neurourol Urodyn. 2014;33(1):17–30. https://doi.org/10.1002/nau.22505.
38. Cui Y, Zong H, Yang C, Yan H, Zhang Y. The efficacy and safety of mirabegron in treating OAB: a systematic review and meta-analysis of phase III trials. Int Urol Nephrol. 2014;46(1):275–84. https://doi.org/10.1007/s11255-013-0509-9.
39. Athanasiou S, Pitsouni E, Grigoriadis T, Zacharakis D, Salvatore S, Serati M. Mirabegron in female patients with overactive bladder syndrome: what's new? A systematic review and meta-analysis. Eur J Obstet Gynecol Reprod Biol. 2020;251:73–82. https://doi.org/10.1016/j.ejogrb.2020.05.018.
40. Chapple C, Sievert KD, MacDiarmid S, Khullar V, Radziszewski P, Nardo C, Thompson C, Zhou J, Haag-Molkenteller C. OnabotulinumtoxinA 100 U significantly improves all idiopathic overactive bladder symptoms and quality of life in patients with overactive bladder and urinary incontinence: a randomised, double-blind, placebo-controlled trial. Eur Urol. 2013;64(2):249–56. https://doi.org/10.1016/j.eururo.2013.04.001.
41. Duthie JB, Vincent M, Herbison GP, Wilson DI, Wilson D. Botulinum toxin injections for adults with overactive bladder syndrome. Cochrane Database Syst Rev. 2011;12:CD005493. https://doi.org/10.1002/14651858.CD005493.pub3.

42. Mohee A, Khan A, Harris N, Eardley I. Long-term outcome of the use of intravesical botulinum toxin for the treatment of overactive bladder (OAB). BJU Int. 2013;111(1):106–13. https://doi.org/10.1111/j.1464-410X.2012.11282.x.
43. Jairam R, Drossaerts J, Marcelissen T, van Koeveringe G, Vrijens D, van Kerrebroeck P. Predictive factors in sacral neuromodulation: a systematic review. Urolog Int. 2022;106(4):323–43. https://doi.org/10.1159/000513937.
44. Siegel S, Noblett K, Mangel J, Griebling TL, Sutherland SE, Bird ET, Comiter C, Culkin D, Bennett J, Zylstra S, Berg KC, Kan F, Irwin CP. Results of a prospective, randomized, multicenter study evaluating sacral neuromodulation with InterStim therapy compared to standard medical therapy at 6-months in subjects with mild symptoms of overactive bladder. Neurourol Urodyn. 2015;34(3):224–30. https://doi.org/10.1002/nau.22544.
45. Amundsen CL, Komesu YM, Chermansky C, Gregory WT, Myers DL, Honeycutt EF, Vasavada SP, Nguyen JN, Wilson TS, Harvie HS, Wallace D, Network PFD. Two-year outcomes of sacral neuromodulation versus onabotulinumtoxinA for refractory urgency urinary incontinence: a randomized trial. Eur Urol. 2018;74(1):66–73. https://doi.org/10.1016/j.eururo.2018.02.011.
46. Gozukara YM, Akalan G, Tok EC, Aytan H, Ertunc D. The improvement in pelvic floor symptoms with weight loss in obese women does not correlate with the changes in pelvic anatomy. Int Urogynecol J. 2014;25(9):1219–25. https://doi.org/10.1007/s00192-014-2368-z.
47. Wing RR, Creasman JM, West DS, Richter HE, Myers D, Burgio KL, Franklin F, Gorin AA, Vittinghoff E, Macer J, Kusek JW, Subak LL. Improving urinary incontinence in overweight and obese women through modest weight loss. Obstet Gynecol. 2010;116(2 Pt 1):284–92. https://doi.org/10.1097/AOG.0b013e3181e8fb60.
48. Leshem A, Shimonov M, Amir H, Gordon D, Groutz A. Effects of bariatric surgery on female pelvic floor disorders. Urology. 2017;105:42–7. https://doi.org/10.1016/j.urology.2017.03.003.
49. Zubieta M, Carr RL, Drake MJ, Bø K. Influence of voluntary pelvic floor muscle contraction and pelvic floor muscle training on urethral closure pressures: a systematic literature review. Int Urogynecol J. 2016;27(5):687–96. https://doi.org/10.1007/s00192-015-2856-9.
50. Hoff Brækken I, Majida M, Engh ME, Bø K. Morphological changes after pelvic floor muscle training measured by 3-dimensional ultrasonography: a randomized controlled trial. Obstet Gynecol. 2010;115(2 Pt 1):317–24. https://doi.org/10.1097/AOG.0b013e3181cbd35f.
51. Dumoulin C, Cacciari LP, Hay-Smith EJC. Pelvic floor muscle training versus no treatment, or inactive control treatments, for urinary incontinence in women. Cochrane Database Syst Rev. 2018;2018(10):CD005654. https://doi.org/10.1002/14651858.CD005654.pub4.
52. Guidance NICE. Urinary incontinence and pelvic organ prolapse in women: management. BJU Int. 2019;123:777–803.
53. Veit-Rubin N, Dubuisson J, Ford A, Dubuisson JB, Mourad S, Digesu A. Burch colposuspension. Neurourol Urodyn. 2019;38(2):553–62. https://doi.org/10.1002/nau.23905.
54. Riss P, Ralph G. Die abdominale Kolposuspension–Der Goldstandard in der Inkontinenztherapie? [Abdominal colposuspension–the gold standard in incontinence therapy?]. Geburtshilfe Frauenheilkd. 1994;54(2):69–74. https://doi.org/10.1055/s-2007-1023555.
55. Burch JC. Urethrovaginal fixation to Cooper's ligament for correction of stress incontinence, cystocele, and prolapse. Am J Obstet Gynecol. 1961;81:281–90. https://doi.org/10.1016/s0002-9378(16)36367-0.
56. Lapitan MC, Cody JD. Open retropubic colposuspension for urinary incontinence in women. Cochrane Database Syst Rev. 2016;2:CD002912. https://doi.org/10.1002/14651858.CD002912.pub6.
57. Cumberlege J. First do no harm: The report of the Independent Medicines and Medical Devices Safety Review. Department of Health and Social; 2020.
58. Brubaker L, Richter HE, Norton PA, Albo M, Zyczynski HM, Chai TC, Zimmern P, Kraus S, Sirls L, Kusek JW, Stoddard A, Tennstedt S, Gormley EA. 5-year continence rates, satisfaction, and adverse events of Burch urethropexy and fascial sling surgery for urinary incontinence. J Urol. 2012;187(4):1324–30. https://doi.org/10.1016/j.juro.2011.11.087.
59. Giammò A, Geretto P, Ammirati E, Manassero A, Squintone L, Vercelli D, Carone R. Urethral bulking with Bulkamid: an analysis of efficacy, safety profile, and predictors of functional outcomes in a single-center cohort. Neurourol Urodyn. 2020;39(5):1523–8. https://doi.org/10.1002/nau.24388.
60. Pai A, Al-Singary W. Durability, safety, and efficacy of polyacrylamide hydrogel (Bulkamid®) in the management of stress and mixed urinary incontinence: three-year follow-up outcomes. Cent Eur J Urol. 2015;68(4):428–33. https://doi.org/10.5173/ceju.2015.647.
61. Peyronnet B, O'Connor E, Khavari R, Capon G, Manunta A, Allue M, Hascoet J, Nitti VW, Gamé X, Gilleran J, Castro-Sader L, Cornu JN, Waltregny D, Ahyai S, Chung E, Elliott DS, Fournier G, Brucker BM. AMS-800 artificial urinary sphincter in female patients with stress urinary incontinence: a systematic review. Neurourol Urodyn. 2019;38(Suppl 4):S28–41. https://doi.org/10.1002/nau.23833.

Diagnosis and Treatment of Pelvic Organ Prolapse

5

Fazlı Demirtürk and Abdulgafur Alim Uçar

5.1 Introduction

Pelvic organ prolapse (POP) is defined as the downward or anterior displacement of one of the pelvic organs from its normal location and is also called urogenital prolapse. Pelvic organ prolapse (POP) is a gynecological problem that affects older women, has a very low mortality rate, causes genitourinary and gastrointestinal system symptoms, and also reduces the quality of life of women by affecting their daily activities. POP involves the prolapse of pelvic organs, such as the bladder, rectum, or uterus, into or outside the vaginal canal. Although the pathophysiology of POP is not fully understood, it is known to be a multifactorial problem in which genetic and environmental factors play a role. POP may be present with symptoms such as pain, pressure sensation, urinary and fecal incontinence, constipation, difficulty in micturition and/or defecation, and difficulty in coitus [1].

The incidence and prevalence of POP vary between 2% and 50%, depending on the type of definition and the differences in the population screened. In routine gynecological cases, POP due to the loss of uterovaginal support tissue is seen in more than 50% of women, while pelvic organ protrusion from the hymen increases with age and is seen between 2% and 12% [2].

Treatment of symptomatic POP is only possible with surgery. The rate of surgery due to POP and the symptoms it causes is given as 11% in the female population. One third of them are candidates for reoperation [3]. The goals of reconstructive surgery in a vaginal vault or uterine prolapse (Fig. 5.1) are to relieve symptoms, reconstruct the anatomy, preserve vaginal capacity for sexual function, and prevent recurrent prolapse. Many operations have been described for the treatment of vaginal vault and uterine prolapse, including both vaginal and abdominal approaches. As a result, an ideal method with high success and low complication rates has not been determined in uterovaginal prolapse surgery [4].

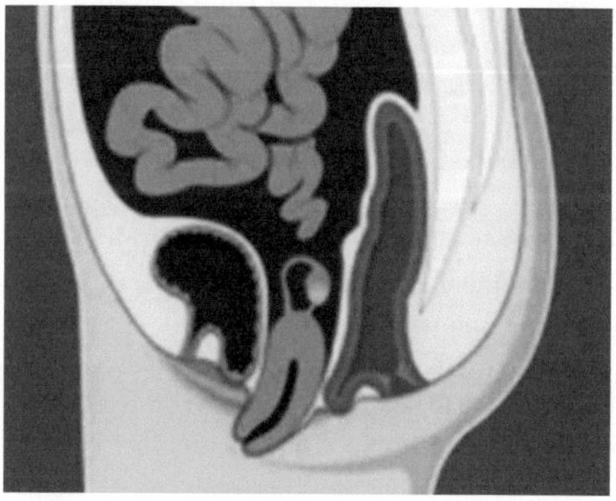

Fig. 5.1 Uterine prolapsus

F. Demirtürk (✉) · A. A. Uçar
Department of Obstetrics and Gynecology, Faculty of Medicine,, Tokat Gaziosmanpaşa University, Tokat, Türkiye

T. Akbayrak, E. Üzelpasaci (eds.), *Physiotherapy and Rehabilitation in Pelvic and Women's Health-Related Problems*, https://doi.org/10.1007/978-3-032-28741-0_5

5.2 Anatomy of the Pelvis

The vagina is a fibromuscular, tube-shaped space extending between the vestibule and the cervix uteri. In an upright woman, the lower one third of the vagina is vertical, while the upper two thirds is nearly horizontal. Normally, the anterior and posterior walls of the vagina are in contact with each other, except for the part held open by the cervix. Normal pelvic support is provided by the pelvic floor muscles and connective tissue connections. The pelvic muscles are essentially the primary support for the pelvic organs; they provide a solid but elastic base with a constant tone at rest. They also provide the ability to create extra contractions when desired, allowing continence and voluntary termination of urinary flow and defecation. The connective tissue (endopelvic fascia) stabilizes the pelvic organs in the correct position and provides optimum support. During relaxation of the pelvic muscles, such as during micturition and defecation, connective tissue connections temporarily suspend the pelvic organs [5].

The endopelvic fascia is a network of connective tissue that surrounds all the pelvic organs and loosely attaches them to the levator ani muscle and the pelvic bones. The peritoneum is located between the pelvic floor muscles and the pelvic organs. The endopelvic fascia consists of collagen, elastin, adipose tissue, a vascular network, and a small amount of smooth muscle. Its fibers blend with the muscular structure of the vagina and the perineal body below [6].

These connective tissue connections stabilize the vagina at three different levels. The first level corresponds to the uterosacral–cardinal ligament complex and provides the primary support for the upper one fourth of the vagina. This ligament complex supports the cervix and upper vagina while ensuring vaginal length and maintaining the upper vaginal axis close to horizontal. Thus, the vagina is held in a position resting on the rectum. There is no other support force to fix the uterus other than the uterosacral–cardinal ligament complex. This allows the uterus to grow without restriction throughout pregnancy [7].

The second level support is provided by the paravaginal connections formed by the endopelvic fascia of the vagina and laterally by the arcus tendineus fasciae pelvis (ATFP) and arcus tendineus rectovaginal. It provides support for the middle half of the vagina. The arcus tendineus fasciae pelvis (ATFP), or "white line," is a robust tendinous arch that begins behind the symphysis pubis and extends along the edge of the fascia of the obturator internus muscle to end at the ischial spine. The connection of the pubocervical fascia to the white line provides support for the lateral vaginal walls. Separation of the pubocervical fascia from this line leads to paravaginal defects. ATFP can be seen with the naked eye as a thickened borderline of the fascia covering the obturatorius internus muscle in the retropubic area with dissection. The part to which the levator ani muscle, which is related to this arch but ends more superiorly and laterally than the pubic bone, is attached is called the arcus tendineus levator ani. In the middle half of the vagina, the endopelvic tissue connections from the anterior lateral vaginal sulci to the ATFP and from the posterior lateral sulci to the arcus tendineus rectovaginal provide the basic support. The third level of support is provided by the perineal body, perineal membrane, superficial and deep perineal muscles, and endopelvic fascia and is responsible for the normal position of the lower one fourth of the vagina and the introitus. The perineal body is critical in protecting the genital hiatus and in anus function. Damage to the perineal body as a result of recurrent traumatic births causes perineal descent and defecation dysfunction [5–7].

5.3 Pathophysiology in Pelvic Organ Prolapse

When the vagina, bladder, and rectum are held in a horizontal plane by the levator plate and pelvic floor muscles, intra-abdominal pressure and pregnancy-related forces are applied perpendicularly to the vagina and pelvic floor, and the pelvic floor muscles respond to these forces with constant tone. With this correct position and appropriate tone, stress on the paravaginal connective tissue is minimized. During acute stress, such as coughing or sneezing, the pelvic floor muscles stabilize the organs through reflex contraction. Additionally, the genital hiatus is narrowed and provides level 3 support [8]. When the pelvic floor muscles become weak due to neuropathic damage or mechanical muscular damage, the endopelvic fascia and its connections become the primary mechanism for vaginal support. Over time, stress becomes dominant over the endopelvic fascial connections and causes loss of normal anatomy through tearing, stretching, or thinning. This leads to changes in the vector forces on the organs, causing pelvic organ prolapse and/or dysfunction [9].

In addition to the ventral suspension of the proximal urethra and bladder base by ligamentous structures, it is also supported by the anterior vagina, which connects to the ATFP laterally. The pubourethral ligament is already formed by the perineal membrane and is the most caudal part of the ATFP, which fixes the distal urethra just below the pubic bone. The anterolateral vaginal connections to the ATFP provide a fixed base for the bladder neck and proximal urethra. In these defects, loss of proximal urethral support (urethral hypermobility) and anterior prolapse (cystocele (Fig. 5.2)) occur, which are associated with stress urinary incontinence (SUI) [10].

The predisposing factors include genetic and racial characteristics. Factors that initiate prolapse are pregnancy, childbirth, hysterectomy, myopathy, and neuropathy. Precipitating factors are obesity, smoking, pulmonary disease, and constipation. Decompensating factors are aging, menopause, extreme thinness, and the use of certain medications [11]. Depending on the combination of risk factors in an individual, prolapse may or may not develop at any time in their life. According to American data, one in nine women undergoes surgery due to pelvic organ prolapse or stress incontinence, and 30% of these women undergo reoperation due to recurrent prolapse [12]. Changing modifiable risk factors (obesity, smoking, chronic constipation, etc.) can reduce the likelihood of developing prolapse. However, increased parity is a risk factor for prolapse, according to the data of the Women's Health Initiative [13]. Hendrix et al. [14] detected varying degrees of prolapse in almost one in five nulliparous women. These data contradict the approach of gynecologists who believe that cesarean delivery prevents prolapse. In light of this information, the goal of reconstructive surgery is to reestablish the proper positions and functions of the vaginal support connections and organs and provide vaginal length while preserving the apex [14].

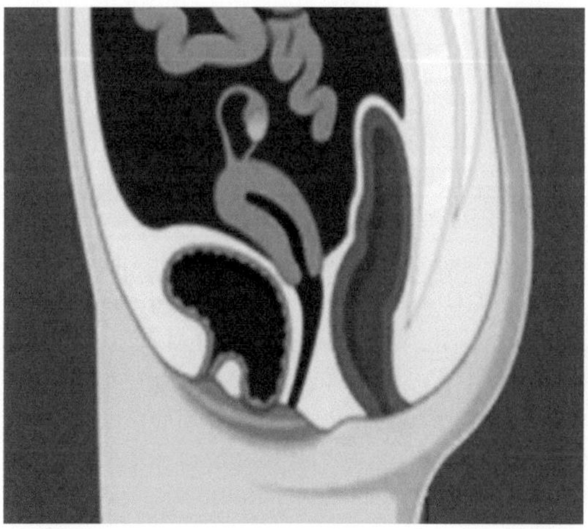

Fig. 5.2 Cystocele

5.4 Diagnosis of Pelvic Organ Prolapse

The primary methods for diagnosing POP are clinical examination and history [15]. The patient's symptoms related to POP and other bowel and urinary functions should be thoroughly documented in the medical history. It is desirable to evaluate risk variables and document the extent of patient disturbance from POP. Both systemic and local explorations (abdominal and pelvic inspections) should be part of the physical examination. Accurate evaluation requires pelvic examination, which includes examining the external genitalia, both at rest and during Valsalva, to examine each pelvic organ prolapse compartment specifically. Because it enables the standardization of analysis and recording of the various POP compartments, the POP-

Quantification (POP-Q) system is recommended. POP-Q provides necessary standardized measurements that can be compared before and after conservative and surgical treatments [16, 17]. To check for prolapse, the examination should be conducted with the bladder empty and the front and posterior vaginal walls retracted using a single-bladed speculum. During maximum Valsalva, six specific locations of the hymen are assessed to evaluate the anterior, posterior, and apical compartments. The genital hiatus, perineal body, and total vaginal length are three further descriptive measurements that are taken separately from the hymen. Total vaginal length is the only measurement that may be taken without Valsalva. Each compartment's prolapse is then categorized according to its relationship to the hymen. The full burden of the condition remains underestimated, even with the simple diagnosis and available treatment choices. The most sensitive symptom that POP patients report is the existence of a vaginal bulge that is visible or palpable at the vaginal opening. In some cases, the patients were asymptomatic, and the bulge was only discovered during pelvic examination; in other cases, the patients would frequently appear with additional overlapping symptoms, such as urinary or defecatory dysfunction. Both patients and their treating physicians face additional challenges as a result of this discrepancy between the symptoms and clinical assessment. Prolapse education is crucial, as is the creation of reliable screening instruments that can be applied to the general public. Chen et al. [18] constructed and validated an online predictor model in a recent study conducted in Austria. Before being used more widely, this model may need to be validated in various populations.

For the initial evaluation of a woman in the early stage of POP (stages I and II), a thorough history and physical examination are sufficient. An assessment of postvoid residual is advised for patients with more severe prolapse to identify voiding dysfunction. A discussion of management options, including surgery if necessary, is warranted if an examination reveals evidence of stress urinary incontinence (SUI). Suppose the patient is considering invasive treatment alternatives, such as surgery. In that case, urodynamic testing can help with counseling regarding the likelihood of SUI following treatment if the patient does not exhibit SUI during examination [19].

Imaging is not required for most patients. However, what imaging could show may be helpful for patients with recurrent POP and defecatory dysfunction. Perineal ultrasonography and dynamic magnetic resonance imaging are two imaging modalities that have been developed and suggested for assessing pelvic organ prolapse (POP). Both modalities are reserved for complex clinical situations and are not yet incorporated into standard clinical evaluation [20].

5.5 Surgical Methods

5.5.1 Anterior Wall Prolapse Repair Anterior Colporrhaphy

Anterior colporrhaphy involves the plication of the fibromuscular layer (pubocervical fascia) of the anterior vaginal wall in the midline. In this way, the endopelvic fascia that has been distended, thinned, or torn is repaired in the midline. Although it has been performed for over a century, few studies indicate that the procedure is successful. The anatomical cure rate varies between 30% and 97% [21]. Weber et al. [22] compared these two procedures in a prospective randomized study by applying "ultralateral plication," in which the dissection is advanced laterally to the pubic ramus and the standard plication. They reported a success rate of 30% (optimal anatomical cure—anterior wall at least 1 cm behind the hymen) after a mean follow-up of 23.3 months after standard anterior colporrhaphy. The success rates for tension-applied polyglactin 910 (absorbable) mesh and ultralateral plication were reported as 42% and 46%, respectively, but no statistically significant difference was found between these rates. In a randomized controlled study by Hiltunen et al. [23], the recurrence rate was lower in anterior colporrhaphy using polypropylene mesh compared to standard repair (6.7% vs. 38.5%; $p < 0.001$). The anatomical cure rate was higher in the polypropylene mesh group, and incontinence symptoms improved in both treatment groups. In mild stress incontinence and urethral hypermobility, bladder neck plication can also be performed during anterior colporrhaphy. However, the success rate after 1 year has been reported as 60%, which is considerably lower than that of Burch colposuspension and sling operations [24]. In women with significant stress incontinence or those at a high risk of developing postoperative de novo stress incontinence due to advanced prolapse, the postoperative success of transvaginal tape (TVT) placement with anterior repair (92%) is significantly higher than that of suburethral plication (56%; $p < 0.01$) [25]. Therefore, in patients with potential stress urinary incontinence, TVT or transobturator sling placement is recommended during anterior repair. Complications of anterior vaginal repair include hemorrhage, cystotomy, changes in bladder function, postoperative dyspareunia, and urethral obstruction. Lateral plication of the endopelvic fascia under the bladder trigone has been reported to cause urethral kinking [26].

5.5.2 Paravaginal Defect Repair

Although there may be many variations of paravaginal defect, it generally occurs when the paravaginal connections are separated from the arcus tendineus. It may also occur when the arcus tendineus is separated from the pelvic sidewall. Determining the presence of a paravaginal defect is very important in evaluating the patient. Performing colporrhaphy with standard anterior plication on such a patient will cause the lateral defect to grow by retracting it medially. Paravaginal defect repair is the reconstruction of the lateral defect formed by separating the lateral fascial connections. It can be performed abdominally, vaginally, or laparoscopically [27].

In the abdominal approach, the retropubic area is dissected with an open incision or laparoscopy, and the bladder and vagina are pushed medially to visualize the arcus tendineus fasciae pelvis on the pelvic sidewall. The dissection is advanced from the inferior part of the pubic bone to the spina ischiadica, and the ATFP can be seen along the thickened lower edge of the obturator fascia. The anterior lateral vaginal sulcus is identified with the help of the finger of the nondominant hand placed in the vagina, and the paravaginal tissue is fixed to the arcus tendineus with five to six nonabsorbable sutures. When the sutures are tied, it can be seen that the lateral vaginal sulcus is elevated. The basic procedure is the same in the repair of the paravaginal defect with the vaginal approach; it is necessary to expose the retropubic area by dissection from the inferior surface of the pubic bone to the spina ischiadica. A retractor is required to retract the bladder medially. After the arcus tendineus is identified by palpation and visualization, it is fixed to the separated pubocervical fascia with five to six sutures. The use of the Capio suture device (Microvasive Endoscopy, Natick, MA) in the vaginal approach may facilitate suture placement. When the cure rates are examined, the success rate in the transabdominal approach is reported as 90–95% [28] and in the transvaginal approach, as 80–85% [22, 29]. Although paravaginal defect repair is a safe and effective method, its success in correcting concurrent stress urinary incontinence is low. Mallipedi et al. [30] reported that urinary incontinence continued in 57% of the patients after a mean follow-up of 1.6 years after paravaginal repair and bladder neck plication in patients with anterior wall prolapse and stress incontinence.

5.5.3 Graft Use

Approximately 30% of surgical treatments for pelvic organ prolapse are performed due to recurrence. Although there is no standard surgical method for approaching these patients, surgeons often use mesh to achieve better results. Some operators even prefer to use mesh during primary repair due to low recurrence rates. Anatomical results are encouraging with the use of nonabsorbable synthetic mesh. Hiltunen et al. [23] compared the use of standard anterior repair with the use of low-weight type 1 polypropylene mesh in randomized postmenopausal women with anterior vaginal prolapse. After 12 months, women who used mesh had a lower recurrence of prolapse (38.5% vs. 6.7%, $p < 0.001$). In a recent study, Nguyen and Burchette [31] compared standard anterior colporrhaphy with polypropylene mesh–assisted repair in 77 women with anterior wall prolapse. One year after surgery, anatomical success and patient satisfaction rates were 55% in the standard colporrhaphy group, whereas these rates were 87% in the mesh group ($p = 0.005$). The mesh erosion rate was reported as 5%. Although anatomical results are encouraging in repair with nonabsorbable synthetic mesh, decisions should be made by considering high vaginal erosion rates, concern about infection, and postoperative pain and dyspareunia [31].

Synthetic meshes have been developed recently due to the unacceptably high erosion rate of traditional meshes. The aim is to bring the erosion rates of vaginally placed meshes to a level comparable to sacrocolpopexy. In recent years, better results and lower erosion rates have been reported in anterior prolapse repair with polypropylene mesh [32]. In these studies, mesh erosion rates ranged from 0% to 6.9%, but not all patients with mesh erosion required surgical intervention. Being older than 70 years has been defined as an independent risk factor for vaginal erosion. In addition, mesh use should be avoided in women with moderate cystoceles. If possible, total hysterectomy and vertical vaginal incision should be avoided in cases where mesh will be placed. In cases where this surgical technique was applied, it was observed that the vaginal erosion rate reached 20% [33].

Finally, the postoperative results of low-weight polypropylene meshes, which typically come with a prosthetic kit for placement, are promising. Today, these low-molecular-weight meshes include Prolift (Gynecare), Apogee (American Medical Systems, Minnetonka, USA), Perigee (American Medical Systems), and Avaulta (Bard Ltd., Mol, Belgium). Sivaslıoğlu [34] randomized 90 women to undergo defect-specific cystocele repair with low-molecular-weight polypropylene mesh placed transobturatorally. At the 12-month follow-up, better anatomical results were achieved using low-molecular-weight polypropylene mesh (72% vs. 91%).

5.5.4 Posterior Wall Prolapse Repair

Posterior vaginal wall prolapse may be due to enterocele, sigmoidocele, rectocele (Fig. 5.3), or a combination of these. The rectovaginal space is a potential space between the rectum and vagina, consisting of areolar tissue and allowing the vagina and rectum to perform their functions independently of each other. The fibromuscular layer surrounding the posterior wall of the vagina is called the rectovaginal fascia or perirectal fascia, which is an extension of the endopelvic fascia. However, as its name suggests, this fascia is relatively weak [35].

In the presence of a healthy pelvic floor, there is minimal load on the connective tissue system because the genital hiatus is closed and the anterior and posterior walls of the vagina are in contact with each other. In this case, the intra-abdominal vector forces are applied equally to the anterior and posterior walls of the vagina and do not cause any increase in load or tension in any tissue since they balance each other. However, when the pelvic floor weakens and the chronic contraction power of the puborectalis muscle decreases, the genital hiatus remains open. In this case, the vaginal walls no longer touch each other, and the increased intra-abdominal pressure overpowers the atmospheric pressure in the vagina, putting a strain on the connective tissues. When perineal body damage is added to this, the rectum and the posterior vaginal wall and the perineal body can be seen to descend with increased abdominal and rectal pressure [35].

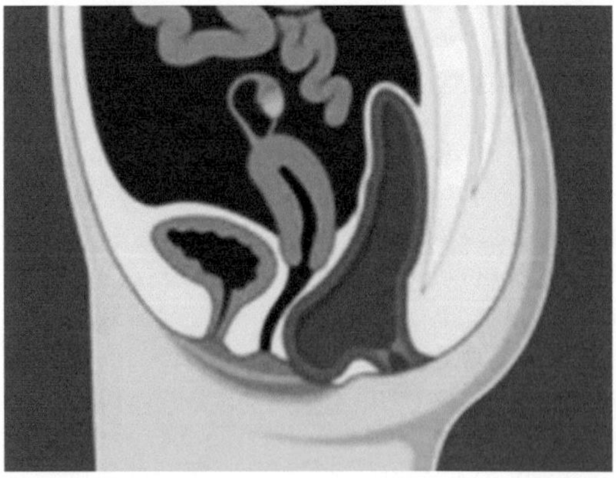

Fig. 5.3 Rectocele

5.5.5 Posterior Colporrhaphy

This procedure aims to narrow the vaginal tube and genital hiatus and create a new support base. In the standard method, after the posterior vaginal mucosa is dissected from the underlying fibromuscular layer, a midline plication is made from the fibromuscular layer proximal to the hymenal ring. The plication of the levator ani muscle can also be added; when individual sutures placed on the posterior muscular side walls are tied in the midline, the levator fascia approaches reciprocally and provides excellent support to the base. Levator ani plication has been associated with postoperative dyspareunia. The bulbocavernosus and perinei transversus muscles are brought closer to the midline in simultaneous perineorrhaphy. In prospective and retrospective studies, the anatomical failure rate has been reported as 25% and the improvement in defecation dysfunction as 75%. However, the rates of severe dyspareunia have been determined to be 12–27% [36].

5.5.6 Side-Specific Defect Repair

Side-specific defect repair was first described and accepted by Richardson [37] in 1993, considering that plication of the rectovaginal fibromuscularis in the midline does not correct the actual anatomical defect. This approach aims to find the defective areas on the rectovaginal septum after dissecting the vaginal epithelium and repair them primarily. A finger placed by the surgeon in the rectum helps find the defective fascial areas. Perineorrhaphy is performed after this repair. A levator fascia suture is not specified in this procedure. The anatomical failure rate has been reported as 8–18%, which is quite close to the standard rate for posterior colporrhaphy. Some publications report fewer cases of postoperative dyspareunia in patients who have undergone side-specific defect repair [38, 39].

5.5.7 Posterior Repair with Mesh

A graft can be used to reinforce the posterior vaginal wall during posterior colporrhaphy or specific defect repair. Mesh placement is done after fibromuscular plication or specific defect repair and is fixed to the levator fascia bilaterally. Late-absorbable or nonabsorbable No. 0 suture material is used [34].

The indication for using mesh in posterior repair is not as straightforward as in anterior repair [34]. However, synthetic meshes are used less frequently. The use of absorbable mesh in posterior repair does not increase treatment success, and its morbidity is not lower than that of nonabsorbable mesh. However, erosion rates are higher in posterior repair than in cystocele (anterior) repair. Sand [40] performed posterior vaginal prolapse repair with and without mesh and compared the anatomical outcomes. There was no significant difference in rectocele recurrence between the group using polyglactin (VICRYL: synthetic and absorbable) mesh and the group not using mesh (7/67 vs. 6/65; relative risk (RR): 1.13; confidence interval (CI): 0.40–3.19).

5.5.8 Abdominal Colpoperineopexy

In this method, which can be preferred when there is a simultaneous apical prolapse with rectocele, the surgeon dissects the avascular area between the vagina and rectum with the abdominal approach—sometimes advancing to the perineal body—and places a mesh between the posterior vaginal wall and the anterior sacral ligament. It is important to note that the mesh should not be placed taut. Cundiff et al. [41] performed colpoperineopexy with an abdominal approach on 19 patients with vaginal vault prolapse and also rectocele and perineal descent. They fixed the mesh to the posterior vaginal wall dissected up to the perineal body. They reported a 100% anatomical success rate after 11 weeks, with stage 0 prolapse rates of 63%, stage 1 prolapse rates of 21%, and stage 2 prolapse rates of 16%. In 12 of these patients, bowel dysfunction was observed, 8 of whom regressed within 11 months. Sullivan et al. [42] placed a total pelvic mesh in 236 patients, extending from the perineal body down to the pubis to support the vagina and bladder laterally in sacrocolpoperineopexy. When the success criterion was taken as no rectal or vaginal prolapse recurrence, they stated the success rate as 100% after 64 months of follow-up. However, 10% of the patients required reoperation due to surgical complications. They reported complete continence in 66 of 78 patients with preoperative fecal incontinence, improvement in 76% of patients with defecation difficulty, dyspareunia in 4 patients, and chronic pelvic pain in 3 patients [42].

5.5.9 Apical Prolapse

As previously mentioned, the uterosacral–cardinal ligament complex provides support for the upper one fourth of the uterus and vagina. If these ligaments tear or thin, prolapse of the uterus or the vaginal apex (vault) in hysterectomized patients may occur. After a hysterectomy, the vaginal apex is formed by merging the pubocervical fascia and the rectovaginal fascia posteriorly. If these two fascias are separated, enterocele (Fig. 5.4) develops [43, 44].

The main approaches described for vault prolapse are vaginal sacrospinous vault suspension and abdominal or laparoscopic sacrocolpopexy. The success rate after abdominal sacrocolpopexy has been reported as 78–100% in follow-ups ranging from 6 months to 3 years [45]. In the study by Hilger et al. [46], the success rate was reported as 74%, and the need for reoperation was 10.5% after an average follow-up period of 13.7 years. In the vaginal approach, uterosacral ligament vault suspension is another method used, like sacrospinous ligament vault suspension, and uterosacral ligament fixation prevents recurrent prolapse of other vaginal segments (especially the anterior segment) since it preserves the vaginal axis in its natural position [47, 48]. Although sacrospinous ligament suspension is quite successful in protecting the vaginal apex, postoperative cystocele formation has been reported as 18–92%. Although iliococcygeal fixation provides more anatomical fixation to the vagina, it causes severe shortening of the vagina because it is more distal to the ischial spines [48]. Uterosacral ligament suspension provides the most normal anatomical axis of the vagina on the pelvic floor muscles. Suspension of the bilateral uterosacral ligaments elevate vaginal corners and also preserves the vaginal length. However, the most frequently reported complication due to the proximity of the ureters to the uterosacral ligament is ureteral injury or kinking. Mallipedi et al. [30] reported this as 2.4%, while Visco et al. [49] reported it as 11%. Intraoperative cystoscopy is a recommended approach by the authors to prevent ureteral injury. During cystoscopy, the sutures

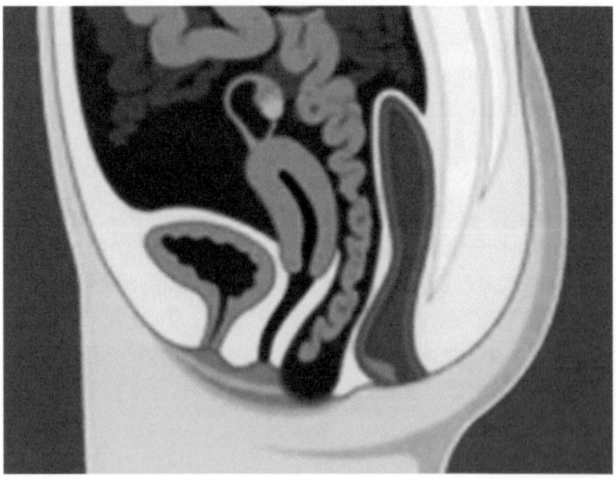

Fig. 5.4 Enterocele

should be removed and reevaluated if clear urine flow is not observed from both ureteral ostia.

5.5.10 Sacrospinous Ligament Fixation

The sacrospinous ligament extends between the lower part of the sacrum, the coccyx, and the ischial spine. It was stated that the sacrospinous ligament extends with the musculus coccygeus; its fibers blend into this muscle, and thus, these two structures form an inseparable whole called the coccygeus–sacrospinal ligament complex. It is palpable and is a triangular fibromuscular structure extending medially and posteriorly from the ischial tuberosity. Behind the sacrospinous ligament are the gluteus maximus muscle and the ischiorectal fossa, and the pudendal vessels and nerves, inferior gluteal vessels, and hypogastric venous plexus located in this fossa are essential structures. Therefore, the surgeon must be familiar with the pararectal anatomy, the sacrospinous ligament, and the surrounding structures [50].

The success rate of the surgical method is 79–100% for apical support, while the anatomical success rate in all vaginal areas varies between 8% and 100% [49]. The superiority of bilateral sacrospinous ligament fixation over unilateral fixation has not been demonstrated. After entering the rectovaginal space, dissection is performed according to the surgeon's dominant hand (usually the right side). The ischial tuberosity and the fibromuscular ligament extending posteromedially are palpated. Late-absorbable or nonabsorbable suture material is placed approximately two fingers medial to the ischial tuberosity and the vaginal apex. Several suture devices have been described to facilitate this procedure, including the Deschamps ligature carrier, Shutt needle punch, Miya hook, Endo Stitch, and Capio devices [51]. Complications of sacrospinous suspension include the general complications of vaginal surgery (infection and damage to adjacent organs). A rectal laceration has been described. Postoperative gluteal pain is also a common complication. Severe pain and motor and sensory damage have been reported as a result of damage to the pudendal and sciatic nerves located immediately above and lateral to the sacrospinous ligament [52]. Life-threatening vascular damage has also been reported. Placing the suture medially on the sacrospinous ligament avoids the pudendal neurovascular structures, but in this case, the inferior gluteal vessels are approached. If bleeding occurs, tight vaginal packing is applied to the bleeding area, and stabilization of the patient is recommended. De novo anterior wall prolapse after sacrospinous fixation has been reported in the literature at rates as high as 92% [49]. The probable reason for this is that the newly formed axis of the vagina is directed more posteriorly compared to the natural form. Primarily, suppose another surgical procedure that elevates the bladder neck is added. In that case, most of the abdominal head is concentrated on the anterior vaginal wall, which leads to anterior descent over time.

5.5.11 Abdominal Sacrocolpopexy

Suspension of the vagina to the sacral promontory via an abdominal approach is a safe and effective approach for uterovaginal prolapse and vaginal eversion. Various materials, including autologous and synthetic grafts, have been used as grafts for sacral colpopexy. Natural materials include fascia lata, rectus fascia, and dura mater. Synthetic materials include polypropylene mesh, polyester fiber mesh, polytetrafluoroethylene mesh, Dacron mesh, and SILASTIC silicone rubber. Culligan et al. [53], in a randomized controlled study, compared the objective anatomical results after sacrocolpopexy operations using cadaver fascia lata graft and polypropylene mesh and showed that repair with Prolene mesh was superior to repair with fascia lata in terms of POP-Q points, POP-Q stages, and objective anatomical success (objective success was found as 91% vs. 68%, $p = 0.007$) [53].

The literature also supports the use of MERSILENE mesh in abdominal sacrocolpopexy. In 61 patients who underwent abdominal sacrocolpopexy, the objective success rate was reported as 91%, the subjective cure rate as 90%, and the complication rate as 15% after a 26-month follow-up [54]. However, using other synthetic materials in abdominal sacrocolpopexy (e.g., Gore-Tex and silicone mesh) is associated with high complication and erosion rates [55].

The normal vaginal axis extends toward the S3–S4 segment of the sacrum. Some authors advocated that the graft be attached to this point. However, Sutton et al. [56] abandoned this approach when they encountered life-threatening bleeding from the presacral vessels at these lower sacrum levels. Therefore, fixing the graft to the anterior ligament extending in front of the sacral promontory at the upper one third of the sacrum increases safety without compromising anatomical results and vaginal function. There are four randomized controlled studies in the literature comparing abdominal sacrocolpopexy with the vaginal approach in pelvic organ prolapse surgery. Sacral colpopexy has also been shown to be superior to vaginal hysterectomy, which also includes anterior and posterior repair [57].

In a comprehensive literature study by Nygaard et al. [58], the success rate of apical prolapse repair ranged from 78% to 100%, and the success rate in all compartments ranged from 58% to 100% after an average follow-up of 6 months to 3 years. Reoperation rates due to recurrent pelvic organ prolapse or stress urinary incontinence were reported as 4.4% (0–18.2%) and 4.9% (1.9–30.9%), respectively [58].

Extensive literature studies on sacrocolpopexy have determined the average mesh erosion rates as 3.4–9%. In studies using type 1 mesh, such as polypropylene, mesh erosion rates are reported as low as 0.5%. In contrast, the erosion rate is reported as 3% for the use of type 3 mesh, such as MERSILENE; 3.4–5.5% for the use of Teflon mesh or Gore-Tex; and 23% for the use of silicone-coated polyester mesh. The mesh erosion rate is higher when a simultaneous hysterectomy is performed than when sacrocolpopexy is performed for vault prolapse. This is thought to be due to the freshness of the incision in the vaginal vault after hysterectomy [58].

Visco et al. [49] retrospectively examined the erosion rates in 273 women who underwent abdominal sacral colpopexy or sacral colpoperineopexy with MERSILENE mesh and reported erosion rates of 3.2% in sacral colpoperineopexy and 4.5% in colpoperineopexy when the graft and sutures were placed abdominally. In sacrocolpoperineopexy, if the mesh placed abdominally is fixed with vaginal sutures, the erosion rate reaches 16%. If both the mesh and fixation sutures are placed vaginally, the erosion rate reaches 40%. Other complications that can be seen, other than mesh erosion, include enterotomy, cystotomy, proctotomy, ureteral damage, and extrafascial tissue infections. Advanced age is the only identified risk factor for ileus or small bowel obstruction. After abdominal sacral colpopexy, 5.9% of patients developed ileus or small bowel obstruction, 1.2% of whom required reoperation due to obstruction. This problem highlights the importance of reperitonization to prevent the small bowel from adhering to the graft [59].

5.5.12 Abdominal Uterosacral Suspension

This is an alternative method to using synthetic grafts. High success rates have been reported when this technique is performed via the vaginal approach. The advantage of abdominal uterosacral suspension over sacrocolpopexy is the use of permanent sutures instead of synthetic mesh. There is no risk of mesh erosion, but the obvious disadvantage is that the durability of the repair is significantly higher when using mesh. The technique is similar to the vaginal approach; after the ureter is visualized, the sacrouterine ligaments are palpated 2 cm posterior and medial to the ischial tuberosity. Six permanent sutures, three to each sacrouterine ligament at the sacrum edge, are passed, and each end of the suture is passed through the anterior and posterior endopelvic fascia of the vaginal cuff and tied with the other end. The vaginal apex can be seen to be elevated toward the sacrum [60].

5.5.13 Uterus Preservation in Uterovaginal Prolapse Surgery

Sacrospinous hysteropexy is an anatomically effective and reliable choice for women who want to preserve their fertility [61].

A retrospective study by Maher et al. [61] compared 34 women who underwent sacrospinous hysteropexy with 36 women who underwent vaginal hysterectomy and sacrospinous fixation, and the hysterectomy group was followed up for an average of 36 months and the hysteropexy group for an average of 26 months. Subjective success rates and patient satisfaction were 86% in the hysterectomized group and 78% in the hysteropexy group ($p = 0.70$). The objective anatomical success rate was 72% in the hysterectomy group and 74% in the hysteropexy group ($p = 1.00$). The mean operative time was 91 min in the hysterectomy group and 59 min in the hysteropexy group ($p < 0.01$). Roovers [62] compared abdominal sacral hysteropexy with vaginal hysterectomy and uterosacral ligament suspension. At 1 year after surgery, the vaginal hysterectomy and uterosacral ligament suspension group had significantly better scores, less discomfort/pain (RR: 7.1; 95% CI: 1.1–13.2), less overactive bladder symptoms (RR: 8.7; 95% CI: 0.5–16.9), and less obstructive voiding dysfunction (RR: 10.3; 95% CI: 0.6–20.1). The abdominal sacral hysterotomy group had more reoperations for recurrent prolapse (RR: 9.0; 95% CI: 1.19–67.85); five women (13%) had reoperations for recurrent cystocele and four women for recurrent uterine prolapse. In contrast, only one patient in the vaginal hysterectomy group required reoperation for vaginal vault prolapse at 1 year after surgery. The operative time was shorter in the sacral hysterotomy group than in the vaginal hysterectomy and uterosacral ligament suspension group (−10 min; 95% CI: −12—8) [62].

5.5.14 Vaginal Approach Comparison with Abdominal Approach

Today, there is little scientific evidence regarding which surgical route is appropriate for advanced uterovaginal or post-hysterectomy vaginal vault prolapse. Two studies in the literature [61, 63] compared abdominal sacrocolpopexy with vaginal sacrospinous ligament suspension. The data showed a lower recurrence rate of vault prolapse in the abdominal sacrocolpopexy group (3/84 vs. 13/85; RR: 0.23; 95% CI: 0.07–0.77), fewer patients with failure to regress prolapse to stage 2 or lower (3/52 vs. 13/66; RR: 0.29; 95% CI: 0.09–0.97), less postoperative dyspareunia (7/45 vs. 22/61; RR: 0.39; 95% CI: 0.18–0.86), and less postoperative stress urinary incontinence (14/47 vs. 28/81; RR: 0.55; 95% CI: 0.32–0.95). However, there was no statistically significant difference in reoperation rates for stress urinary incontinence (RR: 0.6; 95% CI: 0.21–1.73).

5.6 Conclusion

POP will continue to exist as a disease that we will need to be more concerned about within the coming years, along with the increase in average life expectancy in society. The high expectations of the aging population regarding quality of life can make more permanent treatments challenging. Since there are insufficient studies to demonstrate significant differences in surgical success and complications between the elderly and younger populations, treatment is recommended for both groups. For many asymptomatic patients, physiotherapy applications, with methods such as pelvic floor exercises, can slow down the progression of the disease. Pessary applications are an effective and safe alternative for many patients. Surgical procedures are also effective and safe for the elderly population. Vaginal colpocleisis is a valuable alternative for individuals who have ended their sexual life. In appropriate cases, vaginal or abdominal reconstructive surgeries are practical and successful in POP treatment. As a result, in POP treatment, the patient's biological age, as well as their functional status, sexual activity, and expectations regarding quality of life, should play a role in determining the treatment to be selected.

References

1. Barber MD. Measuring pelvic organ prolapse: an evolution. Int Urogynecol J. 2024;35(5):967–76. https://doi.org/10.1007/s00192-024-05798-0. Epub 2024 May 10.
2. Hadizadeh-Talasaz Z, Khadivzadeh T, Mohajeri T, Sadeghi M. Worldwide prevalence of pelvic organ prolapse: a systematic review and meta-analysis. Iran J Public Health. 2024;53(3):524–38. https://doi.org/10.18502/ijph.v53i3.15134. PMID: 38919293; PMCID: PMC11194659.
3. Pizzoferrato AC, Sallée C, Thubert T, Fauconnier A, Deffieux X. Value of pelvic examination in women with pelvic organ prolapse: a systematic review. Int J Gynaecol Obstet. 2024;167(2):573–97. https://doi.org/10.1002/ijgo.15697. Epub 2024 May 22.
4. Qin Y, Liu J, Wu J. Advancements in surgical treatment for pelvic organ prolapse. Asian J Surg. 2024;47(7):3218–9. https://doi.org/10.1016/j.asjsur.2024.03.061. Epub 2024 Apr 10.
5. Bordoni B, Sugumar K, Leslie SW. Anatomy, Abdomen and Pelvis, Pelvic Floor. 2023 July 17. In: StatPearls [Internet]. Treasure Island (FL): StatPearls Publishing; 2024 Jan.
6. Eggleton JS, Cunha B. Anatomy, Abdomen and Pelvis, Pelvic Outlet. 2023 Aug 14. In: StatPearls [Internet]. Treasure Island (FL): StatPearls Publishing; 2024 Jan.
7. Shao P, Ai Z, Li H, Guo R, Wang Y. Understanding the anatomy of pelvic fascia: implications for regional anesthesia. Minerva Anestesiol. 2024; https://doi.org/10.23736/S0375-9393.24.18290-9. Epub ahead of print.
8. DeLancey JO, Mastrovito S, Masteling M, Horner W, Ashton-Miller JA, Chen L. A unified pelvic floor conceptual model for studying morphological changes with prolapse, age, and parity. Am J Obstet Gynecol. 2024;230(5):476–484.e2. https://doi.org/10.1016/j.ajog.2023.11.1247. Epub 2023 Nov 29. PMID: 38036167; PMCID: PMC11210379.
9. MJJ v V, Gudde AN, van der Kruit M, MPC v L, Rasing L, FADTG W, Roovers JP, Guler Z, PHJ K. An improved understanding of the pathophysiology of pelvic organ prolapse: a 3D in vitro model under static and mechanical loading conditions. Adv Healthc Mater. 2024;13(8):e2302905. https://doi.org/10.1002/adhm.202302905. Epub 2024 Jan 26. PMID: 38219051; PMCID: PMC11469184.
10. Cosgriff L, Ramanathan A, Iglesia CB. Pelvic floor disorders and sexual function: a review. Obstet Gynecol Clin N Am. 2024;51(2):241–57. https://doi.org/10.1016/j.ogc.2024.02.001. Epub 2024 Apr 4.
11. Pecorella G, Sparic R, Morciano A, Babovic I, Panese G, Tinelli A. Fortifying the foundation: assessing the role of uterine ligament integrity in uterine prolapse and beyond. Arch Gynecol Obstet. 2024;310(5):2333–43. https://doi.org/10.1007/s00404-024-07732-7. Epub 2024 Sept 20.
12. Florence E, Limtrakul N, Sanchez S, Montoya TI, Maldonado PA. Aversion to Mesh Use in Pelvic Floor Surgery in a Latina Population at the U.S.-Mexico Border. Urogynecology (Phila). 2024;30(1):17–25. https://doi.org/10.1097/SPV.0000000000001375. Epub 2023 May 29.
13. Pecorella G, Morciano A, Sparic R, Tinelli A. Literature review, surgical decision making algorithm, and AGREE II-S comparison of national and international recommendations and guidelines in pelvic organ prolapse surgery. Int J Gynaecol Obstet. 2024;167(2):560–72. https://doi.org/10.1002/ijgo.15614. Epub 2024 May 17.
14. Hendrix SL, Clark A, Nygaard I, Aragaki A, Barnabei V, McTiernan A. Pelvic organ prolapse in the Women's Health Initiative: gravity and gravidity. Am J Obstet Gynecol. 2002;186(6):1160–6. https://doi.org/10.1067/mob.2002.123819.
15. Abrams P, Andersson KE, Birder L. Members of Committees; Fourth international consultation on incontinence.Fourth international consultation on incontinence recommendations of the international scientific committee: evaluation and treatment of urinary incontinence, pelvic organ prolapse, and fecal incontinence. Neurourol Urodyn. 2010;29:213.
16. Hall AF, Theofrastous JP, Cundiff GW, Harris RL, Hamilton LF, Swift SE, Bump RC. Interobserver and intraobserver reliability of the proposed international continence society, Society of Gynecologic Surgeons, and American Urogynecologic Society pelvic organ prolapse classification system. Am J Obstet Gynecol. 1996;175(6):1467–71. https://doi.org/10.1016/s0002-9378(96)70091-1.
17. Shen L, Yang J, Bai X, Sun Z. Analysis of the current status of pelvic floor dysfunction in urban women in Xi'an City. Ann Palliat Med. 2020;9(3):979–84. https://doi.org/10.21037/apm-20-784.
18. Chen Z, Mikhail SM, Buttini M, Mowat A, Hartel G, Maher C. Online prediction tool for female pelvic floor dysfunction: development and validation. Int Urogynecol J. 2022;33(11):3025–33. https://doi.org/10.1007/s00192-021-04985-7.
19. Nager CW, Brubaker L, Litman HJ, Zyczynski HM, Varner RE, Amundsen C, Sirls LT, Norton PA, Arisco AM, Chai TC, Zimmern P, Barber MD, Dandreo KJ, Menefee SA, Kenton K, Lowder J, Richter HE, Khandwala S, Nygaard I, Kraus SR, Johnson HW, Lemack GE, Mihova M, Albo ME, Mueller E, Sutkin G, Wilson TS, Hsu Y, Rozanski TA, Rickey LM, Rahn D, Tennstedt S, Kusek JW, Gormley EA. A randomized

trial of urodynamic testing before stress-incontinence surgery. N Engl J Med. 2012;366(21):1987–97. https://doi.org/10.1056/NEJMoa1113595.
20. Lakeman MM, Zijta FM, Peringa J, Nederveen AJ, Stoker J, Roovers JP. Dynamic magnetic resonance imaging to quantify pelvic organ prolapse: reliability of assessment and correlation with clinical findings and pelvic floor symptoms. Int Urogynecol J. 2012;23(11):1547–54. https://doi.org/10.1007/s00192-012-1772-5.
21. Balsamo R, Uricchio F, Costantini E, De Sio M, Illiano E, Arcaniolo D, Domizio S, D'Afiero A. Anterior colporrhaphy and sacrospinous hysteropexy in women with pelvic organ prolapse: urodynamic findings and functional outcomes. Eur J Obstet Gynecol Reprod Biol. 2022;271:255–9. https://doi.org/10.1016/j.ejogrb.2022.02.027. Epub 2022 Feb 24.
22. Weber AM, Walters MD, Piedmonte MR, Ballard LA. Anterior colporrhaphy: a randomized trial of three surgical techniques. Am J Obstet Gynecol. 2001;185(6):1299–304.; discussion 1304–6. https://doi.org/10.1067/mob.2001.119081.
23. Hiltunen R, Nieminen K, Takala T, Heiskanen E, Merikari M, Niemi K, Heinonen PK. Low-weight polypropylene mesh for anterior vaginal wall prolapse: a randomized controlled trial. Obstet Gynecol. 2007;110(2 Pt 2):455–62. https://doi.org/10.1097/01.AOG.0000261899.87638.0a.
24. Capobianco G, Sechi I, Muresu N, Saderi L, Piana A, Farina M, Dessole F, Virdis G, De Vita D, Madonia M, Petrillo M, Sotgiu G. Native tissue repair (NTR) versus transvaginal mesh interventions for the treatment of anterior vaginal prolapse: systematic review and meta-analysis. Maturitas. 2022;165:104–12. https://doi.org/10.1016/j.maturitas.2022.07.013. Epub 2022 Aug 3.
25. Meschia M, Pifarotti P, Spennacchio M, Buonaguidi A, Gattei U, Somigliana E. A randomized comparison of tension-free vaginal tape and endopelvic fascia plication in women with genital prolapse and occult stress urinary incontinence. Am J Obstet Gynecol. 2004;190(3):609–13. https://doi.org/10.1016/j.ajog.2003.09.027.
26. Link G, van Dooren IM, Wieringa NM. The extended reconstruction of the pubocervical layer appears superior to the simple plication of the bladder adventitia concerning anterior colporrhaphy: a description of two techniques in an observational retrospective analysis. Gynecol Obstet Investig. 2011;72(4):274–80. https://doi.org/10.1159/000328741. Epub 2011 Oct 12.
27. Huang S, Lv Q, Li Y, Meng Q, Li M. A modified technique for paravaginal repair of cystocele with paravaginal defect: a retrospective study. Eur J Obstet Gynecol Reprod Biol. 2022;269:108–13. https://doi.org/10.1016/j.ejogrb.2021.12.028. Epub 2021 Dec 28.
28. Wang R, Tulikangas PK, Sappenfield EC. The impact of preoperative pain on outcomes after vaginal reconstructive surgery and perioperative pelvic floor muscle training. Urogynecology (Phila). 2023;29(12):930–7. https://doi.org/10.1097/SPV.0000000000001361. Epub 2023 Apr 26.
29. Kalis V, Kovarova V, Rusavy Z, Ismail KM. Transobturator cystocele repair of level 2 paravaginal defect. Int Urogynecol J. 2020;31(11):2435–8. https://doi.org/10.1007/s00192-020-04337-x. Epub 2020 June 3.
30. Mallipeddi PK, Steele AC, Kohli N, Karram MM. Anatomic and functional outcome of vaginal paravaginal repair in the correction of anterior vaginal wall prolapse. Int Urogynecol J Pelvic Floor Dysfunct. 2001;12(2):83–8. https://doi.org/10.1007/s001920170070.
31. Nguyen JN, Burchette RJ. Outcome after anterior vaginal prolapse repair: a randomized controlled trial. Obstet Gynecol. 2008;111(4):891–8. https://doi.org/10.1097/AOG.0b013e31816a2489.
32. Wu X, Jia Y, Sun X, Wang J. Tissue engineering in female pelvic floor reconstruction. Eng Life Sci. 2020;20(7):275–86. https://doi.org/10.1002/elsc.202000003. PMID: 32647506; PMCID: PMC7336160.
33. Deffieux X, de Tayrac R, Huel C, Bottero J, Gervaise A, Bonnet K, Frydman R, Fernandez H. Vaginal mesh erosion after transvaginal repair of cystocele using Gynemesh or Gynemesh-soft in 138 women: a comparative study. Int Urogynecol J Pelvic Floor Dysfunct. 2007;18(1):73–9. https://doi.org/10.1007/s0192-005-0041-2. Epub 2006 Jan 4.
34. Sivaslioglu AA, Unlubilgin E, Dolen I. A randomized comparison of polypropylene mesh surgery with site-specific surgery in the treatment of cystocoele. Int Urogynecol J Pelvic Floor Dysfunct. 2008;19(4):467–71. https://doi.org/10.1007/s00192-007-0465-y.
35. Oh S, Choi S, Lee SY, Jeon MJ. Posterior repair versus no posterior repair for posterior vaginal wall prolapse resolved under simulated apical support at the time of native tissue apical suspension. Int Urogynecol J. 2021;32(8):2203–9. https://doi.org/10.1007/s00192-021-04728-8. Epub 2021 Feb 26.
36. Shen SH, Chen JW, Liu MZ, Peng L, Chen YZ, Shen H, Luo DY. Modified posterior colporrhaphy: a better technique to improve sexual function in women with vaginal laxity. Int J Surg. 2024;110(4):2435–7. https://doi.org/10.1097/JS9.0000000000001057. PMID: 38215253; PMCID: PMC11019970
37. Richardson AC. The rectovaginal septum revisited: its relationship to rectocele and its importance in rectocele repair. Clin Obstet Gynecol. 1993;36(4):976–83. https://doi.org/10.1097/00003081-199312000-00022.
38. Kilic D, Guler T, Gokbel I, Gokbel DA, Ceylan DA, Sivaslioglu A. Effects of isolated posterior vaginal wall prolapse on lower urinary tract symptoms. J Gynecol Obstet Hum Reprod. 2021;50(4):102095. https://doi.org/10.1016/j.jogoh.2021.102095. Epub 2021 Feb 13.
39. Winkelman WD, Macharia A, Bharadwa S, Bharadwaj M, Hacker MR, Rosenblatt PL. Composite out-

comes after posterior Colporrhaphy with and without biologic graft augmentation. Female Pelvic Med Reconstr Surg. 2021;27(2):e414–7. https://doi.org/10.1097/SPV.0000000000000949. PMID: 32910081; PMCID: PMC8903065.
40. Sand PK, Koduri S, Lobel RW, Winkler HA, Tomezsko J, Culligan PJ, Goldberg R. Prospective randomized trial of polyglactin 910 mesh to prevent recurrence of cystoceles and rectoceles. Am J Obstet Gynecol. 2001;184(7):1357–62.; discussion 1362–4. https://doi.org/10.1067/mob.2001.115118.
41. Cundiff GW, Harris RL, Coates K, Low VH, Bump RC, Addison WA. Abdominal sacral colpoperineopexy: a new approach for correction of posterior compartment defects and perineal descent associated with vaginal vault prolapse. Am J Obstet Gynecol. 1997;177(6):1345–53; discussion 1353–5. https://doi.org/10.1016/s0002-9378(97)70074-7.
42. Sullivan ES, Longaker CJ, Lee PY. Total pelvic mesh repair: a ten-year experience. Dis Colon Rectum. 2001;44(6):857–63. https://doi.org/10.1007/BF02234709.
43. Lua-Mailland LL, Wallace SL, Khan FA, Kannikal JJ, Israeli JM, Syan R. Review of vaginal approaches to apical prolapse repair. Curr Urol Rep. 2022;23(12):335–44. https://doi.org/10.1007/s11934-022-01124-7. Epub 2022 Nov 10.
44. Geoffrion R, Larouche M. Guideline No. 413: surgical management of apical pelvic organ prolapse in women. J Obstet Gynaecol Can. 2021;43(4):511–523.e1. https://doi.org/10.1016/j.jogc.2021.02.001. Epub 2021 Feb 3.
45. Chan CYW, Fernandes RA, Yao HH, O'Connell HE, Tse V, Gani J. A systematic review of the surgical management of apical pelvic organ prolapse. Int Urogynecol J. 2023;34(4):825–41. https://doi.org/10.1007/s00192-022-05408-x. Epub 2022 Dec 3.
46. Hilger WS, Poulson M, Norton PA. Long-term results of abdominal sacrocolpopexy. Am J Obstet Gynecol. 2003;189(6):1606–10; discussion 1610-1. https://doi.org/10.1016/j.ajog.2003.10.689.
47. Lee W, Tam J, Kobashi K. Surgery for apical vaginal prolapse after hysterectomy: abdominal sacrocolpopexy. Urol Clin North Am. 2019;46(1):113–21. https://doi.org/10.1016/j.ucl.2018.08.006.
48. Okcu NT, Gürbüz T, Uysal G. Comparison of patients undergoing vaginal hysterectomy with sacrospinous ligament fixation, laparoscopic hysterectomy with sacrocolpopexy and abdominal hysterectomy with sacrocolpopexy in terms of postoperative quality of life and sexual function. J Gynecol Obstet Hum Reprod. 2021;50(4):101977. https://doi.org/10.1016/j.jogoh.2020.101977. Epub 2020 Nov 6.
49. Visco AG, Weidner AC, Barber MD, Myers ER, Cundiff GW, Bump RC, Addison WA. Vaginal mesh erosion after abdominal sacral colpopexy. Am J Obstet Gynecol. 2001;184(3):297–302. https://doi.org/10.1067/mob.2001.109654.
50. Jelovsek JE, Barber MD, Brubaker L, Norton P, Gantz M, Richter HE, Weidner A, Menefee S, Schaffer J, Pugh N, Meikle S; NICHD Pelvic Floor Disorders Network. Effect of uterosacral ligament suspension vs sacrospinous ligament fixation with or without perioperative behavioral therapy for pelvic organ vaginal prolapse on surgical outcomes and prolapse symptoms at 5 years in the OPTIMAL randomized clinical trial. JAMA 2018 319(15):1554–1565. doi:https://doi.org/10.1001/jama.2018.2827. PMID: 29677302; PMCID: PMC5933329.
51. Zhang W, Cheon WC, Zhang L, Wang X, Wei Y, Lyu C. Comparison of the effectiveness of sacrospinous ligament fixation and sacrocolpopexy: a meta-analysis. Int Urogynecol J. 2022;33(1):3–13. https://doi.org/10.1007/s00192-021-04823-w. Epub 2021 June 3. PMID: 34081163; PMCID: PMC8739324.
52. Goh JTW, Ganyaglo GYK. Sacrospinous fixation: review of relevant anatomy and surgical technique. Int J Gynaecol Obstet. 2023;162(3):842–6. https://doi.org/10.1002/ijgo.14751. Epub 2023 Mar 20.
53. Culligan PJ, Blackwell L, Goldsmith LJ, Graham CA, Rogers A, Heit MH. A randomized controlled trial comparing fascia lata and synthetic mesh for sacral colpopexy. Obstet Gynecol. 2005;106(1):29–37. https://doi.org/10.1097/01.AOG.0000165824.62167.c1.
54. Limb J, Wood K, Weinberger M, Miyazaki F, Aboseif S. Sacral colpopexy using mersilene mesh in the treatment of vaginal vault prolapse. World J Urol. 2005;23(1):55–60. https://doi.org/10.1007/s00345-004-0457-1. Epub 2004 Nov 11.
55. Begley JS, Kupferman SP, Kuznetsov DD, Kobashi KC, Govier FE, McGonigle KF, Muntz HG. Incidence and management of abdominal sacrocolpopexy mesh erosions. Am J Obstet Gynecol. 2005;192(6):1956–62. https://doi.org/10.1016/j.ajog.2005.02.062.
56. Sutton GP, Addison WA, Livengood CH 3rd, Hammond CB. Life-threatening hemorrhage complicating sacral colpopexy. Am J Obstet Gynecol. 1981;140(7):836–7. https://doi.org/10.1016/0002-9378(81)90750-x.
57. Campagna G, Vacca L, Panico G, Caramazza D, Lombisani A, Natale F, Scambia G, Ercoli A. Clinical, anatomical and perioperative outcomes of abdominal sacral colpopexy using autologous fascia: a systematic review of the literature. J Gynecol Obstet Hum Reprod. 2023;52(8):102635. https://doi.org/10.1016/j.jogoh.2023.102635. Epub 2023 July 25.
58. Nygaard IE, McCreery R, Brubaker L, Connolly A, Cundiff G, Weber AM, Zyczynski H, Pelvic Floor Disorders Network. Abdominal sacrocolpopexy: a comprehensive review. Obstet Gynecol. 2004;104(4):805–23. https://doi.org/10.1097/01.AOG.0000139514.90897.07.
59. Hanes CR 2nd. Vaginal sacral colpopexy: a natural orifice approach to a gold standard procedure. J Minim Invasive Gynecol. 2018;25(1):47–52. https://doi.org/10.1016/j.jmig.2017.06.009. Epub 2017 June 20.

60. Zakhari A, Nguyen DB, Smith JP, Mansour FW, Krishnamurthy S. vNOTES hysterectomy, adnexectomy, and uterosacral ligament suspension: a walk-through guide. J Minim Invasive Gynecol. 2022;29(10):1134–5. https://doi.org/10.1016/j.jmig.2022.06.023. Epub 2022 July 2.
61. Maher CF, Cary MP, Slack MC, Murray CJ, Milligan M, Schluter P. Uterine preservation or hysterectomy at sacrospinous colpopexy for uterovaginal prolapse? Int Urogynecol J Pelvic Floor Dysfunct. 2001;12(6):381–4.; discussion 384–5. https://doi.org/10.1007/s001920170017.
62. Roovers JP, van der Vaart CH, van der Bom JG, van Leeuwen JH, Scholten PC, Heintz AP. A randomised controlled trial comparing abdominal and vaginal prolapse surgery: effects on urogenital function. BJOG 2004 111(1):50–56. doi:https://doi.org/10.1111/j.1471-0528.2004.00001.x.
63. Benson JT, Lucente V, McClellan E. Vaginal versus abdominal reconstructive surgery for the treatment of pelvic support defects: a prospective randomized study with long-term outcome evaluation. Am J Obstet Gynecol. 1996;175(6):1418–21.; discussion 1421–2. https://doi.org/10.1016/s0002-9378(96)70084.

6 Diagnosis and Treatment of Menstrual Disorders

Zuhal Yapici Coskun and Gurkan Bozdag

6.1 Introduction

Menstrual cycle refers to regular cyclic changes in the female reproductive system due to ovulation and hormonal changes that prepare the system for pregnancy. This hormonal cyclicity results in cyclic vaginal bleeding called menstruation [1]. Menstruation starts with menarche (starting cyclic vaginal menstrual bleeding) at puberty around 12.4 years of age, depending on the ethnicity, and ceases at approximately 48.8 years old with menopause [2, 3].

6.2 What Is the Definition of Menstrual Disorders?

We should first define a normal menstrual cycle before we go into the details of menstrual disorders. The definition of a normal menstrual cycle differs between age groups. The first age group is adolescents between the ages of 10 and 19 in a phase of life between childhood and adulthood [4]. During this period of life, there is a transition to adult body features. Secondary sexual characteristics emerge and develop, the musculoskeletal system gains strength, the maturation of reproductive system continues, and psychosocial maturation is provided. As hypothalamic–pituitary–ovarian axis maturity is not fully achieved yet, the menstrual regularity is not established in the first years of menarche due to anovulation [2]. The menarche is expected to occur within 3 years following thelarche or until 15 years of age [5].

Besides regularity, duration, amount, and abnormal pattern of bleeding disorders, the menstrual cycle may be accompanied by pain and general discomfort. The pain disorders encountered during menstruation are the most common cause for adolescent girls to apply to gynecology clinics. Primary dysmenorrhea is the menstrual pain without an underlying pelvic pathology, whereas in secondary dysmenorrhea, there is a defined organic cause and pelvic pathology [6]. This complaint is also encountered in the reproductive-age adult female population. The physiological and psychological discomfort during the last days of the menstrual cycle is defined as premenstrual syndrome (PMS). Premenstrual syndrome (PMS) is a complex disorder with psychological and physical complaints occurring during the luteal phase of the menstrual cycle [6].

These conditions can significantly impact a woman's health, causing physical, emotional, and psychological distress. The diagnosis of menstrual disorders generally involves a combi-

Z. Yapici Coskun (✉)
Department of Obstetrics and Gynecology, Ministry of Health Ankara Bilkent City Hospital, Ankara, Türkiye

G. Bozdag
Bahceci Health Group, IVF Center, Istanbul, Türkiye

T. Akbayrak, E. Üzelpasaci (eds.), *Physiotherapy and Rehabilitation in Pelvic and Women's Health-Related Problems*, https://doi.org/10.1007/978-3-032-28741-0_6

nation of clinical assessment, medical history evaluation, laboratory tests, and imaging studies.

6.2.1 Menstrual Bleeding Disorders

Disorders related to the menstrual cycle may include irregularity, excess amount, and duration of menstrual bleeding.

Primary amenorrhea is the lack of menarche menstrual bleeding in ≥15-year-old adolescent girls with developed secondary sexual characteristics within 3 years after thelarche (onset of breast budding and development) or in ≥13-year-old girls without development of secondary sexual characteristics [7]. Secondary amenorrhea is defined as the cessation of previously regular menses for 3 months or the cessation of already irregular menstrual cycles for at least 6 months [8].

Normal menstruation in adolescents is expected to last for 2–7 days, with an interval of 21–45 days and an amount between 30 and 80 ml per cycle. Cycle intervals longer than 3 months of period should be further evaluated for adolescent girls [2]. The most common cause of menstrual disorders in the adolescent period is the immaturity of the hypothalamic–pituitary–ovarian axis, followed by endocrine disorders, pregnancy, and coagulopathies. Endocrinological causes include hyperandrogenic anovulatory pathologies such as polycystic ovary syndrome, congenital adrenal hyperplasia, thyroid disorders, hyperprolactinemia, hypothalamic or pituitary dysfunctions, primary ovarian insufficiency, medications, and genital infections. Anatomical problems such as genital tract malformations, uterine lesions, and malignancies may also cause menstrual disorders [2, 6].

In the adult female population, the definitive terms for normal menstruation differ from those of the adolescent group. Normal menstruation in adolescents is expected to last for ≤8 days, with an interval of 24–38 days and an amount between 30 and 80 ml per cycle with a variation of shortest to longest days for 18–25 years at ≤9 days, 26–41 years at ≤7 days, and 42–45 years at ≤9 days [9].

The etiology of menstrual bleeding disorders in women is classified systematically, and some definitive terms are abandoned to facilitate standardization and communication between clinicians and patients. The PALM-COEIN (polyp, adenomyosis, leiomyoma, malignancy and hyperplasia, coagulopathy, ovulatory dysfunction, endometrial, iatrogenic, and not yet classified) classification system for abnormal uterine bleeding has been introduced by the International Federation of Gynecology and Obstetrics (FIGO). Terminologies such as menorrhagia, metrorrhagia, hypermenorrhea, and hypomenorrhea are abandoned [10, 11]. The accepted terminology for menstrual disorders includes:

Frequent: Menstrual bleeding that occurs in <24 days of interval

Infrequent: Menstrual bleeding that occurs in >38 days of interval

Absent: Primary or secondary amenorrhea

Prolonged menstrual bleeding: Menstrual bleeding periods lasting >8 days

Intermenstrual bleeding: Cyclic intermenstrual bleeding can be seen just following ovulation due to a sudden decrease in blood estradiol levels. Acyclical intermenstrual bleeding can occur due to benign (cervical or endometrial infection, polyp, or intracavitary fibroids) or malignant lesions of the female genital system [12].

6.2.1.1 Evaluation and Diagnostic Tools for Menstrual Disorders

Clinical assessment includes gathering information about the patient's menstrual history, symptoms, and accompanying health problems. Clinician questions about the regularity, frequency, duration, and volume of menstruation; menstrual pain and associated symptoms (e.g., bloating, headaches, or mood changes); and any patterns of irregular bleeding help guide the diagnostic process [9, 10]. Potential contributing factors, such as stress, diet, exercise habits that may cause hypothalamic–pituitary–ovarian axis dysfunction, and the presence of conditions like polyendocrine metabolic ovarian syndrome (PMOS), formerly known as polycystic ovary syndrome (PCOS), thyroid disorders, or obesity should also be considered [13]. Family history of menstrual or reproductive disorders and genetic predispositions can play a role in the development of certain conditions [14].

The patient's gynecological history (fibroids, endometriosis, PCOS, etc.), including previous pregnancies, contraceptive use, and any prior surgeries, should also be asked. The clinical assessment also involves a physical examination to check for signs of systemic or reproductive abnormalities.

Laboratory tests are often performed to evaluate potential hormonal imbalances or underlying health conditions. Blood tests are typically conducted to assess the hormone levels, including thyroid function tests, prolactin, and androgens, in order to detect conditions like hypothyroidism, hyperprolactinemia, or PCOS. Additionally, testing for levels of luteinizing hormone (LH), follicle-stimulating hormone (FSH), serum estradiol, and progesterone levels can provide insights into the integrity of the menstrual cycle and the function of the hypothalamic–pituitary–ovarian axis. In women with suspected bleeding disorders, clotting factor tests or a complete blood count (CBC) may be recommended to rule out conditions such as von Willebrand disease or thrombocytopenia, which can contribute to abnormal bleeding [9, 10, 15].

Imaging studies are often used to visualize the reproductive organs and identify any structural abnormalities that may be contributing to menstrual disturbances. Pelvic ultrasound is one of the most commonly used imaging techniques, as it allows for the detection of conditions like uterine fibroids, polyps, endometrial hyperplasia, or ovarian cysts. In cases of suspected endometriosis, transvaginal ultrasound or even laparoscopy may be required to visualize the presence of endometrial tissue outside the uterus. For women with suspected fibroids or uterine abnormalities, magnetic resonance imaging (MRI) can provide a more detailed view of the uterus and surrounding tissues. MRI is particularly helpful for assessing the size and location of fibroids, which can influence treatment decisions. In cases of severe pelvic pain or suspected malignancy, additional imaging modalities like computed tomography (CT) scans may be necessary to rule out other potential causes [10, 14, 15].

Hysteroscopy, another diagnostic tool, involves the insertion of a small camera through the cervix to directly visualize the uterine cavity. This technique is useful for diagnosing conditions such as uterine polyps, fibroids, and endometrial hyperplasia, and it can also be used for therapeutic purposes, such as the removal of polyps or the biopsy of suspicious tissue [10, 14].

6.2.1.2 Management of Menstrual Bleeding Disorders

6.2.1.2.1 Amenorrhea/Irregular Menstrual Bleeding

Primary amenorrhea is a lack of menarche menstrual bleeding in ≥15-year-old adolescent girls with developed secondary sexual characteristics within 3 years after thelarche (onset of breast budding and development) or in ≥13-year-old girls without development of secondary sexual characteristics [7]. Secondary amenorrhea is defined as the cessation of previously regular menses for 3 months or the cessation of already irregular menstrual cycles for at least 6 months [8]. The management algorithm for amenorrhea depends on etiological factors. Hypothalamic–pituitary–ovarian axis immaturity, endocrine disorders, and anatomical problems such as genital tract malformations should be treated accordingly. As we noted before, potential contributing factors, such as stress, diet, exercise habits, and the presence of conditions like PMOS, thyroid disorders, adrenal gland disorders, or obesity, should also be considered and treated with a multidisciplinary approach accordingly [13].

6.2.1.2.2 Abnormal Uterine Bleeding

Management of menstrual bleeding disorders is dependent on the etiopathogenesis. In the case of abnormal uterine bleeding, the hemodynamic stability of the patient should be ensured. The emergency treatment options include IV conjugated equine estrogen, combined oral contraceptives, progestins, and tranexamic acid for suitable patients without contraindications [14].

Intrauterine foley catheter (26 F infused with 30 ml saline) is reported to be effective for acute abnormal uterine bleeding management [14, 16, 17].

Long-term treatment options include levonorgestrel intrauterine system (IUD), cyclic or continuous progestin therapy, combined oral contraceptives (COCs), tranexamic acid, or nonsteroidal anti-inflammatory drugs (NSAIDs) [14].

In cases of coagulopathies, a special evaluation is warranted. For the patients with von Willebrand disease, desmopressin should be used by intranasal, intravenous, or subcutaneous route with caution due to fluid retention and hyponatremia risk. Nonsteroidal anti-inflammatory drugs (NSAIDs) should not be used in platelet function disorders due to their negative effect on platelet aggregation and production of clotting factors [14, 18].

Surgical treatment requirement is also dependent on the patient's stability, underlying pathology, response to previous nonsurgical management, and fertility plan.

In cases of structural abnormalities such as fibroids or small (<1.5 cm) polypoid lesions without symptomatology, we can follow up with the patient unless any symptomatology emerges, and the pathologic lesion expands in size or outgrows.

Dilatation and curettage should be performed for patients with suspicion of intrauterine pathology to define the pathology and rule out malignant or premalignant endometrial pathologies. Hysteroscopy is also useful for the definitive diagnosis and treatment of structural pathologies distorting the endometrial cavity, such as submucous myoma uteri and endometrial polyps.

The surgical management of fibroids depends on the localization of the lesion: hysteroscopic resection, myomectomy via laparoscopy or laparotomy incision, uterine artery embolization, MR-guided focused ultrasound surgery, and hysterectomy [19].

Hysterectomy is the surgical procedure of choice for heavy menstrual bleeding that does not respond to medical or conservative treatment options [14, 15].

6.2.1.2.3 Premenstrual Syndrome (PMS)

Premenstrual syndrome (PMS) is defined as a complex psychological and somatic bundle of complaints occurring during the luteal phase of the menstrual cycle, and hormonal oscillations and fluctuations, as well as serotonin and neurotransmitters, are implicated in physiological and psychological changes causing premenstrual syndrome [20].

The global prevalence ranges from 12% to 98% across different ethnic and cultural groups [21]. Clinical symptoms include abdominal and lower back pain, headache, nausea, constipation, weight gain, breast swelling and tenderness, anxiety, mood changes (e.g., irritability, anger, restlessness, and crying outbursts), and impaired daily functioning [22]. Dysregulation of neurotransmitters, neurosteroids, and hypothalamic–pituitary–ovarian axis products is implicated in the etiopathogenesis [23].

The evaluation and diagnosis process needs a multidisciplinary approach. The team usually includes gynecology, psychiatry, endocrinology, clinical psychology, physiotherapy, and rehabilitation professionals. Treatment for PMS and its severe form, premenstrual dysphoric disorder (PMDD), includes pharmacological and nonpharmacological interventions. Selective serotonin reuptake inhibitors (SSRIs) are the first-line pharmacological treatment [24, 25]. Other options include oral contraceptives, calcium supplements, and vitamin D. Non-pharmacological treatments include lifestyle modifications, such as dietary adjustments, stress management, cognitive behavioral therapy, mindfulness-based exercises, aerobic activities, and yoga, which have shown efficacy in improving patient well-being [26, 27].

6.2.1.2.4 Dysmenorrhea

Dysmenorrhea refers to painful menstrual bleeding and has a prevalence of 50–90% among women of reproductive age, negatively affecting daily functioning and quality of life [28, 29]. Primary dysmenorrhea occurs without underlying pathology and is often linked to prostaglandin release by endometrial cells [30–32]. Secondary dysmenorrhea is associated with underlying pathologies, such as endometriosis, adenomyosis, or uterine abnormalities.

Treatment includes patient education, lifestyle changes, supportive therapies, and pharmacological interventions. Secondary dysmenorrhea may require surgical treatment if conservative approaches fail. Pharmacological options include nonsteroidal anti-inflammatory drugs (NSAIDs), acetaminophen, hormonal contraceptives, and magnesium [28]. Non-pharmacological interventions include heat application, dietary modifications, exercise, acupuncture, transcutaneous electrical nerve stimulation (TENS), and behavioral counseling [33, 34]. Physiotherapy techniques, such as isometric exercises, massage therapy, yoga, electrotherapy, connective tissue manipulation, stretching, kinesiotape, and relaxation exercises, have demonstrated efficacy in reducing menstrual pain by modulating prostaglandins, tumor necrosis factor (TNF), and interleukin levels [35, 36].

6.3 Conclusion

In conclusion, the diagnosis and management of menstrual disorders requires a comprehensive and multifaceted approach that includes a detailed medical history, physical examination, laboratory tests, and imaging studies. Accurate diagnosis is essential for guiding treatment decisions and improving patient outcomes. A combination of clinical expertise and diagnostic tools allows healthcare providers to identify the underlying causes of menstrual irregularities and develop personalized treatment plans to address each patient's unique needs. By carefully assessing hormonal imbalances, structural abnormalities, and systemic conditions, clinicians can provide effective care for women suffering from menstrual disorders.

References

1. Thiyagarajan DK, Basit H, Jeanmonod R. Physiology, menstrual cycle. In: StatPearls [Internet]. Treasure Island: StatPearls Publishing; 2024. PMID: 29763196. Last Update: 27 Sept 2024.
2. ACOG Committee Opinion No. 651: menstruation in girls and adolescents: using the menstrual cycle as a vital sign. Obstet Gynecol. 2015;126(6):e143–6.
3. Davis SR, Baber RJ. Treating menopause—MHT and beyond. Nat Rev Endocrinol. 2022;18(8):490–502. https://doi.org/10.1038/s41574-022-00685-4. Epub 2022 May 27. PMID: 35624141.
4. https://www.who.int/health-topics/adolescent-health. Accessed date 23 Dec 2024.
5. Reindollar RH, Byrd JR, McDonough PG. Delayed sexual development: a study of 252 patients. Am J Obstet Gynecol. 1981;140:371–80.
6. Deligeoroglou E, Creatsas G. Menstrual disorders. Endocr Dev. 2012;22:160–70. https://doi.org/10.1159/000331697. Epub 2012 Jul 25. PMID: 22846527.
7. Seppä S, Kuiri-Hänninen T, Holopainen E, Voutilainen R. Management of endocrine disease: diagnosis and management of primary amenorrhea and female delayed puberty. Eur J Endocrinol. 2021;184(6):R225–42. https://doi.org/10.1530/EJE-20-1487. PMID: 33687345.
8. Klein DA, Paradise SL, Reeder RM. Amenorrhea: a systematic approach to diagnosis and management. Am Fam Physician. 2019;100(1):39–48. PMID: 31259490.
9. Jain V, Munro MG, Critchley HOD. Contemporary evaluation of women and girls with abnormal uterine bleeding: FIGO systems 1 and 2. Int J Gynaecol Obstet. 2023;162(Suppl 2):29–42. https://doi.org/10.1002/ijgo.14946. PMID: 37538019; PMCID: PMC10952771.
10. Munro MG, Critchley HO, Broder MS, Fraser IS, FIGO Working Group on Menstrual Disorders. FIGO classification system (PALM-COEIN) for causes of abnormal uterine bleeding in nongravid women of reproductive age. Int J Gynaecol Obstet. 2011;113(1):3–13. https://doi.org/10.1016/j.ijgo.2010.11.011. Epub 2011 Feb 22. PMID: 21345435.
11. Fraser IS, Critchley HO, Broder M, Munro MG. The FIGO recommendations on terminologies and definitions for normal and abnormal uterine bleeding. Semin Reprod Med. 2011;29(5):383–90. https://doi.org/10.1055/s-0031-1287662.

12. Kaunitz MA. Abnormal uterine bleeding in nonpregnant reproductive-age patients: terminology, evaluation, and approach to diagnosis, Literature review current through. 2024. https://www.uptodate.com/contents/abnormal-uterine-bleeding-in-nonpregnant-reproductive-age-patients-terminology-evaluation-and-approach-to-diagnosis. Accessed date 23 Dec 2024.
13. Huhmann K. Menses requires energy: a review of how disordered eating, excessive exercise, and high stress Lead to menstrual irregularities. Clin Ther. 2020;42(3):401–7. https://doi.org/10.1016/j.clinthera.2020.01.016. Epub 2020 Mar 2. PMID: 32139174.
14. ACOG committee opinion no. 557: management of acute abnormal uterine bleeding in nonpregnant reproductive-aged women. Obstet Gynecol. 2013;121(4):891–6. https://doi.org/10.1097/01.AOG.0000428646.67925.9a. PMID: 23635706.
15. Lebduska E, Beshear D, Spataro BM. Abnormal uterine bleeding. Med Clin North Am. 2023;107(2):235–46. https://doi.org/10.1016/j.mcna.2022.10.014. Epub 2022 Dec 26. PMID: 36759094.
16. James AH, Kouides PA, Abdul-Kadir R, Dietrich JE, Edlund M, Federici AB, et al. Evaluation and management of acute menorrhagia in women with and without underlying bleeding disorders: consensus from an international expert panel. Eur J Obstet Gynecol Reprod Biol. 2011;158:124–34.
17. Hamani Y, Ben-Shachar I, Kalish Y, Porat S. Intrauterine balloon tamponade as a treatment for immune thrombocytopenic purpura induced severe uterine bleeding. Fertil Steril. 2010;94:2769.e13–5.
18. Kadir RA, Lukes AS, Kouides PA, Fernandez H, Goudemand J. Management of excessive menstrual bleeding in women with hemostatic disorders. Fertil Steril. 2005;84:1352–9.
19. De La Cruz MS, Buchanan EM. Uterine fibroids: diagnosis and treatment. Am Fam Physician. 2017;95(2):100–7. PMID: 28084714.
20. Takeda T. Premenstrual disorders: premenstrual syndrome and premenstrual dysphoric disorder. J Obstet Gynaecol Res. 2023;49(2):510–8. https://doi.org/10.1111/jog.15484. Epub 2022 Nov 1. PMID: 36317488.
21. Gudipally PR, Gyanendra K. Sharma premenstrual syndrome. StatPearls Publishing; 2024.
22. Tiranini L, Nappi RE. Recent advances in understanding/management of premenstrual dysphoric disorder/premenstrual syndrome. Fac Rev. 2022;11:11. https://doi.org/10.12703/r/11-11.eCollection2022.
23. Rapkin AJ. Pathophysiology of premenstrual syndrome and premenstrual dysphoric disorder. Menopause Int. 2012;18(2):52–9.
24. Marjoribanks J, et al. Selective Serotonin Reuptake inhibitors for premenstrual syndrome. Cochrane Database Sysyt Rev. 2013;2013(6):CD001396.
25. Hofmeister S, Bodden DS. Premenstrual syndrome and premenstrual dysphoric disorder. Am Fam Physician. 2016;94(3):236–40.
26. Liguori F, Saraiello E, Calella P. Premenstrual syndrome and premenstrual dysphoric disorder's impact on quality of life, and the role of physical activity. Medicina (Kaunas). 2023;59(11):2044. https://doi.org/10.3390/medicina59112044. PMID: 38004093; PMCID: PMC10673441.
27. Ranga M, Dev K. The effect of yoga therapy in premenstrual syndrome: a systematic review and meta-analysis of randomised controlled trials. J Obstet Gynaecol Can. 2024;46(10):102579. https://doi.org/10.1016/j.jogc.2024.102579. Epub 2024 Jun 12. PMID: 38871120.
28. Nagy H, Carlson K, Khan MAB. Dysmenorrhea [Updated 2023 Nov 12]. In: StatPearls [Internet]. Treasure Island: StatPearls Publishing; 2024. Available from: https://www.ncbi.nlm.nih.gov/books/NBK560834/
29. McKenna KA, Fogleman CD. Dysmenorrhea. Am Fam Physician. 2021;104(2):164–70. PMID: 34383437.
30. Ferries-Rowe E, Corey E, Archer JS. Primary dysmenorrhea: diagnosis and therapy. Obstet Gynecol. 2020;136(5):1047–58.
31. Proctor M, Farquhar C. Diagnosis and management of dysmenorrhoea. BMJ. 2006;332(7550):1134–8.
32. Coco AS. Primary dysmenorrhea. Am Fam Physician. 1999;60(2):489–96. PMID: 10465224.
33. Shetty GB, Shetty B, Mooventhan A. Efficacy of acupuncture in the management of primary dysmenorrhea: a randomized controlled trial. J Acupunct Meridian Stud. 2018;11(4):153–8.
34. Elboim-Gabyzon M, Kalichman L. Transcutaneous electrical nerve stimulation (TENS) for primary dysmenorrhea: an overview. Int J Women's Health. 2020;12:1–10. https://doi.org/10.2147/IJWH.S220523. PMID: 32021488; PMCID: PMC6955615.
35. López-Liria R, Torres-Álamo L, Vega-Ramírez FA, García-Luengo AV, Aguilar-Parra JM, Trigueros-Ramos R, Rocamora-Pérez P. Efficacy of physiotherapy treatment in primary dysmenorrhea: a systematic review and meta-analysis. Int J Environ Res Public Health. 2021;18(15):7832. https://doi.org/10.3390/ijerph18157832. PMID: 34360122; PMCID: PMC8345570.
36. Barcikowska Z, Rajkowska-Labon E, Grzybowska ME, Hansdorfer-Korzon R, Zorena K. Inflammatory markers in dysmenorrhea and therapeutic options. Int J Environ Res Public Health. 2020;17(4):1191. https://doi.org/10.3390/ijerph17041191.

Diagnosis and Treatment of Sexual Dysfunction

7

Süleyman Eserdağ and Emrah Yakut

7.1 Introduction

Sexuality is an important element in human life that affects the quality of life beyond the biological reproductive function. For this reason, problems related to sexuality can negatively affect social relationships. Erectile dysfunction (ED) and premature ejaculation (PE) are the most common sexual dysfunctions in men. Female sexual dysfunctions (FSDs) encompass a wide range of disorders that impair sexual response, desire, arousal, or orgasm or cause pain during sexual activity. These disorders can be multifaceted, influenced by physical, psychological, and relational factors.

7.2 Female Sexual Dysfunctions (FSDs)

According to the fifth edition of the *DSM* by the American Psychiatric Association (APA) in 2013, FSD includes [1]:

- Genito-pelvic pain/penetration disorder (GPPPD)
- Female sexual arousal/interest disorder (FSAID)
- Female orgasmic disorder (FOD)

For each diagnosis, symptoms must be experienced 75–100% of the time, last for at least 6 months, and cause significant distress.

7.2.1 Genito-pelvic Pain/ Penetration Disorder (GPPPD)

It is not easy for clinicians to distinguish between vaginismus and dyspareunia problems due to overlapping symptoms. That is why, in the *DSM-5* classification, vaginismus and dyspareunia were classified under the category of "genito-pelvic pain and penetration disorder" (GPPPD), which describes persistent or recurrent difficulty/ pain during sexual intercourse or penetration attempts. Both conditions involve many organic, psychological, cultural, and interpersonal relationship factors.

7.2.1.1 Vaginismus

Vaginismus is a common sexual dysfunction characterized by involuntary pelvic floor muscle spasms that prevent vaginal penetration [2]. This can occur during sexual intercourse, gynecological examinations, or tampon insertion.

S. Eserdağ (✉)
Department of Obstetrics and Gynecology, Faculty of Medicine, Altınbaş University, Istanbul, Türkiye

Hera Clinic, Istanbul, Türkiye
e-mail: suleyman@eserdag.com

E. Yakut
Department of Urology, Faculty of Medicine, Yuksek Ihtisas University, Ankara, Türkiye

T. Akbayrak, E. Üzelpasaci (eds.), *Physiotherapy and Rehabilitation in Pelvic and Women's Health-Related Problems*, https://doi.org/10.1007/978-3-032-28741-0_7

Vaginismus may have a psychological origin but can also be exacerbated by organic factors such as inflammation or infections. It is estimated that vaginismus affects approximately 2–6% of women, making it a relatively common condition. Diagnostic criteria include subjective reports of muscle spasms and an inability to achieve vaginal penetration despite adequate lubrication [3].

7.2.1.2 Definition

The DSM-5 diagnostic criteria for GPPPD include difficulty with at least one of the following [1]

- Vaginal penetration during intercourse
- Marked vulvovaginal or pelvic pain during vaginal intercourse or penetration attempts
- Marked fear or anxiety about vulvovaginal or pelvic pain in anticipation of, during, or as a result of vaginal penetration
- Marked tensing or tightening of the pelvic floor muscles during attempted vaginal penetration

Normally, the vaginal muscles under conscious control contract involuntarily during intercourse. In vaginismus, the problem is not limited to these contractions; many couples with this issue also exhibit behaviors such as avoiding sexual intercourse. According to a recent consensus, it can also be described as persistent or recurrent difficulties of the woman in allowing vaginal entry of a penis, finger, and/or any object despite her expressed wish to do so.

In vaginismus, contractions occur in the pelvic floor muscles surrounding the urethra, vagina, and anus. These contractions are voluntary in maintaining urine and feces retention, while involuntary contractions also occur during orgasm. The involuntary contractions in vaginismus are spastic contractions that are the opposite of the rhythmic contractions during orgasm. Depending on the severity of vaginismus, these involuntary contractions may not be limited to the vagina but can be widespread throughout the body, particularly in the lumbar, inguinal, gluteal, and inner thigh regions, and even in the face.

The International Classification of Diseases (ICD)-11 categorizes vaginismus as a "sexual pain-penetration disorder" under HA20. According to the ICD-11, sexual pain-penetration disorder is characterized by at least one of the following [4]:

1. Marked and persistent or recurrent difficulties with penetration, including due to involuntary tightening or tautness of the pelvic floor muscles during attempted penetration
2. Marked and persistent or recurrent vulvovaginal or pelvic pain during penetration
3. Marked and persistent or recurrent fear or anxiety about vulvovaginal or pelvic pain in anticipation of, during, or due to penetration

In severe vaginismus, reactions such as fear of death, pushing away the partner, crying, and screaming are commonly observed, alongside involuntary physical responses like sweating, tachycardia, hyperventilation, nausea, vomiting, and fainting.

7.2.1.3 Prevalence

Epidemiological studies showing its prevalence in populations are scarce, and it is believed that factors such as cultural values attributed to sexuality, the importance of sexuality, and perceptions of sexual dysfunction play a significant role in its frequency in Eastern cultures. In Western societies, the most common sexual issue is a lack of sexual desire, while vaginismus is a much rarer problem compared to Eastern societies. Although the exact cause is not known, the prevalence of vaginismus in clinics ranges from 5% to 17% [5]. Studies have reported a 6.2% prevalence in Morocco and 8% in Iran [6].

7.2.1.4 Types of Vaginismus

Like other sexual dysfunctions, vaginismus is classified into primary, secondary, situational, and generalized types. Primary (lifelong) vaginismus occurs in individuals who have never engaged in sexual intercourse, while secondary (acquired) vaginismus occurs in those who have previously engaged in sexual intercourse but can no longer do so. The most common cause of secondary vaginismus is past trauma, such as difficult childbirth, abortion, sexual abuse, rape, violence, or relational trauma.

Situational vaginismus occurs when the issue arises only in certain environments or with specific partners but does not occur in other settings or with other partners. If the sexual problem occurs independently of the environment and during all sexual activities, it is referred to as generalized vaginismus.

7.2.1.5 Etiology

The etiology of vaginismus is multifactorial, often rooted in a combination of psychological, cultural, and physical factors. Fear of penetration, trauma, anxiety about sexual performance, and negative sexual experiences can contribute to its development [7]. Organic factors, such as genital infections, pelvic floor dysfunction, or anatomical abnormalities, should also be considered potential contributors.

7.2.1.5.1 Psychological Factors

Lack of sexual information, incorrect beliefs about sexuality (sexual myths), negative and exaggerated stories heard about the first sexual experience, and past sexual traumas can cause vaginismus. Fears related to pain expectations and hypersensitivity to erotic touch are also among the causes of vaginismus [8].

Vaginismus can also present as an "unconscious defense mechanism." Although the exact cause cannot be determined, potential reasons can be identified. It is generally seen as a disorder influenced by social, cultural, psychological, and physiological factors, particularly childhood sexual trauma and religious conservatism.

In a study, it was demonstrated that women with vaginismus have a lower pain threshold, which decreases further in more severe grades of the condition. This pain may exacerbate their avoidance of sexual intercourse [9].

Patients with vaginismus have negative beliefs about sexual intercourse, known as "maladaptive cognitions," which lead to negative emotions and automatic physical responses. Common cognitive distortions include beliefs that "the vaginal structure is narrow, the partner's penis is too large, there will be excessive pain and bleeding during the first intercourse, the hymen is closed, or the canal is obstructed." Myths such as "penis captivus," believing the penis will damage the urethra or enter the anus, are also common. The inexperience of the partner in sexual matters can further exacerbate the anxiety in women.

7.2.1.5.2 Organic Factors

When the genito-pelvic pain is described as burning, widespread rather than localized, and spontaneous rather than provoked, organic factors are considered more likely in the etiology. Structural or other organic abnormalities must be ruled out prior to treatment [7]. Possible organic causes include congenital anomalies of the hymen (Fig. 7.1b), vaginal atrophy, vaginal surgeries or intravaginal radiation, adhesions, uterine prolapse, vulvar vestibulitis syndrome (VVS), endometriosis, infections, vaginal lesions and tumors, and sexually transmitted diseases (STDs).

7.2.1.6 Genital Examination and Grading

The experience of the initial gynecological examination on a gynecological table can be difficult for patients. After establishing a doctor-patient trust relationship, providing detailed information about the examination, assuring that no instruments will be used, and providing positive reinforcement can significantly reduce anxiety.

Gynecological examination and a detailed anamnesis taken upon the first admission have an important impact on the management of therapy and treatment success [10]. Grading of vaginismus is also based on the patient's history and gynecological evaluation. In 1978, Lamont classified vaginismus into four levels [11], which were later expanded by Dr. Pacik to five levels in 2010 [12]. In first-degree vaginismus, known as pelvic floor spasm, the patient can be relaxed enough for the examination with encouragement. In second-degree vaginismus, the patient does not relax during the examination, and pelvic floor contractions are observed. In third-degree vaginismus, the patient tries to avoid the examination by lifting her hips. In fourth-degree vaginismus, the patient raises her hips, withdraws completely,

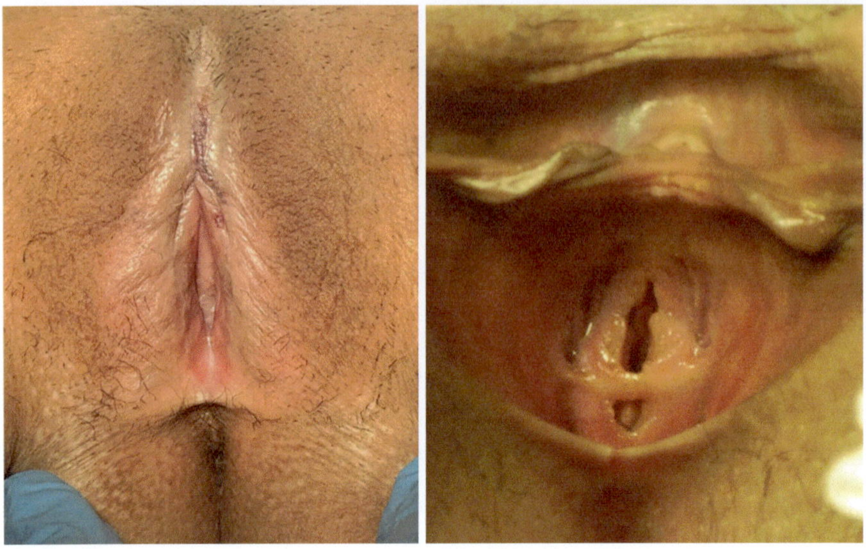

Fig. 7.1 Vulvar pathologies can cause genito-pelvic pain/penetration disorder (GPPPD). (**a**) Vulvar lichen sclerosus with perineal and clitoral adhesions (left) and (**b**) septate hymen (right)

or covers herself, contracting all body muscles, and does not allow any physical contact during the examination. Dr. Pacik describes fifth-degree vaginismus as a visceral reaction resulting from adrenaline discharge, which may include symptoms such as tachycardia, tremors, hyperventilation, uncontrolled crying, fainting, gagging, nausea or vomiting, and even a desire to attack the doctor.

The level of vaginismus is crucial for planning treatment methods. Instead of using the term "gynecological examination" for patients, it might be more appropriate to use "gynecological assessment" or "gynecological evaluation." During the assessment, the vulva is examined visually first, followed by gentle retraction of the labia majora to inspect the vestibulum and hymenal structures. Then, a gentle penetration with the pinky finger into the vagina is performed to observe the patient's openness to suggestions. The level of muscle spasm and reactions are assessed. It is important to determine whether the hymen is anatomically intact and, if so, its anatomical structure, the presence of inflammation or hyperesthesia in the vestibulum, and the absence or presence of vaginal or vulvar lesions or infections.

Table 7.1 The new classification system of vaginismus based on a gynecological examination, the "Eserdag classification"

First grade	The patient tolerates the examiner's index finger insertion into the vaginal canal, and involuntary vaginospasm is felt by the examiner
Second grade	The patient tolerates insertion of the examiner's little finger to vaginal entry with difficulty and some anxiety
Third grade	The patient demonstrates fear, cannot tolerate the examiner's finger in her vagina, and only allows the examiner to touch her vestibulum and vulva
Fourth grade	The patient demonstrates tremendous fear, anxiety, and embarrassment; sometimes cries and elevates her buttocks; constricts her thighs; withdraws herself; contracts all her muscles (sometimes even her chin and toes); and does not allow the examiner even to touch her vulva or allows it with difficulty

We use our own grading system in our clinics for vaginismus classification, which is entirely based on genital examination (Table 7.1). It is easy to apply and practical, providing guidance in terms of the patient's openness to suggestion [13].

7.2.1.7 Differential Diagnosis

Many couples experiencing penetration problems come to clinics complaining of "inability to have intercourse" or "pain during intercourse." Through Internet research, many come across terms like "vaginismus" or "dyspareunia" for the first time in their lives. Sexual penetration issues can develop depending on the patient's biological or psychological relationship with themselves, their partner, or the couple's relationship. Therefore, it would be incorrect to immediately diagnose every couple who cannot have intercourse with vaginismus. A definitive diagnosis must be made through a detailed history and a gynecological examination.

All couples experiencing an inability to engage in sexual intercourse, like all other sexual dysfunctions, should be treated from a "biopsychosocial" perspective, adopting a holistic approach. It may not always be easy to determine whether the pain causes the spasm or the spasm causes the pain. Generally, in vaginismus patients, the spasm is related to a fear of feeling pain, which can lead to pain. Sometimes, intercourse may not progress to the point of experiencing pain. Therefore, the presence of penetration pain is not essential for the diagnosis of vaginismus. In dyspareunia patients, there is real pain felt during intercourse, leading to spasm as a result. Vaginismus is more centrally originated, while dyspareunia is more peripherally originated.

Vaginismus is often confused with a superficial dyspareunia condition known as "vulvar vestibulitis syndrome" (VVS). Vulvar vestibulitis syndrome is characterized by hyperesthesia in the vestibule due to inflammation. Vestibular hyperemia may sometimes be present. The diagnosis is made by applying gentle pressure with a cotton-tipped swab on the vestibule (Q-tip test). In cases where there is excessive pain during the application, "pain mapping" is performed. In the etiology of VVS, recurrent fungal infections, other vaginal infections, Human Papilloma Virus (HPV), and urogenital inflammatory conditions play a role. It can be quite difficult to differentiate between partial vaginismus and the VVS group based on pain history and clinical findings.

Vaginismus can also be confused with sexual desire disorders. Sometimes, these two issues coexist. Sexual desire problems associated with vaginismus generally improve on their own after treatment. However, if there is a primary sexual desire disorder or aversion and associated inability to engage in intercourse, the therapies may take longer.

7.2.1.8 Management

The management of vaginismus begins with a detailed history that includes medical, social, and psychological questions. Subsequently, an overview of the treatment is provided, and a patient-physician trust relationship is established. This is followed by a gynecological evaluation. For patients who are excessively responsive and insecure and have intense anxiety, it is crucial to first relax them through general therapy before starting vaginismus treatment. Treatments should progress step by step.

Treatment approaches for vaginismus are individualized and often involve a multidisciplinary approach. Cognitive-behavioral therapy (CBT) is the cornerstone of treatment, addressing underlying fears and anxieties. Pelvic floor physical therapy is also beneficial, aimed at relaxing the muscles and improving muscle coordination. In some cases, the use of dilators can help in desensitizing the vagina to penetration [14]. Pharmacological treatments are typically not recommended as a first-line approach, but they may be considered in cases where psychological factors are less prominent.

7.2.1.9 Cognitive-Behavioral Approaches

Systematic desensitization techniques with cognitive-behavioral therapies are the gold standard in the treatment of vaginismus. Cognitive therapy for vaginismus includes cognitive restructuring, sexual education, therapy, and home assignments [10]. Sexual education is the first step of the treatment. For women with prevalent sexual myths and cognitive distortions, it is essential to replace incorrect thoughts with correct ones through sexual and psycho-education and cognitive restructuring. Therapies should be conducted with couples whenever possible, as many men also lack information and experience. Simultaneously, other sexual disorders may coexist. In cognitive therapies, anatomical and physiological information regarding female and male genital organs, including sexuality, the first night, hymen, and vagina, is provided.

In behavioral approaches for vaginismus, mirror, massage, and breathing exercises are prominently used. Various sizes of plastic, glass, or metal dilators; finger exercises; Kegel exercises; and progressive muscle relaxation are other behavioral methods employed.

7.2.1.10 Psychodynamic Approaches

Psychoanalysis conceptualizes vaginismus as a conversion disorder caused by unresolved preoedipal or oedipal conflicts from early childhood, a severe neurotic reaction that is difficult to resolve [15]. According to Freud's ego psychology, human sexual pleasure, which is a connected and interrelated experience, is nourished by the "id," the unconscious part of the psyche working according to the pleasure principle. The id's orientation toward this pleasure is perceived as a danger by another mental apparatus, the "ego." The disturbance of the ego causes anxiety in the person, who then resorts to "sexual inhibition" to escape this anxiety. In other words, sexual inhibitions serve as a defense mechanism to relieve anxiety. Furthermore, the "superego," another significant psychological component that increases anxiety, nourished by religion, morality, and traditional laws, also plays a crucial role.

In vaginismus patients, if there is a history of sexual trauma, such as abuse, rape, or incest, in the detailed history taken during the first session, it needs to be examined further. Including a woman with a history of abuse and sexual desire problems in short-term treatment programs is not a correct approach. In such cases, psychodynamic therapies can be applied by psychiatrists or psychotherapists.

7.2.1.11 Surgical Methods

If the hymen structurally blocks the vaginal entrance, this can complicate or make the treatment impossible. In cases where the hymen is rigid, high-edged, cribriform, or septate, hymenotomy or hymenectomy surgeries may become necessary. On the other hand, in patients who cannot tolerate penetration exercises during treatment or experience pain due to sensitivity at vaginal entry, surgical methods may be preferred to facilitate treatment.

Furthermore, patients diagnosed with vaginismus may encounter vulvar vestibulitis issues as the treatment progresses. In our observations, "vulvar vestibulectomy" surgeries in such patients effectively resolve the pain problem. In cases where there are no physical issues, empirical hymen surgeries performed solely to meet patient expectations tend to cause more harm than good. Therefore, unnecessary surgical procedures should be avoided.

For patients with increasing spasms due to hymenal anomalies, we recommend providing sexual therapy even after hymenectomy or hymenotomy.

7.2.1.12 Hypnotherapy

Hypnotherapy is a treatment method aimed at accessing unconscious thoughts and creating a state of "awareness." Under hypnosis, past experiences that caused negative emotional states can be resolved. Relaxation and comfort can be achieved through the given suggestions. With the anesthetic effect of hypnosis, the pain threshold can be raised. The ego, weakened over time, can be strengthened. Patient compliance with the treatment can be increased, and the treatment duration can be shortened. Hypnotherapy and ego-oriented therapy have been reported to provide effective results in the treatment of vaginismus [16]. Hypnosis can also be used as a complementary, supportive method in many sexual dysfunctions in both women and men.

7.2.1.13 Acupuncture Treatment

As a form of Chinese folk medicine, thousands of years old, acupuncture has been approved by the World Health Organization for its effectiveness in treating 150 different diseases. Acupuncture treatment for vaginismus is a supportive method that addresses the anxiety and pain that cause an inability to engage in sexual intercourse. It enhances the effectiveness of cognitive and behavioral treatments. Through acupuncture treatment, the body produces its natural painkillers. Acupuncture treatment also helps in correcting depression and a lack of self-confidence in vaginismus, increasing relaxation and comfort. It is especially a complementary method in the treatment of resistant and highly anxious vaginismus patients. However, acupuncture alone will not be effective without concurrent sexual therapy.

7.2.1.14 Botulinum Toxin Injection

For the first time, botulinum toxin injection was applied to a vaginismus patient by Mitchell F. Brin in 1997 and presented as a case report [17]. The application generally involves injecting 100–200 IU of botulinum toxin type A at the 2–4–8-10 o'clock positions. To avoid incontinence risks, care should be taken to stay away from the urethra or anal sphincter. Simultaneously, local anesthetic (bupivacaine) injections and the removal of the hymen in a triangular shape from the 3 and 9 o'clock positions (limited hymenectomy) are also recommended by Dr. Pacik [18].

Vaginal botulinum toxin application can also be performed to relieve spasm in cases of "hypertonic vagina," a different condition from vaginismus.

7.2.1.15 Eye Movement Desensitization and Reprocessing (EMDR)

Eye movement desensitization and reprocessing (EMDR) is a psychological therapy method. It addresses traumas that prevent the balanced functioning of the right and left lobes of the brain through eye movements. It provides quick results in a short time, reduces the effects of trauma, desensitizes against past negative experiences, enhances life quality, and instills positive beliefs about oneself [19].

7.2.1.16 Medical Treatments

Due to its anxiolytic effect, benzodiazepines like diazepam can be used in treatments. However, it has been reported that antidepressants and tranquilizers are ineffective and can even worsen the sexual issue by impairing arousal and orgasm functions due to their side effects [20]. In vaginismus treatments, water-based lubricating gels or creams and topical anesthetic substances can be used. However, attempts at intercourse under spinal, epidural, or general anesthesia can cause additional sexual trauma and are never recommended.

On the other hand, in cases of premature ejaculation in male partners or secondary conditions, medications like paroxetine or dapoxetine can be prescribed. For erectile dysfunction issues, phosphodiesterase type 5 (PDE5) inhibitors may also be recommended.

7.2.1.17 Dyspareunia

Although vaginismus and dyspareunia have been merged in the category of GPPPD, they have different features and management methods. Symptoms of dyspareunia affect psychology, body image, partner relationships, general social life, and even fertility. Over time, it can lead to sexual desire, arousal, and orgasm problems. Factors like young age, low educational level, urinary symptoms, emotional issues, stress, and a decrease in household income of more than 20% have been found to be significant risk predictors.

7.2.1.18 Definition

Dyspareunia is defined as persistent or recurrent pain during sexual intercourse, regardless of adequate lubrication. It can be classified into two types: superficial dyspareunia (pain occurring at the entry of the vagina) and deep dyspareunia (pain occurring within the pelvis).

7.2.1.19 Prevalence

The lifetime prevalence of dyspareunia ranges from 10% to 20% of women. The prevalence of chronic dyspareunia, defined as pain occurring for at least 6 months, is about 7% in the general population [21].

7.2.1.20 Anamnesis

The first step in correct diagnosis is taking a detailed anamnesis. It can be challenging for many women to discuss sexual issues. Therefore, patients should be reassured, a complete doctor-patient trust relationship should be established, and no judgment should be made during consultations. Initially, a general medical and surgical history is taken, followed by a gynecological and obstetric history, and finally a detailed sexual history with open-ended questions. If the pain started later, it could be due to an infection, vulvar vestibulitis, or sexual trauma. If penetration is difficult, vulvodynia or vaginismus may be underlying. If there is insufficient arousal or lubrication, this could be due to negative partner relationships, stress, or personal psychological factors. Questions asked should include whether the complaint increased over time or started suddenly, how it affected the patient, if it was provoked/spontaneous, if it intensified at certain times, if it was associated with the menstrual cycle, and if there was partner support for marriage and treatment. The McGill Pain Questionnaire can be used to facilitate the process. Then, a genital examination is performed.

7.2.1.21 Genital Examination

Genital examination is very important for diagnosis and treatment. Especially for patients with vaginismus and sexual discomfort, the genital examination process can be more challenging. Prior to the genital examination, explaining what to expect during it can be comforting for the patient. Depending on the severity of the problem, symptoms such as embarrassment, sweating due to sympathetic discharge, trembling, dizziness, vasovagal syncope, and nausea may often be observed. The examination should include only external inspection, and if the patient permits, the genital area can be pulled open for vestibular inspection. Again, if the patient permits, the pinky or index finger can be gently inserted into the vaginal canal. For patients with severe vaginismus or advanced pelvic hypertonicity, attempting to insert a speculum, use dilators, or perform bimanual touch or an anal touch can create additional trauma.

For vulvar vestibulitis (vestibulodynia), which is one of the main causes of superficial dyspareunia, sensitivity to the vestibular region is diagnostic during the "Q-tip test."Various skin conditions, like lichen sclerosus, can be easily diagnosed through external genital examination (Fig. 7.1a). A biopsy may be necessary for a definitive diagnosis and exclusion of malignancy.

If deep dyspareunia is suspected to be due to pelvic internal pathologies, a vaginal evaluation by speculum and manual palpation is crucial. After a short wait to allow the patient to relax, the urethra, bladder, vaginal walls, cervix, and adnexa are examined individually with one finger. Nodules associated with endometriosis are checked. If the patient permits, a two-finger examination can be performed to gather more detailed information. A thin, plastic speculum lubricated with gel can also be used for the examination, allowing for the assessment of sexually transmitted diseases.

7.2.1.22 Diagnostic Imaging

Transabdominal or transvaginal ultrasonography and pelvic MR imaging are important to rule out organic pathologies.

7.2.1.23 Pathophysiology

In vulvodynia, multiple factors are involved, generally suggesting neuropathic pathways. Localized vulvar pain is due to neurogenic inflammation, where inflammatory peptides, prostaglandins, and cytokines activate afferent nerves, subsequently stimulating the spinal cord. Impulses are then transported to the central nervous system via sympathetic afferent nerves and return with efferent fibers, completing the pain loop. "Allodynia" (pain from stimuli that should not be painful) in vaginismus and "hyperalgesia" (= hyperesthesia, or excessive response to mild pain) observed in vestibulodynia can be explained by this hypothesis.

7.2.1.24 Etiology

The issue in dyspareunia is generally due to an organic pathology, but it can sometimes be psychological in origin. However, even if it is not primarily psychological, it can lead to different psychological and relationship problems over time. The pain during sexual intercourse can be superficial and deep (Table 7.2).

Table 7.2 Etiology of dyspareunia (superficial and deep pain)

Superficial pain
Inflammatory/dermatologic
Provoked vestibulodynia (PVD) Lichen sclerosus, lichen planus, and other inflammatory skin diseases Granuloma fissuratum Chemical irritants (soaps, douches, etc.) and vulvar dermatitis Skin allergies (condom, semen, and pads)
Superficial infectious
Recurrent vulvovaginal candidiasis Sexually transmitted infections (herpes and trichomoniasis)
Neoplastic
Paget disease Vulvar and vaginal intraepithelial neoplasms and premalignant lesions Pelvic neoplasms (cervical, uterine, ovarian, and colon)
Neurological
Postherpetic neuralgia Nerve compression or injury (pudendal nerve or genitofemoral nerve entrapment) Neuroma
Traumatic
Female genital mutilation Obstetric lacerations and episiotomy scars
Structural (anatomical)
Congenital abnormalities of the hymen (imperforate hymen and septate hymen) Müllerian agenesis
Latrogenic
Genital operations (Bartholin cyst excision, vaginoplasty, labiaplasty, and vaginal hysterectomy) Cancer treatments: chemotherapy and radiation
Hormonal
Genitourinary syndrome (GUS) of menopause Lactational amenorrhea Anorexia nervosa Hyperprolactinemia Oophorectomy
Psychogenic
Vaginismus Female sexual arousal/interest disorder (FSAID) Other psychopathologies (somatization, depression, and Obsessive Compulsive Disorder (OCB))

(continued)

Table 7.2 (continued)

Superficial pain
Deep pain
Endometriosis Leiomyoma Ovarian mass Pelvic adhesions Pelvic congestion syndrome Pelvic malignancies Chronic pelvic pain Skeletal and muscular diseases Gastrointestinal diseases (Irritable Bowel Syndrome (IBS) and inflammatory bowel diseases) Pelvic organ prolapse (POP) Uterine retroversion
Deep infectious
Pelvic inflammatory disease (PID) UTI

7.2.1.24.1 Infections

Vaginitis, cervicitis, endometritis, urinary tract infections (UTIs), and pelvic inflammatory disease (PID) are infection-related causes of dyspareunia. Asymptomatic vaginal candida infections, Herpes Simplex Virus (HSV), and bacterial vaginosis are reasons for sexual pain. Vaginal and cervical culture tests are important to check for infections. If growth occurs, the first step in treatment is to address the infection.

7.2.1.25 Vaginismus

Most patients with vaginismus cannot even attempt sexual penetration, so they do not experience pain at all. However, some can attempt and experience pain due to involuntary muscular spasms.

7.2.1.26 Dyspareunia and Vaginismus Pain Cycle (Dr. Eserdag Model)

Although the *DSM-5* states that vaginismus and dyspareunia overlap and should be evaluated together, in my view, these two criteria are quite different. Vaginismus is an issue of involuntary muscle contraction due to intense anxiety, preventing intercourse or making it very difficult. Anxiety causes contraction, which, in turn, causes pain, creating a vicious cycle. Dyspareunia is more about real pain felt during intercourse, resulting in contraction and worsening pain. In other words, in vaginismus, allodynia (interpreting pain where there should not be) is present, while in dyspareunia, hyperesthesia (increased reaction to painful stimuli, or sensory nerve hypersensitivity) is more pronounced. Vaginismus is more centrally driven, while dyspareunia is more peripherally driven. In vaginismus treatment, reducing anxiety and changing the learned wrong behavior through systematic desensitization help break the vicious cycle, whereas in dyspareunia, the organic problem can turn into a psychological one over time. This can lead to "negative conditioning," anxiety, depression, and pelvic hypertonicity, which require psychological support and pelvic rehabilitation exercises after hyperesthesia treatment.

In our study, we emphasized the importance of a gynecological examination before starting vaginismus treatment. After the examination, the exact reason for the inability to engage in sexual intercourse will be identified—whether pain initiates muscle spasms or vice versa. Any congenital or acquired anatomical abnormalities that may obstruct intercourse will be detected. Moreover, the severity of vaginismus, which has five different levels, is crucial for treatment planning.

7.2.1.27 Vulvar Vestibulitis (Vestibulodynia and Provoked Vestibular Vulvodynia)

Vulvar vestibulitis is a common cause of superficial dyspareunia but is often overlooked by gynecologists. Characterized by hypersensitivity of the vestibular area, it may be triggered by chronic infections, HPV, mechanical irritation, or prolonged use of birth control pills.

It was first described by Friedrich in 1987 as [22]:

(a) Severe pain on vestibular touch or attempted vaginal entry
(b) Tenderness to pressure localized within the vulvar vestibule
(c) No evidence of physical findings except for varying degrees of erythema

In 1988, Friedrich added that symptoms must be present for at least 6 months and be of moderate to severe intensity. In 1991, Goetsch refined a test to measure the tenderness to pressure using a cotton swab applied to six designated sites [23]. Sometimes, vestibular hyperemia is present (Fig. 7.2), but it is not mandatory in patients with vulvar vestibulitis.

The examination should also check for infections or irritations in this region. A complete evaluation requires "pain mapping," with the patient rating pain levels from 0 (none) to 10 (worst) at positions 2-4-6-8-10 on a visual analog scale. A culture test can be performed to check for asymptomatic fungal infections. The patient's complaints and a positive Q-tip test can lead to a diagnosis of "vestibulodynia."

Initial treatment involves avoiding irritants. Conservative approaches include lubricants, anesthetic creams, and medications. Vestibular hyaluronic acid injection is also a promising management option in provoked vestibulodynia

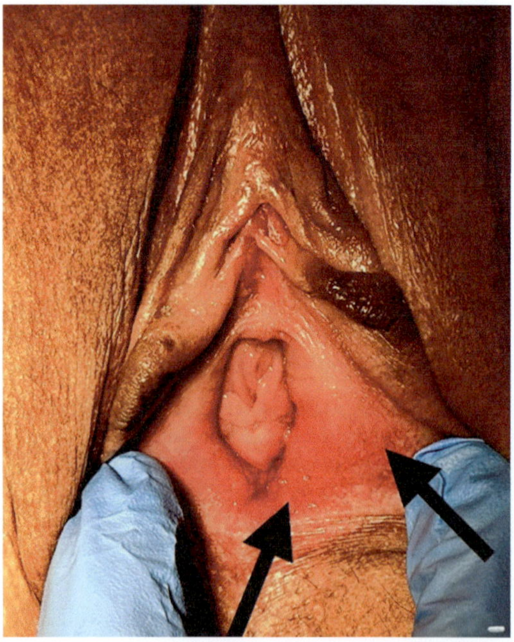

Fig. 7.2 Marked vestibular hyperemia in a vulvar vestibulitis patient

[24]. In resistant cases, surgical excision of the vestibular mucosa (partial vulvar vestibulectomy operation) can be performed. It is also recommended to send the excised tissue for pathological examination, particularly to investigate histological findings related to HPV. A study reports that cellular changes associated with HPV were detected in the vestibular mucosa of women with superficial dyspareunia and vulvar vestibulitis [25]. Additionally, pelvic floor rehabilitation and psychological support are essential after surgery.

7.2.1.28 Vulvodynia

Vulvodynia refers to widespread vulvar pain lasting at least 3 months, often described as burning. It can be provoked or spontaneous. Treatment includes avoiding irritants, antidepressants, pelvic physiotherapy, and nerve blocks. Surgical intervention is limited to provoked vestibular vulvodynia. Capsaicin, botulinum toxin, and interferon can be considered as second-line options [26].

7.2.1.29 Vulvovaginal Atrophy

Vaginal atrophy due to estrogen deficiency is common in postmenopausal women, characterized by dryness, loss of elasticity, and pain. Topical estrogens are effective, with CO_2 laser and radiofrequency treatments as alternatives.

7.2.1.30 Lack of Sufficient Lubrication

In reproductive-age women, decreased lubrication is often due to a lack of sexual arousal, while in menopause, estrogen deficiency is the primary cause. Hormonal, vascular, or neurological factors may also contribute. Topical estrogens and regenerative methods are effective treatments.

7.2.1.31 Postpartum Dyspareunia

Postpartum pain can result from perineal trauma, increased prolactin levels, or postpartum depression. Treatments include lubricants, surgical correction of scars, and pelvic rehabilitation.

7.2.1.32 Endometriosis and Deep Pain

Ectopic endometrial tissue can cause deep dyspareunia, especially during intercourse. Treatment options include hormonal therapies and laparoscopic surgery.

7.2.1.33 Management

Management strategies for female GPPPD are varied and should be tailored to the underlying cause (Table 7.3). For instance, treating infections or hormonal imbalances can alleviate symptoms. Pelvic floor physical therapy and behavioral interventions are effective for managing pain due to muscle spasm or tension. For psychological contributors, cognitive-behavioral therapy or sex therapy is often recommended. In refractory cases, surgical interventions may be necessary. Furthermore, sexual dysfunctions of male partners should not be ignored. Spouses should be questioned for sexual dysfunction and included in the treatment process [27].

7.2.2 Female Sexual Arousal/Interest Disorder (FSAID)

Sex is one of the most fulfilling human activities, offering excitement, pleasure, and satisfaction. Sexual arousal is often confused with desire, though these are entirely different concepts. Arousal typically precedes desire in the sexual

Table 7.3 Management of the female genito-pelvic pain/penetration disorder (GPPPD)

Cognition
Verbal suggestions and encouragement
Sexual awareness exercises
Information about genital anatomy and physiology
Motivational and positive thinking methods
Information about coitus, reproduction, and contraception
Exercises
Mirror exercises
Breathing techniques
Sensate focus and genital massage
Pelvic floor muscle and Kegel exercises
Progressive relaxation
Progressive finger and vaginal trainer exercises
Main treatment methods
Pelvic floor physiotherapy
Psychological managements
Surgical interventions
Pharmacological agents
Botulinum toxin injections

cycle, yet they are interconnected. Sometimes, desire influences arousal, and other times, arousal impacts desire—they may even occur simultaneously. Arousal is the body's response to sexual stimuli (visual, auditory, tactile, mental, physical, etc.), preparing it for sexual intercourse. It involves a series of physical, hormonal, neurological, and psychological changes that begin and intensify before any sexual activity (intercourse, masturbation, foreplay, and coitus) and progress throughout the body. With the continuation of stimuli, arousal strengthens and moves toward orgasm in the cycle [28].

7.2.2.1 Prevalence

This process varies greatly, with the duration of each phase and transitions between them depending on a combination of physical, medical, psychological, social, and partner-related factors. These variations also occur differently each time. Physical changes during arousal include vaginal lubrication and tumescence, clitoral erection and enlargement, cervical and uterine elevation, vulvar and labial congestion, breast firmness, nipple erection, and tachycardia.

7.2.2.2 Definition

According to the diagnostic criteria for FSAID in the *DSM-5* [1], a lack of or significantly reduced sexual interest/arousal is manifested by at least three of the following, occurring for a minimum of 6 months and leading to significant distress:

- Sexual interest: Absent/reduced frequency of sexual thoughts, fantasies, or desire
- Sexual initiation: No or significantly reduced initiation of sexual activity and typically unresponsive to the partner's attempts to initiate
- Sexual excitement/pleasure during sexual activity: Absence or significantly reduced excitement or pleasure during sexual activity in most or all sexual encounters
- Sexual excitement/pleasure in response to sexual cues: Absence or significant reduction of sexual excitement/pleasure in response to internal or external sexual cues (e.g., erotic thoughts and visual sexual cues)
- Genital or nongenital sensations during sexual activity: Absence or significant reduction in genital or nongenital sensations during sexual activity in most or all sexual encounters

7.2.2.3 Prevalence

Arousal disorders affect 12.2–17% of women, and hypoactive sexual desire disorder (HSDD) affects 7.3–23%, varying based on factors such as age, cultural background, and reproductive status [29, 30].

7.2.2.4 Diagnosis

Diagnosis of FSAID involves anamnesis, including medical, sexual, and psychological history (reviewing illnesses, surgeries, medications, and hormonal levels and evaluating sexual background and psychological factors) and gynecological examination (identifying issues like vaginal atrophy, infections, inflammations, or pelvic muscle problems).

7.2.2.5 Etiology

The etiology of FSAID is complex and may include biological, psychological, and relational factors. Hormonal changes, such as those associated with menopause or postpartum, can impact sexual desire and arousal. Psychological factors like stress, depression, anxiety, and relationship issues play significant roles. Additionally, medical conditions such as diabetes, cardiovascular diseases, and thyroid dysfunctions can contribute to desire and arousal difficulties. Desire is mostly a psychological process, whereas arousal is a neurovascular response, so issues affecting the genito-pelvic nervous system or blood flow (e.g., surgery and radiotherapy) can impair it.

7.2.2.6 Cultural Factors

Early life experiences and societal views on femininity and sexuality play a significant role in the development of sexual issues in women. For instance, ingrained gender biases, such as favoring male offspring, can lead to systemic challenges for women, ultimately shaping their adult sexual identity and behavior. This societal conditioning can impose restrictive roles, such as being "silent," compliant to male desires, and unable to assert one's own sexual needs.

7.2.2.7 Psychological Factors

Psychological barriers, including a lack of trust in a partner, past trauma, false beliefs, and personality traits (e.g., perfectionism), can impact desire and arousal. For example, a woman who enjoys masturbation but cannot engage in a relationship, even with someone she is attracted to, may need to be evaluated for physical causes. Partners of women with desire or arousal problems may also harbor incorrect beliefs, such as *"She doesn't love me or doesn't find me attractive."* Solving these misconceptions requires open communication.

7.2.2.8 Sexual Myths

Sexual myths and prejudices contribute significantly to desire and arousal disorders. Women raised with taboos, such as considering sexuality as shameful or sinful, may develop distorted views about their own sexual function. These myths promote unrealistic standards, instill anxiety, and hinder healthy sexual function.

7.2.2.9 Management

As with other FSDs, the management of FSAIDs should be individualized for the patient with a multidisciplinary approach, and it includes cognitive and behavioral sexual therapies as the gold standard. Cognitive management includes providing information regarding sexuality, sexual function, and anatomy, as well as psychoeducation. Behavioral therapies focus on relaxation techniques and sexual exercises. Rebuilding the partner relationship is also essential. By addressing both individual and relational factors, treatment enhances both sexual health and the overall relationship.

Hormonal therapies, such as estrogen or testosterone replacement, may be beneficial if hormonal deficiencies are identified, especially in the postmenopausal term. Psychotherapy, particularly CBT or sex therapy, is effective in addressing underlying psychological issues. Lifestyle modifications, such as stress management, exercise, and yoga, are also recommended. In some cases, medications like phosphodiesterase type 5 inhibitors (commonly used for erectile dysfunction) may be considered off-label to improve genital arousal. Vaginal laser [31], platelet-rich plasma (PRP) [32], and vaginal radiofrequency [33] applications can also alleviate vaginal dryness problems in menopause and enhance sexuality.

7.2.3 Female Orgasmic Disorder (FOD)

In women, orgasm is a sudden, transient, and intense sensation of pleasure that temporarily alters consciousness. It typically involves involuntary rhythmic contractions of the pelvic striated muscles, along with uterine and perianal contractions, and is accompanied by myotonia, which resolves sexually induced vasocongestion. This results in a feeling of well-being and relaxation.

Women's orgasms vary according to biological, physiological, sociocultural, and personal factors. Female orgasm begins with rhythmic contractions in the outer one-third of the vaginal muscles. These contractions are accompanied by sensations in the pelvic area and a strong feeling of pleasure perceived by the brain's pleasure centers. The intensity and frequency of these contractions differ from person to person. During orgasm, the vagina widens further, its length increases, and uterine contractions occur. Typically, 3–10 contractions are experienced, lasting 3–15 s. Orgasms are categorized as clitoral or vaginal, though the clitoris is always considered a core organ.

Female orgasms can be induced through erotic stimulation of various genital or nongenital areas. Conscious awareness is not a prerequisite; orgasms can also occur during sleep.

7.2.3.1 Definition

Female orgasmic disorder (FOD) is defined as the inability to achieve orgasm or a significant delay or reduction in the intensity of orgasm during sexual activity. Complete inability to orgasm is also termed “anorgasmia.”

Diagnosis of FOD is clinical, based on criteria in the *DSM-5* [1]:

- Delayed, infrequent, or absent orgasm or markedly decreased intensity of orgasm after a normal sexual arousal phase on all or almost all occasions of sexual activity
- Distress or interpersonal problems due to orgasmic dysfunction
- No other disorder or substance that exclusively accounts for the orgasmic dysfunction

Symptoms must have been present for at least 6 months.

Because the type of stimulation that triggers orgasm varies widely, clinicians must use clinical judgment to determine whether the woman’s response is deficient, based on her age, sexual experience, and the adequacy of the sexual stimulation she receives.

7.2.3.2 Prevalence

Orgasm disorders are the second most common cause of female sexual dysfunction, affecting 20% of women. Studies suggest that orgasm disorders affect 11–41% of women, with 18.4% experiencing orgasm solely during intercourse, while 36.6% require clitoral stimulation to achieve orgasm [34].

7.2.3.3 Types

It can be primary (lifelong), secondary (acquired), situational, and general.

- *Primary or Lifelong Orgasm Disorder*
  This condition occurs when a person has never experienced an orgasm. It applies to cases where there has been no attempt to achieve orgasm or no orgasm despite adequate stimulation and sexual interaction. While feelings of arousal and pleasure may exist, orgasm does not occur.
- *Secondary Orgasm Disorder*
  This condition involves difficulty in achieving orgasm or an inability to orgasm in situations where it was previously possible. Secondary orgasm disorders are often linked to hypoactive sexual desire disorder (HSDD), past pelvic surgeries, or medication effects.
- *Situational Orgasm Disorder*
  Individuals can orgasm in specific situations or environments but fail to do so in different contexts. Factors like habits, religious beliefs, familial influences, crowded settings, lighting, noise, fear of being noticed, and different scents may contribute.
- *General Orgasm Disorder*
  This refers to an inability to orgasm despite adequate stimulation at any moment and in any situation.

Several sexual response models have been proposed for women. Kaplan’s model highlights that sexual desires, such as thoughts and fantasies, are necessary for initiating subsequent phases like arousal and orgasm. This model has been instrumental in defining hypoactive desire disorder and advancing research in this area. Sexual activity in women can be initiated by internal desires, a partner’s physical stimulation, emotional intimacy, or cognitive motivation. Female sexual response phases—desire, arousal, and orgasm—are interconnected and overlapping.

Hormones such as testosterone, dopamine, estrogen, and norepinephrine exhibit positive feedback effects between the phases of desire and arousal. The parasympathetic nervous system is activated between the arousal and plateau phases. Oxytocin also positively affects orgasm. Nitric oxide, vasoactive intestinal peptide (VIP), serotonin, acetylcholine, prostaglandins, substance P, neuropeptides, progesterone, and prolactin also play roles in these stages.

A young woman trying to explore her body may initially attempt to orgasm through clitoral stimulation, using her hand or objects for rhythmic and circular stimulation. This typically occurs between the ages of 16 and 20.

If a woman achieves orgasm during the early stages of her sexual life, subsequent orgasms may become easier. However, if she never experiences orgasm, even with adequate stimulation, this is classified as primary orgasm disorder (anorgasmia). It is often linked to a history of trauma or sexual abuse.

7.2.3.4 Disorders in the Intensity and Duration of Orgasm

The quality of orgasm is influenced by numerous factors, including an individual's previous orgasmic experiences. Fears and misconceptions are primary factors affecting orgasm quality.

While a small proportion of women can regularly achieve high-quality, rhythmic, and consecutive orgasms, this is not common. Even healthy individuals may experience a low frequency of such orgasms, which can affect the quality of relationships, self-esteem, and mental health.

Women who orgasm once often do not lose sexual arousal, allowing them to continue sexual activity and experience multiple orgasms. Clitoral and vaginal orgasm disorders are evaluated separately. For instance, a woman may be able to achieve clitoral orgasms but not vaginal ones.

7.2.3.5 Etiology

The causes of FOD are varied and include the patient's own factors, partner and couple factors, environmental factors, chronic diseases, and certain medications (Table 7.4). Orgasm disorders occur in both men and women, but they are more prevalent in women.

7.2.3.6 Management

Management of FOD begins with a thorough history taking to identify causes. Rapidly developed disorders may require addressing biological causes. For long-term or lifelong issues, psychosexual causes are prioritized. Treatment approaches for FOD are individualized and may include cognitive-behavioral therapy (CBT), psychosexual therapy, mindfulness meditation therapy (MMT), pelvic physiotherapy, and hormone replacement therapy (HRT). Sensate focus exercises, masturbation, and other behavioral techniques are used to enhance sexual function and reduce anxiety around orgasm.

Medications in male partners, like selective serotonin reuptake inhibitors (SSRIs), may be used to manage performance anxiety or premature orgasm, in conjunction with behavioral therapy.

Table 7.4 Etiology of female orgasmic disorder (FOD)

Patient factors
Lack of sexual knowledge
Lack of sexual communication with partner
Lack of trust
High self-control
Subconscious guilt
Sexual phobias and/or taboos
Fear of pregnancy
Performance anxiety
Age and attractiveness concerns
Menopause and aging
Homosexuality
Vaginal looseness
Poor body image
STDs
Unhealthy or unintended sexual practices in the past
Partner and couple factors
Premature ejaculation and/or erectile dysfunction
Insufficient foreplay and short stimulation
Communicational or relational problems
Marital conflicts
Partner discrepancy
Domestic violence, discord, and oppression
Partner's sexual inexperience
Monotony in sexual life
Environmental factors
Economic problems and stressful life
Rigid religious, cultural, and moral aspects
Disasters
Substance and alcohol dependency: individuals who rely on substances for orgasm may be unable to achieve orgasm without them
Diseases
Cancer
Obesity
Type 1 and type 2 diabetes
Hypertension
High LDL and low HDL cholesterol
Psychogenic disorders
Substance addiction (alcohol, drugs, and smoking)
Neurological disorders (multiple sclerosis, spinal cord injury, etc.)
Chronic infections (vaginitis and cystitis)
Hormonal diseases (hypothyroidism and hyperthyroidism, high prolactin (PRL), low E2, and reduced testosterone)
Medications
High-dose corticosteroids
Chemotherapy and radiotherapy
Antihypertensives (alpha blockers, calcium channel blockers, and diuretics)
Central nervous system medications (tranquilizers)
Chemotherapeutic agents (busulfan, chlorambucil, and cyclophosphamide)
Hormonal medications (antiandrogens)
Antidepressants (fluoxetine, paroxetine, and sertraline)

Key Treatment Steps

- Sexual education
- Counseling
- Guided self-exploration
- Cognitive-behavioral therapy
- Masturbation training (manual or with vibrators)
- Stress management techniques
- Kegel exercises

Further measures include hormonal treatments, treating underlying infections, and lifestyle changes like exercise and balanced diets.

Additionally, different surgical and nonsurgical genital procedures, including vaginal laser applications and aesthetic and functional genital surgeries, can enhance genital appearance, increase stimulation, and boost comfort and self-confidence [35].

7.2.3.7 Medications

Drug therapies for general FSD are summarized in Table 7.5

Recommended supplements and herbs for orgasm support include cacao, saffron, garlic, cinnamon, and ginseng.

Table 7.5 Medications recommended for the treatment of FSD [36]

Agent/class	Formulation and mechanism of action	Evidence-based dosage	Primary indications
Menopausal hormone therapy (MHT)	Systemic estrogen (oral or transdermal), combined with progestogen when the uterus intact; restores genital trophism; enhances lubrication and blood flow; local estrogen improves mucosal integrity	Oral estradiol 0.5–1 mg/day; transdermal 25–50 μg/day; vaginal estradiol 10–25 μg maintenance 2–3×/week	Genitourinary Syndrome of Menopause (GSM)-related sexual pain, lubrication impairment, estrogen deficiency–related arousal issues. The FDA recently approved it
Progesterone (systemic or vaginal)	Oral micronized or vaginal progesterone for endometrial protection with systemic estrogen; neurosteroid metabolites may indirectly influence sexual function	Oral or vaginal route by micronized progesterone 100–200 mg/day	Adjunct to estrogen therapy, allowing safe treatment of GSM and estrogen-related dysfunction
Androgens (transdermal testosterone)	Transdermal formulations increasing central sexual motivation via dopaminergic pathways	~300 μg/day (studied dose)	HSDD in postmenopausal women
Vaginal DHEA(prasterone)	Prasterone is vaginal dehydroepiandrosterone (DHEA), a precursor hormone converted locally into estrogens and androgens within vaginal tissues	Insert using a small applicator similar to a suppository.6.5 mg vaginal insert once daily at bedtime	Postmenopausal women with vaginal dryness, dyspareunia, or genital arousal problems, especially those who prefer non-estrogen-labeled therapies
Tibolone	Steroid metabolized to estrogenic, progestogenic, and androgenic metabolites; tissue-selective	2.5 mg/day orally	Improves desire, arousal, lubrication
Ospemifene	SERM with estrogen-agonist vaginal actions, improving mucosal thickness and lubrication	60 mg/day orally	Dyspareunia, vaginal dryness (FDA-approved)

(continued)

Table 7.5 (continued)

Agent/class	Formulation and mechanism of action	Evidence-based dosage	Primary indications
Bupropion	NDRI enhancing dopamine/norepinephrine activity, increasing desire and arousal	150–300 mg/day orally	HSDD; antidepressant-associated dysfunction
Flibanserin	5-HT1A agonist/5-HT2A antagonist, resulting in the lowering of serotonin in the brain as well as an effect on increasing norepinephrine and dopamine neurotransmitters	100 mg/day orally at bedtime	FDA-approved for premenopausal HSDD ("female Viagra") [36]
Alprostadil (topical PGE1)	Increases genital blood flow via smooth muscle relaxation	Topical cream, apply before intercourse(limited benefit)	Arousal difficulties in postmenopausal women, mostly indicated in erectile dysfunction
Sildenafil	PDE5 inhibitor enhancing nitric oxide–mediated smooth muscle relaxation	50–100 mg orally (off-label)	Arousal disorder, especially vascular or SSRI-related
Apomorphine	Short-acting dopamine agonist	3 mg sublingual(not first-line)	Enhances desire and arousal; limited regional usage
Phentolamine mesylate	Nonselective α1/α2 antagonist improving genital blood flow	40 mg/day oral/topical(off-label)	Arousal disorder in postmenopausal women on HRT
Bremelanotide	MC4R agonist augmenting central desire pathways	1.75 mg SC, 45 min before sexual activity	FDA-approved for premenopausal HSDD

Recommended supplements and herbs for orgasm support include maca root (*Lepidium meyenii*), *Panax ginseng* (ginseng), saffron (*Crocus sativus*), *Tribulus terrestris*, and *Ginkgo biloba*

7.3 Male Sexual Dysfunction

Common sexual dysfunctions in men can be listed as follows [37, 38]:

1. Erectile dysfunction
2. Premature ejaculation
3. Low sexual desire disorder in men

7.3.1 Erectile Dysfunction

Erectile dysfunction is considered erectile dysfunction if one or more of the following conditions, such as significant difficulty in achieving an erection during sexual intercourse, difficulty in maintaining an erection until sexual intercourse is completed, and a significant decrease in the erection level, have persisted for at least 6 months [38].

Erectile dysfunction is a very common problem. Most men experience problems with erections at some point in their lives, especially when they are under stress or have a serious illness. If this problem persists for a long time, medical help should be sought. It has been found that 30% of men between the ages of 40 and 70 have some form of erectile dysfunction. The incidence and severity of erectile dysfunction increase with advancing age. Smoking and alcohol consumption, high blood pressure, diabetes, hyperlipidemia, heart disease, depression, and drugs used to treat these diseases are risk factors for erectile dysfunction [39].

7.3.1.1 Diagnosis of Erectile Dysfunction

Evaluation is required to diagnose erectile dysfunction in men. It should include a detailed medical and psychosexual history, a standard inquiry form questioning erectile functions, physical examination, and laboratory and radiological tests when necessary [40]. Figure 7.3 summarizes the standard baseline evaluation algorithm for a patient presenting with erectile dysfunction [40].

A detailed medical and psychosexual history is the most important part of the diagnostic evaluation. Taking the history in a comfortable environment and making the patient feel comfortable while explaining their complaints will make it easier to reach the diagnosis more quickly. The history should also include questioning the quality of erection, the presence of nocturnal erections, the duration of erectile dysfunction, the presence and duration of ejaculation, the level of sexual desire, the level of sexual intercourse in

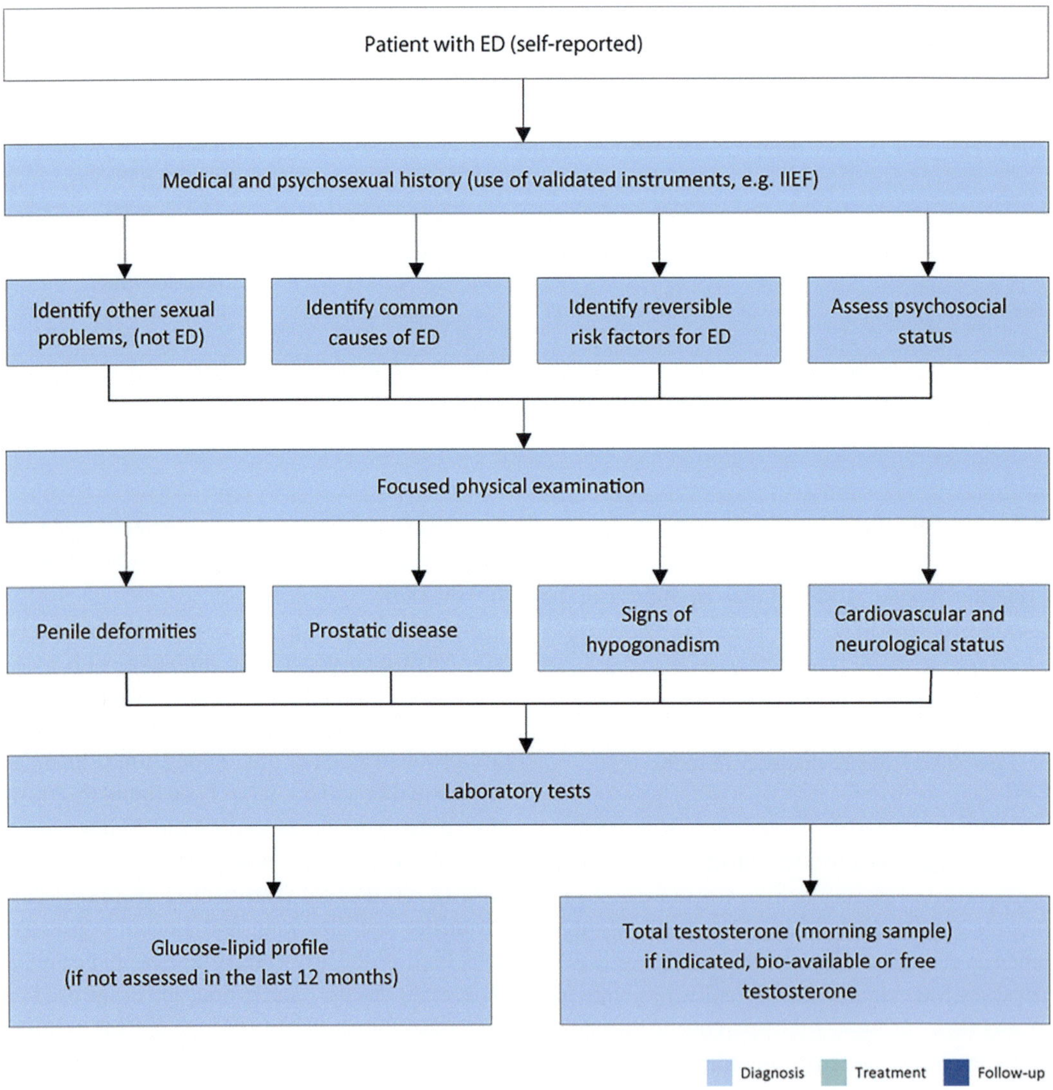

Fig. 7.3 Standard basic evaluation algorithm for a patient presenting with erectile dysfunction [41]

previous relationships, and the sexual functions of the female partner [42]. An idea can be obtained about the etiological type of erectile dysfunction with the findings obtained during the history. For example, the presence of nocturnal erections, a sudden onset of erectile dysfunction, concomitant psychological factors such as anxiety or performance-related fears, and sexual dysfunction in the female partner are suggestive of a psychogenic etiology. In contrast, the absence of nocturnal erections, a gradual progression of symptoms over time, and the presence of systemic problems such as aging, diabetes mellitus, and vascular disease are more indicative of an organic cause of erectile dysfunction [43].

During physical examination, breasts, hair distribution, testicles, and penis, which are organs that can examine genitourinary, endocrine, vascular, and neurological system diseases, should be examined carefully [44]. During the physical examination of the urogenital organs, the presence of Peyronie's disease in the penis, the presence of a precancerous or cancerous penile cancer, the presence of benign or malignant prostate disease in rectal examination, and the presence of hypogonadism by measuring the volume of the testicles can be easily detected. In addition, when an endocrine disease is suspected, thyroid gland examination, femoral and pedal pulsation in case of vascular disease, and genital and perineal sensation in case of a neurological disorder should be examined. A blood pressure and pulse measurement should be performed in patients who have not had a cardiological examination in the last 3–6 months [40].

Erectile functions can also be evaluated with inquiry forms. The most commonly used accredited inquiry form is the International Index of Erectile Function (IIEF). It evaluates five functions: erectile function, orgasm function, sexual desire, sexual intercourse satisfaction, and general satisfaction, with 15 questions [45]. According to the answers obtained with the IIEF-6 question shown in Table 7.6, if the total score is <10, severe erectile dysfunction is indicated; with a score between 11 and 16, moderate erectile dysfunction; with a score between 17 and 21, mild-to-moderate erectile dysfunction; and a score between 22 and 25 indicates the presence of mild erectile dysfunction, while a total score of ≥26 indicates normal erectile functions [45].

Table 7.6 International Index of Erectile Function (IIEF) domains of male sexual function [46]

Domain	Total score range	Item in each domain
Erectile function	1–30	Q1: ability to achieve an erection
		Q2: frequency of erections hard enough for penetration
		Q3: frequency of penetration
		Q4: ability to maintain an erection after penetration
		Q5: ability to maintain erection to sexual intercourse completion
		Q15: confidence in getting and maintaining erection
Orgasmic function	0–10	Q9: frequency of ejaculation
		Q10: frequency of orgasm
Sexual desire	2–10	Q11: frequency of sexual desire
		Q12: level of sexual desire
Intercourse satisfaction	0–15	Q6: frequency of attempted sexual intercourse
		Q7: satisfaction of sexual intercourse
		Q8: enjoyment of sexual intercourse
Overall satisfaction	2–10	Q13: satisfaction with sex life
		Q14: satisfaction with sexual relationship with partner

7.3.1.2 Laboratory Tests for Erectile Dysfunction

Tests requested in accordance with the European Urology Association Guidelines for patients presenting with impaired erectile function should include complete blood count, urinalysis, fasting glucose level, lipid profile, and serum testosterone level and other specific tests when necessary. After a detailed history, physical examination, and, if necessary, laboratory examination, advanced tests can be carried out to make a more definitive diagnosis according to the etiology of erectile dysfunction, and treatment options can be started without resorting to more advanced diagnostic methods.

In cases presenting with complaints of decreased sexual desire and nocturnal erections, the initial test should be to measure serum total testosterone level. In cases where the serum total testosterone level is borderline, the biologically active testosterone level should be determined by measuring serum albumin and free testosterone levels when making treatment decisions. Testosterone replacement therapy should be administered in cases with low serum testosterone levels. Additional laboratory tests include the measurement of prostate-specific antigen (PSA), luteinizing hormone (LH), and prolactin [40].

7.3.1.3 Radiological Examinations in Erectile Dysfunction

The etiology of erectile dysfunction can be determined by recording the severity and duration of nocturnal erections during sleep with the help of a device attached to the penis [47]. This test is called the nocturnal penile tumescence (NPT) test. While a vascular or neurological disorder is considered in the presence of a decrease in the frequency and severity of nocturnal erections, a diagnosis of psychogenic erectile dysfunction can be made in the presence of normal nocturnal erections (at least 60% rigidity lasting longer than 10 m) obtained in the NPT test [40].

Another test used in erectile dysfunction is the intracavernosal injection and stimulation test. It is the injection of a pharmacological agent such as papaverine or prostaglandin E1 into the cavernosal bodies and the subsequent observation of erection by visual or manual penile stimulation [48]. The test is considered normal if there is a rigid erection achieved within 10 m after the injection and lasting for at least 15 m. Failure to achieve adequate erection despite intracavernosal injection (arterial origin) or short duration of erection (venous insufficiency) suggests a vascular-induced erectile dysfunction. Significant side effects associated with intracavernosal injections include penile fibrosis, ecchymosis, and, rarely, priapism, which may necessitate urgent medical intervention [48]. Penile color Doppler ultrasonography provides information about the arterial and venous hemodynamic structure of the penis. Peak systolic blood flow velocity in both cavernosal arteries was 30 cm/sec. While a value above indicates a normal arterial system, end-diastolic blood flow is 3 cm/sec. A value below and a resistive index (RI) >0.8 indicate the presence of normal venous function. In the presence of abnormal findings, vascular system disease is considered [48].

The localization of arterial insufficiency suspected by penile color Doppler ultrasonography is best demonstrated by arteriography performed with the help of opaque material. Arterial insufficiency due to trauma in young men can be diagnosed with arteriography and can be corrected with arterial neovascularization surgery. Again, the diagnosis and localization of venous insufficiency suspected by penile color Doppler ultrasonography is best demonstrated by cavernosometry and cavernosography. By determining the localization of venous collaterals with cavernosography, venous surgery can be performed in appropriate cases [49].

7.3.1.4 Treatment for Erectile Dysfunction

The choice of treatment method in male sexual dysfunctions depends on the organic or psychogenic nature of the cause. If a young patient has an erection during sleep, his physical examination and blood/urine tests are normal, and his general condition is good, the cause is most likely psychogenic. In such a case, the help of clinicians specialized in sexual therapy should be sought. Interviews may be held in which the patient's partner also participates. In cases of erectile dysfunction (ED), premature ejaculation (PE), or sexual reluctance due to organic causes, cause-specific treatment can be applied.

Many hormonal factors play a role in the pathophysiology of ED. Hyperprolactinemia, thyroid dysfunction, and hypogonadism are the most common hormonal disorders that cause ED.

Studies have concluded that the incidence of low testosterone levels in men over the age of 40 with ED complaints is between 20% and 40% [50]. Testosterone replacement should be performed in men suffering from ED and hypogonadism. It is known that in ED cases with untreated hypogonadism, the response to other treatments used is not complete [51, 52].

Increased prolactin levels have been found to be associated with loss of libido and ED, especially in men. Increased prolactin levels are observed due to medication or functional adenomas of the anterior lobe of the pituitary gland. Oral prolactin inhibitors should be used first in the treatment of individuals with prolactinoma. In cases with large adenomas, it is recommended to remove the adenoma with surgery and then continue treatment with oral prolactin inhibitors if necessary. In cases with high serum prolactin levels and complaints of ED, magnetic resonance imaging should be performed. In general terms, it can be said that medical treatment should continue throughout life. Especially in cases with macroadenoma, complaints due to hyperprolactinemia recur when dopamine agonists are discontinued [53].

The physiopathology of the relationship between thyroid dysfunction and ED has not been fully demonstrated. However, it has been stated that hypothyroidism or hyperthyroidism is more common in men with ED. It is not necessary to routinely evaluate thyroid dysfunction in the ED approach.

7.3.1.5 Phosphodiesterase Type 5 (PDE5) Inhibitors

The first-line treatment for erectile dysfunction worldwide is PDE5 inhibitors. Studies on the use of PDE5 inhibitors have shown significant improvement in erectile function compared to placebo [54].

In a meta-analysis investigating the effectiveness of PDE5 inhibitors, according to the results of studies evaluating the effectiveness of sildenafil, the rate of successful sexual intercourse was found to be 69% (52–85%), and this rate was significantly higher than the 35.5% (19–68%) rate obtained in the placebo group. The common result of four studies evaluating successful relationship attempts was stated to be an increase of 34.4% [55].

When the studies evaluating the effectiveness of vardenafil were examined, it was seen that the rate of successful sexual intercourse was 68% with the use of vardenafil. This rate was found to be 35% in the placebo group. In two studies evaluating the increase in successful sexual intercourse, an increase of 33.2% was observed [56].

When the results of studies evaluating the contribution of tadalafil to successful sexual intercourse were evaluated, the rate of successful sexual intercourse in the tadalafil group was found to be 69%, and this rate was found to be significantly higher than the 33% rate obtained in the placebo group. In a study evaluating the increase in the frequency of successful sexual intercourse compared to the beginning, it was found that there was a 35.1% increase with the use of tadalafil [57]. In the study on avanafil in men with mild-to-moderate ED, patients were given 50-100-200 mg of avanafil or placebo. It was determined that patients showed significant improvement in all termination criteria with avanafil use compared to placebo after 12 weeks of treatment [58].

In the study conducted with udenafil, it was stated that a 91% success rate was achieved with 100- and 200-mg doses for vaginal penetration. It has been shown to be effective and safe in both diabetic patients and those with hypertension receiving multiple medical treatments [59]. In a study on single daily dose use of udenafil, 25-, 50-, and 75-mg doses were used, and a significant improvement was found compared to placebo [60].

In a study with lodenafil, 40- and 80-mg doses were compared with placebo, and the 80-mg dose was shown to be significantly more effective than both the 40-mg dose and placebo [61].

One of the most criticized aspects of treatment with PDE5 inhibitors is the inability to provide spontaneous sexual intercourse. In studies on this situation, it has been observed that this is achieved with daily use of tadalafil. Tadalafil can be used daily, thanks to its longer serum half-life than other PDE5 inhibitors. In this way, it is thought that a more natural sexual intercourse experience can be achieved, and this can provide a complete cure for ED [55, 62]. Chronic, low-dose PDE5 inhibitor therapy may be recommended for patients with difficult-to-treat diabetes, postprostatectomy ED, or post-radiotherapy ED or patients who do not respond to precoital PDE5 inhibitor use [63].

Although all PDE5 inhibitors have been shown to be effective in placebo-controlled studies, studies comparing different active ingredients are quite limited. The results obtained from comparative studies are far from revealing a clear conclusion, but it can be said that tadalafil is more preferred in these studies with its prolonged duration of action [64]. PDE5 inhibitors are well-tolerated in the treatment of ED. The most commonly reported side effects are headache, hot flushes, nasal congestion, nasopharyngitis, and dyspepsia. A less common but more serious side effect is priapism. Visual disturbances and hearing loss have also been reported with PDE5 inhibitors.

7.3.1.6 Other Pharmacological Treatments

L-arginine is the precursor of nitric oxide (NO) synthesis. In a study, L-arginine was given to 20 men for 2 weeks, and while six of the 15 men who completed the study achieved improvement in erection, no improvement was observed in nine [65]. High-dose L-arginine achieved 31% success in terms of successful sexual intercourse in the group with complete ED. No side effects have been observed with the use of L-arginine. However, a 10% decrease in blood pressure was observed in some patients, but it was stated that it had no clinical significance.

Apomorphine is a centrally acting dopamine receptor agonist. It is effective on the paraventricular nucleus, medial preoptic area, amygdala, and stria terminalis. Both testosterone and NO-dependent erection are achieved with apomorphine [66]. It is known that apomorphine reaches measurable levels in plasma within 10 m after taking the developed sublingual form and reaches its maximum plasma concentration within 1 h. Although apomorphine demonstrated a statistically significant improvement in erectile function compared with placebo, it was subsequently withdrawn from the European market. This decision was largely driven by evidence showing that sildenafil was significantly more effective than apomorphine, with approximately 94–95% of patients expressing a preference for sildenafil therapy [67].

Yohimbine is obtained from a tree called yohimbehe, which grows in Central Africa. Its first clinical use was in combination with papaverine for the treatment of ED. Until the introduction of sildenafil and other PDE5 inhibitors, yohimbine was one of the most commonly used drugs for the treatment of ED [68]. Yohimbine is a centrally acting alpha-2 receptor blocker. Its activity on presynaptic receptors is 50 to 100 times greater than its activity on postsynaptic receptors. Yohimbine also acts peripherally on the alpha-2 receptors of the penile arteries. Alpha-2 receptors in the presynaptic area eliminate the erection-suppressing effects of sympathetic alpha-1 receptors. Thus, the onset of erection becomes easier. In addition, yohimbine also has a relaxing effect on the smooth muscles in the corpus cavernosum [69]. Yohimbine is well-absorbed when taken orally, and its plasma half-life is 0.25–2.5 h. The majority of it is metabolized by the liver, and only 1% is excreted in the urine. The dose used in clinical studies is 5–15 mg three times a day. In clinical studies conducted with yohimbine, its effectiveness was observed at rates of up to 71%. A meta-analysis showed that there was a significant improvement with yohimbine compared to placebo. Side effects seen with yohimbine include symptoms of anxiety, nausea, restlessness, agitation, insomnia, tachycardia, diarrhea, and mania due to increased sympathetic activity. Another effect seen with the use of yohimbine is increased blood pressure. Caution should be exercised, especially in individuals receiving antihypertensive treatment. The use of yohimbine is contraindicated in patients who have recently had a myocardial infarction, in cases of hypertension that are difficult to treat, and in cases of severe liver failure [70].

7.3.1.7 Stem Cell Treatment

Stem cells are the main cells that form organs and tissues in the human body. These cells, which have not yet differentiated, have the ability to renew themselves, multiply continuously, and transform into other cell types. Although studies on the use of stem cells for ED treatment have focused on cavernous nerve (CN) damage and neurogenic ED, the subject has also been examined with experimental studies in models related to diabetes mellitus, metabolic syndrome, radiation damage, and aging. Rat blastocysts showed higher intracavernous pressure and better neurofilament staining than the embryonic stem cell (ESC) control group, and the curative effect of stem cell therapy in neurogenic ED was emphasized. The authors of the study suggested that the exact mechanism of action of stem cells is unknown, but they support axonal spread in the lesion area; increase the production of growth factors such as brain-derived neurotrophic factor (BDNF), nerve growth factor, and neurotrophin-3; and also act by reducing demyelination [71]. Albersen et al. evaluated [72] erectile function and penile histology by inducing CN in rats to which they administered stem cells obtained from adipose tissue intracavernosally after 4 weeks [72]. It was shown that significantly higher intracavernous pressure, less fibrosis, and better penile smooth muscle tissue ratio were detected in the treatment group compared to the control group. In another study, Xu et al. created micro-tissue from stem cells derived from fat cells in a rat model and injected this tissue intracavernosally, and they detected an improvement in intracavernous pressure and tissue histology [73]. In conclusion, although stem cell studies have been conducted on ED, which occurs due to almost all etiological reasons, the main problem is the lack of clinical studies on humans. Both cost, difficulties in obtaining stem cells, and ethical issues seem to lead to this situation.

7.3.2 Premature Ejaculation

In 1970, Masters and Johnson defined PE as "the inability to delay ejaculation," which fails to bring the woman to orgasm in 50% of relationships, and cited it as a cause of female anorgasmia [74]. Waldinger et al. reported the intravaginal ejaculation delay time, which is an objective method for the definition of PE (intravaginal ejaculation latency time (IELT)) in 1994 [75]. In 2000, the American Psychiatric Association defined PE in the *Diagnostic and Statistical Manual of Mental Disorders-IV-Text Revision (DSM-IV-TR)* as "persistent or repeated occurrence with minimal sexual stimulation, without the person willing. In the DSM-IV-TR, premature ejaculation (PE) was defined as persistent or recurrent ejaculation occurring with minimal sexual stimulation before, on, or shortly after penetration and before the individual wishes it, resulting in marked personal distress or interpersonal difficulties. The European Association of Urology (EAU) further describes PE as a male sexual dysfunction characterized by the inability to delay ejaculation sufficiently during vaginal intercourse, leading to negative personal consequences, including distress, frustration, and avoidance of sexual intimacy.

PE that begins with the first sexual intercourse and continues in all subsequent sexual intercourses is called primary or lifelong PE. PE that has a normal ejaculation time and occurs later is called secondary or acquired PE [76]. Many studies have shown that IELT measured with a stopwatch is under 1 min in 90% of the cases and between 1 and 2 min in 10% of the cases [77].

According to the International Society of Sexual Medicine report, PE is defined as "always, almost always, ejaculation within 1 min before, during, or after vaginal penetration, inability to delay ejaculation during almost every vaginal penetration; and negative personal effects such as anxiety, distress, disappointment, and loss of self-confidence in sexual intercourse." It is defined as "a sexual dysfunction that creates consequences" [78].

PE as a male sexual dysfunction according to the 2013 guidelines of the International Society for Sexual Medicine (ISSM) [79]:

(a) Lifelong PE, starting from the first sexual experience, when ejaculation always and almost always occurs before vaginal penetration or within about 1 min after vaginal penetration; acquired PE is defined as ejaculation delay time frequently decreasing to 3 min or less after a period of normal ejaculatory function.
(b) Inability to delay ejaculation at all or almost all vaginal entrances.
(c) It is defined as having negative personal consequences such as sadness, distress, disappointment, and loss of self-confidence in sexual intercourse.

Since PE is defined differently among experts and scientific institutions, it is very difficult to collect epidemiological data on PE worldwide and meta-analyze these data. For this reason, the prevalence of PE is not known clearly.

7.3.2.1 Diagnosis of Premature Ejaculation

Medical and sexual history are sufficient for the diagnosis of PE. With a good sexual history, lifelong and acquired PE can be diagnosed, and a differential diagnosis of other types of PE can be made. When taking a clinical history, diabetes, neuropathy, trauma, urogenital infections, previous surgical operations, and medications used should be questioned. Urination and ejaculation (nocturnal emissions) characteristics, educational status, psychological traumas, sexual fears, and beliefs should be questioned. Whether PE is acquired throughout life or later, whether it occurs with a partner or in special situations, and its continuity are questioned. It is especially necessary to learn the time of ejaculation. "How long is the time between penetration and ejaculation during sexual intercourse?" Determination of the intravaginal ejaculatory latency time (IELT) begins with a detailed clinical history. During the evaluation of premature ejaculation (PE), information should be obtained regarding the degree of sexual stimulation required to trigger ejaculation, the impact of the condition on sexual satisfaction, interpersonal relationships, and quality of life, as well as any previous or current treatments used for PE. In addition, alcohol consumption, substance use, and recreational drug use should be assessed. The diagnostic work-up of PE is based on a comprehensive sexual history, objective assessment of IELT by stopwatch measurement when feasible, and the use of validated diagnostic questionnaires. Several validated instruments are available for this purpose and are summarized in Table 7.7 [80].

There is no need for physical examination for men diagnosed with lifelong PE through history. In men with acquired PE, physical examination should be performed based on the etiological target. In the presence of comorbid conditions such as ED, physical examination should be performed. In the evaluation of men with PE, by performing vascular, endocrine, and nervous system examinations, conditions that cause PE or sexual dysfunction, such as chronic diseases, endocrinopathy, autonomic neuropathy, Peyronie's disease, urethritis, or prostatitis, can be detected. In the evaluation of a man with PE, laboratory and physiological tests should be performed according to the history and physical examination findings; they are not routinely recommended. A serum Thyroid-Stimulating Hormone (TSH) level below 0.2 μU/mL indicates the presence of hyperthyroidism. Two- or four-cup tests can be performed in men with suspected prostatitis [81].

7.3.2.2 Treatment for Premature Ejaculation

7.3.2.2.1 Topical Anesthetics

There are many studies showing that they delay the time of ejaculation by reducing the sensitivity of the glans penis. In addition, using more than the appropriate amount may cause loss of erection as it will increase the numbness too much.

As a topical anesthetic, lidocaine can be applied 20–30 min before sexual intercourse. However, attention should be paid to the dose of the drug used here. When using topical anesthetics, a condom must be used to prevent the medicine from affecting the vagina. Long-term application may lead to ED [82]. In one study, ejaculation time was prolonged from 1.67 min to 1.95 min in the placebo group and from 1.49 min to 8.45 min in the treatment group [83]. For premature ejaculation, the topical, water-soluble mixture contains 7.5 mg lidocaine and 2.5 mg prilocaine and is applied as a spray to the glans penis 10 min before sexual intercourse. Since it is less absorbed through the keratinized glans skin, penile numbness and ED are less common.

7.3.2.2.2 Selective Serotonin Reuptake Inhibitors (SSRIs)

Selective serotonin reuptake inhibitors (SSRIs) are among the most commonly preferred drugs in the treatment of premature ejaculation. However, when using antidepressants for this purpose,

Table 7.7 English version of the Premature Ejaculation Diagnostic Tool (PEDT) questionnaire [81]

Tool for Assessing Premature Ejaculation

This is a questionnaire to help identify men who may have a problem with ejaculating too soon during sexual activity. Even if you do not have difficulties, please answer all the questions.

- Please mark ☒ the box that best represents your answer for each of the questions below.
- Please mark <u>only one box</u> for each question.
- Remember there are no right or wrong answers to these questions.
- While your experiences may change from time to time, what we're interested in here is your general experience with intercourse.

Definition:
<u>Ejaculation</u> here refers to ejaculation (release of semen) after penetration (when your penis enters your partner)

	Not difficult at all	Somewhat difficult	Moderately difficult	Very difficult	Extremely difficult
1. How difficult is it for you to delay ejaculation?	☐ 0	☐ 1	☐ 2	☐ 3	☐ 4

	Almost never or never 0%	Less than half the time 25%	About half the time 50%	More than half the time 75%	Almost always or always 100%
2. Do you ejaculate before you want to?	☐ 0	☐ 1	☐ 2	☐ 3	☐ 4
3. Do you ejaculate with very little stimulation?	☐ 0	☐ 1	☐ 2	☐ 3	☐ 4

	Not at all	Slightly	Moderately	Very	Extremely
4. Do you feel frustrated because of ejaculating before you want to?	☐ 0	☐ 1	☐ 2	☐ 3	☐ 4
5. How concerned are you that your time to ejaculation leaves your partner sexually unfulfilled?	☐ 0	☐ 1	☐ 2	☐ 3	☐ 4

patients and their relatives should be informed about the possible side effects of these drugs. It should be emphasized that antidepressants may cause discomfort in the first days, that it takes some time for their effects to appear, and that they are not addictive.

The effectiveness and safety of SSRIs in delaying ejaculation have been demonstrated in many well-controlled, evidence-based meta-analyses, and their role in the first-line treatment of lifelong and acquired PE has been proven. Not all SSRIs delay ejaculation, and their effects in delaying ejaculation depend on their effects on the 5-HT receptor [80].

The first drugs used in the treatment of PE are paroxetine and clomipramine. Citalopram, fluoxetine, fluvoxamine, and sertraline, which have similar pharmacological effects, are the most commonly used drugs in the treatment of PE. According to studies, SSRI drugs increase intravaginal ejaculation latency time (IELT) by 2.6 to 13.2 times [80].

While the effectiveness of paroxetine in prolonging IELT was found to be greater than that of uoxetine, clomipramine, and sertraline, sertraline was found to be more effective than uoxetine, and the effectiveness of clomipramine was found to be similar to that of uoxetine and sertraline [76]. No difference was found between dose and response among the most commonly prescribed SSRIs, paroxetine, sertraline, fluoxetine, citalopram, and clomipramine. Citalopram was found to be less effective than these four drugs, and fluvoxamine was found to be ineffective in the treatment of PE.

The effectiveness of SSRIs in the treatment of PE can begin within a few days, but receptor insensitivity occurs after 1–2 weeks. Therefore, long-acting SSRIs are used daily. Studies on taking SSRIs as needed before intercourse are limited. It has been shown that clomipramine, a tricyclic antidepressant and norepinephrine and serotonin reabsorption inhibitor, prolongs IELT when taken 3–5 h before intercourse, although it remains lower than during daily use [76].

The most common side effects are weakness, drowsiness, yawning, nausea, vomiting, dry mouth, diarrhea, and sweating, which are usually mild and disappear after 2–3 weeks. They have also been reported to cause sexual dysfunctions such as decreased libido, anorgasmia, anejaculation, and ED [76].

Dapoxetine: It is a new, well-tolerated, effective, short-acting SSRI and is suitable for use on demand in the treatment of PE [76]. Dapoxetine, like other SSRIs, shows its effect by blocking serotonin reabsorption transporters [84]. Many studies have shown that dapoxetine prolongs IELT and is also effective when taken as the first dose 1–3 h before intercourse. Dapoxetine at doses of 30 mg and 60 mg has been shown to increase intravaginal ejaculatory latency time (IELT) by approximately 2.5-fold and 3-fold, respectively. In men with a baseline IELT of less than 30 seconds, the improvement was even more pronounced, with IELT increasing by approximately 3.5-fold and 4-fold, respectively [85]. In another study, it was found that 30 and 60 mg of dapoxetine taken 1–2 h before intercourse increased IELT in the first dose, helped control ejaculation, reduced stress, and increased satisfaction. Dapoxetine has similar effectiveness in lifelong and acquired PE [86]. Side effects associated with dapoxetine treatment are dose-related, and nausea, diarrhea, headache, and fatigue are the most commonly reported side effects.

7.3.2.2.3 Phosphodiesterase Type 5 (PDE5) Inhibitors

Men with PE are also likely to have ED. While PE and ED may occur together due to performance anxiety, PE may also develop due to the necessity of premature ejaculation due to ED. In both cases, PDE5 inhibitors can be used in treatment.

Although sildenafil does not prolong IELT, it increases self-confidence, ejaculation control, and sexual satisfaction; it also reduces anxiety and the refractory period for the second erection after ejaculation. When combined with sildenafil, paroxetine, and sertraline, it prolongs IELT more than an SSRI alone. Additionally, sildenafil significantly prolongs IELT when combined with SSRIs and behavioral therapy or with behavioral therapy alone [87]. Vardenafil has been reported to prolong IELT and improve results. In men with lifelong PE, the time to ejaculation by vibroejaculation in a laboratory environment was investigated for sildenafil, tadalafil, and vardenafil, and only vardenafil was found to prolong the ejaculation time due to vibro-stimulation [88]. In another study, it was shown that the combination of tadalafil and fluoxetine significantly prolonged IELT compared to tadalafil, fluoxetine, and placebo [89].

7.3.3 Low Sexual Desire Disorder

Low sexual desire disorder in men is considered to be a condition in which sexual thoughts or fantasies and desire for sexual activity are constantly or recurrently low or absent and persist for at least 6 months [74]. The existence of sexual desire depends on some variables: biological factors, sexual experiences, self-esteem, the presence of a suitable partner, and a good relationship with the partner in nonsexual areas. Difficulties in one or more of these variables may reduce sexual desire [90]. An Australian study involving

8517 men found low desire to be the most common sexual difficulty (24.9%). Around 17.1% of men reported low desire for at least 1 month in the last year [91]. As men get older, erectile and orgasmic problems, as well as a lack of sexual desire, become more common due to psychological changes and medical factors. However, education has a protective effect in terms of sexual difficulties. While the prevalence of low sexual desire is rare (2%) under the age of 55, it is approximately 7% in those aged 55 and over. In men under the age of 45, 4–11% reported low desire in at least half of their sexual activities. Erectile difficulties, seen in 63.2% of men with low sexual desire, are the most common accompanying sexual problem [91].

Boys generally learn about sexuality through masturbation between the ages of 10 and 16 [92]. Adolescents and young men can easily and largely autonomously engage in sexual experiences with their partners. In other words, they do not need the help of their partners for sexual desire, arousal, and orgasm. Premature ejaculation, the most common sexual problem, does not generally negatively affect sexual desire. Men's sexual socialization and these early learning experiences may result in sexual dysfunction and decreased sexual desire with aging and the aging of their relationships [93].

It is thought that 20% of the entire population has decreased sexual desire disorder. In cases where sexual desire has decreased, possible organic conditions should be excluded, and the patient's psychological state and sexual knowledge should be reviewed. Existing psychiatric disorders should be treated. Decreased sexual desire increases people's distress and causes difficulties between partners. Most studies have shown that sexual desire decreases with age. However, interestingly, the degree of complaint about decreased sexual desire also decreases with age. Culture also affects sexual desire. Overly strict attitudes about sexuality can cause a decrease in sexual desire. Sexual reluctance can affect the frequency of sexual intercourse. There is no frequency of sexual intercourse defined as sexual "normality." There are many factors that affect the frequency of sexual intercourse: Age, equality, intercourse process, time, relationship status, reproductive purpose, and use of birth control methods are some of them. Since decreased sexual desire can be caused by a wide variety of reasons, a detailed evaluation is needed before starting sexual therapy. In some cases, a urology examination may also be needed.

7.4 Conclusion

Since male and female sexual dysfunction can stem from multiple causes, it requires a multidisciplinary and holistic approach to treatment. Treatments may involve psychiatrists, gynecologists, urologists, psychologists, family counselors, sociologists, and physiotherapists. Humans are biopsychosocial beings and should be evaluated from different perspectives. Instead of adopting a dogmatic approach to a single method, combining various methods will yield higher treatment success in a shorter time.

References

1. American Psychiatric Association. Diagnostic and statistical manual of mental disorders. 5th ed. Arlington: American Psychiatric Publishing; 2013. p. 423–44.
2. Cherner RA, Reissing ED. A comparative study of sexual function, behavior, and cognitions of women with lifelong vaginismus. Arch Sex Behav. 2013;42:1605–14.
3. Borg C, Peters LM, Weijmar-Schultz W, de Jong PJ. Vaginismus: heightened harm avoidance and pain catastrophizing cognitions. J Sex Med. 2012;9(2):497–506.
4. World Health Organization. International classification of diseases, 11th revision (ICD-11). Geneva: World Health Organization; 2019. Retrieved from https://icd.who.int/
5. Spector I, Carey M. Incidence and prevalence of the sexual dysfunctions: a critical review of the empirical literature. Arch Sex Behav. 1990;19:389–96.
6. Crowley T, Goldmeier D, Hiller J. Diagnosing and managing vaginismus. BMJ (Clin Res Ed). 2009;338:b2284. https://doi.org/10.1136/bmj.b2284.
7. Lahaie MA, Boyer SC, Amsel R, et al. Vaginismus: a review of the literature on the classification/diagnosis, etiology, and treatment. Women's Health (Lond Engl). 2010;6(5):705–19.

8. Jeng CJ. The pathophysiology and etiology of vaginismus. Taiwan J Obstet Gynecol. 2004;43:10–5.
9. Eserdağ S, Sevinc T, Tarlacı S. Do women with vaginismus have a lower threshold of pain? Eur J Obstet Gynecol Reprod Biol. 2021;258:189–92. https://doi.org/10.1016/j.ejogrb.2020.12.059.
10. Eserdağ S, Anğın AD. Importance of gynecological assessment for the treatment of vaginismus as a predictive value. J Obstet Gynaecol Res. 2021;47(7):2537–43.
11. Lamont JA. Vaginismus. Am J Obstet Gynecol. 1978;131:633–6.
12. Pacik PT, Babb CR, Polio A, Nelson CE, Goekeler CE, Holmes LN. Case series: redefining severe grade 5 vaginismus. Sex Med. 2019;7(4):489–97.
13. Eserdağ S, Zülfikaroglu E, Akarsu S, Micozkadıoglu S. Treatment outcome of 460 women with vaginismus. Eur J Surg Sci. 2011;2(3):73–9.
14. Eserdağ S, Ezberci Akgün M, Şükrü Gürbüz F. Outcomes of vaginismus therapy assessed by penetrative intercourse, psychiatric symptoms, and marital satisfaction. J Sex Marital Ther. 2023;49(4):412–9.
15. Coppini A. A case of primary vaginismus. Int Forum Psychoanal. 1999;8(1):49–52.
16. Lemke W. Utilizing hypnosis and ego-state therapy to facilitate healthy adaptive differentiation in the treatment of sexual disorders. Am J Clin Hypn. 2005;47(3):179–89.
17. Brin Mitchell F, et al. Treatment of vaginismus with botulinum toxin injections. Lancet. 1997;349(9047):252–3.
18. Pacik PT. Vaginismus: review of current concepts and treatment using Botox injections, bupivacaine injections, and progressive dilation with the patient under anesthesia. Aesth Plast Surg. 2011;35:1160–4.
19. Torun F. Vajinismusun EMDR Yöntemi ile Tedavisi: Iki Olgu Sunumu [Treatment of vaginismus with EMDR: a report of two cases]. Turk Psikiyatri Derg. 2010;21(3):243–8.
20. Yetkin N. Vaginismus. Sex Funct Disord Monogr Ser, Türk Psikiyatri Dizini. 1999;3:26–9.
21. Brotto LA, Liao M. Dyspareunia in women: prevalence, risk factors, and treatment options. J Sex Med. 2014;11(7):1694–703.
22. Bergeron S, Binik YM, Khalifé S, Pagidas K, Glazer HI. Vulvar vestibulitis syndrome: reliability of diagnosis and evaluation of current diagnostic criteria. Obstet Gynecol. 2001;98(1):45–51.
23. Masheb RM, Nash JM, Brondolo E, Kerns RD. Vulvodynia: an introduction and critical review of a chronic pain condition. Pain. 2000;86(1–2):3–10.
24. Eserdağ S, Akdag Özkok B, Süphan Ersahin S, Zeynep Yilmaz E. Vestibular hyaluronic acid injection in provoked vestibulodynia patients and its effect on pain and sexual function: a preliminary report. Eur J Obstet Gynecol Reprod Biol. 2023;280:64–7.
25. Eserdağ S, Kurban D, Kiseli M, Alan M, Alan Y. The histopathological results of vestibulectomy specimens in localized provoked vulvodynia in Turkey. Pan Afr Med J. 2020;37:267. https://doi.org/10.11604/pamj.2020.37.267.21240.
26. Goldstein AT, Pukall CF, Brown C, Bergeron S, Stein A, Kellogg-Spadt S. Vulvodynia: assessment and treatment. J Sex Med. 2016;13(4):572–90.
27. Eserdağ S, Kurban D, Yakut E, Mishra PC. Insights into the vaginismus treatment by cognitive behavioral therapies: correlation with sexual dysfunction identified in male spouses of the patients. J Fam Reprod Health. 2021;15(1):61–9.
28. Basson R. The female sexual response: a different model. J Sex Marital Ther. 2000;26(1):51–65.
29. Bancroft J, Loftus J, Long S. Distress about sex: a national survey of women in heterosexual relationships. Arch Sex Behav. 2003;32:193–208.
30. Dunn K, Croft P, Hackett G. Sexual problems: a study of the prevalence and need for health care in the general population. Fam Pract. 1998;15:519–24.
31. Paraiso MFR, Ferrando CA, Sokol ER, Rardin CR, Matthews CA, Karram MM, Iglesia CB. A randomized clinical trial comparing vaginal laser therapy to vaginal estrogen therapy in women with genitourinary syndrome of menopause: the VeLVET trial. Menopause. 2020;27(1):50–6.
32. Waghe T, Acharya N, Karnik M, Mohammad S, Patel NA, Gemnani R. Role of platelet-rich plasma in genitourinary syndrome of menopause. Cureus. 2024;16(1):e53316.
33. Gueldini de Moraes AV, Costa-Paiva L, da Costa Machado H, Maciel TF, Mariano FV, Pedro AO. Comparison of the effect of noninvasive radiofrequency with vaginal estrogen and vaginal moisturizer in the treatment of vulvovaginal atrophy in postmenopausal women: a randomized clinical trial. Menopause. 2024;31(4):288–302. https://doi.org/10.1097/GME.0000000000002169.
34. Rellini AH, Clifton J. Female orgasmic disorder. Adv Psychosom Med. 2011;31:35–56. https://doi.org/10.1159/000327315.
35. Eserdağ S, editor. Aesthetic and functional female genital surgery. New York: Springer; 2023. https://doi.org/10.1007/978-3-031-16019-6.
36. Prabhu SS, Hegde S, Sareen S. Female sexual dysfunction: a potential minefield. Ind J Sex Transmit Dis AIDS. 2022;43(2):128–34. https://doi.org/10.4103/ijstd.ijstd_56_22.
37. C INCESU. Dsm-5 ve Cinsel İşlev Bozuklukları. Arch Neuropsych/Nöropsikiyatri Arşivi. 2011;48
38. Edition, F., Diagnostic and statistical manual of mental disorders. Am Psychiatric Assoc, 2013. 21(21): p. 591–643.
39. Martin C, et al. Current and emerging therapies in premature ejaculation: where we are coming from, where we are going. Int J Urol. 2017;24(1):40–50.
40. Hatzimouratidis K, Hatzimouratidis K, Eardley I, Giuliano F, Moncada I, Salonia A. Guidelines on male sexual dysfunction: erectile dysfunction and premature ejaculation. Reply to Pero Bokarica's letter to the editor re: European Association of Urology Website. https://uroweb.org/guideline/

male-sexual-dysfunction/. Updated 2015. Eur Urol. 2015;68(4):e78.
41. Salonia A, et al. European Association of Urology guidelines on sexual and reproductive health—2021 update: male sexual dysfunction. Eur Urol. 2021;80(3):333–57.
42. Melman A, Fogarty J, Hafron J. Can self-administered questionnaires supplant objective testing of erectile function? A comparison between the International Index of Erectile Function and objective studies. Int J Impot Res. 2006;18(2):126–9.
43. Kendirci M, et al. Prevalence of male pelvic dysfunction: results from the Turkish society of andrology male sexual health study group. Andrology. 2014;2(2):219–24.
44. Ghanem HM, Salonia A, Martin-Morales A. SOP: physical examination and laboratory testing for men with erectile dysfunction. J Sex Med. 2013;10(1):108–10.
45. Rosen RC, et al. Development and evaluation of an abridged, 5-item version of the International Index of Erectile Function (IIEF-5) as a diagnostic tool for erectile dysfunction. Int J Impot Res. 1999;11(6):319–26.
46. Glina S, et al. Efficacy and safety of flexible-dose oral sildenafil citrate (Viagra®) in the treatment of erectile dysfunction in Brazilian and Mexican men. Int J Impot Res. 2002;14(2):S27–32.
47. Kessler WO. Nocturnal penile tumescence. Urol Clin N Am. 1988;15(1):81–6.
48. Sikka SC, et al. Standardization of vascular assessment of erectile dysfunction. J Sex Med. 2013;10(1):120–9.
49. Glina S, Ghanem H. SOP: corpus cavernosum assessment (cavernosography/cavernosometry). J Sex Med. 2013;10(1):111–4.
50. Köhler TS, et al. Prevalence of androgen deficiency in men with erectile dysfunction. Urology. 2008;71(4):693–7.
51. Chiang H-S, et al. Testosterone gel monotherapy improves sexual function of hypogonadal men mainly through restoring erection: evaluation by IIEF score. Urology. 2009;73(4):762–6.
52. Hwang T-S, et al. Combined use of androgen and sildenafil for hypogonadal patients unresponsive to sildenafil alone. Int J Impot Res. 2006;18(4):400–4.
53. Tsertsvadze A, et al. Oral phosphodiesterase-5 inhibitors and hormonal treatments for erectile dysfunction: a systematic review and meta-analysis. Ann Intern Med. 2009;151(9):650–61.
54. Andersson KE. PDE5 inhibitors–pharmacology and clinical applications 20 years after sildenafil discovery. Br J Pharmacol. 2018;175(13):2554–65.
55. Hackett GI. Patient preferences in treatment of erectile dysfunction: the continuing importance of patient education. Clin Cornerstone. 2005;7(1):57–64.
56. Huang SA, Lie JD. Phosphodiesterase-5 (PDE5) inhibitors in the management of erectile dysfunction. Pharm Ther. 2013;38(7):407.
57. Porst H, et al. Long-term safety and efficacy of tadalafil 5 mg dosed once daily in men with erectile dysfunction. J Sex Med. 2008;5(9):2160–9.
58. Goldstein I, et al. A randomized, double-blind, placebo-controlled evaluation of the safety and efficacy of avanafil in subjects with erectile dysfunction. J Sex Med. 2012;9(4):1122–33.
59. Moon DG, et al. A therapeutic confirmatory study to assess the safety and efficacy of Zydena®(Udenafil) for the treatment of erectile dysfunction in male patients with diabetes mellitus. J Sex Med. 2011;8(7):2048–61.
60. Zhao C, et al. Efficacy and safety of once-daily dosing of udenafil in the treatment of erectile dysfunction: results of a multicenter, randomized, double-blind, placebo-controlled trial. Eur Urol. 2011;60(2):380–7.
61. Glina S, et al. Efficacy and tolerability of lodenafil carbonate for oral therapy in erectile dysfunction: a phase II clinical trial. J Sex Med. 2009;6(2):553–7.
62. Fusco F, et al. A new era in the treatment of erectile dysfunction: chronic phosphodiesterase type 5 inhibition. BJU Int. 2010;105(12):1634–9.
63. Sung HH, Lee SW. Chronic low dosing of phosphodiesterase type 5 inhibitor for erectile dysfunction. Korean J Urol. 2012;53(6):377–85.
64. Porst H, Hell-Momeni K, Büttner H. Chronic PDE-5 inhibition in patients with erectile dysfunction–a treatment approach using Tadalafil once-daily. Expert Opin Pharmacother. 2012;13(10):1481–94.
65. Zorgniotti A, Lizza E. Effect of large doses of the nitric oxide precursor, L-arginine, on erectile dysfunction. Int J Impot Res. 1994;6(1):33–6.
66. Andersson K-E, Steers WD. The pharmacological basis of sexual. In: Erectile dysfunction: issues in current pharmacotherapy; 1998. p. 97.
67. Porst H. Oral pharmacotherapy of erectile dysfunction. In: Standard practice in sexual medicine; 2006. p. 75–93.
68. de Saenz Tejada I. Mechanisms for the regulation of penile smooth muscle contractility. In: World Book of Impotence; 1992. p. 39.
69. Freitas F, et al. Yohimbine relaxes the human corpus cavernosum through a non-adrenergic mechanism involving the activation of K+ ATP-dependent channels. Int J Impot Res. 2009;21(6):356–61.
70. Ernst E, Pittler M. Yohimbine for erectile dysfunction: a systematic review and meta-analysis of randomized clinical trials. J Urol. 1998;159(2):433–6.
71. Bochinski D, et al. The effect of neural embryonic stem cell therapy in a rat model of cavernosal nerve injury. BJU Int. 2004;94(6):904–9.
72. Albersen M, et al. Injections of adipose tissue-derived stem cells and stem cell lysate improve recovery of erectile function in a rat model of cavernous nerve injury. J Sex Med. 2010;7(10):3331–40.
73. Xu Y, et al. Therapeutic potential of adipose-derived stem cells-based micro-tissues in a rat model of postprostatectomy erectile dysfunction. J Sex Med. 2014;11(10):2439–48.
74. Master VA, Turek PJ. Ejaculatory physiology and dysfunction. Urol Clin N Am. 2001;28(2):363–76.

75. Waldinger MD, et al. An empirical operationalization study of DSM-IV diagnostic criteria for premature ejaculation. Int J Psychiatry Clin Pract. 1998;2(4):287–93.
76. Godpodinoff ML. Premature ejaculation: clinical subgroups and etiology. J Sex Marital Ther. 1989;15(2):130–4.
77. Gur S, Sikka S. The characterization, current medications, and promising therapeutics targets for premature ejaculation. Andrology. 2015;3(3):424–42.
78. Althof SE, et al. International Society for Sexual Medicine's guidelines for the diagnosis and treatment of premature ejaculation. J Sex Med. 2010;7(9):2947–69.
79. Serefoglu EC, et al. An evidence-based unified definition of lifelong and acquired premature ejaculation: report of the second international society for sexual medicine ad hoc committee for the definition of premature ejaculation. Sex Med. 2014;2(2):41–59.
80. Waldinger MD. Treatment of premature ejaculation. In: The textbook of clinical sexual medicine; 2017. p. 283–8.
81. Gallo L. The prevalence of an excessive prepuce and the effects of distal circumcision on premature ejaculation. Arab J Urol. 2017;15:140–7.
82. Hisasue S-i. The drug treatment of premature ejaculation. Transl Androl Urol. 2016;5(4):482.
83. Pu C, et al. Topical anesthetic agents for premature ejaculation: a systematic review and meta-analysis. Urology. 2013;81(4):799–804.
84. Modi NB, et al. Pharmacokinetic, pharmacodynamic, and electrocardiographic effects of dapoxetine and moxifloxacin compared with placebo in healthy adult male subjects. J Clin Pharmacol. 2009;49(6):634–42.
85. McMahon CG, et al. Efficacy and safety of dapoxetine for the treatment of premature ejaculation: integrated analysis of results from five phase 3 trials. J Sex Med. 2011;8(2):524–39.
86. Porst H, et al. Baseline characteristics and treatment outcomes for men with acquired or lifelong premature ejaculation with mild or no erectile dysfunction: integrated analyses of two phase 3 dapoxetine trials. J Sex Med. 2010;7(6):2231–42.
87. McMahon CG, et al. Efficacy of sildenafil citrate (Viagra) in men with premature ejaculation. J Sex Med. 2005;2(3):368–75.
88. Gökçe A, et al. The effects of three phosphodiesterase type 5 inhibitors on ejaculation latency time in lifelong premature ejaculators: a double-blind laboratory setting study. BJU Int. 2011;107(8):1274–7.
89. Mattos RM, Marmo Lucon A, Srougi M. Tadalafil and fluoxetine in premature ejaculation: prospective, randomized, double-blind, placebo-controlled study. Urol Int. 2008;80(2):162–5.
90. Hatzimouratidis K, et al. Guidelines on male sexual dysfunction: erectile dysfunction and premature ejaculation. Eur Urol. 2010;57(5):804–14.
91. Quinta Gomes AL, Nobre PJ. Prevalence of sexual problems in Portugal: results of a population-based study using a stratified sample of men aged 18 to 70 years. J Sex Res. 2014;51(1):13–21.
92. Bancroft J, Herbenick D, Reynolds M. Masturbation as a marker of sexual development. In: Sexual development in childhood; 2003. p. 156–85.
93. McCarthy B, McDonald D. Assessment, treatment, and relapse prevention: male hypoactive sexual desire disorder. J Sex Marital Ther. 2008;35(1):58–67.

Diagnosis and Treatment of Colorectoanal Dysfunctions

8

Muhammed Bahaddin Durak, Cem Simsek, and Hatice Yasemin Balaban

8.1 Introduction

Functional disorders of the gastrointestinal system (FGIDs) are the most common diagnoses in gastroenterology and account for at least 40% of all referrals to gastroenterologists. Since 1990, FGIDs have been classified based on organ regions (i.e., esophageal, gastroduodenal, bowel, biliary, and anorectal) by the Roma Foundation. The last version is Roma IV, which was developed by using the Delphi method and published in 2016 [1]. Roma IV consensus reports updated the diagnostic criteria for FGIDs and aimed to reduce stigmatization of the patients.

Historically, FGIDs were defined as conditions that had no organic basis. However, this definition has evolved with an increasing understanding of these conditions, and the current hypothesis is that they arise from the alterations in brain–gut communication. The morphological and physiological abnormalities that have been identified in patients with FGIDs include motility disturbance, visceral hypersensitivity, altered mucosal and immune function, altered gut microbiota, and altered central nervous system processing.

The current chapter focuses on selected topics on functional bowel disorders (FBDs) (namely irritable bowel syndrome (IBS) and functional constipation) and functional anorectal disorders (namely fecal incontinence and functional anorectal pain) (Table 8.1).

Table 8.1 Roma IV functional bowel and anorectal disorders' classification

C. Functional bowel disorders	F. Functional anorectal disorders
C1. Irritable bowel syndrome (IBS) C2. Functional constipation C3. Functional diarrhea C4. Functional abdominal bloating/distension C5. Unspecified functional bowel disorder C6. Opioid-induced constipation	F1. Fecal incontinence F2. Functional anorectal pain Fa. *Levator ani syndrome* Fb. *Unspecified functional anorectal pain* Fc. *Proctalgia fugax* F3. Functional defecation disorders Fa. *Inadequate defecatory propulsion* Fb. *Dyssynergic defecation*

M. B. Durak (✉) · C. Simsek · H. Y. Balaban
Department of Gastroenterology, Faculty of Medicine, Hacettepe University, Ankara, Türkiye
e-mail: ybalaban@hacettepe.edu.tr

T. Akbayrak, E. Üzelpasaci (eds.), *Physiotherapy and Rehabilitation in Pelvic and Women's Health-Related Problems*, https://doi.org/10.1007/978-3-032-28741-0_8

8.2 Functional Bowel Disorders

8.2.1 Colonic Motor and Sensory Function

Each day, 1200–1500 mL of ileal content enters the colon, and 200–400 mL is excreted as stool. The colon can increase its fluid absorption fivefold when required, but this ability is greatly impaired when transit is accelerated. The human colon consists of circular and longitudinal muscles. The smooth muscle cells of the colon do not contract as individual cells but in a large coordinated assembly called a syncytium that shows spontaneous oscillatory mechanical and electrical activity. The myogenic activity identified in the human colon includes rhythmic motor patterns and a slower pattern. When slow waves reach a threshold for contractions, they create peristaltic waves that mix the stool and push it forward. Slow waves occur throughout the human colon at a frequency of 2–4/min and are created by interstitial Cajal cells (ICCs), which are the pacemakers of the colon muscles [2, 3]. The direct neuronal control of colonic motility is mediated mostly by the enteric nervous system (ENS). The nerve cell bodies of the ENS are located in plexuses of the myenteric ganglia (Auerbach's plexus) that lie between the longitudinal and the circular muscle layers of the muscularis externa or in the submucosal ganglia that lie between the muscle and mucosa.

8.2.2 Irritable Bowel Syndrome (IBS)

8.2.2.1 Definition

Irritable bowel syndrome (IBS) is an FGID characterized by *chronic abdominal pain and altered bowel habits*. IBS accounts for one third of FGIDs and is reported to affect 11% of the global population, with 21% of the North American population and 7% of Asians affected [4]. It is the seventh most common diagnosis by primary care physicians [5]. IBS is associated with other conditions, including fibromyalgia, chronic fatigue syndrome, and psychiatric disorders, including major depression, anxiety, and somatization [6, 7].

Abdominal pain in IBS is usually described as a cramping sensation with variable intensity and periodic exacerbations. The pain is frequently related to defecation (may decrease or increase with defecation). Emotional stress and meals may exacerbate the pain. Patients with IBS also frequently report abdominal bloating and increased gas production in the form of flatulence or belching [8]. Abdominal pain that is constant or unrelated to defecation or induced by menstruation, urination, or physical activity is unlikely to be explained by IBS. Pain does not interrupt midnight sleep.

Altered bowel habits include diarrhea, constipation, or periodic combinations of both. Diarrhea is usually presented as frequent loose stools of small to moderate volume. Bowel movements generally occur during waking hours, most often in the morning or after meals. Most bowel movements are preceded by lower abdominal cramping pain, urgency, and a sensation of incomplete evacuation or tenesmus. Large-volume diarrhea, bloody stools, nocturnal diarrhea, and greasy stools are not associated with IBS. Stools are often hard and may be described as pellet-shaped. Patients may also experience tenesmus even when the rectum is empty. About half of all patients with IBS complain of mucus discharge with the stool. Bloating and abdominal distension are not diagnostic criteria for IBS but are present in 60% of patients.

8.2.2.2 Pathophysiology

Psychological disorders are seen in 70% of IBS patients, with IBS symptom severity correlating with an increased number of psychosocial factors (anxiety, sleep problems, and somatic symptoms) [9]. Traditional theories for pathophysiology visualize IBS as a three-part complex of *altered gastrointestinal (GI) motility, visceral hyperalgesia, and psychopathology* [10]. More recently, it has been understood that IBS is a disorder of gut–brain interaction, and as such, theories inch closer to a unifying mechanism, though with multiple underlying etiologies. The gut–brain connection is the key to understanding IBS.

Altered gastrointestinal (GI) motility is detectable in some patients with IBS and includes increased frequency and irregularity of luminal contractions, prolonged transit time in constipation-predominant IBS, and an exaggerated motor response to meal ingestion in diarrhea-predominant IBS [11].

Visceral hypersensitivity (increased sensation in response to stimuli) is a frequent finding in IBS patients. In particular, mechano- and chemosensitivity of the gut may lead to abnormal gut peptide release and change afferent and efferent signaling [12]. *The gut–brain axis* communicates bidirectionally. The gastrointestinal system sends afferent signals to the central nervous, spinal, and vagal systems, while, in return, their efferent signals influence intestinal secretion, motility, visceral sensation, and the immune system. Neuron sensitization and neuroimmune activation cause multiple up- and downstream effects, including the triggering of pain receptors that lead to visceral hypersensitivity [13].

Intestinal inflammation is characterized by alterations in particular immune cells and markers in some patients with IBS. An infectious enteritis, suspected clinically based on a history of an acute diarrheal illness, may precede the onset of IBS symptoms [14]. It has been shown that the fecal microbiota composition in individuals with IBS differs from that in healthy controls and varies according to the predominant symptom. Small intestinal bacterial overgrowth (SIBO) is associated with an increased number and/or type of bacteria in the upper gastrointestinal tract. However, data reporting an association between IBS and SIBO has been conflicting [15, 16].

The role of food in the pathophysiology of IBS is not clear and might stem from food intolerance or sensitivity [18]. Between 45 and 60% of IBS patients report worsening symptoms after eating, and some perceive intolerance to certain foods [17]. However, immunoglobulin (Ig) E–related food allergies are not more common in IBS. Another theory for IBS suggests that symptoms may be related to impaired absorption of carbohydrates. This theory originated from studies in inflammatory bowel disease (IBD) and was extended to IBS. Accordingly, the symptoms of IBS or IBD were suggested to develop by fermentable oligo-, di-, and monosaccharides and polyols (FODMAPs) in the distal small bowel and colon, where their fermentation leads to increased intestinal permeability and, possibly, inflammation [18]. Furthermore, 12.4% of IBS patients have biological evidence of gluten/wheat sensitivity [19]. Several studies suggest some overlap between celiac disease and IBS. Almost 87% of patients with IBS having antigliadin antibody (AGA) responded to a gluten-free diet [20, 21]. Besides gluten, other components of wheat may also induce local gut inflammation independent of gluten [22].

8.2.2.3 Diagnosis

IBS should be suspected in patients with chronic abdominal pain and altered bowel habits (constipation and/or diarrhea). A clinical diagnosis of IBS requires the fulfillment of symptom-based diagnostic criteria and a limited evaluation to exclude underlying organic disease [23]. The Rome IV criteria [24] for the diagnosis of IBS require that patients have had recurrent abdominal pain on average at least 1 day per week during the previous 3 months, which is associated with a change in stool frequency or appearance. The four subtypes of IBS are classified based on the patient's reported predominant bowel habit on days with abnormal bowel movements as follows:

- IBS-D (diarrhea-predominant; stools are watery and loose in >25% of defecations, and stools are hard or lumpy in <25% of defecations)
- IBS-C (constipation-predominant; >25% of bowel movements are hard or lumpy, and <25% of bowel movements are watery and loose)
- IBS-M (mixed diarrhea and constipation; >25% of bowel movements are hard or lumpy, and >25% of bowel movements are watery and loose)
- IBS-U (unclassified; the symptoms cannot be categorized into one of the above three subtypes)

8.2.2.4 Management

Alarm symptoms should be examined to rule out underlying organic structural disorders. *Alarm symptoms* include blood in the stool or positive occult blood in stool, involuntary weight loss, anemia, chronic diarrhea (>4 weeks), a history of colon cancer in first-degree relatives, and new-onset IBS symptoms over the age of 45. The medication history should be questioned about medications that can cause constipation or diarrhea.

In the presence of alarm symptoms, a colonoscopy is performed to rule out underlying organic pathology. Ultrasonography (USG) and cross-sectional imaging are performed in selected cases to rule out structural pathology. In patients who meet the diagnostic criteria for IBS and do not have alarm features, it is not routine to perform any additional tests beyond the initial evaluation. This limited diagnostic approach can exclude organic disease in more than 95% of patients. In the absence of alarm symptoms, inflammatory markers (leukocyte and C-reactive protein (CRP)), thyroid function tests, and serum calcium levels should be checked. In diarrhea-predominant or mixed-type IBS, autoantibodies to exclude celiac disease, stool tests for giardia, and fecal calprotectin for inflammatory bowel disease are also recommended. In patients with severe constipation resistant to dietary changes and osmotic laxative therapy, physiological tests (anorectal manometry and balloon expulsion test) are performed to exclude dyssynergic defecation. In a meta-analysis of 14 studies involving 4204 individuals, 2278 (54%) of whom met the diagnostic criteria for IBS, 4% of the patients had celiac disease. In patients with IBS symptoms and CRP levels ≤ 0.5 or calprotectin levels ≤ 40 μg/g, the probability of IBD was reported as $\leq 1\%$. The physical examination is usually normal in patients with IBS. However, patients may have mild abdominal tenderness to palpation. In patients with constipation, a rectal examination may be useful in identifying dyssynergic defecation.

8.2.2.5 Treatment

Patients should be informed that IBS is a chronic disease, although it is not associated with an increased risk of malignancy. The clinician should include the patient in treatment decisions and set a realistic expectation with consistent targets. The patient should understand that diet and lifestyle changes are essential parts of treatment and that medications have limited effects for controlling symptoms. If there are mild and intermittent symptoms without impairment in the quality of life, lifestyle and diet changes rather than pharmacological agents are recommended. Pharmacological therapy is recommended as an adjunctive treatment for patients with mild to moderate symptoms not responding to lifestyle change and for patients with severe symptoms affecting quality of life.

A careful dietary history may reveal symptom patterns associated with specific foods. Underlying visceral hypersensitivity may exacerbate the discomfort experienced after consumption of gas-producing foods. Therefore, IBS patients may benefit from the elimination of *gas-producing foods* (e.g., beans, onions, celery, carrots, raisins, bananas, apricots, prunes, Brussel sprouts, wheat germ, bagels, and pretzels), alcohol, and caffeine. A diet low in fermentable oligo-, di-, and monosaccharides and polyols (*FODMAPs*) is recommended for IBS patients who experience abdominal bloating or pain despite a gas-producing food elimination diet [25]. Low-FODMAP diet education should be provided by a trained dietitian to avoid unnecessary dietary restrictions and follow a nutrient-rich diet. Low-FODMAP education consists of initially eliminating FODMAPs from the diet for 6–8 weeks, followed by gradually rechallenging foods rich in fermentable carbohydrates following the resolution of symptoms to determine individual tolerance to specific fermentable carbohydrates [26]. Patients with known lactose intolerance should have a lactose-restricted diet. A trial of a lactose-free diet is also recommended for patients with persistent abdominal bloating despite the elimination of gas-producing foods in the diet. Gluten has been shown to alter intestinal barrier function in patients with IBS-D [28]. Non-celiac gluten sensitivity (NCGS) has been suggested as a mechanism for IBS symptoms, but the evidence supporting gluten avoidance is conflicting. Symptomatic improvement associated with a gluten-free diet may be due to the reduction of fructans and not the removal of gluten protein [27, 28]. Fibers can increase stool bulk and may also change the gut microbiome to decrease gases produced by fermentation. *Soluble fiber* should be offered to patients with IBS, and psyllium has been shown to improve both constipation and diarrhea. However, insoluble fiber (e.g., bran) should be avoided since it is not significantly better than placebo in improving symptoms and can cause bloating.

Pharmacological treatment is chosen based on control of symptoms. The pain is perceived as the bowel wall is stretched more than normal when the bowel wall tension is aggravated by stimulation of noradrenergic and serotonergic neurons in the posterior horn of the spinal cord. *Spasmolytics* (otilonium, pinaverium, and alverine) relax intestinal smooth muscle and are the first-line drugs for controlling abdominal pain. Tricyclic antidepressants (*TCAs*) or selective serotonin reuptake inhibitors (*SSRIs*) are recommended for patients unresponsive to spasmolytics. TCAs are also the most effective drugs for the control of pain originating from the distension in the rectosigmoid region. *Peppermint oil* is recommended for IBS-D and IBS-M and functional dyspepsia due to its smooth muscle relaxation, reduction of visceral hypersensitivity, and anti-inflammatory effects. Peppermint oil is also effective for bloating, distension, and moderate pain.

The first choice for diarrhea is 1200 mg/day *rifaximin* in three divided doses for 14 days. It has high tolerability and is effective in improving diarrhea but has a high recurrence rate. It can be administered once more when symptoms recur. Loperamide and ondansetron are alternative options for diarrhea in patients who do not respond to rifaximin. *Loperamide* acts by binding to the opioid receptor (agonist). It blocks L-type calcium channels and reduces bowel movements. *Ondansetron* is a 5-hydroxytryptamine (5HT3) receptor antagonist. It reduces stool frequency, consistency, and urgency and is also effective for pain. Bile acid sequestrants (cholestyramine) are recommended for patients with persistent diarrhea despite antidiarrheals. The rationale for using bile acid sequestrants in patients with IBS-D is that functional diarrhea and bile acid malabsorption are present in up to 50% of these patients. Bile acids stimulate colonic secretion and motility, causing diarrhea.

A high-fiber diet is recommended for constipation. *Soluble psyllium/ispaghula husk* is recommended rather than insoluble fibers such as bran. Another reason for not preferring wheat bran is that it contains fructans, increasing colonic gas production. Polyethylene glycol (PEG) is recommended for patients who have failed with soluble fiber (e.g., psyllium/ispaghula). However, side effects such as bloating and abdominal discomfort limit the use of PEG. Lubiprostone, linaclotide, and plecanatide are alternative options for patients with persistent constipation despite PEG therapy.

8.2.3 Functional Constipation

The symptoms of constipation include hard stools, excessive straining, infrequent bowel movements (<3 per week), a sense of incomplete evacuation, or the use of manual maneuvers to facilitate defecation. Constipation is the most common digestive complaint in the general population and is associated with substantial economic costs [29]. The prevalence of chronic constipation increases with age, most dramatically in patients >65 years of age. Approximately 26% of males and 34% of females have symptoms of constipation in patients >65 years of age [30].

8.2.3.1 Diagnosis

Constipation is described as difficult defecation, hard stools, or a decrease in the frequency of defecation by patients. Rome IV functional constipation diagnostic criteria are as follows, and these symptoms must have been present for the last 6 months, and diagnostic criteria must have been met for the last 3 months:

I. At least two of the following are required:
   - More than 25% of defecations require straining.
   - More than 25% of defecations are hard or lumpy stools (Bristol stool scale 1 and 2).
   - More than 25% of defecations are a feeling of incomplete evacuation.
   - More than 25% of defecations are a feeling of anorectal obstruction.
   - More than 25% of defecations require digital manipulation to facilitate defecation.
   - Less than three defecations per week.

II. Soft defecation without laxative use is rare.

III. IBS diagnostic criteria are not met.

The initial evaluation of patients who present with chronic constipation should include a careful history and physical examination to identify secondary causes of constipation and alarm features that warrant additional evaluation for organic disease. Several diseases that impair colonic motility affect organs outside the gastrointestinal tract. Secondary causes of constipation should be ruled out before a functional constipation diagnosis is made, and these causes include but are not limited to systemic diseases (diabetes mellitus, hypothyroidism, hypoparathyroidism, or pregnancy) or neurological disorders (multiple sclerosis, Parkinson's disease, Chagas disease, autonomic neuropathy, spinal cord injury, or intestinal pseudo-obstruction). As in IBS, in the presence of alarm symptoms, colonoscopy and, in selected cases, abdominal ultrasonography and cross-sectional imaging are performed. After all these conditions are excluded, functional constipation is diagnosed.

Functional constipation is divided into three broad categories:

- *Normal transit* constipation (59%), most of which is IBS-C
- *Slow transit* constipation (13%)
- *Defecation disorder* (25%)

Patterns of radiopaque marker movement may be used to identify the subgroup of functional constipation. The radiopaque marker study is commonly performed by measuring the movement of radiopaque markers through the gut. After radiopaque markers are swallowed, their passage through the colon is monitored by abdominal radiographs. For routine clinical purposes, a single capsule with 24 markers is administered on day 1 and followed by a single radiograph on day 6 (after 120 h). In patients with slow transit constipation, transit in the right colon or left colon is delayed. Markers progress normally through the proximal colon and then stagnate in the rectum in those with outlet delay in defecatory disorder.

Slow transit and defecation disorder are concomitantly present in 3% of patients with functional constipation. Patients with *normal transit constipation* may misperceive bowel frequency and often exhibit increased psychosocial distress. Patients have less than one per week of frequent defecation, usually accompanied by abdominal pain and bloating, in *slow transit constipation.* These patients do not respond to laxatives and fiber, and their symptoms usually begin at puberty and increase over time.

8.2.3.2 Treatment

8.2.3.2.1 Non-pharmacological Treatment

It should be explained that irregular bowel habits are common in the healthy general population and that their symptoms are not worrisome. The concerns of patients about the symptoms are an indication for appropriate investigation to reassure them. A fiber-rich diet, adequate fluid intake, and physical activity are recommended as the initial treatment. Daily consumption of 30–40 grams of fiber, including whole grain bread, unrefined cereals, and plenty of fruits and vegetables, is recommended. Raw bran consumption can also be added to breakfast or meals.

8.2.3.2.2 Pharmacological Treatment

Osmotic laxatives are administered if the non-pharmacological treatment has failed. Stimulant laxatives should be reserved for patients who do not respond to osmotic laxatives. *Osmotic laxatives* contain sugars (polyethylene glycol, sorbitol, magnesium hydroxide, and cellulose) and ions that are poorly absorbed. It is recommended to consume them with plenty of water. *Stimulant laxatives* have a rapid onset of action and often cause abdominal distension. They increase intestinal and colonic motility, stimulating water, electrolyte, and prostaglandin secretion into the lumen. Stimulant laxatives include anthraquinones (cascara, aloe, and senna), diphenylmethanes (bisacodyl and sodium picosulfate), and castor oil. *Glycerin suppositories* draw fluid into the rectum by osmotic action, stimulate sigmoid and rectal motility, and have a lubricating effect. *Surgical treatment* should be considered for patients with severe constipation unresponsive to medical treatment and for those who meet the following five criteria.

- The patient has chronic and severe symptoms resulting from constipation unresponsive to medical treatment.
- The patient must have slow colonic transit constipation.
- Imaging and manometric studies should rule out colonic pseudo-obstruction.
- Anal manometry, defecation, and balloon expulsion testing should show that there is no pelvic floor dysfunction.
- The patient should not have significant abdominal pain (i.e., not have IBS-C).

8.3 Functional Defecation Disorders

The functions of the anal canal include providing fecal continence, controlling defecation, perceiving rectal content, holding it voluntarily or involuntarily, and controlling its expulsion. The evacuation of intestinal contents is achieved by the coordinated work of the colon, rectum, and anus. The disorders that result from dysfunctions of these units are classified by Roma IV as fecal incontinence, functional anorectal pain (levator ani syndrome, unspecified anorectal pain, and proctalgia fugax), and functional defecation disorders (dyssynergic defecation and inadequate defecatory propulsion) (Table 8.1). Diagnostic evaluations of motor function disorders include anorectal manometry, balloon expulsion tests, and colon transit time, while endoanal USG and magnetic resonance (MR) defecography are used to evaluate structural disorders.

8.3.1 Anorectal Anatomy and Innervation

Layers of the intestinal wall that include the smooth muscle, mucosa, and connective tissue can collectively be regarded as a viscoelastic body. Under the combined influence of enteric neuronal and myogenic mechanisms, smooth muscle can generate both active contractions and active relaxations. The internal anal sphincter (IAS) is a thickened band of smooth muscle with a relatively high spontaneous tone that is in continuity with the circular smooth muscle of the rectum. By contrast, the external anal sphincter (EAS) is a striated muscle and is located distal to but partially overlying the internal sphincter. EAS also has a high resting tone and, unlike IAS, can be influenced by voluntary efforts to help maintain continence.

The *anorectal junction is formed by the longitudinal muscle of the rectum, the levator ani* muscle, and the proximal margins of the *IAS and EAS*. The *puborectalis and levator ani muscles* are important in maintaining continence and defecation. These striated muscles form part of the pelvic floor, and their constant tone serves to pull the rectum anteriorly and elevate it, thereby reducing the anorectal angle. The basic structure that keeps the anal canal closed is the *IAS, EAS, and puborectalis muscle*, a component of the levator ani. Additionally, the angle between the rectum and pelvis floor is the anorectal angle, and it contributes to keeping the anal canal closed. The angle of the anorectal junction is 70–90° at rest and 110–130° when the puborectalis muscle is voluntarily contracted. The puborectalis muscle begins at the symphysis pubis, passes around the anorectal junction, and ends by attaching to the symphysis pubis. When the puborectalis muscle contracts, the anorectal junction is pulled toward the symphysis pubis. This mechanical effect prevents the entry of stool into the upper anal canal.

8.3.2 Defecation

During the pre-defecatory phase, high-amplitude propagating contractions (HAPCs) occur in a characteristic sequence. The first ones start in the proximal colon, with each successive sequence originating slightly more distal than the preceding one. These first priming sequences do not evoke conscious sensation but successively propel content distally. In the 15 min leading up to defecation, a dramatic increase occurs in the frequency of these propagating sequences, which leads to a strong, conscious defecatory urge. These final sequences generate the forces necessary to fill and distend the rectum with semisolid fecal matter. When stool or gas enters the rectum, the *rectal wall is stretched*, thereby activating an enteric descending inhibitory reflex *(rectoanal inhibitory reflex (RAIR))* that causes transient relaxation of the internal anal sphincter. RAIR can be demonstrated and tested by balloon distention of the rectum, and its presence reflects the integrity of enteric neural pathways. Voluntary contraction of the EAS is required to maintain continence while deciding how best to handle intraluminal contents (feces or gas). Suppression of the urge to defecate at this time results in temporary storage of the contents in the rectum. If the processes just described give rise to the urge to defecate and the social circumstances are appropriate, the full defecation process is activated. This involves a combination of pelvic reflexes coordinated in the medulla and pons. Rectal distention by stool stimulates complete relaxation of the IAS via enteric reflexes, and the stool moves into the upper anal canal, heightening the sense of urge. Postural changes and straining facilitate the defecation process in several ways. Sitting or squatting causes descent of the anorectal junction, and straining produces further rectal descent. Both activities serve to increase the anorectal angle, thereby reducing resistance to outflow. At this point, if the person wishes to proceed to expel stool, EAS is relaxed voluntarily. At the same time, *the puborectalis muscle is relaxed* (further increasing the anorectal angle), the levator ani muscles contract, the perineum descends further, and stool is funneled into the anal canal and expelled by increasing strain-induced intrarectal pressure.

8.3.3 Fecal Incontinence

8.3.3.1 Definition

Fecal incontinence is the involuntary discharge of rectal contents from the anus. Fecal incontinence is observed in cases where the structural and functional integrity of the anal sphincters responsible for providing normal continence, pelvic floor muscles, pudendal nerve function, rectal compliance, and rectal sensation are impaired.

8.3.3.2 Prevalence

The incidence of fecal incontinence varies according to gender and age. In a study conducted in the adult population in the United States, the prevalence of fecal incontinence was reported to be 3% between the ages of 20 and 29 and 16% over the age of 70 [31].

8.3.3.3 Types of Fecal Incontinence

There are three clinical subtypes of fecal incontinence [32].

(i) *Passive Incontinence*: Patients are not aware that they are leaking stool. They become aware of their leakage when they feel wetness in their pelvic region or when they smell an unpleasant odor. The underlying cause is pudendal nerve pathology.

(ii) *Urge Incontinence*: The patient feels the need to go to the toilet urgently. Despite making an active effort to hold the stool, it leaks before reaching the toilet. EAS defect is present.

(iii) *Fecal Leakage*: A condition in which a person unknowingly passes a small amount of liquid or soft stool following normal defecation. The underlying mechanism is a loss or decrease in sensitivity of the rectum and dyssynergic defecation disorder.

8.3.3.4 Fecal Incontinence Causes and Risk Factors

Fecal incontinence may be due to dysfunction of anal sphincters, rectal dysfunction, congenital problems, structural deformities, or inflammatory (colitis, proctitis, and radiation), metabolic (diabetes mellitus), musculoskeletal (systemic sclerosis and myotonic dystrophy), neurological (Parkinson, spinal cord traumas, and myotonic dystrophy), psychological, or functional diseases [33].

8.3.3.5 History and Physical Examination

A detailed history should be taken, and possible causes and risk factors should be investigated. Physical examination is done to evaluate the anorectal region, fecal residue around the anus, skin irritation due to itching, skin infections, hemorrhoids, fistula, and anal fissure. A rectal examination can determine the resting, squeezing, and relaxing pressures of the anal sphincter and whether there is a rectal content, mass, or tumor.

8.3.3.6 Diagnosis

High-Resolution Anorectal Manometry Examination Today, the first diagnostic test that should be performed in patients with fecal incontinence is the high-resolution manometry *(HRM)* examination [34]. Decreased resting anal sphincter pressure, impaired squeeze pressure indicating anal hypocontractility, abnormal rectal sensitivity, and hypo/hypersensitivity are the pathological findings detected in HRM in patients with fecal incontinence.

Transrectal Ultrasonography or Endoanal Ultrasonography Transrectal ultrasonography *(TRUS), or endoanal ultrasonography,* is a simple, well-tolerated, and widely used method that is considered the gold standard for the investigation of the integrity of the IAS. Information is obtained about the presence of IAS defects and atrophy. In the presence of IAS atrophy, the thickness of the internal sphincter is less than 1 mm [35]. The most common causes of EAS pathologies are injuries that develop due to damage to the sphincter innervation during vaginal delivery in women.

Magnetic Resonance Imaging Magnetic resonance imaging *(MRI)* is a highly sensitive method for demonstrating EAS defects and scarring [36]. The use of *MR defecography* is becoming increasingly widespread. In addition to important functional disorders related to the defecation process, it also allows the determination of various structural abnormalities, such as rectocele and intussusception, associated with fecal incontinence and other pelvic floor disorders.

8.3.4 Functional Anorectal Pain

8.3.4.1 Definition

Levator ani syndrome and unspecified anorectal pain are characterized by chronic and long-lasting anorectal pain. They occur in organic or functional conditions affecting the anorectum, bladder, reproductive system, pelvic floor muscles, and the innervation of these muscles. Thus, anorectal pain can have organic causes such as anal fissure, endometriosis, and pelvic inflammatory diseases, as well as functional causes such as levator ani syndrome, proctalgia fugax, and unspecified anorectal pain [37].

Proctalgia fugax is characterized by pain that lasts seconds or minutes and occurs once a month or less frequently. Although the underlying mechanism is not fully explained, excessive contractions of the smooth muscles of the large intestine and anal canal have been observed. In hereditary *proctalgia fugax* disease, there is constipation and hypertrophy of the IAS [38]. Pudendal nerve compression or neuralgia plays a role in the pathogenesis of proctalgia fugax [39]. *Levator ani syndrome* is characterized by pelvic floor muscle spasms, increased resting anal canal pressure, and rectoanal coordination disorder, as in dyssynergic defecation disorder. On rectal examination, the levator ani muscle is tight and painful in levator ani syndrome.

8.3.4.2 Diagnosis

(i) **Levator Ani Syndrome**

Persistent or recurrent rectal discomfort and tenderness of the levator ani muscle palpation are hallmarks of levator ani syndrome, so the levator ani muscle is not tender in unspecified pain. According to the Rome IV criteria, for the diagnosis of levator ani syndrome, patients must meet all of the following criteria within the last 3 months, and the symptoms must have started at least 6 months before the diagnosis [40]:

- Chronic or recurrent rectal pain.
- Episodes last at least 30 min.
- Exclusion of other causes of rectal pain.
- Tenderness occurs during posterior traction of the puborectalis muscle.

Patients who meet all of the criteria for levator ani syndrome, except tenderness during posterior traction of the puborectalis muscle, are classified as having unspecified functional anorectal pain, according to the Rome IV criteria.

(ii) **Proctalgia Fugax**

Proctalgia fugax is characterized by recurrent pain episodes localized in the rectum, not associated with defecation. Episodes usually occur suddenly, during the day or at night, and once a month. Stress may provoke attacks of pain. The pain is characterized by cramping, spasm, or stabbing pain that does not spread, lasts an average of 15 min, and passes on its own [41]. There is no anorectal pain between attacks. Other pelvic floor symptoms, such as painful defecation, may also be reported. In coccydynia, patients complain of pain in the coccyx while sitting, especially when leaning back and pain when standing up and standing for long periods. Pain may radiate to the pelvic floor. Coccydynia is diagnosed by rectal examination, which shows tenderness and pain when the coccyx is moved, although adjacent structures are not tender.

Some diagnostic tests are necessary to exclude a structural disorder or identify the underlying disorder. Evaluation with rectosigmoidoscopy and anal manometry is recommended in the differential diagnosis of levator ani syndrome. Rectosigmoidoscopy helps exclude anal fissures, hemorrhoids, and chronic proctosigmoiditis (due to inflammatory bowel disease or ischemia). However, the procedure should be performed under anesthesia, i.e., sedation, because it can cause intense pain. Pelvic MRI helps identify perirectal abscesses or fistulas. Additionally, MR defecography detects anal canal relaxation disorder; paradoxical contraction of the puborectalis muscle, or defecation disorders; and conditions such as rectocele and intussusception.

8.3.4.3 Treatment

Psychological problems such as depression and anxiety may coexist in patients with levator ani syndrome and must be treated accordingly. There is limited data to guide management in patients with proctalgia fugax [42]. The pain episodes are typically brief, and prevention is not possible. Since symptomatic episodes are brief and infrequent and do not usually require specific treatment [40], most patients with mild and infrequent symptoms are advised to be reassured and informed. Severe or frequent symptoms are experienced by just a small percentage of patients for whom sitz baths and treatment with topical antispasmodics may be helpful.

8.3.5 Dyssynergic Defecation

8.3.5.1 Definition and Subtypes

According to the Rome IV criteria, functional defecation disorders include inadequate defecatory propulsion and dyssynergic defecation. Functional defecation disorders are the underlying cause in 25% of patients with functional constipation. Moreover, dyssynergic defecation disorder has been detected in IBS-C and slow transit constipation by anorectal manometry. Since the majority of patients with functional defecation disorders have dyssynergic defecation, this section is focused on it.

The diagnosis of functional defecation disorder is based on the fulfillment of functional constipation and/or IBS-C diagnostic criteria and the additional presence of two of the following three parameters, which indicates incomplete evacuation during repeated defecation attempts:

- Abnormal balloon expulsion test
- Abnormal anorectal failure to evacuate pattern (on electromyography (EMG) or anal manometry)
- Impaired rectal emptying on imaging

8.3.5.2 Pathophysiology

Defecation normally involves coordinated relaxation of the puborectalis and external anal sphincter muscles, increased intra-abdominal pressure, and inhibition of colonic segmentation activity. Normally, the anal sphincter should relax when the patient strains by contracting the abdominal muscles, but in dyssynergic defecation, adequate relaxation is not achieved. Dyssynergic defecation occurs when the puborectalis and external anal sphincter muscles fail to relax or contract inappropriately. This causes the anorectal angle to narrow and the anal canal pressure to increase, thus making evacuation less effective. It can also occur due to anatomical disorders (such as rectocele) if the anal sphincter contracts paradoxically during defecation (straining) or if the perineum moves downward greater than normal due to weakness in the pelvic floor muscles. Since patients cannot completely empty the rectum, they often require excessive straining and may often resort to manual maneuvers to facilitate defecation.

8.3.5.3 Diagnosis

In patients diagnosed with functional constipation, if symptomatic improvement is not achieved despite lifestyle changes and laxatives, dyssynergic defecation is suspected, and it is diagnosed with a balloon expulsion test and/or anal manometry studies. When necessary, magnetic resonance defecography is applied to detect the anatomical disorder that may cause defecation disorders.

Pelvic floor dyssynergia is divided into four subgroups by high-resolution manometry (HRM):

- *Type I:* Increased intrarectal pressure *AND* paradoxical contraction in the anal canal
- *Type II:* Decreased intrarectal pressure *AND* paradoxical contraction in the anal canal
- *Type III:* Increased intrarectal pressure *AND* normal anal sphincter pressure (no sphincter relaxation)
- *Type IV:* Decreased intrarectal pressure *AND* normal anal sphincter pressure (no sphincter relaxation)

Rectal Examination Rectal prolapse can be detected when the patient strains. A digital rectal examination should be performed to evaluate the patient for fecal impaction, anal stricture, or rectal mass. The perianal area should be examined for scarring, fistula, fissure, and external hemorrhoids. An open or asymmetric anal opening may suggest a neurological disorder impairing sphincter function. Difficulty inserting a finger into the anal canal may indicate increased anal sphincter pressure. The tenderness on palpation of the pelvic floor as it passes the posterior aspect of the rectum may suggest pelvic floor spasm.

Normally, the perineum descends 1–4 cm during straining. When the patient is in the left lateral position, the perineum descending below the plane of the ischial tuberosity (i.e., >4 cm) usually suggests excessive perineal descent. Lack of descent may indicate failure of the pelvic floor muscles to relax during defecation, while excessive perineal descent may indicate *descending perineum syndrome*. Patients with descending perineum syndrome strain excessively and cannot fully defecate due to a failure to straighten the anorectal angle. This excessive descent of the perineum may result in injury to the sacral nerves from stretching and decreased rectal sensation and, ultimately, lead to incontinence due to denervation.

Anorectal Manometry Anorectal manometry is used for evaluating the functions of anal sphincters. The differential diagnosis of anal sphincter dysfunction and rectoanal coordination disorders is based on anorectal manometry, which measures the pressures created in the anal canal by the contraction and relaxation of anal sphincters. However, it cannot evaluate the contractions of the puborectalis muscle. HRM is a recently developed and universally used test that analyzes the pelvic floor and distal rectum muscles better.

Anorectal manometry systems have two different types: aqueous- and solid-state. It provides detailed information about both the anal canal and the distal rectum. The solid-state catheter anorectal manometry system reflects the functions of the anal sphincter with high accuracy. Before the procedure, the details of the procedure should be explained to the patient, and they should be asked to be comfortable and relaxed. If there is residual urine or a feeling of defecation, the bladder and bowel should be emptied. Enema is not routinely recommended but can be applied in patients with constipation, in whom manometry should be performed 1 h after the enema. During manometric examination, patients should be in the left lateral position with the hips and knees flexed. Then, a flexible catheter is advanced from the anal canal to the rectum, and the parameters listed below are evaluated during the anorectal manometry [43]:

- *Anal canal resting pressure* shows the involuntary function of the anal canal at rest. Anal canal resting pressure is under the control of the IAS (80%) and EAS (20%). The patient is asked not to strain or squeeze the anal canal for 30 s. The average resting pressure of the anal canal is measured.
- *Squeeze pressures and endurance* show the voluntary function during squeezing. The squeeze pressure analyzes the contraction of the EAS. The patient is asked to squeeze the anal canal for 5 s, and the process is repeated three times at 30-s intervals. Endurance of squeeze pressure shows the fatigue slope of the EAS. For this measurement, the patient is asked to squeeze the anal sphincter for 30 s.
- *Straining (pushing pressure)* analyzes whether there is an increase in the intrarectal pressure and a decrease in the anal canal pressure. The patient is asked to strain as if defecating, three times for 5 s with 30-s intervals.
- *Rectal sensitivity measurement* detects the minimum volume for initial sensation and the maximal tolerable volume. The balloon at the tip of the manometry catheter is placed into the rectum and is inflated at 10-ml intervals until it reaches the maximal tolerable volume.
- *Rectoanal inhibitory reflex (RAIR)* shows the rectoanal coordination reflex during rectal distension. A balloon is inflated with 30 ml of air to create tension in the rectum, and the response of IAS is examined. The normal response of the IAS to the given air is relaxation. RAIR is not seen in aganglionic conditions (Hirschsprung's disease), rectal resection, ileal pouch, anal anastomosis, anal hypotony, and megarectum.
- *Anal canal and rectum pressures, with the push maneuver*, evaluate the rectoanal coordination during simulated defecation.
- *The cough maneuver* is used to evaluate the damage to the sacral reflex arc. The patient is asked to cough twice at 30-s intervals. The contraction response of the EAS to the sudden increase in abdominal pressure during coughing is evaluated. The normal response of EAS to coughing is contraction, and the pressure increase at EAS should be greater than the increase in rectal pressure.
- *Balloon expulsion test:* After the anorectal manometry procedure, another catheter with a balloon at its tip is placed in the rectum in the position where the manometry catheter was placed. The balloon at the tip of the catheter is inflated with 50 ml of water, and the patient is seated on the bed. The stopwatch is pressed, and the patient is expected to expel the balloon by straining as if defecating. If the balloon cannot be expelled in less than a minute, it is considered an abnormal balloon expulsion test.

8.3.5.4 Treatment

Since dyssynergic defecation is a functional disease of the anal sphincters and pelvic floor muscles, its treatment is based on retraining of these striated muscles. *Biofeedback* is used to achieve the coordinated contraction and relaxation of the pelvic floor and anal sphincters during defecation. The indications for biofeedback are (1) constipation (related to anismus), (2) urinary incontinence, and (3) fecal incontinence.

Before starting biofeedback, the patient is shown their own normal manometric and electromyography (EMG) findings. After initial education on the pathological contraction, he/she is asked to correct this trace. For this biofeedback training, a 50-mL balloon is placed into the rectum of the patient, who is asked to defecate it. If the person starts to obtain images close to normal, the biofeedback device gives sensory or visual signals. Each session lasts approximately 45 min and requires 30 to 35 defecation attempts. If EAS relaxation can be achieved without images ten times during two sessions, biofeedback treatment is terminated. The successful response to treatment is usually obtained by one to three biofeedback sessions per week for 4–8 weeks [5, 11]. The biofeedback devices that the patient can apply at home also provide further results. For successful biofeedback application in neurogenic fecal incontinence, EAS innervation must be partially intact, and rectal distension must be, to some extent, perceived by the patient.

8.4 Conclusion

In conclusion, functional bowel diseases and defecatory disorders are common conditions that impact the quality of life and can be challenging for clinicians during diagnosis. Although they are historically defined as conditions without an organic basis, the definition and understanding of their pathogenesis have been evolving. Dyssynergic defecation is characterized by constipation with excessive straining, a sense of inadequate evacuation, and digital stimulation of bowel movements. The paradoxical contraction or insufficient relaxation of the pelvic floor and/or insufficient propulsive forces during attempted defecation are the main pathophysiological findings. Diet modifications and lifestyle changes are the mainstays of treatment, and biofeedback therapy is effective in patients with dyssynergic defecation.

References

1. Drossman DA, Hasler WL. Rome IV-functional GI disorders: disorders of gut-brain interaction. Gastroenterology. 2016;150:1257–61. https://doi.org/10.1053/j.gastro.2016.03.035.
2. Everhart JE, Ruhl CE. Burden of digestive diseases in the United States part II: lower gastrointestinal diseases. Gastroenterology. 2009;136:741–54. https://doi.org/10.1053/j.gastro.2009.01.015.
3. Lovell RM, Ford AC. Global prevalence of and risk factors for irritable bowel syndrome: a meta-analysis. Clin Gastroenterol Hepatol. 2012;10:712–721, e714. https://doi.org/10.1016/j.cgh.2012.02.029.
4. Canavan C, West J, Card T. The epidemiology of irritable bowel syndrome. Clin Epidemiol. 2014;6:71–80. https://doi.org/10.2147/CLEP.S40245.
5. Chang L, Lembo A, Sultan S. Spotlight: IBS treatment. Gastroenterology. 2022;163:153. https://doi.org/10.1053/S0016-5085(22)00537-6.
6. Chey WD, Kurlander J, Eswaran S. Irritable bowel syndrome: a clinical review. JAMA. 2015;313:949–58. https://doi.org/10.1001/jama.2015.0954.
7. Longstreth GF, Thompson WG, Chey WD, Houghton LA, Mearin F, Spiller RC. Functional bowel disorders. Gastroenterology. 2006;130:1480–91. https://doi.org/10.1053/j.gastro.2005.11.061.
8. Simren M, Palsson OS, Whitehead WE. Update on Rome IV criteria for colorectal disorders: implications for clinical practice. Curr Gastroenterol Rep. 2017;19:15. https://doi.org/10.1007/s11894-017-0554-0.
9. Nicholl BI, Halder SL, Macfarlane GJ, Thompson DG, O'Brien S, Musleh M, J MB. Psychosocial risk markers for new onset irritable bowel syndrome--results of a large prospective population-based study. Pain. 2008;137:147–55. https://doi.org/10.1016/j.pain.2007.08.029.
10. Spiegel B. Gravity and the gut: a hypothesis of irritable bowel syndrome. Am J Gastroenterol. 2022;117:1933–47. https://doi.org/10.14309/ajg.0000000000002066.
11. Agrawal A, Houghton LA, Reilly B, Morris J, Whorwell PJ. Bloating and distension in irritable bowel syndrome: the role of gastrointestinal transit. Am J Gastroenterol. 2009;104:1998–2004. https://doi.org/10.1038/ajg.2009.251.
12. Nozu T, Kudaira M, Kitamori S, Uehara A. Repetitive rectal painful distention induces rectal hypersensitivity in patients with irritable bowel

syndrome. J Gastroenterol. 2006;41:217–22. https://doi.org/10.1007/s00535-005-1748-z.
13. Tang HY, Jiang AJ, Wang XY, Wang H, Guan YY, Li F, Shen GM. Uncovering the pathophysiology of irritable bowel syndrome by exploring the gut-brain axis: a narrative review. Ann Transl Med. 2021;9:1187. https://doi.org/10.21037/atm-21-2779.
14. Porcari S, Ingrosso MR, Maida M, Eusebi LH, Black C, Gasbarrini A, Cammarota G, Ford AC, Ianiro G. Prevalence of irritable bowel syndrome and functional dyspepsia after acute gastroenteritis: systematic review and meta-analysis. Gut. 2024;73:1431–40. https://doi.org/10.1136/gutjnl-2023-331835.
15. Crouzet L, Gaultier E, Del'Homme C, Cartier C, Delmas E, Dapoigny M, Fioramonti J, Bernalier-Donadille A. The hypersensitivity to colonic distension of IBS patients can be transferred to rats through their fecal microbiota. Neurogastroenterol Motil. 2013;25:e272–82. https://doi.org/10.1111/nmo.12103.
16. Quigley EMM, Murray JA, Pimentel M. AGA clinical practice update on small intestinal bacterial overgrowth: expert review. Gastroenterology. 2020;159:1526–32. https://doi.org/10.1053/j.gastro.2020.06.090.
17. Arsie E, Coletta M, Cesana BM, Basilisco G. Symptom-association probability between meal ingestion and abdominal pain in patients with irritable bowel syndrome. Does somatization play a role? Neurogastroenterol Motil. 2015;27:416–22. https://doi.org/10.1111/nmo.12510.
18. Zhang J, Yu P, Xu Y, Lu XY, Xu Y, Hang J, Zhang Y. Efficacy and safety of a low-FODMAP diet in combination with a gluten-free diet for adult irritable bowel syndrome: a systematic review and meta-analysis. Dig Dis Sci. 2024; https://doi.org/10.1007/s10620-024-08671-8.
19. Ahmed A, Dixit K, Singh A, Agarwal A, Mehtab W, Prasad S, Rajput MS, Chauhan A, Agarwal A, Mehta S, Ahuja V, Shouche Y, Dhotre D, Makharia GK. Sieving out non-celiac gluten sensitivity amongst patients with irritable bowel syndrome. Dig Liver Dis. 2024;56:451–7. https://doi.org/10.1016/j.dld.2023.10.014.
20. Bierla JB, Cukrowska B, Skrzydlo-Radomanska B, Prozorow-Krol B, Kurzeja-Miroslaw A, Cichoz-Lach H, Laskowska K, Sowinska A, Majsiak E. The occurrence of gluten-related antibodies, sensitization to selected food allergens, and antibodies against intrinsic factor in adult patients with diarrhea-predominant irritable bowel syndrome. J Pers Med. 2023;13 https://doi.org/10.3390/jpm13071165.
21. Wahnschaffe U, Schulzke JD, Zeitz M, Ullrich R. Predictors of clinical response to gluten-free diet in patients diagnosed with diarrhea-predominant irritable bowel syndrome. Clin Gastroenterol Hepatol. 2007;5:844–50.; quiz 769. https://doi.org/10.1016/j.cgh.2007.03.021.
22. Van den Houte K, Bercik P, Simren M, Tack J, Vanner S. Mechanisms underlying food-triggered symptoms in disorders of gut-brain interactions. Am J Gastroenterol. 2022;117:937–46. https://doi.org/10.14309/ajg.0000000000001812.
23. Smalley W, Falck-Ytter C, Carrasco-Labra A, Wani S, Lytvyn L, Falck-Ytter Y. AGA clinical practice guidelines on the laboratory evaluation of functional diarrhea and diarrhea-predominant irritable bowel syndrome in adults (IBS-D). Gastroenterology. 2019;157:851–4. https://doi.org/10.1053/j.gastro.2019.07.004.
24. Mearin F, Lacy BE, Chang L, Chey WD, Lembo AJ, Simren M, Spiller R. Bowel Disorders. Gastroenterology. 2016; https://doi.org/10.1053/j.gastro.2016.02.031.
25. Chey WD, Hashash JG, Manning L, Chang L. AGA clinical practice update on the role of diet in irritable bowel syndrome: expert review. Gastroenterology. 2022;162:1737–1745 e1735. https://doi.org/10.1053/j.gastro.2021.12.248.
26. YA MK, Alder A, Anderson W, Wills A, Goddard L, Gulia P, Jankovich E, Mutch P, Reeves LB, Singer A, Lomer MC, Gastroenterology Specialist Group of the British Dietetic A. British dietetic association evidence-based guidelines for the dietary management of irritable bowel syndrome in adults. J Hum Nutr Diet. 2012;25:260–74. https://doi.org/10.1111/j.1365-277X.2012.01242.x.
27. Biesiekierski JR, Newnham ED, Irving PM, Barrett JS, Haines M, Doecke JD, Shepherd SJ, Muir JG, Gibson PR. Gluten causes gastrointestinal symptoms in subjects without celiac disease: a double-blind randomized placebo-controlled trial. Am J Gastroenterol. 2011;106:508–14; quiz 515. https://doi.org/10.1038/ajg.2010.487.
28. Verdu EF, Huang X, Natividad J, Lu J, Blennerhassett PA, David CS, McKay DM, Murray JA. Gliadin-dependent neuromuscular and epithelial secretory responses in gluten-sensitive HLA-DQ8 transgenic mice. Am J Physiol Gastrointest Liver Physiol. 2008;294:G217–25. https://doi.org/10.1152/ajpgi.00225.2007.
29. Sethi S, Mikami S, Leclair J, Park R, Jones M, Wadhwa V, Sethi N, Cheng V, Friedlander E, Bollom A, Lembo A. Inpatient burden of constipation in the United States: an analysis of national trends in the United States from 1997 to 2010. Am J Gastroenterol. 2014;109:250–6. https://doi.org/10.1038/ajg.2013.423.
30. Higgins PD, Johanson JF. Epidemiology of constipation in North America: a systematic review. Am J Gastroenterol. 2004;99:750–9. https://doi.org/10.1111/j.1572-0241.2004.04114.x.
31. Ditah I, Devaki P, Luma HN, Ditah C, Njei B, Jaiyeoba C, Salami A, Ditah C, Ewelukwa O, Szarka L. Prevalence, trends, and risk factors for fecal incontinence in United States adults, 2005-2010. Clin Gastroenterol Hepatol. 2014;12:636–643 e631–632. https://doi.org/10.1016/j.cgh.2013.07.020.
32. Rao SS, American College of Gastroenterology Practice Parameters C. Diagnosis and manage-

ment of fecal incontinence. American College of Gastroenterology practice parameters committee. Am J Gastroenterol. 2004;99:1585–604. https://doi.org/10.1111/j.1572-0241.2004.40105.x.
33. Sbeit W, Khoury T, Mari A. Diagnostic approach to faecal incontinence: what test and when to perform? World J Gastroenterol. 2021;27:1553–62. https://doi.org/10.3748/wjg.v27.i15.1553.
34. Scott SM, Carrington EV. The London classification: improving characterization and classification of anorectal function with anorectal Manometry. Curr Gastroenterol Rep. 2020;22:55. https://doi.org/10.1007/s11894-020-00793-z.
35. Engin G. Endosonographic imaging of anorectal diseases. J Ultrasound Med. 2006;25:57–73. https://doi.org/10.7863/jum.2006.25.1.57.
36. Thanaracthanon P, Sasiwimonphan K, Sunthornram A, Harisinghani MG, Chulroek T. Diagnostic performance of dynamic MR defecography in assessment of dyssynergic defecation. Abdom Radiol (NY). 2023;48:3458–68. https://doi.org/10.1007/s00261-023-04010-z.
37. Hananel N, Gordon PH. Re-examination of clinical manifestations and response to therapy of fissure-in-ano. Dis Colon Rectum. 1997;40:229–33. https://doi.org/10.1007/BF02054993.
38. Atkin GK, Suliman A, Vaizey CJ. Patient characteristics and treatment outcome in functional anorectal pain. Dis Colon Rectum. 2011;54:870–5. https://doi.org/10.1007/DCR.0b013e318217586f.
39. Takano M. Proctalgia fugax: caused by pudendal neuropathy? Dis Colon Rectum. 2005;48:114–20. https://doi.org/10.1007/s10350-004-0736-3.
40. Rao SS, Bharucha AE, Chiarioni G, Felt-Bersma R, Knowles C, Malcolm A, Wald A. Functional anorectal disorders. Gastroenterology. 2016; https://doi.org/10.1053/j.gastro.2016.02.009.
41. Jeyarajah S, Chow A, Ziprin P, Tilney H, Purkayastha S. Proctalgia fugax, an evidence-based management pathway. Int J Color Dis. 2010;25:1037–46. https://doi.org/10.1007/s00384-010-0984-8.
42. Lacy BE, Weiser K. Common anorectal disorders: diagnosis and treatment. Curr Gastroenterol Rep. 2009;11:413–9. https://doi.org/10.1007/s11894-009-0062-y.
43. Carrington EV, Heinrich H, Knowles CH, Rao SS, Fox M, Scott SM, International Anorectal Physiology Working Party G. Methods of anorectal manometry vary widely in clinical practice: results from an international survey. Neurogastroenterol Motil. 2017;29:e13016. https://doi.org/10.1111/nmo.13016.

Diagnosis and Treatment of Common Problems During Pregnancy and Postpartum Period

9

Atakan Tanaçan and Osman Onur Özkavak

9.1 Introduction

Pregnancy and the postpartum period represent a critical juncture in the lives of many women. This period, which is accompanied by substantial physical and psychological effects, has the potential to result in the development of certain unique problems. When a pregnant woman presents to a health professional with a complaint, a special approach is required. In order to differentiate between physiologic and pathologic conditions in these patients, to perform appropriate diagnostic tests, and to apply the right treatments, it is important to be familiar with the anatomic and physiologic changes in pregnancy and to be able to correctly evaluate the benefit-harm balance for both diagnostic tests and treatment options.

A. Tanaçan (✉)
Department of Perinatology, Ministry of Health Ankara Bilkent City Hospital, Ankara, Türkiye

Department of Obstetrics and Gynecology, Ministry of Health Ankara Bilkent City Hospital, Ankara, Türkiye

O. O. Özkavak
Department of Perinatology, Ministry of Health Ankara Bilkent City Hospital, Ankara, Türkiye

9.2 Pelvic Region Anatomy During Pregnancy and Postpartum Period

During pregnancy, pelvic bones undergo adaptations to enhance mobility, particularly in the sacroiliac joint and pubic symphysis, in order to accommodate the growing fetus and prepare for delivery [1]. The hormonal changes during pregnancy cause the pelvic ligaments to loosen. Relaxin plays a significant role in the preparation of the pelvis for childbirth by increasing the elasticity of pelvic connective tissues during pregnancy [2]. Furthermore, progesterone enhances the elasticity of connective tissue during pregnancy, thereby facilitating the expansion of the pelvic organs. However, this process can also result in connective tissue weakness and a reduction in pelvic floor support, which may give rise to a number of associated complications. While this relaxation makes the pelvis more flexible and favorable for delivery, it can also result in loss of stability and pain. The pelvic floor muscles play a critical role in supporting the growing uterus and other pelvic organs. As pregnancy progresses, the load on these muscles increases, which can lead to functional changes. Additionally, the enlarging uterus exerts pressure on adjacent organs, including the bladder, rectum, and intestines, during pregnancy. Such pressure may result in the development of urinary and gastrointestinal symptoms. Moreover, the pressure exerted by the expanding uterus on the venous sys-

T. Akbayrak, E. Üzelpasaci (eds.), *Physiotherapy and Rehabilitation in Pelvic and Women's Health-Related Problems*, https://doi.org/10.1007/978-3-032-28741-0_9

tem has the potential to impact venous return, particularly in the lower extremities. Consequently, this may result in the formation of vulvar and lower extremity varices [3].

As gestation progresses, the pelvic floor muscles experience an increase in load due to the augmented weight of the pregnancy. As a consequence of increased tension, loss of elasticity and functional weakness may occur in the pelvic muscles. The tone of the pelvic floor muscles may be diminished as a consequence of hormonal fluctuations. This may consequently elevate the probability of incontinence during pregnancy. During vaginal delivery, there is a significant degree of tension in the pelvic floor muscles, which may result in the development of trauma in these muscles. The traumas, in addition to the recovery period that follows, may lead to a reduction in muscle strength and functionality in the pelvic floor muscles during the postpartum period [4]. A decline in muscle strength may contribute to the development of long-term complications, including postpartum pelvic organ prolapse, stress incontinence, and sexual dysfunction [5].

9.3 Common Problems During Pregnancy and Systematic Approach to These Problems

When a pregnant patient presents with a symptom, it requires a specialized approach from anamnesis to imaging techniques. In this chapter, we aimed to describe the common women's health and pelvic health problems in pregnant women and in the puerperium with a systematic approach to pelvic health assessment and management. The most common problems that require pregnant women to consult a health institution were discussed in detail, and other common problems in pregnancy and postpartum periods were discussed by dividing them into related systems.

9.3.1 Nausea and Vomiting

History The first thing that comes to mind in a pregnant woman presenting with nausea and vomiting, especially in the first trimester, is pregnancy-induced nausea and vomiting. However, this is a diagnosis of exclusion. The pattern of nausea and vomiting, the times of the day at which it is more frequent, and the presence of accompanying findings should be questioned. Gushing, nausea, and vomiting accompanied by a severe headache may be associated with conditions that increase intracranial pressure, such as intracranial hemorrhage [6]. In the presence of nausea and vomiting with new onset and especially unilateral abdominal pain, there may be a pathology such as acute appendicitis or ovarian torsion in a patient with a history of ovarian cyst [7, 8]. The presence of diarrhea and fever may indicate gastroenteritis [9]. Symptoms such as groin pain, dysuria, pollakiuria, and accompanying flank pain suggest urinary tract infection [10]. Prolonged nausea and vomiting, especially in the first half of the pregnancy, may be considered pregnancy-related nausea and vomiting [11].

Physical Examination The vital signs of the patient should be evaluated. The presence of hypotension may indicate dehydration. In addition, an abdominal examination should be performed in a patient with abdominal pain, and the presence of guarding, abdominal tenderness, and rebound tenderness should be investigated [12].

Imaging Fetal status should be determined by ultrasound (USG). USG is also useful in the diagnosis of conditions such as acute appendicitis or ovarian torsion. Magnetic resonance imaging (MRI) is a safe imaging method in pregnancy for further investigation. In suspected intracranial hemorrhage, brain tomography can be used with the consent of the patient and/or relatives according to the laws of the country [13].

Laboratory A complete blood count, electrolytes, liver and kidney function tests, and complete urinalysis should be evaluated in necessary cases. Leukocytosis may be seen in conditions such as acute appendicitis, torsion, or gastroenteritis. Hemoconcentration findings may be observed due to dehydration. Electrolyte disturbances, deterioration in liver and kidney function tests, and the presence of ketones in urine may be detected in cases of hyperemesis gravidarum requiring hospitalization [14]. Stool parasite examination may be useful in patients with gastroenteritis [15].

Treatment Treatment should be directed toward the cause. Surgical treatment should be performed in cases such as ovarian torsion and acute appendicitis. Appropriate antibiotherapy should be given for gastroenteritis and urinary tract infections. In cases of severe nausea and vomiting due to pregnancy, restriction of oral intake, appropriate fluid-electrolyte replacement, and antiemetic treatment are performed [16].

9.3.2 Abdominal Pain

Abdominal pain is a frequent cause of hospital admission at any stage of pregnancy. It can be attributed to either physiological conditions or life-threatening emergencies.

History The time of onset, location, change over time, and the presence of accompanying findings should be carefully questioned. The obstetric history of the patient should also be questioned, and the gestational week should be calculated according to the last menstrual period. In the presence of acute-onset bilateral groin pain, abortion is considered if there is accompanying vaginal bleeding. If the pain is unilateral, the possibility of ectopic pregnancy comes to the fore. This possibility is even stronger in patients with previous ectopic pregnancy. If the pain is accompanied by nausea and vomiting and increases and decreases over time, ovarian torsion may be considered. The presence of gastrointestinal system findings accompanying the pain directs the physician to the possibility of gastroenteritis, and the presence of urinary system findings directs the physician to the possibility of urinary system infection. In the later stages of pregnancy, pain in the epigastric region may be associated with serious conditions such as severe preeclampsia and hemolysis, elevated liver enzymes, and low platelet (HELLP) syndrome. In addition, cyclic pain may be a sign of preterm or term labor. Sudden onset of severe and widespread abdominal pain and associated vaginal bleeding in the second half of pregnancy may be a symptom of a life-threatening condition such as placental abruption. In the presence of foul-smelling vaginal discharge and fever, pelvic inflammatory disease or infective conditions such as chorioamnionitis should be considered [17, 18].

Physical Examination Accurate assessment of the patient's vital signs is very important. The presence of hypotension and tachycardia is seen in cases that may be associated with severe bleeding, such as ectopic pregnancy or abortion, while the presence of hypertension is often associated with preeclampsia, HELLP syndrome, or placental abruption. In the presence of peritoneal irritation signs on abdominal examination, ectopic pregnancy rupture and ovarian torsion requiring emergency surgery should be investigated. In addition, if there is a continuously contracted uterus on palpation, care should be taken in terms of placental abruption. Uterine tenderness and the presence of fever may indicate chorioamnionitis [17].

A vaginal examination should be performed in every pregnant woman presenting with abdominal pain. Conditions such as bleeding and discharge are investigated in a speculum examination. In addition, cervical patency should be evaluated by vaginal examination in suspected labor. Evaluation of the presence of uterine contractions with a cardiotocogram helps the diagnosis in patients with threatened preterm labor [19].

Imaging Fetal status should be evaluated by USG. Although placental abruption may give USG findings in some cases, it is not always useful to exclude this diagnosis. Evaluation of the adnexal areas and other abdominal organs is useful to rule out pathologies such as ovarian torsion and acute appendicitis. Evaluation of the gallbladder and kidneys will also be useful. MRI or CT can be used in necessary cases in consultation with the patient [20].

Laboratory Complete blood count, liver and kidney function tests, and complete urinalysis are the first laboratory tests to be performed in pregnant women presenting with abdominal pain. Elevated liver and kidney function tests and thrombocytopenia may be associated with hypertensive diseases of pregnancy, while infectious conditions such as pyelonephritis or chorioamnionitis are suspected in the presence of severe leukocytosis. Urinalysis should be evaluated for urinary tract infection. Coagulation tests and fibrinogen should be checked in placental abruption [21].

Treatment Except for the pathologies described in the previous section, in hypertensive cases of pregnancy, delivery or follow-up may be planned according to the gestational week and severity of the disease [22]. In the presence of chorioamnionitis, broad-spectrum antibiotherapy and termination of pregnancy or delivery should be planned according to the gestational week [23]. In the presence of threatened miscarriage, rest and follow-up are recommended. In placental abruption, an emergency cesarean section should be performed immediately in the presence of a viable fetus, but in cases of fetal loss, vaginal delivery can be performed with close follow-up of the maternal condition. In the presence of threatened preterm labor, tocolysis, neuroprotective magnesium sulfate administration, and antenatal corticosteroid administration for fetal lung maturity should be considered in appropriate patients [24].

9.3.3 Vaginal Bleeding

In a pregnant woman presenting with vaginal bleeding, the gestational week, the amount of bleeding, and accompanying findings will be diagnostically useful.

History Characteristics of the symptoms, such as the amount of vaginal bleeding, color, and accompanying pain, may help the diagnosis. Vaginal bleeding in the form of spotting accompanied by groin pain in early pregnancy is considered in favor of the miscarriage threat, while vaginal bleeding in the form of spotting accompanied by unilateral severe pain is considered in favor of ectopic pregnancy. In the presence of spotting vaginal bleeding in the later gestational period, etiologic causes such as the threat of preterm delivery and placenta previa are considered in the foreground, while large amounts of vaginal bleeding accompanied by pain may be caused by conditions leading to serious maternal and fetal mortality, such as placental abruption [25]. In addition, the blood groups of the patient and her partner should be determined in terms of Rhesus (Rh) incompatibility [26].

Physical Examination The amount of bleeding and the presence of pregnancy material in the vagina should be evaluated by speculum examination. In addition, the presence of acute abdomen, uterine contraction, and tenderness in patients in advanced gestational weeks should be investigated by abdominal examination. A digital examination should be performed to evaluate cervical patency in patients at advanced gestational weeks, but the presence of placenta previa should be excluded by USG before this examination. In patients with pain and mild vaginal bleeding, fetal well-being and the presence of contractions should be assessed by cardiotocography [27].

Imaging Ultrasonography is preferred as the first imaging method. Fetal status and retroplacental areas should be carefully examined. In addition, in suspected placenta previa, the relationship between the placenta and cervix should be evaluated by transvaginal ultrasound. Transvaginal cervical length measurement is also useful in cases of threatened preterm labor [28]. In patients who describe unilateral abdominal pain and spotting in early pregnancy, the presence of a conglomerated mass adjacent to the ovary and free fluid in the Douglas suggests ectopic pregnancy [29].

Laboratory A complete blood count, maternal blood group, and coagulation parameters should be evaluated. Beta-HCG should be evaluated in cases without an intrauterine gestational sac [29].

Treatment Treatment of related conditions has been described in the previous sections. In cases of Rh incompatibility, administration of anti-D immunoglobulin to the mother is very important to prevent maternal sensitization [30]. In the presence of placenta previa, delivery should be performed by cesarean section [31].

9.3.4 Gastroesophageal Reflux

Gastroesophageal reflux is a common complaint in pregnant women, especially in the second half of pregnancy, due to decreased gastrointestinal motility caused by hormones and the compressive effect of the growing uterus [32]. In this case, patients are usually relieved with lifestyle changes, proton pump inhibitors, and antacids [33].

9.3.5 Constipation

Another problem caused by decreased gastrointestinal motility is constipation. This may be caused by the physiological effects of pregnancy or by iron preparations routinely used during pregnancy [34]. In this case, lifestyle changes such as a fibrous diet, drinking more fluids, and defecation training are recommended. In patients who do not benefit from this, the use of laxatives may be useful [35].

9.3.6 Hemorrhoids

Another condition that can be frequently encountered in pregnant women due to increasing constipation and pelvic venous stasis in advanced gestational age is hemorrhoids [36]. This condition can sometimes be painful enough to limit the life of the pregnant woman. The diagnosis is made by inspection and rectal examination. Although warm sitz baths and medical treatment are usually beneficial, surgical treatment may be required in rare cases [37].

9.3.7 Urinary Tract Infection

Urinary tract infection is the most common bacterial infection in pregnancy. Acute cystitis for lower urinary tract infection, acute pyelonephritis for upper urinary tract infection, and asymptomatic bacteriuria are included in the definition of urinary tract infection [38]. Due to the physiologic changes of pregnancy, urinary tract infections are more common in pregnant women. The ureteral dilatation seen in pregnancy facilitates the exit of bacteria from the bladder to the kidney, and the risk of pyelonephritis increases with the pressure on the bladder and ureter with the growth of the uterus [38]. It has been reported that 11–26% of women are diagnosed and treated for urinary tract infections during pregnancy [39]. Escherichia coli is the most common pathogen seen in both symptomatic and asymptomatic bacteriuria [38]. Previous history of urinary tract infection, gestational diabetes, and low socioeconomic status are among the risk factors [39]. There is a significant association between maternal urinary tract infection, including asymptomatic bacteriuria, and adverse pregnancy outcomes. Untreated urinary tract infection is associated with preterm delivery, low birth weight, preeclampsia, and increased perinatal mortality [38]. In asymptomatic bacteriuria, the diagnosis is made by positive bacterial growth in urine culture despite the absence of symptoms of urinary tract infection. In treatment, antibiotics are given according to the microorganism isolated in the culture. The most commonly used drugs include beta-lactams, nitrofurantoin, and fosfomycin [40, 41].

9.3.8 Hydronephrosis

Maternal hydronephrosis, especially on the right side, is common in pregnancy due to uterine compression and the progesterone effect [42]. In this condition, the patient usually presents with right flank pain. Urinary tract infection due to urinary stasis accompanies a significant proportion of cases. The diagnosis can be easily made with urinary system ultrasonography. In severe cases, double j stenting provides significant relief. However, nephrostomy may be required in some cases [43].

9.3.9 Urinary Incontinence

Urinary incontinence is the involuntary leakage of urine. It is frequently observed in women and especially in pregnant women. The prevalence of urinary incontinence in pregnancy has been reported to be 40% [44]. It causes individual morbidity, loss of quality of life, and socioeconomic costs. Risk factors include obesity, increased parity, mode of delivery, family history, medical comorbidity and drug use, and heavy exercise [45]. The first step in treatment is lifestyle modification, pelvic floor exercises, weight loss, and topical vaginal estrogen therapy if necessary. Surgery can be applied in cases unresponsive to treatment [46].

9.3.10 Vaginal Discharge

In pregnant women, an increase in vaginal discharge draws attention. In some patients, this condition can reach a disturbing level and it can sometimes be confused with leakage of amniotic fluid due to rupture of membranes. A pregnant woman presenting with vaginal discharge should be examined with a speculum to determine whether there is amniotic fluid leakage, and the amount, color, and odor of the discharge should be evaluated; if necessary, a smear should be performed. Cervicovaginal culture may also be taken in cases deemed necessary. The most common cause of discharge other than physiologic discharge in pregnant women is bacterial vaginosis and is treated with metronidazole [47]. Since it is very important to exclude the presence of pelvic inflammatory disease or chorioamnionitis in a pregnant woman presenting with vaginal discharge, these diagnoses should be kept in mind when evaluating patients.

9.3.11 Fibroid Degeneration or Torsion

The majority of fibroids in pregnancy are asymptomatic. With fibroid degeneration, the patient may experience pain, leukocytosis, fever, peritoneal symptoms, and nausea and vomiting. Fibroid degeneration is seen especially in fibroids larger than 5 cm and is most common in the late first trimester and early second trimester [48]. When fibroids are torsioned, they may also give clinical findings like fibroid degeneration. Stalked fibroids are at risk of torsion. Fibroids are detected by ultrasound examination. The presence of pain after ballottement examination with an ultrasound probe supports the diagnosis of fibroid degeneration or fibroid torsion. Painful fibroids are treated with analgesics. The first choice is paracetamol derivatives. In severe pain, short-term opioids or nonsteroidal anti-inflammatory drugs may be used [49].

9.3.12 Uterine Incarceration

Uterine incarceration is diagnosed ultrasonographically after the first trimester when the cervix is displaced anteriorly and the uterus is located below the sacrum, toward the posterior pelvis. It occurs in one in 3000 pregnancies [50]. Patients especially present with pain at the end of the first trimester and the beginning of the second trimester. It may manifest itself with pelvic discomfort and pelvic fullness. Frequent urination, dysuria, a feeling of incomplete emptying, and urinary retention may also be seen. Conservative management consists of knee-chest positioning and manual reduction. Colonoscopic reduction and use of pessaries are also thought to be useful [51].

9.3.13 Low Back Pain and Pelvic Girdle Pain

Pain in the lower back and pelvic girdle is a problem observed in approximately half of pregnant women. Lumbar pain, described as low back pain, develops in the region of the lumbar vertebrae and sacrum, while pelvic girdle pain is felt between the posterior iliac crest and gluteal fold. Lumbar pain tends to worsen in the postpartum period, while pelvic girdle pain tends to be more severe during pregnancy. The two conditions can be differentiated with the posterior pain provocation test. This test is positive for pelvic girdle pain and negative for lumbar pain [52]. Early recognition and treatment of these two conditions is important for patient comfort during pregnancy and the postpartum period. Methods such as posture training, avoiding sitting and standing in the same position for a long time, using back support while sitting, and using a pillow between the legs while lying down are useful in preventing the development of these pains [53]. Patients also benefit from physiotherapy, acupuncture, and medical treatments [53].

9.3.14 Muscle Cramps

Between 30% and 50% of pregnant women complain of muscle cramps, which are sudden, painful contractions in the legs, especially in the last trimester [54]. These patients are often accompanied by restless leg syndrome, which is defined as a feeling of discomfort in the legs against immobility and a desire to move the legs [55]. Identifiable causes of muscle cramps include various vitamin and mineral deficiencies, especially vitamin D deficiency and magnesium and calcium deficiency [55]. These cramps can have a serious impact on the lives of patients, leading to reduced mobility and even depression. A diet rich in these vitamins and minerals and vitamin D, calcium, and magnesium replacements is recommended in cases where necessary [56].

9.3.15 Carpal Tunnel Syndrome

Carpal tunnel syndrome is an entrapment neuropathy that occurs especially in the last trimester of pregnancy but can be seen at any stage [57]. Fluid retention and local edema due to hormonal changes during pregnancy are thought to be responsible for this pathology. Patients present with periodic discomfort in the hands and tingling, especially in the first three fingers. The desire to shake hands, especially at night, is a very specific finding for this condition. Although this problem is usually relieved after delivery, there are studies showing that symptoms may persist up to 6 months postpartum in a significant proportion of patients [58]. Nonsurgical methods such as angle stabilization or local steroid injection are generally useful in treatment. However, surgical treatment under regional anesthesia may be required in rare cases [59].

9.3.16 Sexual Problems

Couples experiencing pregnancy are often reluctant to consult a health professional about their sexual problems [60]. Health professionals often ignore patient education on this issue. Studies have shown a slight decrease in sexual activity in the first trimester of pregnancy, followed by a significant decrease in the last trimester. If there is no high-risk pregnancy such as threatened preterm labor or placenta previa, couples should be told that sexual restriction during pregnancy is unnecessary [61].

9.4 Common Problems in the Postpartum Period

9.4.1 Breast Engorgement

It presents with pain, swelling, and fever due to milk retention in the breasts in the early postpartum period. It may cause patients to discontinue breastfeeding early and may also cause the development of serious conditions, such as breast abscess, as a predisposing condition for the development of infection. It usually resolves in a short time with warm application, massage, and expressing milk. Paracetamol for fever and pain palliation relieves the majority of patients. However, if fever and other findings persist, ultrasonographic evaluation, culture in necessary cases, and antibiotherapy should not be delayed [62].

9.4.2 Uterine Involution

Especially in the first 3 days postpartum, patients complain of lower abdominal pain that increases during breastfeeding. This pain is defined as uterine involution pain and is more pronounced during breastfeeding due to increased oxytocin. Multiparous patients tend to experience uterine involution pain more often. After excluding other causes by physical examination and imaging, patients with such a complaint should be informed, and medical treatment should be provided in necessary cases. A Cochrane analysis has shown that nonsteroidal anti-inflammatory drugs are the group of drugs that relieve the symptoms of medical patients the most [63].

9.4.3 Postpartum Endometritis

Postpartum endometritis is an important cause of postpartum fever and uterine tenderness. The infection is usually polymicrobial and is defined as an infection of the decidua. Cesarean section poses a greater risk for the development of postpartum endometritis than vaginal delivery. The infection is usually limited to the uterus and responds well to antibiotherapy [64]. However, in cases where treatment is delayed, serious complications such as peritonitis, pelvic septic thrombophlebitis, or sepsis may develop. Therefore, patients in the postpartum period should be warned that they should be urgently admitted to the hospital in case of fever, foul-smelling discharge, or abdominal pain [64].

9.4.4 Urinary Retention

Urinary retention may develop after all deliveries, whether vaginal or cesarean. Forceps use and epidural analgesia are factors that increase the risk of urinary retention. Impaired function of the pudendal nerve is thought to be the etiology [65]. Medical treatment and antibiotic prophylaxis are not recommended. Bladder catheterization is recommended. Retention is considered to be eliminated when the residual urine after urination is less than 150 ml [66].

9.4.5 Wound Site Infection

Especially obese patients and diabetic pregnant women are candidates for wound infection after cesarean section. One of the major risk factors for wound site infection is cesarean section [67]. Approximately 2% of all cesarean deliveries are at risk of developing a wound infection [68]. Patients usually present 3–7 days after the operation with complaints of redness, increased temperature, and discharge from the wound. In earlier wound site infections, different microorganisms are active, and symptoms such as fever and malaise tend to be more severe. Factors such as regular training of personnel, attention to sterility, prophylactic antibiotic use, and care in wound closure are useful in preventing these infections [69]. In a patient presenting with a wound infection, a wound culture should be obtained and antibiotherapy should be started without waiting for the results. The antibiotherapy regimen can then be revised according to the culture results. Surgical treatments such as wound debridement and secondary suturing may be required in some cases.

Necrotizing fasciitis is the most important complication after wound infection. Necrotic tissues should be surgically debrided, broad-spectrum antibiotics should be used, and patients should be closely monitored and supported hemodynamically [70].

9.4.6 Urinary and Fecal Incontinence

Especially patients with operative vaginal delivery and anal sphincter injury are at risk for urinary and fecal incontinence [71, 72]. The presence of these findings in the postpartum period should be questioned in all patients. Although these problems are usually transient, they may persist in some patients and may require treatment. The first approach in treatment is pelvic floor muscle exercises. Medical treatment should be added for patients who do not benefit from these methods. The approach to urinary incontinence in the postpartum period is the same as in nonpregnant patients [73].

9.4.7 Pubic Symphysis Diastasis

Separation of the symphysis pubis by more than 1 cm is considered pathologic. Clinical manifestations include suprapubic pain, tenderness, swelling, edema, and pain radiating to the legs, buttocks, and back [74]. Pain increases with weight-bearing, walking, and climbing stairs. It usually occurs within 48 h after birth, but there are cases that begin 6 months after birth. The diagnosis is made with characteristic examination findings and ultrasonography [75].

9.4.8 Coccydynia

The coccyx is the bone structure at the bottom of the sacrum. Risk factors include obesity. Although there are many factors in its etiology, the most common causes are related to trauma [76]. Injury can be seen during labor. Especially with difficult labor and the use of forceps during labor, the pressure applied to the coccyx may increase. This may cause coccyx pain and fractures [77].

9.4.9 Hemorrhoids

Hemorrhoids are defined as the downward displacement of the anal pads, causing venous pooling. It can be seen in one third of postpartum patients [36]. The main symptoms are burning, itching, pain, and bleeding. The best-known risk factor is constipation. The primary objective of treatment is to alleviate the symptoms. Surgical treatment can be performed if necessary [78].

9.5 Conclusion

Pregnancy and the postpartum period are unique periods with their own problems. It is very important that women who present with any complaint during this period are evaluated by healthcare providers who have sufficient knowledge in this field and under appropriate conditions. Identifying risk factors and implementing the necessary prevention strategies can help prevent some important women's health problems that may start during pregnancy or the postpartum period and continue throughout life. It is important to pass this period with as few problems as possible in order to ensure that women prepare for motherhood in a healthier way, both psychologically and physically.

References

1. Alperin M, Lawley DM, Esparza MC, Lieber RL. Pregnancy-induced adaptations in the intrinsic structure of rat pelvic floor muscles. Am J Obstet Gynecol. 2015;213(2):191.e1–7.
2. Aldabe D, Ribeiro DC, Milosavljevic S, Dawn Bussey M. Pregnancy-related pelvic girdle pain and its relationship with relaxin levels during pregnancy: a systematic review. Eur Spine J. 2012;21(9):1769–76.
3. Fan CM. Venous pathophysiology. Semin Intervent Radiol. 2005;22(3):157–61.
4. Kearney R, Miller JM, Ashton-Miller JA, DeLancey JOL. Obstetric factors associated with levator ani muscle injury after vaginal birth. Obstet Gynecol. 2006;107(1):144–9.
5. Friedman S, Blomquist JL, Nugent JM, McDermott KC, Muñoz A, Handa VL. Pelvic muscle strength after childbirth. Obstet Gynecol. 2012;120(5):1021–8.
6. Sharma S, Hashmi MF, Davidson CL, Kumar A. Intracranial hypertension. In: StatPearls [Internet]. Treasure Island: StatPearls Publishing; 2025 [cited 2025 Mar 29]. Available from: http://www.ncbi.nlm.nih.gov/books/NBK507811/.
7. Moris D, Paulson EK, Pappas TN. Diagnosis and management of acute appendicitis in adults: a review. JAMA. 2021;326(22):2299–311.
8. Bridwell RE, Koyfman A, Long B. High risk and low prevalence diseases: ovarian torsion. Am J Emerg Med. 2022;56:145–50.
9. Graves NS. Acute gastroenteritis. Prim Care. 2013;40(3):727–41.
10. Chu CM, Lowder JL. Diagnosis and treatment of urinary tract infections across age groups. Am J Obstet Gynecol. 2018;219(1):40–51.
11. Liu C, Zhao G, Qiao D, Wang L, He Y, Zhao M, et al. Emerging Progress in nausea and vomiting of pregnancy and hyperemesis gravidarum: challenges and opportunities. Front Med [Internet]. 2022 [cited 2025 Mar 28];8. Available from: https://www.frontiersin.org/journals/medicine/articles/10.3389/fmed.2021.809270/full.
12. Zachariah SK, Fenn M, Jacob K, Arthungal SA, Zachariah SA. Management of acute abdomen in pregnancy: current perspectives. Int J Women's Health. 2019;11:119–34.
13. Wiles R, Hankinson B, Benbow E, Sharp A. Making decisions about radiological imaging in pregnancy. 2022 [cited 2025 Mar 28]; Available from: https://www.bmj.com/content/377/bmj-2022-070486.
14. Jansen LAW, Koot MH, Van't Hooft J, Dean CR, Bossuyt PMM, Ganzevoort W, et al. The windsor definition for hyperemesis gravidarum: a multistakeholder international consensus definition. Eur J Obstet Gynecol Reprod Biol. 2021;266:15–22.
15. Potters I, Bottieau E, Yansouni CP, Cnops L, Cox H, Vereecken H, et al. The case for parasitological stool microscopy. Clin Microbiol Infect. 2022;28(10):1310–2.

16. Lowe SA, Steinweg KE. Review article: management of hyperemesis gravidarum and nausea and vomiting in pregnancy. Emerg Med Australas. 2022;34(1):9–15.
17. Tita ATN, Andrews WW. Diagnosis and management of clinical chorioamnionitis. Clin Perinatol. 2010;37(2):339–54.
18. Marcinkowski KA, Mehta V, Mercier R, Berghella V. Pelvic inflammatory disease in pregnancy: a systematic review focusing on perinatal outcomes. Am J Obstet Gynecol MFM. 2022;4(4):100643.
19. Iams JD. National Institute of Child Health and Human Development Maternal-Fetal Medicine Units Network. What have we learned about uterine contractions and preterm birth? The HUAM Prediction Study. Semin Perinatol. 2003;27(3):204–11.
20. Dempsey PJ, Delaney FT, Geoghegan T, Lawler L, Bolster F. MR imaging of acute abdominal pain in pregnancy. Br J Radiol. 2022;95(1136):20211114.
21. Hill MG, Brighton A, Burgess W. Placental abruption leading to disseminated intravascular coagulation: a clinical case and short review. AJOG Glob Rep. 2023;3(3):100247.
22. Obstetricians AC of Gynecologists. Gestational hypertension and preeclampsia: ACOG practice bulletin, number 222. Obstet Gynecol. 2020;135(6):e237–60.
23. Committee opinion no. 712: intrapartum management of intraamniotic infection. Obstet Gynecol. 2017;130(2):e95–101.
24. American College of Obstetricians and Gynecologists' Committee on Practice Bulletins—Obstetrics. Practice bulletin no. 171: management of preterm labor. Obstet Gynecol. 2016;128(4):e155–64.
25. Young JS, White LM. Vaginal bleeding in late pregnancy. Emerg Med Clin North Am. 2019;37(2):251–64.
26. de Winter DP, Kaminski A, Tjoa ML, Oepkes D. Hemolytic disease of the fetus and newborn: systematic literature review of the antenatal landscape. BMC Pregnancy Childbirth. 2023;23(1):12.
27. David AL, Spencer RN. Clinical assessment of fetal well-being and fetal safety indicators. J Clin Pharmacol. 2022;62(S1):S67–78.
28. Reicher L, Fouks Y, Yogev Y. Cervical assessment for predicting preterm birth-cervical length and beyond. J Clin Med. 2021;10(4):627.
29. Mullany K, Minneci M, Monjazeb R, Coiado OC. Overview of ectopic pregnancy diagnosis, management, and innovation. Womens Health (Lond). 2023;19:17455057231160349.
30. McBain RD, Crowther CA, Middleton P. Anti-D administration in pregnancy for preventing Rhesus alloimmunisation. Cochrane Database Syst Rev. 2015;2015(9):CD000020.
31. Jain V, Bos H, Bujold E. Guideline no. 402: diagnosis and management of pacenta previa. J Obstet Gynaecol Can. 2020;42(7):906–917.e1.
32. Rey E, Rodriguez-Artalejo F, Herraiz MA, Sanchez P, Alvarez-Sanchez A, Escudero M, et al. Gastroesophageal reflux symptoms during and after pregnancy: a longitudinal study. Am J Gastroenterol. 2007;102(11):2395–400.
33. Altuwaijri M. Evidence-based treatment recommendations for gastroesophageal reflux disease during pregnancy: a review. Medicine (Baltimore). 2022;101(35):e30487.
34. Bradley CS, Kennedy CM, Turcea AM, Rao SSC, Nygaard IE. Constipation in pregnancy: prevalence, symptoms, and risk factors. Obstet Gynecol. 2007;110(6):1351–7.
35. Body C, Christie JA. Gastrointestinal diseases in pregnancy: nausea, vomiting, hyperemesis gravidarum, gastroesophageal reflux disease, constipation, and diarrhea. Gastroenterol Clin N Am. 2016;45(2):267–83.
36. Rao SSC, Qureshi WA, Yan Y, Johnson DA. Constipation, hemorrhoids, and anorectal disorders in pregnancy. Am J Gastroenterol. 2022;117(10S):16–25.
37. Saleeby RG, Rosen L, Stasik JJ, Riether RD, Sheets J, Khubchandani IT. Hemorrhoidectomy during pregnancy: risk or relief? Dis Colon Rectum. 1991;34(3):260–1.
38. Ansaldi Y, Martinez de Tejada Weber B. Urinary tract infections in pregnancy. Clin Microbiol Infect. 2023;29(10):1249–53.
39. Johnson CY, Rocheleau CM, Howley MM, Chiu SK, Arnold KE, Ailes EC. Characteristics of women with urinary tract infection in pregnancy. J Womens Health (Larchmt). 2021;30(11):1556–64.
40. Glaser AP, Schaeffer AJ. Urinary tract infection and bacteriuria in pregnancy. Urol Clin North Am. 2015;42(4):547–60.
41. Kalinderi K, Delkos D, Kalinderis M, Athanasiadis A, Kalogiannidis I. Urinary tract infection during pregnancy: current concepts on a common multifaceted problem. J Obstet Gynaecol. 2018;38(4):448–53.
42. Beydoun SN. Morphologic changes in the renal tract in pregnancy. Clin Obstet Gynecol. 1985;28(2):249–56.
43. Hosny M, Chan K, Ibrahim M, Sharma V, Vasdev N. The management of symptomatic hydronephrosis in pregnancy. Cureus. 2024;16(1):e52146.
44. Dinç A. Prevalence of urinary incontinence during pregnancy and associated risk factors. Low Urin Tract Symptoms. 2018;10(3):303–7.
45. Hage-Fransen MAH, Wiezer M, Otto A, Wieffer-Platvoet MS, Slotman MH, Nijhuis-van der Sanden MWG, et al. Pregnancy- and obstetric-related risk factors for urinary incontinence, fecal incontinence, or pelvic organ prolapse later in life: a systematic review and meta-analysis. Acta Obstet Gynecol Scand. 2021;100(3):373–82.
46. Moossdorff-Steinhauser HFA, Berghmans BCM, Spaanderman MEA, Bols EMJ. Prevalence, incidence and bothersomeness of urinary incontinence in pregnancy: a systematic review and meta-analysis. Int Urogynecol J. 2021;32(7):1633–52.
47. Yudin MH, Money DM. No. 211-screening and management of bacterial vaginosis in pregnancy. J Obstet Gynaecol Can. 2017;39(8):e184–91.

48. Coutinho LM, Assis WA, Spagnuolo-Souza A, Reis FM. Uterine fibroids and pregnancy: how do they affect each other? Reprod Sci. 2022;29(8):2145–51.
49. Roberts WE, Fulp KS, Morrison JC, Martin JN. The impact of leiomyomas on pregnancy. Aust N Z J Obstet Gynaecol. 1999;39(1):43–7.
50. Shnaekel KL, Wendel MP, Rabie NZ, Magann EF. Incarceration of the gravid uterus. Obstet Gynecol Surv. 2016;71(10):613–9.
51. Dierickx I, Van Holsbeke C, Mesens T, Gevers A, Meylaerts L, Voets W, et al. Colonoscopy-assisted reposition of the incarcerated uterus in mid-pregnancy: a report of four cases and a literature review. Eur J Obstet Gynecol Reprod Biol. 2011;158(2):153–8.
52. Katonis P, Kampouroglou A, Aggelopoulos A, Kakavelakis K, Lykoudis S, Makrigiannakis A, et al. Pregnancy-related low back pain. Hippokratia. 2011;15(3):205–10.
53. Ribeiro Lira SO, Soares de Sousa VP, Viana E de SR. Therapeutic exercise versus other modalities for prevention and treatment of low back, pelvic girdle, and lumbopelvic pain during pregnancy: a review protocol. PLoS One. 2022;17(9):e0274471.
54. Garrison SR, Korownyk CS, Kolber MR, Allan GM, Musini VM, Sekhon RK, et al. Magnesium for skeletal muscle cramps. Cochrane Database Syst Rev. 2020;9(9):CD009402.
55. Luo L, Zhou K, Zhang J, Xu L, Yin W. Interventions for leg cramps in pregnancy. Cochrane Database Syst Rev. 2020;2020(12):CD010655.
56. Singh J, Kaur M, Rasane P, Kaur S, Kaur J, Sharma K, et al. Nutritional management and interventions in complications of pregnancy: a systematic review. Nutr Health. 2023;32(1):81–93. https://doi.org/10.1177/02601060231172545.
57. Weimer LH. Neuromuscular disorders in pregnancy. Handb Clin Neurol. 2020;172:201–18.
58. Turgut F, Cetinşahinahin M, Turgut M, Bölükbaşi O. The management of carpal tunnel syndrome in pregnancy. J Clin Neurosci. 2001;8(4):332–4.
59. Bland JDP. Carpal tunnel syndrome in pregnancy. Muscle Nerve. 2023;68(4):345–7.
60. Alizadeh S, Hedyeh R, Hamid A-M, Ozgoli G. Prevalence of female sexual dysfunction during pregnancy in Eastern Mediterranean Regional Office Countries (EMRO): a systematic review and meta-analysis. J Matern Fetal Neonatal Med. 2022;35(25):6654–62.
61. MacPhedran SE. Sexual activity recommendations in high-risk pregnancies: what is the evidence? Sex Med Rev. 2018;6(3):343–57.
62. Zakarija-Grkovic I, Stewart F. Treatments for breast engorgement during lactation. Cochrane Database Syst Rev. 2020;9(9):CD006946.
63. Deussen AR, Ashwood P, Martis R, Stewart F, Grzeskowiak LE. Relief of pain due to uterine cramping/involution after birth. Cochrane Database Syst Rev. 2020;10(10):CD004908.
64. Chaim W, Bashiri A, Bar-David J, Shoham-Vardi I, Mazor M. Prevalence and clinical significance of postpartum endometritis and wound infection. Infect Dis Obstet Gynecol. 2000;8(2):77–82.
65. Mulder FEM, Hakvoort RA, Schoffelmeer MA, Limpens J, Van der Post JAM, Roovers JPWR. Postpartum urinary retention: a systematic review of adverse effects and management. Int Urogynecol J. 2014;25(12):1605–12.
66. Nutaitis AC, Meckes NA, Madsen AM, Toal CT, Menhaji K, Carter-Brooks CM, et al. Postpartum urinary retention: an expert review. Am J Obstet Gynecol. 2023;228(1):14–21.
67. Hamel MS, Tuuli M. Prevention of postoperative surgical site infection following cesarean delivery. Obstet Gynecol Clin N Am. 2023;50(2):327–38.
68. Carter EB, Temming LA, Fowler S, Eppes C, Gross G, Srinivas SK, et al. Evidence-based bundles and cesarean delivery surgical site infections: a systematic review and meta-analysis. Obstet Gynecol. 2017;130(4):735–46.
69. Sarsam SE, Elliott JP, Lam GK. Management of wound complications from cesarean delivery. Obstet Gynecol Surv. 2005;60(7):462–73.
70. Allaw F, Wehbe S, Kanj SS. Necrotizing fasciitis: an update on epidemiology, diagnostic methods, and treatment. Curr Opin Infect Dis. 2024;37(2):105–11.
71. Lukacz ES, Lawrence JM, Contreras R, Nager CW, Luber KM. Parity, mode of delivery, and pelvic floor disorders. Obstet Gynecol. 2006;107(6):1253–60.
72. Larsson C, Hedberg CL, Lundgren E, Söderström L, TunÓn K, Nordin P. Anal incontinence after caesarean and vaginal delivery in Sweden: a national population-based study. Lancet. 2019;393(10177):1233–9.
73. Von Aarburg N, Veit-Rubin N, Boulvain M, Bertuit J, Simonson C, Desseauve D. Physical activity and urinary incontinence during pregnancy and postpartum: a systematic review and meta-analysis. Eur J Obstet Gynecol Reprod Biol. 2021;267:262–8.
74. Stolarczyk A, Stępiński P, Sasinowski Ł, Czarnocki T, Dębiński M, Maciąg B. Peripartum pubic symphysis diastasis-practical guidelines. J Clin Med. 2021;10(11):2443.
75. Seidman AJ, Siccardi MA. Postpartum pubic symphysis diastasis. In: StatPearls [Internet]. Treasure Island: StatPearls Publishing; 2025 [cited 2025 Mar 29]. Available from: http://www.ncbi.nlm.nih.gov/books/NBK537043/.
76. Maigne JY, Rusakiewicz F, Diouf M. Postpartum coccydynia: a case series study of 57 women. Eur J Phys Rehabil Med. 2012;48(3):387–92.
77. Guo F, Yang Z, Tang L, Ming F, Guo Y, Zhu Y. An intrapartum coccygeal fracture: an easily missed buttock pain. Eur J Obstet Gynecol Reprod Biol. 2019;236:259–60.
78. Lohsiriwat V. Treatment of hemorrhoids: a coloproctologist's view. World J Gastroenterol. 2015;21(31):9245–52.

10 Diagnosis and Treatment of Infertility

Onur Ince and Sezcan Mumusoglu

10.1 Introduction

The desire to reproduce, form a family, and give birth is a fundamental survival instinct deeply rooted in human nature [1]. This essential function relies on "fertility," which is defined as the ability to conceive and carry a pregnancy to a live birth. Impairment of fertility constitutes a significant medical condition that affects couples worldwide, imposing physical and emotional stress on individuals and creating economic burdens for society [2, 3]. This condition compromises all four dimensions of health as defined by the World Health Organization (WHO): physical, mental, emotional, and social well-being.

The inability to reproduce encompasses two primary conditions: *infertility* and *sterility*. *Infertility* is broadly defined as the inability to conceive despite regular, unprotected intercourse for a specified duration. In contrast, sterility refers to a permanent inability to conceive, often due to irreversible physiological factors.

To further delineate reproductive potential, specific metrics such as *fecundity* and *fecundability* are employed.

O. Ince (✉)
Department of Obstetrics and Gynecology, Faculty of Medicine, Hacettepe University, Ankara, Türkiye

S. Mumusoglu
SM Clinic, Ankara, Türkiye

- *Fecundity* is the biological capacity to conceive and achieve a live birth within a single menstrual cycle.
- *Fecundability* represents the probability of achieving a pregnancy within one menstrual cycle.

In humans, cyclic fecundability is approximately 20–25%, significantly lower compared to other species [4]. This natural limitation becomes more pronounced with age and varies across individuals, making the decline in fecundity over time a key factor in infertility evaluation.

10.2 Diagnosing Infertility

10.2.1 Theoretical Perspective

The primary goal of infertility diagnosis is to identify individuals or couples who may benefit from targeted interventions to enhance fecundity. If such interventions can improve cyclic fecundity at an acceptable cost to both patients and society, diagnosing and treating infertility becomes a justified approach. Validated predictive models—such as those incorporating female age, duration of infertility, semen analysis, and prior pregnancy history—are available to estimate baseline fecundity (e.g., Hunault et al.) [5]. However, a critical limitation remains: the absence of universally validated models that pre-

T. Akbayrak, E. Üzelpasaci (eds.), *Physiotherapy and Rehabilitation in Pelvic and Women's Health-Related Problems*, https://doi.org/10.1007/978-3-032-28741-0_10

dict the degree of fecundity improvement across different treatment modalities, patient ages, clinical scenarios, and infertility indications [6]. This gap hinders the ability to accurately assess the impact of specific treatments on cyclic fecundity, particularly in complex and individualized cases.

10.2.2 Diagnostic Criteria Across Guidelines

Due to the challenges in defining infertility solely based on fecundity rates, no universally accepted definition of infertility exists. Instead, clinical guidelines provide slightly varying criteria grounded in evidence-based data and clinical traditions. Although definitions vary slightly, they share fundamental principles that agree on timely evaluation, early assessment for high-risk individuals, and inclusive access to fertility treatments.

The International Committee for Monitoring Assisted Reproductive Technologies (ICMART) defines infertility as a disease characterized by the failure to achieve a clinical pregnancy after 12 months of regular, unprotected sexual intercourse or an impairment of an individual's reproductive capacity, either alone or with a partner. This definition acknowledges that infertility may result from factors beyond reproductive disease and introduces the concept of functional impairment leading to disability [7].

The American Society for Reproductive Medicine (ASRM), in its latest committee opinion, expands upon the ICMART definition by including a broader range of factors contributing to infertility [8]. According to ASRM, infertility encompasses not only the inability to achieve a successful pregnancy based on medical, sexual, and reproductive history, age, physical findings, and diagnostic testing but also the need for medical intervention, such as the use of donor gametes or embryos to achieve pregnancy. ASRM recommends infertility evaluation after 12 months of regular, unprotected intercourse for women under the age of 35, and after 6 months for women aged 35 and older, in the absence of any known reproductive impairment. Furthermore, ASRM underscores that access to infertility care should not be denied or delayed based on relationship status, gender identity, or sexual orientation, promoting an inclusive and patient-centered approach to fertility treatment.

The National Institute for Health and Care Excellence (NICE) defines infertility as the inability to conceive after 1 year of regular, unprotected vaginal intercourse in the absence of known reproductive health issues [9]. For women attempting conception through artificial insemination with partner or donor sperm, further clinical assessment and investigation are recommended after six unsuccessful cycles. NICE guidelines emphasize the need for early referral to specialist care in cases where the woman is aged 36 years or older or when known clinical risk factors for infertility are present, such as a history of pelvic inflammatory disease, endometriosis, or prior medical treatments that may impact reproductive function, including cancer therapies. Additionally, NICE advises specialized fertility care for individuals with chronic viral infections, such as HIV, hepatitis B, and hepatitis C, to ensure safe and appropriate treatment options. Alongside clinical assessments, NICE highlights the importance of addressing lifestyle and sexual history factors that may influence fertility outcomes, advocating for a comprehensive and individualized approach to infertility care.

10.3 Evaluation of Infertility

10.3.1 Initiation of Infertility Evaluation

The timing and criteria for initiating an infertility evaluation according to different clinical guidelines were outlined in the "Diagnosing Infertility" section. Infertility is a multifactorial condition that requires a comprehensive assessment of both partners to identify potential underlying causes and determine appropriate management strategies. The primary goals of infertility evaluation include:

- Identifying correctable causes of infertility
- Developing individualized treatment plans based on specific patient characteristics
- Assessing overall reproductive potential to optimize conception outcomes

10.3.2 Components of the Infertility Evaluation

A comprehensive infertility evaluation includes *history-taking, physical examination,* and *diagnostic testing* for both partners.

10.3.2.1 History and Physical Examination

10.3.2.1.1 Female Partner

History
A detailed history provides critical insights into potential causes of infertility [10]:

- *Reproductive History:* Menstrual cycle patterns, presence of ovulatory dysfunction symptoms (e.g., oligomenorrhea, amenorrhea), history of pregnancy and pregnancy outcomes, prior sexually transmitted infections (STIs), and pelvic inflammatory disease (PID).
- *Gynecological History:* Contraceptive use, history of pelvic surgeries, symptoms indicative of endometriosis (e.g., dysmenorrhea, dyspareunia), and abnormal uterine bleeding.
- *Sexual History:* Presence of dyspareunia, vaginismus, or sexual dysfunctions affecting fertility. Frequency and timing of intercourse in relation to ovulation, as well as the use of lubricants that may impair sperm motility [11].
- *Lifestyle Factors:* Smoking, alcohol consumption, recreational drug use, excessive exercise, and nutritional status. Both obesity (Body mass index [BMI] $\geq$ 30) and being underweight can negatively impact fertility [12, 13].
- *Medical History:* Chronic conditions and endocrine disorders such as diabetes, thyroid disorders, polycystic ovary syndrome (PCOS), hyperprolactinemia, hirsutism, autoimmune diseases, and prior exposure to gonadotoxic agents (chemotherapy, radiation) should be assessed.
- *Family History:* A familial predisposition to infertility, early menopause, or congenital anomalies may suggest underlying genetic factors.

Physical Examination
A focused physical assessment helps identify *anatomical and hormonal factors* affecting fertility:

- *General Examination:* Evaluation of BMI, signs of androgen excess (hirsutism, acne), and thyroid dysfunction.
- *Pelvic Examination and Ultrasound:* Assessment of the *uterus and ovaries* to identify structural abnormalities, ovarian reserve markers (e.g., antral follicle count), or other gynecological conditions contributing to infertility.

10.3.2.1.2 Male Partner

History
A detailed history includes:

- Previous testicular trauma or surgeries, history of cryptorchidism, infections such as mumps orchitis, and lifestyle factors including smoking, alcohol use, or exposure to environmental toxins.
- Symptoms of erectile dysfunction or ejaculatory abnormalities and any history of previous paternity should also be documented.
- Lifestyle Habits: Smoking, alcohol use, recreational drug use, and occupational or environmental exposure to toxins (e.g., heat, pesticides, heavy metals) that may impact spermatogenesis or hormonal balance.

Physical Examination
A focused physical examination identifies potential anatomic or hormonal issues. Examination of the external genitalia for abnormalities such as varicocele, testicular size and consistency, and

signs of hypogonadism, such as gynecomastia or reduced body hair, is essential.

10.3.2.2 Diagnostic Testing

10.3.2.2.1 Ovulatory Status

Evaluating ovulatory function is a crucial first step in the infertility assessment, as ovulatory dysfunction is a leading cause of female infertility. Regular menstrual cycles within a 21–35-day range generally indicate ovulation, whereas irregular cycles, oligomenorrhea, or amenorrhea necessitate further investigation. Several diagnostic methods are available to assess ovulatory function. Serum progesterone measurement is a widely used method, with a luteal phase serum progesterone level greater than 3 ng/mL confirming ovulation, while lower levels suggest anovulation [14]. Another common approach involves the use of luteinizing hormone (LH) predictor kits, which detect the mid-cycle LH surge preceding ovulation. Although convenient, these kits have a false-positive rate of approximately 7%, particularly in women with PCOS, leading to potential misinterpretation of results [15, 16]. For a more direct evaluation, serial transvaginal ultrasound monitoring can provide visualization of follicular development and corpus luteum formation, offering a reliable assessment of ovulation. However, this method is time-consuming and costly, which limits its routine use. Traditional approaches such as basal body temperature charting, endometrial biopsy, and histological dating are no longer recommended due to their limited accuracy in predicting ovulation timing and clinical utility [16, 17].

10.3.2.2.2 Ovarian Reserve Testing

Ovarian reserve testing is essential for predicting ovarian response to gonadotropin stimulation and guiding treatment decisions in infertility management. However, unlike chronological age, ovarian reserve tests do not directly predict cyclic fecundity rates. Assessing ovarian reserve is particularly important for women over 35 years of age or those with risk factors such as a history of ovarian surgery, chemotherapy, or genetic conditions associated with diminished ovarian reserve, such as FMR1 mutation [6, 16]. The most commonly used biochemical markers for ovarian reserve assessment include *anti-Müllerian hormone (AMH), day-3 follicle-stimulating hormone (FSH),* and *estradiol* levels. AMH is a widely accepted and reliable indicator of ovarian reserve, with levels below 1.2 ng/mL suggesting a diminished ovarian reserve [18]. Day-3 FSH and estradiol levels also provide insight into ovarian reserve, with elevated FSH levels indicating diminished ovarian function. When multiple FSH measurements are available, the highest value is considered prognostic, with threshold values ranging between 10 and 25 IU/L [10, 19]. However, FSH is considered less reliable than AMH for assessing ovarian reserve [20, 21].

In addition to biochemical tests, ovarian reserve can also be evaluated using transvaginal ultrasonography to determine the *antral follicle count (AFC),* which reflects the number of small antral follicles measuring 2–10 mm and correlates closely with AMH levels [22]. According to NICE guidelines, a total AFC above 16 is associated with a high ovarian response to stimulation, while a count below 4 indicates a poor response [9]. Other tests, such as *inhibin B, the clomiphene challenge test, ovarian volume,* and *ovarian blood flow measurement,* are no longer recommended for routine clinical use due to their limited predictive value.

10.3.2.2.3 Tubal Patency, Uterine, and Cervical Factor Evaluation

Evaluation of tubal patency is a fundamental component of the initial infertility workup in couples. Commonly used methods include *hysterosalpingography (HSG), sonohysterography (SHG),* and *laparoscopy with chromopertubation. HSG* involves the introduction of a radiopaque contrast medium (either oil- or water-based) through the cervix into the uterine cavity, allowing real-time visualization of the fallopian tubes via fluoroscopy. While HSG demonstrates high sensitivity and positive predictive value for detecting distal tubal disease, it presents an approximate 15.9% false-positive rate in diagnosing proximal tubal occlusion due to tubal spasm, necessitating additional confirmatory testing in cases of suspected obstruction [6, 23]. *SHG,* which involves the infusion of sterile saline into the uterine cavity under ultrasound guidance, serves as an effective method for detecting intrauterine abnormalities. A variant of this procedure, known as *hysterosalpingo-contrast sonography (HyCoSy),* utilizes agitated saline injection to evaluate tubal patency. The visualization of free fluid in the pouch of Douglas after uterine infusion indicates that at least one fallopian tube is patent. Although HyCoSy was initially considered less accurate than HSG for tubal evaluation, studies have demonstrated its comparable reliability in low-risk patients [10, 24]. Invasive techniques such as laparoscopy with chromopertubation are generally reserved for selected cases where other diagnostic methods fail to provide definitive findings or in patients with suspected endometriosis or pelvic adhesions.

The uterine factor evaluation primarily relies on *transvaginal ultrasonography (TVUS)*, which provides a comprehensive assessment of the myometrium and endometrial cavity, allowing for the detection of structural abnormalities such as fibroids, adenomyosis, and endometrial polyps. Advanced imaging techniques, including *three-dimensional ultrasound* and *magnetic resonance imaging (MRI)*, are utilized when congenital uterine anomalies such as septate, bicornuate, or didelphic uteri are suspected. Although HSG can provide information about the uterine cavity, its sensitivity for detecting subtle lesions is limited. For further evaluation of acquired intrauterine conditions such as polyps, fibroids, and adhesions, SHG offers superior diagnostic accuracy compared to HSG and conventional TVUS, with reported sensitivity and specificity rates of 93–94% and 81%, respectively [25]. Hysteroscopy remains the gold standard for the direct visualization and treatment of intrauterine pathologies, allowing for concurrent therapeutic intervention.

Cervical factor evaluation involves clinical examination to identify abnormalities such as cervical stenosis or chronic cervicitis. Historically, the *postcoital test (PCT)* was used to assess cervical mucus quality and sperm interaction; however, due to its low reproducibility and limited predictive value, it is no longer recommended for routine use in modern infertility evaluation [26, 27].

10.3.2.2.4 Semen Analysis and Advanced Male Fertility Testing

The initial step in the evaluation of male infertility is *semen analysis*, which should be performed after an abstinence period of 2–5 days to ensure accurate results. This analysis assesses key semen parameters, including volume (≥1.4 mL), sperm concentration (≥16 million/mL), total sperm count (≥39 million per ejaculate), progressive motility (≥30%), total motility (≥42%), and normal morphology (≥4%) in accordance with the 2021 WHO guidelines [28]. If abnormalities are detected, further investigations such as hormonal and genetic evaluations may be warranted to determine underlying causes [29].

Sperm DNA fragmentation testing is utilized to assess the integrity of sperm DNA, as higher fragmentation levels have been associated with decreased chances of natural conception and lower success rates in intrauterine insemination (IUI) [30]. However, the strength of this correlation remains insufficient to justify routine use in the initial assessment of infertile couples. Accordingly, recent guidelines from the ASRM and the American Urological Association (AUA) do not recommend sperm DNA fragmentation testing as a standard component of initial male fertility evaluation [29].

In cases of severe oligospermia or azoospermia, *genetic testing*, including *karyotype analysis and Y-chromosome microdeletion testing*, is recommended to identify potential genetic causes such as Klinefelter syndrome or Y-chromosome microdeletions [31]. For further assessment of abnormalities detected during semen analysis or physical examination, imaging studies can provide additional diagnostic insights. Scrotal ultrasound is useful in evaluating testicular pathology, epididymal cysts, and varicocele, while transrectal ultrasound is employed to assess the ejaculatory ducts and seminal vesicles in men with low semen volume or azoospermia, helping to identify possible structural abnormalities contributing to infertility.

10.4 Causes and Treatment of Infertility

Infertility is a medical condition that affects approximately one in seven couples [32]. According to a UK-based study conducted by Datta in 2016, which included 15,000 men and women, infertility—defined as the inability to conceive despite 1 year of unprotected intercourse—was reported by one in eight women and one in ten men aged 16–74 years [33]. The 2013 NICE guidelines attribute infertility to various factors: ovulatory disorders account for approximately 25% of cases, tubal damage for 20%, uterine or peritoneal anatomical abnormalities for 10%, and male-related factors for about 30% [9, 32, 34, 35]. It is important to note that infertility may result from a combination of factors in both partners.

Infertility is a multifaceted condition that demands a structured and individualized management strategy. The choice of treatment should be based on the identified etiology, the couple's prognosis, and their personal preferences, including the consideration of empirical treatment when no definitive cause is found. Management options generally include lifestyle modifications, pharmacological interventions, surgical corrections, and assisted reproductive technologies (ARTs).

The causes and management of infertility in both men and women are outlined below.

10.4.1 Ovulatory Disorders

10.4.1.1 Causes

Ovulatory dysfunction is a common cause of infertility, accounting for approximately 25% of cases [35]. It is characterized by irregular or absent ovulation, which prevents the release of a mature oocyte necessary for fertilization. Among the various causes, PCOS is the most prevalent, contributing to nearly 70% of ovulatory dysfunction cases. PCOS is an endocrine disorder marked by irregular menstrual cycles, hyperandrogenism, and polycystic ovarian morphology, often accompanied by insulin resistance and metabolic disturbances that further impair reproductive function. Another significant cause is hypothalamic dysfunction, which occurs due to stress, excessive physical activity, or eating disorders. These factors suppress the secretion of gonadotropin-releasing hormone (GnRH), leading to decreased levels of LH and FSH, ultimately disrupting ovarian function. Hyperprolactinemia, characterized by elevated prolactin levels, can also interfere with ovulation by inhibiting GnRH secretion. This condition is frequently linked to pituitary adenomas or the use of medications such as antipsychotics and antidepressants. Additionally, thyroid disorders, including both hyperthyroidism and hypothyroidism, are known to cause menstrual irregularities and ovulatory dysfunction.

10.4.1.2 Treatment

10.4.1.2.1 Lifestyle Modifications

Lifestyle modifications play a crucial role in optimizing natural fertility and improving the success of medical treatments by facilitating the restoration of ovulatory cycles. Achieving a healthy body weight is a key component, as both obesity (BMI > 30 kg/m^2) and being underweight (BMI < 18.5 kg/m^2) are associated with ovulatory dysfunction and decreased fertility [36, 37]. Weight management through a balanced diet and regular physical activity is strongly recommended for women experiencing anovulation, particularly those with PCOS. In women with PCOS, even a modest weight reduction of 5–10% can restore ovulation in more than half of cases within 6 months, making it a cost-effective and low-risk intervention [38]. Lifestyle changes not only improve reproductive outcomes but also enhance metabolic and cardiovascular health, which is particularly important for long-term well-being in women with endocrine disorders such as PCOS.

10.4.1.2.2 Ovulation Induction Therapies

For women who do not respond to lifestyle interventions alone, pharmacological ovulation induction is the next step in management.

Letrozole

Letrozole, an aromatase inhibitor, is now considered the first-line pharmacologic treatment for ovulation induction in women with PCOS [39]. By inhibiting aromatase activity, letrozole reduces estradiol production, which in turn leads to increased FSH secretion and enhanced follicular growth. Letrozole has been demonstrated to achieve higher ovulation and live birth rates compared to clomiphene citrate, particularly in women with obesity or clomiphene resistance [40]. A large multicenter, randomized controlled trial comparing letrozole and clomiphene citrate in women with PCOS reported a significantly higher cumulative live birth rate (27.5% vs. 19.1%, $P = 0.007$) and ovulation rate (61.7% vs. 48.3%, $P < 0.001$) with letrozole, while the rates of pregnancy loss and adverse events remained comparable between the two groups [40]. Letrozole offers several advantages over clomiphene citrate, including a lower risk of multifollicular development, reducing the incidence of multiple pregnancies, and a shorter half-life, which minimizes its antiestrogenic effects on the endometrium. Despite its effectiveness, letrozole is not currently approved by the US Food and Drug Administration (FDA) for ovulation induction, though it is widely used off-label in clinical practice.

Clomiphene Citrate

Clomiphene citrate has long been a standard treatment for ovulation induction, particularly in women with WHO class 2 anovulation. It acts by competitively binding to estrogen receptors, thereby blocking the negative feedback of estrogen on the hypothalamus and pituitary, leading to increased secretion of gonadotropins and subsequent follicular development. Clomiphene remains a widely used and effective option; however, it has limitations, particularly in obese women and those with PCOS, where its efficacy is lower compared to letrozole [40]. Additionally, clomiphene's antiestrogenic effects can negatively impact the endometrium and cervical mucus, potentially impairing implantation and reducing pregnancy success rates [41–43]. These limitations have led to a preference for letrozole in recent years.

Metformin

Metformin is used as an adjunct therapy in the management of anovulatory infertility, particularly in women with PCOS who exhibit insulin resistance. By improving insulin sensitivity, metformin can indirectly enhance ovulatory function and menstrual regularity. Although metformin alone is less effective in achieving ovulation and pregnancy compared to first-line agents such as clomiphene citrate or letrozole, its combination with these agents has been shown to improve ovulation rates and overall reproductive outcomes [39, 44]. A clinical study involving 626 women with PCOS-related anovulatory infertility demonstrated that live birth rates were significantly higher in women treated with a combination of clomiphene and metformin (27%) compared to those receiving clomiphene alone (23%) or metformin alone (7%) [45].

Gonadotropin Therapy

Gonadotropin therapy serves as a second-line treatment for anovulatory infertility, particularly in cases where oral agents such as clomiphene citrate or letrozole have failed. Gonadotropins directly stimulate ovarian follicular development by acting on the FSH and LH receptors in the ovaries. Low-dose step-up regimens are preferred to minimize the risks associated with treatment, including ovarian hyperstimulation syndrome (OHSS) and multiple gestations. Although gonadotropin therapy has been associated with higher live birth rates compared to oral agents, it requires careful monitoring through ultrasound and hormone measurements to optimize outcomes and reduce complications. A Cochrane meta-analysis comparing the effectiveness of clomiphene citrate and gonadotropins for live birth and ongoing pregnancy rates found that clomiphene citrate was significantly less effective, with a pooled odds ratio of 0.64 (95% CI: 0.41–0.98), indicating a clear advantage of gonadotropin therapy in achieving successful pregnancies [46]. Furthermore, a randomized controlled trial comparing letrozole and human menopausal gonadotropin (HMG) for ovulation induction in women with clomiphene-resistant PCOS revealed comparable clinical pregnancy rates between the two groups (22.9%

vs. 27.1%, $P > .05$), suggesting that gonadotropins remain a valuable treatment option when oral agents fail to induce ovulation [47].

Laparoscopic Ovarian Drilling (LOD)

LOD is a surgical intervention that serves as an alternative treatment for women with PCOS who are resistant to conventional ovulation induction therapies. This minimally invasive procedure aims to reduce ovarian androgen production, thereby restoring normal follicular development and improving ovulation rates. LOD has been shown to yield comparable pregnancy rates to gonadotropin therapy while offering the advantage of a lower risk of OHSS and multiple pregnancies. However, its role in infertility management is limited by its invasive nature and the potential for postoperative adhesions, which may further impair fertility in some cases.

A Cochrane meta-analysis comparing the effectiveness of letrozole and laparoscopic ovarian drilling for achieving clinical pregnancy reported a pooled odds ratio (OR) of 1.69 (95% CI: 0.96–2.97, $P = 0.07$), indicating a trend favoring letrozole over LOD, although the difference did not reach statistical significance [48]. Despite these findings, LOD remains a viable option in select cases, particularly in women with contraindications to medical therapy or those who have failed multiple cycles of ovulation induction with oral agents and gonadotropins. Patient selection should be carefully considered, weighing the benefits of improved ovulatory function against the potential risks associated with surgical intervention.

Other Interventions

Other interventions for ovulatory dysfunction include pulsatile GnRH therapy, dopamine agonists, and ART, each tailored to specific underlying causes. Pulsatile GnRH therapy is particularly effective in women with WHO class 1 anovulation, such as those with hypothalamic amenorrhea, as it mimics the physiological release of GnRH to stimulate ovulation. Another therapeutic option is the use of dopamine agonists, such as bromocriptine and cabergoline, which are primarily indicated for hyperprolactinemic anovulation. By reducing elevated prolactin levels, these agents help restore the hypothalamic-pituitary-ovarian axis and facilitate ovulation in affected individuals. For women who do not achieve pregnancy with first- or second-line therapies, ART such as in vitro fertilization (IVF) and intracytoplasmic sperm injection (ICSI) provide highly effective alternatives. ART is particularly recommended for women with WHO class 3 anovulation, where ovarian reserve is diminished, or in cases where other treatment modalities have failed to achieve successful conception.

10.4.2 Age-Related Decline in Ovarian Function

Ovarian reserve refers to the quantity and quality of a person's remaining oocytes, playing a critical role in reproductive potential. The quantitative aspect of ovarian reserve, best estimated through AMH levels and AFC, provides valuable information about the remaining reproductive lifespan, the onset of irregular menstrual cycles, and ultimately, the timing of menopause. In contrast, the qualitative aspect, predominantly defined by age, reflects the progressive decline in oocyte competence, leading to an increased risk of aneuploidy and implantation failure, which collectively reduce the probability of achieving a successful pregnancy at a given time [49, 50]. This dual decline in both oocyte quality and quantity contributes to age-related infertility, making it a significant concern for women who delay childbearing. As age advances, the cumulative effects of diminished ovarian reserve and declining oocyte quality pose substantial challenges in achieving and maintaining pregnancy, underscoring the importance of early fertility counseling and appropriate reproductive planning for women at risk of age-related fertility decline.

10.4.3 Tubal Factor Infertility

Tubal factor infertility occurs when structural or functional abnormalities of the fallopian tubes impair the transport of sperm and oocytes or prevent the capture of ovulated oocytes due to pelvic adhesions. The most significant risk factor for tubal infertility is a history of sexually transmitted infections (STIs) and pelvic inflammatory disease (PID), which can lead to tubal scarring and obstruction [51, 52]. Other potential etiologies include endometriosis, post-surgical adhesions following abdominal or pelvic surgeries, salpingitis isthmica nodosa, and hydrosalpinx, all of which can compromise tubal function and reduce the likelihood of natural conception [53].

The treatment approach for tubal infertility is guided by factors such as the severity and location of the tubal pathology, as well as the patient's age, ovarian reserve, and access to ART such as IVF. In cases of bilateral tubal obstruction, IVF is often considered the first-line treatment due to its superior per-cycle pregnancy rates and shorter time to pregnancy compared to surgical options. Most IVF pregnancies occur within a year, whereas surgical interventions, although capable of achieving high cumulative pregnancy rates, generally require a longer time to result in live births [54].

However, surgical interventions remain a valid option for select patients, particularly younger women or those who prefer surgery due to ethical or financial concerns related to IVF. Procedures such as fimbrioplasty, which involves the removal of fimbrial adhesions, and neosalpingostomy, which creates a new tubal opening, are commonly performed for distal tubal obstructions. In cases of proximal occlusion, tubal catheterization and microsurgical reanastomosis can be considered to restore tubal patency and improve fertility outcomes.

Hydrosalpinx, a condition characterized by fluid accumulation within the fallopian tubes, has been shown to negatively impact IVF success by releasing embryotoxic fluid that interferes with implantation. Surgical management, including laparoscopic salpingectomy or proximal tubal occlusion, has been demonstrated to significantly enhance IVF outcomes. According to a 2020 Cochrane review, salpingectomy prior to ART likely increases the clinical pregnancy rate compared to no surgical intervention (RR 2.02, 95% CI 1.44–2.82), with rates improving from approximately 19% to a range between 27% and 52%. Similarly, proximal tubal occlusion may increase clinical pregnancy rates from 12% to between 21% and 74% (RR 3.21, 95% CI 1.72–5.99). However, the review highlighted insufficient evidence regarding live birth rates and surgical complications, emphasizing the need for further high-quality research to fully evaluate long-term fertility outcomes and procedural safety [55].

For women seeking fertility restoration after tubal sterilization, microsurgical tubal reanastomosis offers a viable option with favorable outcomes, especially for those under the age of 40. A study by Gordts et al. (2009) reported cumulative intrauterine pregnancy rates of 81% in women under 36 years, 67% in women aged 36–40, and 50% in women aged 40–43, with a notable decline to 12.5% in those over 43 [56]. Similarly, Malacova et al. (2015) found that cumulative live-delivery rates reached 52% within 10 years of reversal, with a 5-year live-delivery rate of approximately 50% in women under 40. However, this rate dropped to 26% in women aged 40–44 [57]. While surgical reanastomosis remains a favorable option for younger patients with good ovarian reserve, IVF may be preferable for older women or those seeking faster conception due to its higher per-cycle success rates.

10.4.4 Uterine Factor Infertility

Uterine factors contribute to infertility by impairing implantation and pregnancy maintenance. Common uterine conditions affecting fertility include fibroids, endometrial polyps, congenital anomalies, and intrauterine adhesions.

10.4.4.1 Uterine Fibroids and Endometrial Polyps

Uterine fibroids, also known as leiomyomas, are benign tumors of the uterine smooth muscle and are commonly found in women of reproductive age. Their impact on fertility depends on their size, location, and number. Submucosal fibroids, which distort the endometrial cavity, have been shown to significantly reduce fecundity and live birth rates in patients undergoing IVF. In contrast, subserosal fibroids, which do not affect the uterine cavity, are not reported to impair fertility outcomes [58, 59].

Recent evidence from a meta-analysis highlights that even non-cavity-distorting intramural fibroids measuring 2–6 cm (classified as FIGO type 3) can have a detrimental effect on live birth rates in IVF cycles, with a 52% reduction in live birth rates compared to women without fibroids (OR: 0.48, 95% CI: 0.36–0.65) [60]. However, this negative impact was not observed in fibroids measuring ≤2 cm. These findings underscore the need for further high-quality research to determine the potential benefits of myomectomy for small non-cavity-distorting intramural fibroids.

Endometrial polyps, defined as localized overgrowths of the endometrial glands and stroma, may contribute to infertility by distorting the uterine cavity and impairing embryo implantation. Evidence supports the beneficial effect of polypectomy on improving fertility outcomes. In a prospective, randomized study by Pérez-Medina et al. (2005), infertile women undergoing IUI were randomized to either hysteroscopic polypectomy or no intervention. The study demonstrated significantly higher pregnancy rates in the group that underwent polypectomy (64 pregnancies, 63%) compared to the control group (29 pregnancies, 28%), with a relative risk (RR) of 2.1 (95% CI 1.5–2.9) [61].

10.4.4.2 Congenital Uterine Anomalies

Congenital anomalies of the uterus, resulting from abnormal Müllerian duct development, are found in approximately 5.5% of the general population and up to 8% of women experiencing infertility or recurrent pregnancy loss [62]. The septate uterus, the most common anomaly, is linked to a higher risk of miscarriage, preterm birth, and fetal growth restriction, though evidence for its association with infertility remains controversial [63]. Studies have shown that hysteroscopic incision of a uterine septum can reduce the risk of miscarriage, with a meta-analysis reporting a significant decrease in spontaneous abortion rates (RR 0.37, 95% CI 0.25–0.55) [62]. However, the benefit of this procedure in asymptomatic women without a history of reproductive failure is less clear and should be individualized following counseling [63]. Conversely, surgical correction of bicornuate or didelphys uteri is generally not recommended due to insufficient data on its efficacy in improving reproductive outcomes [64]. Until further evidence becomes available, a cautious approach is advised.

10.4.4.3 Intrauterine Adhesions and Synechiae

Intrauterine adhesions, also known as Asherman's syndrome, are caused by the formation of fibrous bands within the uterine cavity, typically following trauma to the endometrium from procedures such as curettage, uterine surgeries, or infections. These adhesions can impair fertility by reducing endometrial receptivity and increasing the risk of recurrent pregnancy loss and menstrual irregularities, including hypomenorrhea and amenorrhea [65].

Hysteroscopic adhesiolysis is the mainstay of treatment and has shown favorable outcomes in improving menstrual function and fertility. Studies indicate that between 92% and 96% of patients with amenorrhea experience the restoration of normal menstrual cycles following hysteroscopic intervention [65]. However, the recurrence of adhesions after treatment remains a significant concern, particularly in severe cases.

To prevent adhesion recurrence after surgery, the application of hyaluronic acid gel barriers has been shown to be effective in reducing adhesion reformation following procedures such as suction dilation and curettage for retained products of conception [66]. Additional postoperative management strategies include the insertion of intrauterine devices (IUDs) or balloon catheters, with or without the use of prophylactic antibiotics, to prevent re-adhesion and promote endometrial healing [67].

10.4.5 Cervical Factor Infertility

Cervical factor infertility results from conditions that hinder sperm passage through the cervix into the uterine cavity, such as abnormalities in cervical mucus production, structural damage, or scarring. These factors can create a barrier to sperm transport, reducing the likelihood of conception. Research indicates that excisional or ablative procedures performed on the cervix can elevate the risk of complications, including cervical stenosis, preterm birth, and low birth weight in offspring.

The management of cervical factor infertility has evolved over time, with IUI being a commonly used approach. IUI, with or without ovarian stimulation, bypasses potential cervical barriers by directly introducing processed sperm into the uterine cavity. However, a Cochrane meta-analysis has reported that IUI does not provide a significant advantage over timed intercourse in cases of cervical factor infertility [68]. This may be due to the difficulty in accurately diagnosing cervical factor infertility, as the traditional postcoital test (PCT), once widely used to evaluate sperm-cervical mucus interaction, has demonstrated considerable variability in interobserver assessments. As a result, the PCT is no longer recommended in routine infertility evaluations due to its low reproducibility and limited clinical utility [69].

10.4.6 Endometriosis

Endometriosis is a prevalent condition among infertile women, affecting approximately 15% of cases according to a WHO study involving 8500 infertile couples [35]. The condition contributes to infertility through several mechanisms, primarily by causing pelvic adhesions that distort normal pelvic anatomy and impede oocyte transport [70, 71]. Inflammatory mediators such as cytokines produced by endometriotic lesions can disrupt ovulation, fertilization, and implantation processes [53]. Additionally, repeated surgical interventions, particularly those targeting ovarian endometriomas, may lead to a decline in ovarian reserve, further complicating fertility outcomes.

The management of endometriosis-related infertility depends on factors such as disease stage, associated symptoms, and the patient's reproductive goals. In cases of mild endometriosis (stage I/II), superovulation combined with IUI is an effective first-line approach, particularly for women under 35 years of age. However, in older patients or those who fail to conceive with IUI, IVF is recommended as a more effective alternative. For advanced endometriosis (stage III/IV), IVF is often considered the primary treatment, as surgical intervention may not significantly improve fertility outcomes and could potentially diminish ovarian reserve, especially in cases requiring endometrioma excision [72, 73].

Ovarian endometriomas are generally managed conservatively during ART cycles unless they obstruct oocyte retrieval or cause significant symptoms. While mild endometriosis has minimal impact on IVF success rates, advanced disease can negatively affect ovarian response and implantation rates; however, ART remains a viable and promising option for these patients [74]. For those not planning immediate conception after surgery, hormonal suppression therapy is recommended to prevent disease recurrence and optimize future fertility potential [75].

10.4.7 Genetic and Immune Factors in Infertility

Genetic abnormalities and autoimmune disorders are recognized as contributing factors to infertility, with studies indicating a higher prevalence of karyotype abnormalities and immune dysfunctions in infertile couples compared to the general population [76, 77]. Common chromosomal aneuploidies associated with female infertility include Turner syndrome (45,X) and fragile X premutation (FMR1 gene abnormalities), both of which can lead to ovarian dysfunction and primary ovarian insufficiency. In men, Klinefelter syndrome (47,XXY) and Y-chromosome microdeletions are frequent genetic causes of infertility, resulting in impaired spermatogenesis and azoospermia.

Autoimmune conditions have also been implicated in infertility, with autoimmune oophoritis presenting as part of polyglandular autoimmune syndromes, leading to ovarian failure. Conditions such as celiac disease and systemic autoimmune disorders, including systemic lupus erythematosus and myasthenia gravis, have been associated with an increased risk of primary ovarian insufficiency [53]. The management of infertility in the context of genetic and autoimmune factors requires a multidisciplinary approach, including genetic counseling, targeted testing, and individualized treatment strategies to optimize reproductive outcomes.

10.4.8 Unexplained Infertility (UI)

UI is diagnosed when a couple is unable to conceive after 12 months of regular, unprotected intercourse despite a comprehensive fertility assessment showing no identifiable abnormalities in ovarian function, fallopian tubes, uterine cavity, cervix, or pelvis, with the female partner being ≤40 years old and having an adequate frequency of intercourse, and the male partner presenting with normal testicular function, genitourinary anatomy, and semen parameters, according to the European Society of Human Reproduction and Embryology (ESHRE) 2023 guidelines on unexplained infertility [78, 79]. Unexplained infertility accounts for approximately 10–20% of infertility cases and is presumed to result from undetected subtle abnormalities in gamete quality, fertilization processes, implantation, or the luteal phase that evade current diagnostic methodologies [80, 81]. Management of UI primarily involves an empirical, stepwise approach, beginning with lower-cost interventions and progressing to advanced ARTs when necessary [6].

10.4.8.1 Expectant Management and Lifestyle Modifications

The Hunault synthesis model is a validated clinical prediction tool used to estimate the probability of spontaneous pregnancy leading to live birth within 1 year in subfertile couples without ovulatory disorders, tubal pathology, or azoospermia. For example, a couple with a female partner aged 30 years, a 2-year history of primary infertility, and a motile sperm percentage of 40% is estimated to have an approximately 30% chance of spontaneous pregnancy leading to live birth within 1 year, equivalent to approximately 3% per month, assuming a constant monthly probability [5]. In younger patients with a shorter duration of infertility and a favorable prognosis, expectant management for 6 months may be considered a reasonable option [82]. However, in patients with a lower probability of natural conception, expectant management may not be an appropriate approach. In support of this, a randomized controlled trial comparing intrauterine insemination with ovarian stimulation (IUI-OS) to expectant management in couples with a Hunault score below 30% demonstrated that IUI-OS significantly increased cumulative live birth rates compared to expectant management, with an RR of 3.41 (95% CI: 1.71–6.79) [83].

Lifestyle modifications play a crucial role in optimizing fertility potential in couples with UI. Obesity has been linked to ovulatory dysfunction, diminished oocyte quality, and lower pregnancy success rates following IVF [36]. These subtle reproductive impairments may contribute to UI, emphasizing the importance of weight loss interventions for overweight and obese women aiming to conceive [9, 84]. Additionally, smoking is known to accelerate ovarian aging and increase the risk of miscarriage [85]. A systematic review and meta-analysis of 98 studies found that active smoking was associated with a 23% increased risk of miscarriage (summary RR = 1.23, 95% CI: 1.16–1.30). Moreover, the risk further increased with the number of cigarettes smoked per day, demonstrating a dose-dependent effect [86].

Beyond smoking cessation, other lifestyle adjustments, such as limiting alcohol intake to fewer than four standard drinks per week and reducing caffeine consumption to below 250 mg daily, are advised for both partners, as these factors have been shown to negatively impact fertility outcomes [6]. Adopting a healthy lifestyle, including a balanced diet and regular physical activity, can enhance the likelihood of conception and improve overall reproductive health.

10.4.8.2 First-Line Treatment: IUI-OS

IUI-OS is the recommended first-line treatment for couples with UI who do not conceive through expectant management or those who have attempted spontaneous conception for an extended period, such as 1–2 years, without seeking clinical consultation [87]. This approach involves the use of ovulation-inducing agents such as clomiphene citrate (CC) or letrozole to stimulate mild ovarian hyperstimulation, leading to the recruitment of multiple follicles, while IUI enhances the chances of fertilization by increasing the concentration of motile sperm in the reproductive tract. Clinical evidence supports the efficacy of this strategy, with a large randomized trial demonstrating significantly higher pregnancy rates in couples undergoing CC-IUI compared to expectant management (31% vs. 9%) in those with a Hunault score below 30% [83]. However, IUI alone has shown limited efficacy, with per-cycle pregnancy rates reported at approximately 4.8%, indicating that its success may rely on its combination with ovarian stimulation to optimize outcomes [88].

Gonadotropin-IUI has been shown to yield higher pregnancy rates compared to CC-IUI, with reported per-cycle live birth rates of 8.7% for CC-IUI and 13.8% for gonadotropin-IUI (RR 1.6, 95% CI 1.0–2.4) in a study involving 330 couples diagnosed with UI, mild male factor infertility, or endometriosis [89]. However, this increased efficacy is accompanied by a higher risk of multiple pregnancies, including twins and triplets. Findings from a network meta-analysis encompassing 26 studies and a total of 5316 women further support these observations. Nonetheless, when the analysis was limited to studies implementing strict cycle cancellation criteria—such as canceling cycles with more than three follicles larger than 14 mm—the efficacy of gonadotropin-IUI and CC-IUI was found to be comparable, with an RR for live birth or ongoing pregnancy rates of 1.20 (95% CI 0.95–1.51) [90]. Given the associated risks of OHSS and high-order multiple gestations, gonadotropin-IUI should be administered using a low-dose regimen and under careful monitoring to minimize potential complications [78].

10.4.8.3 Second-Line Treatment: IVF

IVF is the most effective treatment for UI, offering the highest pregnancy rates within the shortest time frame, with an approximate live birth rate of 40% per cycle. IVF enables better embryo selection and provides the option of single embryo transfer (SET), which significantly reduces the risk of multiple pregnancies. It is generally recommended for couples who do not achieve conception after several cycles of intrauterine insemination (IUI). According to the latest Cochrane meta-analysis, IVF has been shown to improve live birth rates compared to IUI with gonadotropins (OR 3.90, 95% CI 2.32–6.57; one RCT; 280 women; low-quality evidence). However, for women with no prior fertility treatment, it may not always be the most appropriate first choice due to its high cost and resource-intensive nature. The same meta-analysis suggests that there may be little or no difference in live birth rates between IVF and two to three cycles of IUI with gonadotropins (OR 1.19, 95% CI 0.87–1.61; three RCTs; 731 women) or even a single cycle of IUI (OR 1.63, 95% CI 0.91–2.92; two RCTs; 221 women), indicating that IVF should be considered judiciously, particularly in younger women with a good prognosis [91].

However, in older women, immediate IVF may provide superior outcomes compared to IUI. A randomized controlled trial involving 154 couples with UI and female partners aged 38–42 years compared two cycles of CC-IUI, two cycles of gonadotropin-IUI, and immediate IVF [92]. The study demonstrated that IVF resulted in higher cumulative pregnancy rates (49% with IVF vs. 21.6% with CC-IUI and 17.3% with gonadotropin-IUI) and higher live birth rates with fewer treatment cycles. This study highlights the benefit of early IVF initiation in older patients with UI, offering improved success rates in a shorter timeframe compared to IUI-based approaches.

10.4.8.4 The Role of Laparoscopy and Alternative Treatments

The role of laparoscopy in the evaluation of UI remains a topic of ongoing debate. Although laparoscopy can identify underlying conditions such as endometriosis and pelvic adhesions in 25% to 35% of women with UI, its impact on clinical management and pregnancy outcomes is not well established [93]. Some clinicians recommend laparoscopic evaluation for women presenting with symptoms suggestive of endometriosis, such as dysmenorrhea or chronic pelvic pain. However, the European Society of Human Reproduction and Embryology (ESHRE) discourages the routine use of diagnostic laparoscopy in UI, citing insufficient evidence to support its benefit in asymptomatic women [78]. Despite this, in cases where laparoscopy is performed, surgical management of minimal to mild endometriosis has been shown to potentially improve fertility outcomes by restoring normal pelvic anatomy and reducing inflammation [94, 95].

Alternative treatments, including antioxidant supplementation, acupuncture, and endometrial scratching, have been explored in the management of UI. However, current evidence does not consistently demonstrate their effectiveness in enhancing fertility outcomes [78]. Psychological support is an essential component of UI management, as infertility often imposes a significant emotional burden on affected couples [78]. Counseling and support services should be offered to help alleviate stress and improve coping strategies, which may indirectly enhance reproductive success.

10.4.9 Male Infertility

10.4.9.1 Causes

Male infertility is a complex condition with multiple etiologies categorized into pre-testicular, testicular, and post-testicular causes. Pre-testicular causes primarily involve hormonal dysfunctions, such as hypogonadotropic hypogonadism, which impair the hypothalamic-pituitary-gonadal axis, leading to inadequate stimulation of the testes. Testicular causes include primary testicular failure, which may result from genetic disorders (e.g., Klinefelter syndrome), varicocele, infections, and environmental exposures to toxins such as heavy metals and radiation. Post-testicular causes involve sperm transport disorders, such as obstructive azoospermia, commonly caused by prior vasectomy, congenital absence of the vas deferens (often associated with cystic fibrosis), or infections leading to scarring of the epididymis, vas deferens, or ejaculatory ducts. Idiopathic male infertility, accounting for approximately 10–20% of cases, remains without a clearly identifiable cause and is believed to result from a combination of genetic and environmental factors.

Semen analysis serves as the cornerstone of male infertility evaluation, providing critical insights into sperm count, motility, and morphology. Azoospermia, the absence of sperm in the ejaculate, can be categorized into obstructive and nonobstructive types. Obstructive azoospermia, which constitutes approximately 40% of cases, is most commonly attributed to previous vasectomy procedures but may also arise from congenital anomalies, infections, or surgical interventions involving the scrotum or inguinal region [96, 97]. Non-obstructive azoospermia, typically resulting from primary testicular failure, is characterized by impaired spermatogenesis and may have underlying genetic, hormonal, or environmental etiologies. Milder abnormalities, such as oligospermia (low sperm count) and asthenospermia (reduced motility), are frequently linked to hormonal imbalances, varicocele, or lifestyle factors, including smoking, excessive alcohol consumption, and obesity.

10.4.9.2 Treatment

The management of male infertility is individualized based on the underlying cause and typically includes lifestyle modifications, medical therapies, surgical interventions, and ART.

10.4.9.2.1 Lifestyle Modifications

Smoking cessation, limiting alcohol and marijuana use, avoiding excessive heat exposure (e.g., saunas, hot tubs), maintaining a healthy weight, and engaging in regular physical activity have all been associated with improvements in semen parameters [98–101]. The use of anabolic steroids and exogenous testosterone should be avoided, as they can suppress spermatogenesis via feedback inhibition on the hypothalamic-pituitary-gonadal axis [102]. Nutritional interventions, particularly adherence to a Mediterranean diet rich in omega-3 fatty acids, antioxidants, and essential vitamins, have been suggested to enhance sperm quality by reducing oxidative stress and improving sperm function [103].

10.4.9.2.2 Hormonal Therapy

In men with hypogonadotropic hypogonadism, gonadotropin therapy with human chorionic gonadotropin (hCG) and FSH can stimulate testicular function and restore spermatogenesis. Clomiphene citrate, a selective estrogen receptor modulator, is often used off-label in cases of idiopathic oligozoospermia or secondary hypogonadism to enhance endogenous gonadotropin secretion. Aromatase inhibitors such as anastrozole may be beneficial in men with low serum testosterone and a low testosterone-to-estradiol ratio, helping to improve hormonal balance and sperm production [102].

10.4.9.2.3 Varicocele Repair

Varicocele is a common and correctable cause of male infertility. Surgical repair, particularly microsurgical varicocelectomy, has been shown to improve semen parameters and spontaneous pregnancy rates in selected patients [104, 105]. However, current evidence does not support varicocele repair in men with subclinical varicoceles or in those with nonobstructive azoospermia [102, 104, 106]. The decision to proceed with surgery should be individualized based on semen analysis findings and the presence of symptoms such as testicular discomfort.

10.4.9.2.4 Surgical Interventions for Obstructive Azoospermia

For men with obstructive azoospermia, reconstructive surgical procedures such as vasovasostomy and vasoepididymostomy can restore sperm transport in cases of prior vasectomy or epididymal obstruction. Transurethral resection of the ejaculatory ducts (TURED) is an effective intervention for men with ejaculatory duct obstruction, resulting in improved semen parameters and sperm retrieval [106].

10.4.9.2.5 Management of Ejaculatory Dysfunction

Men with retrograde ejaculation can benefit from sympathomimetic medications, which promote antegrade ejaculation. In cases of anejaculation, penile vibratory stimulation and electroejaculation may aid sperm retrieval. When conservative measures fail, sperm can be retrieved directly from the testis or epididymis for use in ART.

10.4.9.2.6 Surgical Sperm Retrieval and ART

For men with severe oligozoospermia or azoospermia, surgical sperm retrieval techniques such as percutaneous epididymal sperm aspiration (PESA), testicular sperm aspiration (TESA), and microdissection testicular sperm extraction (micro-TESE) can be performed. Micro-TESE, in particular, is preferred for men with nonobstructive azoospermia due to its higher sperm retrieval rates and lower risk of testicular damage [107]. Once sperm is obtained, ICSI offers the highest chance of fertilization, even in cases of severe male factor infertility.

10.4.9.2.7 Empirical Medical Therapy for Idiopathic Male Infertility

In idiopathic male infertility, empirical treatments such as antioxidants, carnitine supplements, and coenzyme Q10 have been explored, but robust evidence supporting their effectiveness remains limited. A Cochrane review indicated a possible improvement in live birth rates with antioxidant use, although the evidence quality remains low [108]. The use of FSH supplementation in idiopathic male infertility has also been investigated, with some studies showing modest improvements in sperm concentration and pregnancy rates [109].

10.4.9.2.8 Genetic Considerations and Counseling

Karyotyping and Y-chromosome microdeletion testing should be performed in men with severe oligozoospermia or azoospermia to identify genetic abnormalities that may impact fertility and offspring health [29, 110]. Men with congenital bilateral absence of the vas deferens (CBAVD) should undergo genetic testing for cystic fibrosis mutations, and their female partners should also be screened to assess reproductive risks [111].

10.5 Conclusion

Infertility is a complex condition that necessitates a thorough, individualized approach for both diagnosis and treatment. As discussed throughout this chapter, clinical evaluation should start with a detailed history, physical examination, and targeted investigations—for both partners—to identify underlying causes such as ovulatory disorders, tubal or uterine pathology, and male factor abnormalities. Unexplained infertility remains a diagnostic challenge, managed primarily through empirical methods and ART. Personalized treatment plans—including lifestyle modification, pharmacologic therapy, surgical intervention, and ART—are essential for improving fertility outcomes. A nuanced understanding of these diverse factors is crucial for informed clinical decision-making and the delivery of effective fertility care.

References

1. Turp AB, et al. Infertility and surrogacy first mentioned on a 4000-year-old Assyrian clay tablet of marriage contract in Turkey. Gynecol Endocrinol. 2018;34(1):25–7.
2. Bahadur A, et al. Anxiety, depression, and quality of life among infertile women: a case-control study. Cureus. 2024;16(3):e55837.
3. Bourrion B, et al. The economic burden of infertility treatment and distribution of expenditures overtime in France: a self-controlled pre-post study. BMC Health Serv Res. 2022;22(1):512.
4. Limiñana-Gras RM. Chapter 13—health and gender perspective in infertility. In: Sánchez-López MP, Limiñana-Gras RM, editors. The psychology of gender and health. San Diego: Academic; 2017. p. 363–400.
5. Hunault CC, et al. Two new prediction rules for spontaneous pregnancy leading to live birth among subfertile couples, based on the synthesis of three previous models. Hum Reprod. 2004;19(9):2019–26.
6. Brady PC, Barbieri RL. Female infertility. In: Strauss JF, et al., editors. Yen & Jaffe's reproductive endocrinology: physiology, pathophysiology, and clinical management. Philadelphia: Elsevier Health Sciences; 2023. p. 548–74.
7. Zegers-Hochschild F, et al. The international glossary on infertility and fertility care, 2017. Fertil Steril. 2017;108(3):393–406.
8. Practice Committee of the American Society for Reproductive Medicine ASFRM, Washington, DC. Definition of infertility: a committee opinion. Fertil Steril. 2023;120(6):1170.
9. National Collaborating Centre for Women's and Children's Health (UK). Fertility: assessment and treatment for people with fertility problems. London: Royal College of Obstetricians & Gynaecologists; 2013.
10. Hizkiyahu R, Buckett W, Tulandi T. Initial investigation of the infertile couple. In: Ariel DKWG, Howles CM, Shoham Z, editors. Textbook of assisted reproductive techniques: volume 2: clinical perspectives. Boca Raton: CRC Press; 2023. p. 400–8.
11. Anderson L, Lewis SE, McClure N. The effects of coital lubricants on sperm motility in vitro. Hum Reprod. 1998;13(12):3351–6.
12. O'Flynn N. Assessment and treatment for people with fertility problems: NICE guideline. Br J Gen Pract. 2014;64(618):50–1.
13. Boutari C, et al. The effect of underweight on female and male reproduction. Metabolism. 2020;107:154229.
14. Wathen NC, Perry L, Lilford RJ, Chard T. Interpretation of single progesterone measurement in diagnosis of anovulation and defective luteal phase: observations on analysis of the normal range. Br Med J (Clin Res Ed). 1984;288(6410):7–9.
15. McGovern PG, et al. Absence of secretory endometrium after false-positive home urine luteinizing hormone testing. Fertil Steril. 2004;82(5):1273–7.
16. Practice Committee of the American Society for Reproductive Medicine. Electronic address AAO and M Practice Committee of the American Society for Reproductive. Fertility evaluation of infertile women: a committee opinion. Fertil Steril. 2021;116(5):1255–65.
17. Guermandi E, et al. Reliability of ovulation tests in infertile women. Obstet Gynecol. 2001;97(1):92–6.
18. Poseidon G, et al. A new more detailed stratification of low responders to ovarian stimulation: from a poor ovarian response to a low prognosis concept. Fertil Steril. 2016;105(6):1452–3.
19. Broekmans FJ, et al. A systematic review of tests predicting ovarian reserve and IVF outcome. Hum Reprod Update. 2006;12(6):685–718.
20. de Vet A, et al. Antimullerian hormone serum levels: a putative marker for ovarian aging. Fertil Steril. 2002;77(2):357–62.
21. Practice Committee of the American Society for Reproductive Medicine. Electronic address AAO and M Practice Committee of the American Society for Reproductive. Testing and interpreting measures of ovarian reserve: a committee opinion. Fertil Steril. 2020;114(6):1151–7.

22. Barbakadze L, Kristesashvili J, Khonelidze N, Tsagareishvili G. The correlations of anti-mullerian hormone, follicle-stimulating hormone and antral follicle count in different age groups of infertile women. Int J Fertil Steril. 2015;8(4):393–8.
23. Rice JP, London SN, Olive DL. Reevaluation of hysterosalpingography in infertility investigation. Obstet Gynecol. 1986;67(5):718–21.
24. Saunders RD, Shwayder JM, Nakajima ST. Current methods of tubal patency assessment. Fertil Steril. 2011;95(7):2171–9.
25. Bittencourt CA, et al. Accuracy of saline contrast sonohysterography in detection of endometrial polyps and submucosal leiomyomas in women of reproductive age with abnormal uterine bleeding: systematic review and meta-analysis. Ultrasound Obstet Gynecol. 2017;50(1):32–9.
26. Jette NT, Glass RH. Prognostic value of the postcoital test. Fertil Steril. 1972;23(1):29–32.
27. Oei SG, et al. Effectiveness of the postcoital test: randomised controlled trial. BMJ. 1998;317(7157):502–5.
28. Organization WH. WHO laboratory manual for the examination and processing of human semen. 6th ed. Geneva: WHO Press; 2021.
29. Schlegel PN, et al. Diagnosis and treatment of infertility in men: AUA/ASRM guideline part I. Fertil Steril. 2021;115(1):54–61.
30. Evenson D, Wixon R. Meta-analysis of sperm DNA fragmentation using the sperm chromatin structure assay. Reprod Biomed Online. 2006;12(4):466–72.
31. Practice Committee of the American Society for Reproductive M. Diagnostic evaluation of the infertile male: a committee opinion. Fertil Steril. 2015;103(3):e18–25.
32. Thonneau P, et al. Incidence and main causes of infertility in a resident population (1,850,000) of three French regions (1988-1989). Hum Reprod. 1991;6(6):811–6.
33. Datta J, et al. Prevalence of infertility and help seeking among 15 000 women and men. Hum Reprod. 2016;31(9):2108–18.
34. Hull MG, et al. Population study of causes, treatment, and outcome of infertility. Br Med J (Clin Res Ed). 1985;291(6510):1693–7.
35. Recent advances in medically assisted conception. Report of a WHO Scientific Group. World Health Organ Tech Rep Ser. 1992;820:1–111.
36. Sermondade N, et al. Female obesity is negatively associated with live birth rate following IVF: a systematic review and meta-analysis. Hum Reprod Update. 2019;25(4):439–51.
37. Zhang Y, et al. Couples' prepregnancy body mass index and time to pregnancy among those attempting to conceive their first pregnancy. Fertil Steril. 2020;114(5):1067–75.
38. Crosignani PG, et al. Overweight and obese anovulatory patients with polycystic ovaries: parallel improvements in anthropometric indices, ovarian physiology and fertility rate induced by diet. Hum Reprod. 2003;18(9):1928–32.
39. Teede HJ, et al. Recommendations from the 2023 international evidence-based guideline for the assessment and management of polycystic ovary syndrome. Fertil Steril. 2023;120(4):767–93.
40. Legro RS, et al. Letrozole versus clomiphene for infertility in the polycystic ovary syndrome. N Engl J Med. 2014;371(2):119–29.
41. CVan Campenhout J, Simard R, Leduc B. Antiestrogenic effect of clomiphene in the human being. Fertil Steril. 1968;19(5):700–6.
42. Pildes RB. Induction of ovulation with clomiphene. Am J Obstet Gynecol. 1965;91:466–79.
43. Adashi EY. Clomiphene citrate-initiated ovulation: a clinical update. In: Seminars in reproductive endocrinology. Copyright© 1986 by Thieme Medical Publishers, Inc; 1986.
44. Sharpe A, et al. Metformin for ovulation induction (excluding gonadotrophins) in women with polycystic ovary syndrome. Cochrane Database Syst Rev. 2019;12(12):CD013505.
45. Legro RS, et al. Clomiphene, metformin, or both for infertility in the polycystic ovary syndrome. N Engl J Med. 2007;356(6):551–66.
46. Brown J, Farquhar C. Clomiphene and other antioestrogens for ovulation induction in polycystic ovarian syndrome. Cochrane Database Syst Rev. 2016;12(12):CD002249.
47. Shi S, et al. Letrozole and human menopausal gonadotropin for ovulation induction in clomiphene resistance polycystic ovary syndrome patients: a randomized controlled study. Medicine (Baltimore). 2020;99(4):e18383.
48. Franik S, et al. Aromatase inhibitors (letrozole) for ovulation induction in infertile women with polycystic ovary syndrome. Cochrane Database Syst Rev. 2022;9(9):CD010287.
49. te Velde ER, Pearson PL. The variability of female reproductive ageing. Hum Reprod Update. 2002;8(2):141–54.
50. Broer, S.L., C.H. Weimar, B.C. Fauser, and F.J. Broekmans, Prognostic testing for ovarian reserve, in Textbook of assisted reproductive techniques: volume 2: clinical perspectives, D.K.W.G. Ariel; Howles, Colin M.; Shoham, Zeev, Editor. 2023, CRC Press: Boca Raton. p. 409–418.
51. Carson SA, Kallen AN. Diagnosis and management of infertility: a review. JAMA. 2021;326(1):65–76.
52. Practice Committee of the American Society for Reproductive M. Role of tubal surgery in the era of assisted reproductive technology: a committee opinion. Fertil Steril. 2015;103(6):e37–43.
53. Kuohung WH, Mark D. In: Connor RF, editor. Female infertility: causes. Wolters Kluwer; 2024.
54. Practice Committee of the American Society for Reproductive Medicine. Electronic address AAO. Role of tubal surgery in the era of assisted reproductive technology: a committee opinion. Fertil Steril. 2021;115(5):1143–50.

55. Melo P, et al. Surgical treatment for tubal disease in women due to undergo in vitro fertilisation. Cochrane Database Syst Rev. 2020;10(10):CD002125.
56. Gordts S, Campo R, Puttemans P, Gordts S. Clinical factors determining pregnancy outcome after microsurgical tubal reanastomosis. Fertil Steril. 2009;92(4):1198–202.
57. Malacova E, et al. Live delivery outcome after tubal sterilization reversal: a population-based study. Fertil Steril. 2015;104(4):921–6.
58. Donnez J, Dolmans MM. Uterine fibroid management: from the present to the future. Hum Reprod Update. 2016;22(6):665–86.
59. Somigliana E, et al. Fibroids and female reproduction: a critical analysis of the evidence. Hum Reprod Update. 2007;13(5):465–76.
60. Erden M, et al. The effect of </=6 cm sized noncavity-distorting intramural fibroids on in vitro fertilization outcomes: a systematic review and meta-analysis. Fertil Steril. 2023;119(6):996–1007.
61. Perez-Medina T, et al. Endometrial polyps and their implication in the pregnancy rates of patients undergoing intrauterine insemination: a prospective, randomized study. Hum Reprod. 2005;20(6):1632–5.
62. Venetis CA, et al. Clinical implications of congenital uterine anomalies: a meta-analysis of comparative studies. Reprod Biomed Online. 2014;29(6):665–83.
63. Practice Committee of the American Society for Reproductive Medicine. Electronic address AAO and M Practice Committee of the American Society for Reproductive. Uterine septum: a guideline. Fertil Steril. 2016;106(3):530–40.
64. Sugiura-Ogasawara M, et al. Uterine anomaly and recurrent pregnancy loss. Semin Reprod Med. 2011;29(6):514–21.
65. Deans R, Abbott J. Review of intrauterine adhesions. J Minim Invasive Gynecol. 2010;17(5):555–69.
66. Hooker AB, et al. Prevalence of intrauterine adhesions after the application of hyaluronic acid gel after dilatation and curettage in women with at least one previous curettage: short-term outcomes of a multicenter, prospective randomized controlled trial. Fertil Steril. 2017;107(5):1223–1231 e3.
67. Lin X, et al. A comparison of intrauterine balloon, intrauterine contraceptive device and hyaluronic acid gel in the prevention of adhesion reformation following hysteroscopic surgery for Asherman syndrome: a cohort study. Eur J Obstet Gynecol Reprod Biol. 2013;170(2):512–6.
68. Helmerhorst FM, et al. Intra-uterine insemination versus timed intercourse for cervical hostility in subfertile couples. Cochrane Database Syst Rev. 2005;2005(4):CD002809.
69. Cohlen B, Bijkerk A, Van der Poel S, Ombelet W. IUI: review and systematic assessment of the evidence that supports global recommendations. Hum Reprod Update. 2018;24(3):300–19.
70. Schenken RS, Asch RH, Williams RF, Hodgen GD. Etiology of infertility in monkeys with endometriosis: luteinized unruptured follicles, luteal phase defects, pelvic adhesions, and spontaneous abortions. Fertil Steril. 1984;41(1):122–30.
71. Practice Committee of the American Society for Reproductive M. Endometriosis and infertility: a committee opinion. Fertil Steril. 2012;98(3):591–8.
72. Vercellini P, et al. Surgery for endometriosis-associated infertility: a pragmatic approach. Hum Reprod. 2009;24(2):254–69.
73. Kostrzewa M, et al. Women's fertility after laparoscopic cystectomy of endometrioma and other benign ovarian tumors—a 24-month follow-up retrospective study. Neuro Endocrinol Lett. 2016;37(4):295–300.
74. Broi MGD, Ferriani RA, Navarro PA. Ethiopathogenic mechanisms of endometriosis-related infertility. JBRA Assist Reprod. 2019;23(3):273–80.
75. Chen I, et al. Pre- and postsurgical medical therapy for endometriosis surgery. Cochrane Database Syst Rev. 2020;11(11):CD003678.
76. Kallen CB, Arici A. Immune testing in fertility practice: truth or deception? Curr Opin Obstet Gynecol. 2003;15(3):225–31.
77. Clementini E, et al. Prevalence of chromosomal abnormalities in 2078 infertile couples referred for assisted reproductive techniques. Hum Reprod. 2005;20(2):437–42.
78. Guideline Group on Unexplained I, et al. Evidence-based guideline: unexplained infertilitydagger. Hum Reprod. 2023;38(10):1881–90.
79. Ray A, Shah A, Gudi A, Homburg R. Unexplained infertility: an update and review of practice. Reprod Biomed Online. 2012;24(6):591–602.
80. Hull MG, et al. The contribution of subtle oocyte or sperm dysfunction affecting fertilization in endometriosis-associated or unexplained infertility: a controlled comparison with tubal infertility and use of donor spermatozoa. Hum Reprod. 1998;13(7):1825–30.
81. Blacker CM, et al. Unexplained infertility: evaluation of the luteal phase; results of the National Center for Infertility Research at Michigan. Fertil Steril. 1997;67(3):437–42.
82. Custers IM, et al. Long-term outcome in couples with unexplained subfertility and an intermediate prognosis initially randomized between expectant management and immediate treatment. Hum Reprod. 2012;27(2):444–50.
83. Farquhar CM, et al. Intrauterine insemination with ovarian stimulation versus expectant management for unexplained infertility (TUI): a pragmatic, open-label, randomised, controlled, two-centre trial. Lancet. 2018;391(10119):441–50.
84. Maxwell C, et al. Guideline no. 391-pregnancy and maternal obesity part 1: pre-conception and prenatal care. J Obstet Gynaecol Can. 2019;41(11):1623–40.
85. Jick, H. and J. Porter, Relation between smoking and age of natural menopause. Report from the Boston Collaborative Drug Surveillance Program, Boston University Medical Center. Lancet, 1977. 1(8026): p. 1354–1355.

86. Pineles BL, Park E, Samet JM. Systematic review and meta-analysis of miscarriage and maternal exposure to tobacco smoke during pregnancy. Am J Epidemiol. 2014;179(7):807–23.
87. Practice Committee of the American Society for Reproductive Medicine. Electronic address AAO and M Practice Committee of the American Society for Reproductive. Evidence-based treatments for couples with unexplained infertility: a guideline. Fertil Steril. 2020;113(2):305–22.
88. Guzick DS, et al. Efficacy of superovulation and intrauterine insemination in the treatment of infertility. National Cooperative Reproductive Medicine Network. N Engl J Med. 1999;340(3):177–83.
89. Peeraer K, et al. Low-dose human menopausal gonadotrophin versus clomiphene citrate in subfertile couples treated with intrauterine insemination: a randomized controlled trial. Hum Reprod. 2015;30(5):1079–88.
90. Danhof NA, et al. IUI for unexplained infertility—a network meta-analysis. Hum Reprod Update. 2020;26(1):1–15.
91. Sunkara SK, et al. In vitro fertilisation for unexplained subfertility. Cochrane Database Syst Rev. 2023;9(9):CD003357.
92. Goldman MB, et al. A randomized clinical trial to determine optimal infertility treatment in older couples: the Forty and Over Treatment Trial (FORT-T). Fertil Steril. 2014;101(6):1574–81.e1-2.
93. Tanahatoe S, Hompes PG, Lambalk CB. Accuracy of diagnostic laparoscopy in the infertility work-up before intrauterine insemination. Fertil Steril. 2003;79(2):361–6.
94. Jin X, Ruiz Beguerie J. Laparoscopic surgery for subfertility related to endometriosis: a meta-analysis. Taiwan J Obstet Gynecol. 2014;53(3):303–8.
95. Tanbo T, Fedorcsak P. Endometriosis-associated infertility: aspects of pathophysiological mechanisms and treatment options. Acta Obstet Gynecol Scand. 2017;96(6):659–67.
96. Jarow JP, Espeland MA, Lipshultz LI. Evaluation of the azoospermic patient. J Urol. 1989;142(1):62–5.
97. Practice Committee of American Society for Reproductive Medicine in collaboration with Society for Male R and Urology. The management of infertility due to obstructive azoospermia. Fertil Steril. 2008;90(5 Suppl):S121–4.
98. Anawalt BD. In: Connor RF, editor. Treatments for male infertility. Wolters Kluwer; 2024.
99. Brinson AK, da Silva SG, Hesketh KR, Evenson KR. Impact of physical activity and sedentary behavior on spontaneous female and male fertility: a systematic review. J Phys Act Health. 2023;20(7):600–15.
100. Wang C, et al. Effect of increased scrotal temperature on sperm production in normal men. Fertil Steril. 1997;68(2):334–9.
101. Kandeel FR, Swerdloff RS. Role of temperature in regulation of spermatogenesis and the use of heating as a method for contraception. Fertil Steril. 1988;49(1):1–23.
102. Schlegel PN. Male infertility. In: Strauss JF, et al., editors. Yen & Jaffe's reproductive endocrinology: physiology, pathophysiology, and clinical management. Philadelphia: Elsevier Health Sciences; 2023. p. 575–86.
103. Salas-Huetos A, et al. Adherence to the Mediterranean diet is positively associated with sperm motility: a cross-sectional analysis. Sci Rep. 2019;9(1):3389.
104. Samplaski MK, et al. Varicocelectomy to "upgrade" semen quality to allow couples to use less invasive forms of assisted reproductive technology. Fertil Steril. 2017;108(4):609–12.
105. Wang J, et al. Inguinal and subinguinal micro-varicocelectomy, the optimal surgical management of varicocele: a meta-analysis. Asian J Androl. 2015;17(1):74–80.
106. Schlegel PN, et al. Diagnosis and treatment of infertility in men: AUA/ASRM guideline part II. Fertil Steril. 2021;115(1):62–9.
107. Bernie AM, Mata DA, Ramasamy R, Schlegel PN. Comparison of microdissection testicular sperm extraction, conventional testicular sperm extraction, and testicular sperm aspiration for nonobstructive azoospermia: a systematic review and meta-analysis. Fertil Steril. 2015;104(5):1099–103.e1-3.
108. de Ligny W, et al. Antioxidants for male subfertility. Cochrane Database Syst Rev. 2022;5(5):CD007411.
109. Attia AM, Abou-Setta AM, Al-Inany HG. Gonadotrophins for idiopathic male factor subfertility. Cochrane Database Syst Rev. 2013;2013(8):CD005071.
110. Anawalt BD. Approach to male infertility and induction of spermatogenesis. J Clin Endocrinol Metab. 2013;98(9):3532–42.
111. McLachlan RI, O'Bryan MK. Clinical review: state of the art for genetic testing of infertile men. J Clin Endocrinol Metab. 2010;95(3):1013–24.

11 Diagnosis and Treatment in Menopause

Doruk Cevdi Katlan and Nebahat Uzunay

11.1 Introduction

Menopause is the permanent standstill of the menstrual cycle due to cessation of hormone production from the ovaries for at least 12 months [1]. The Greek words *men*, meaning "month," and *pausis*, meaning "pause," were combined and named menopause [2]. The age of menopause varies depending on the health condition, dietary habits, and socioeconomic status of the individual; however, most women start to go through menopause between 45 and 56 years of age. The average age of natural menopause in the United States is 51 years [3, 4]. Considering the average life expectancy, it can be claimed that women spend approximately 40% of their lives (at least 30 years of life) after menopause [3].

11.2 Diagnosis

As women age, the total number of follicles in the ovaries decreases as a result of the ovulation of some of the follicles and atresia of the others. Therefore, the number of granulosa cells, the primary production site of estradiol (E2), inhibin B, and anti-Mullerian hormone (AMH), also decreases. When the inhibitory effect of E2 and inhibin B on gonadotropins disappears, follicle stimulating hormone (FSH) and luteinizing hormone (LH) production increases [1]. The increase in FSH is thought to be due to the decrease in inhibin B rather than E2. During the transition to menopause, E2 production fluctuates with FSH levels and can reach even higher concentrations than in women of reproductive age, while progesterone levels are lower [4]. With the decrease in E2 levels, menstrual cycles become irregular due to an imbalance in endometrial proliferation and secretion phases. First, the follicular phase shortens and the irregularity appears as frequent menstruation (polymenorrhea) and then as infrequent menstruation (oligomenorrhea) with prolongation of the follicular phase. With such anovulatory cycles, abnormal uterine bleeding may develop. As the process progresses, the cycles become longer and longer, resulting in amenorrhea [1].

In early menopause, testosterone levels do not change significantly. Thus, a relative increase in the ratio of testosterone to estrogen may occur, leading to symptoms of androgen excess [1]. The decrease in sex hormone-binding globulin (SHBG) production with menopause also leads to higher levels of free or unbound estrogen and testosterone [4]. Since some E2 can be produced by aromatization of testosterone secreted from the adrenal glands, menopausal symptoms other than menstrual cessation may not be evident in some women [1].

D. C. Katlan (✉) · N. Uzunay
Department of Obstetrics and Gynecology, Istanbul Training and Research Hospital, Istanbul, Türkiye

T. Akbayrak, E. Üzelpasaci (eds.), *Physiotherapy and Rehabilitation in Pelvic and Women's Health-Related Problems*, https://doi.org/10.1007/978-3-032-28741-0_11

Apart from the natural process, surgical procedures such as bilateral oophorectomy, endometriosis, cancer chemotherapy (especially with alkylating agents), radiation, chronic diseases such as HIV-AIDS, and antiestrogenic drugs can also lead to menopause [5]. Approximately 5% of women develop "early natural menopause" between the ages of 40 and 45, and 1% develop "primary ovarian failure" before the age of 40 [6]. In two prospective cohort studies investigating the effect of ethnicity, natural menopause was found to occur earlier in women of Hispanic origin and later in Japanese American women compared to white women [6].

More than 80% of women experience menopausal symptoms, although the frequency and severity vary according to the individual. Factors such as diet, smoking, ethnicity, comorbid medical problems, exercise, socioeconomic background, and body mass index can affect the severity and frequency of these symptoms [1].

In women over 45 years of age, the diagnosis of "menopausal transition" or "perimenopause" is based on a change in menstrual cycles, independent of symptoms such as hot flashes, sleep disturbance, depression, vaginal dryness, or sexual dysfunction [5]. Although serum FSH concentration is not required to make the diagnosis, a serum FSH concentration ≥25 IU/L indicates a possible menopausal transition [7]. It should be kept in mind that pelvic surgeries may temporarily increase FSH levels, and thus, it should be evaluated at least 3 months after such surgeries [5]. Similarly, E2 levels <20 pg/mL with increased FSH may suggest menopause [8].

There is no reliable marker to predict the timing of the final menstrual period (FMP) for women in menopausal transition. The AMH level has a strong correlation with "time to menopause," especially in older women, with higher sensitivity in women over 51 years of age than in women under 48 years of age [9]. Furthermore, the strong correlation of AMH with the number of early antral follicles makes the test easily reproducible. AMH levels decline with age, reaching below detectable levels about 5 years after menopause [10].

Clinical and endocrinologic findings during the transition to menopause have been described in the light of data from numerous studies. The largest of these studies is the Study of Women's Health Across the Nation (SWAN), which followed more than 3000 women between the ages of 42 and 52 for 15 years. The aim of the study was to predict the age of menopause in women of different ethnic backgrounds and to reveal the psychological, neurological, biochemical, and hormonal changes during menopause. Following the efforts of the World Health Organization (WHO) and the Council of Affiliated Menopause Societies (CAMS) in the last decade of the twentieth century, using data from all these studies, the Stages of Reproductive Aging Workshop (STRAW) was convened in 2001 in the United States with the participation of the American Society for Reproductive Medicine (ASRM), the National Institute on Aging (NIA), the National Institute of Child Health and Human Development (NICHD), and the North American Menopause Society (NAMS) to define changes in reproductive status from reproductive years to menopause and thus to develop a staging system. This system was revised as STRAW+10 in 2012 and is considered to be the gold standard for defining the menopausal process [5].

In this staging system, using the final menstrual period (FMP), menstrual cycle, hormonal levels, and symptoms, the menopause process is divided into three main periods: reproductive, menopausal transition, and postmenopausal. By dividing the reproductive period into three stages—"early," "peak," and "late"—and the menopausal transition and postmenopausal periods into two stages—"early" and "late"—a total of seven phases/stages centered on the final menstrual period were defined. FMP defines the boundary between menopausal transition and postmenopausal periods and is referred to as stage 0. This staging system makes it easier for patients and clinicians to assess the reproductive potential and the need for contraception and hormone therapy. FSH, inhibin B, AMH levels, and antral follicle count (AFC) values, which are endocrine criteria of STRAW+10, are accepted as being more supportive rather than diagnostic

[5, 11]. The AFC value is obtained by counting follicles with a diameter of 2–10 mm in the ovaries on ultrasonographic examination. This number does not change throughout the menstrual cycle. It correlates well with chronological age and reflects the size of immature follicular reserve. The main characteristics of this staging system are summarized in Table 11.1 based on the aforementioned studies [5, 11].

The reproductive period is divided into stages also called "−5," "−4," and "−3," corresponding to "early," "peak," and "late" stages, respectively. The menopausal transition period is similarly divided into stages, also called "−2" and "−1," and the postmenopausal period is classified into stages also called "+1" and "+2," corresponding to "early" and "late" stages of each period in the same order. Stage 0 marks the late menopausal transition–early postmenopausal boundary [5].

To summarize the main features of these stages:

Stage −5: It is the early stage of the reproductive period, starting with menarche. It usually takes several years for menstrual cycles to become regular, leading to variations in their duration depending on the individual. FSH, AMH, inhibin B levels, and AFC are normal.

Stage −4: It is the peak phase of the reproductive period, when fertility is the highest. Its duration is similarly variable during which menstrual cycles are regular. FSH, AMH, inhibin B levels, and AFC are normal.

Stage −3: It is the late stage of the reproductive period, again of variable duration. This is the period when women begin to notice changes in menstrual cycles and when fertility begins to decline. Endocrine changes have already started before the menstrual cycle changes significantly. This stage is subdivided into two substages: "−3b" and "−3a," with "−3b" being the earlier of these two.

In stage "−3b," menstrual cycles are regular, and FSH levels are normal; however, AMH, inhibin B levels, and AFC start to decrease. In stage "−3a," FSH levels, which are monitored between the second and fifth days of the cycle initiation, start to increase and become more variable. FSH levels exceeding two standard deviations above the mean value of women aged 25–30 years are generally considered to be high. Most clinicians use 10 mIU/ml as a cut-off value. E2 levels may be normal or elevated at this substage. Generally, a value of ≥80 pg/ml is considered to be high. If E2 level is elevated, FSH and E2 levels should be evaluated simultaneously, as this may suppress FSH. A single high FSH level is sufficient to define stage −3 and does not need to be repeated. However, in women aged 40–45 years with regular menstrual cycles, FSH level, which is found to be within normal limits, may vary by 30% in subsequent cycles. Therefore, if the first FSH value is normal, a second test is recommended. AMH, inhibin B levels, and AFC are low. Cycles are ovulatory, but with the shortening of the follicular phase, changes in cycle duration and menstrual quantity begin. Luteinizing hormone (LH) levels start to increase later than FSH levels.

Stage −2: It is the early stage of the menopausal transition period during which the variability in the length of menstrual cycles becomes marked. Persistent differences of 7 days or more in the length of consecutive cycles arise. FSH levels monitored between the second and fifth days of the cycle initiation are uneven but continue to rise. AMH levels and AFC are also low. Similar to previous ones, the duration of this stage is also variable.

Stage −1: It is the late stage of the menopausal transition period, which is characterized by more than two missed menstrual cycles or amenorrhea lasting more than 60 days. FSH levels continue to increase; values exceeding 25 IU/L are detected on a random day of the cycle and cycles become anovulatory. AMH levels and AFC are also low in this stage, which lasts 1–3 years on average. It is the stage when vasomotor symptoms start to appear.

Stage 0: Stage 0 is the FMP, which marks the late menopausal transition–early postmenopausal boundary.

Table 11.1 Characteristics of the main periods of menopausal process [5, 11]

Period			Stage	Duration	Menstrual cycle	FSH	INH. B	AMH	AFC	Symptom
Menarche										
1.1.1.Reproductive		Early	−5	Variable	Variable to regular					
		Peak	−4	Variable	Regular					
		1.Late	−3b	Variable	Regular	↓		↓	↓	
			−3a	Variable	Minor changes in duration/amount	Variable	↓	↓	↓	
1.Menopausal transition	1.Perimenopausal	Early	−2	Variable	Variable duration persistent ≥1 week variation of consecutive cycle duration	↑ Variable	↓	↓	↓	
		Late	−1	1–3 years	Amenorrhea ≥2 months	↑ (>25 IU/L)	↓	↓	↓	Vasomotor symptoms
Final menstrual period (FMP) (stage 0)										
1.1.1.Postmenopause	1.1.	1.1.Early	+1a	1 year	–	↑ Variable	↓	↓	↓↓	Vasomotor symptoms
			+1b	1 year	–	↑ Variable	↓	↓	↓↓	Vasomotor symptoms
			+1c	3–6 years	–	Stable	↓↓	↓↓	↓↓	
		Late	+2	Remaining lifespan	–					Genitourinary syndrome

INH B inhibin B, *AFC* antral follicle count, *IU/L* international unit

Stage +1: It is the early stage of the postmenopausal period. This stage is subdivided into three substages: "+1a," "+1b," and "+1c."

Stage +1a is the first year of amenorrhea after the final menstrual period. During this stage, FSH continues to increase, while E2, AMH, inhibin B levels, and AFC gradually decrease. It marks the end of the formerly called "perimenopause," which is accepted to begin at stage −2.

In stage +1b, FSH continues to increase and E2 continues to decrease. AMH, inhibin B levels, and AFC are very low. This similarly limited 1-year period is the stage when vasomotor symptoms are frequently experienced.

This 2-year period of stage +1a and +1b is followed by stage +1c, which lasts for 3–6 years. At this stage, FSH and E2 remain stable.

Stage +2: It is the late stage of the postmenopausal period. This is the stage of the somatic aging process, which includes the remaining life span. FSH and E2 levels do not change significantly. However, years after menopause, in very old women, further decrements of particularly FSH levels may be detected. Symptoms of vaginal dryness and genitourinary atrophy become more common during this stage.

In the STRAW+10 statement, the fixed reference point is the time of last menstrual bleeding. Therefore, the age range of each stage is determined accordingly and is variable. Similarly, each stage may not necessarily occur in all women or in the same chronological order. This makes the staging system difficult to implement for every single individual. To exemplify, it is inconvenient to apply this to women with premature ovarian failure, polycystic ovary syndrome (PCOS), or hypothalamic amenorrhea, or who have undergone endometrial ablation or hysterectomy, since their transitional process is different [5, 12]. In this group of women, it is recommended to measure FSH levels for diagnostic purposes [12].

It is accepted that nonsmoking women can safely use oral contraceptives until the age of menopause. Since these women will not have irregular bleeding or vasomotor symptoms, it is difficult to determine the transition to menopause. In these women, the hypothalamic-pituitary axis is suppressed by high doses of estrogen. Therefore, measurement of serum FSH level under oral contraceptive therapy will not give a reliable result. For these cases, to diagnose menopause, it is recommended to measure serum FSH level after cessation of the drug for 2–4 weeks [13, 14].

For women who have undergone hysterectomy or endometrial ablation, menstrual bleeding cannot be used as a criterion for menopausal transition. In this group, it is also recommended to measure FSH levels, but this time, at least 3 months post-surgery.

In these exceptional women, a serum FSH level >25 IU/L, especially concomitant with hot flashes, suggests late menopausal transition (stage −1). But, in postmenopausal women (stage +1, +2), FSH levels are usually expected to be in the range of 70–100 IU/L [5, 7, 15].

Although for women older than 45 years, the aforementioned staging system may be applicable for the probable diagnosis of menopausal transition, human chorionic gonadotropin (β-HCG), prolactin (PRL), and thyroid-stimulating hormone (TSH) measurements should be ordered to exclude other causes of menstrual cycle dysfunction in women aged 40–45 years. However, for women under 40 years of age with irregular menses and menopausal symptoms, the diagnosis may be primary ovarian failure.

Menopausal transition, on average, begins at 47 years of age, but timing is variable. Therefore, for women over 45 years of age with irregular menstrual cycles presenting with menopausal symptoms, such as hot flushes, sleep disturbances, new-onset depression, cognitive changes (forgetfulness, difficulty in remembering words, brain fog, etc.), genitourinary menopausal syndrome (symptoms and signs caused by hypoestrogenic changes in labia, clitoris, vagina, urethra, and bladder, formerly called vulvovaginal atrophy), joint pain, breast tenderness, increased menstrual migraine headaches, and decreased sexual desire and function, further diagnostic evaluation is not recommended. These women are likely accepted to be in the menopausal transition [5, 11, 16–22]. However, it should be kept in mind that the presence of all these symptoms is not obligatory, or not all women may experience them with the same severity [11].

11.3 Treatment

Hormone replacement therapy (HRT) is highly effective in young postmenopausal women to prevent long-term degenerative diseases such as osteoporotic fractures, cardiovascular diseases, diabetes mellitus, and possible cognitive impairment with vasomotor symptoms [23]. The initial 5 years of treatment are considered to be safe in healthy individuals, provided that it is started before the age of 60 and/or within the first 10 years after menopause [24]. Studies have shown that oral estradiol (E2) slows the progression of atherosclerosis when started within 6 years after menopause, contrary to its initiation at 10 or more years postmenopausal. Similarly, early initiation of HRT may improve insulin action and possibly help to prevent Alzheimer's disease [10].

The primary indication for HRT is to treat moderate to severe vasomotor symptoms. Vasomotor symptoms such as hot flushes and night sweats can occur in two-thirds of menopausal women and can persist for years, affecting the quality of life. The most effective treatment is estrogen HRT with or without progestogen [25]. Their prevalence among women experiencing natural menopause in the United States is 50–82% [26].

Among younger women, the most common reason for initiation of HRT is to improve vasomotor symptoms; however, reducing the risk of osteoporosis is the primary aim in the older age group [26]. There is no standardized duration for HRT. The duration of treatment is determined individually by keeping the dose at the lowest that improves the symptoms.

Treatment of menopause can be classified under several headings [1]:

- Hormonal drug therapy:
  - (a) Systemic hormonal therapy
  - (b) Selective estrogen receptor modulators (SERMs)
  - (c) Local hormonal therapy
- Nonhormonal drug therapy
- Non-drug treatment

11.3.1 Hormonal Drug Therapy

Hormonal drug therapy may be administered either as systemic or local therapy or can be done by SERMs [1].

11.3.1.1 Systemic Hormonal Therapy

Systemic hormonal therapy can be applied continuously or intermittently by tablets, sprays, gels, vaginal rings, or transdermal patches. It can be organized as "estrogen alone," "estrogen-progestin combination," "estrogen-bazedoxifene combination," or "progestin alone" regimens [26]. The American College of Obstetrics and Gynecology (ACOG) recommends the use of progesterone/progestagen in combination with oral estrogen as HRT to prevent endometrial hyperplasia/cancer in women with a uterus. For these women, the incidence of endometrial hyperplasia with "estrogen alone" HRT is approximately 30% at 1 year. Bazedoxifene, a selective estrogen receptor modulator, can be used as an alternative to progesterone to reduce the risk of endometrial hyperplasia and cancer [27].

Systemic hormonal therapy should be used for the shortest duration and at the lowest effective dose, as estrogen therapy alone increases the risk of deep venous thromboembolism and stroke. Although the absolute increased risk in early menopausal women is minimal, combination HRT is also associated with an increased risk of breast cancer. Therefore, caution should be exercised with regard to the duration and dose of therapy [28].

Estrogen-containing HRT is associated with a two- to fivefold increased risk of venous thromboembolism. Studies suggest that natural progesterone does not increase the risk of venous thromboembolism, whereas synthetic progestins (e.g., medroxyprogesterone acetate) do. The use of estrogen alone has been associated with a 1.2–1.5-fold relative risk compared to nonusers. It has been suggested that this increased risk may be due to the prothrombotic effect of orally administered estrogen through hepatic induction. The prothrombotic effect is probably related to the "first-pass" effect of high amounts of estrogen through the liver [29].

Studies comparing oral and transdermal estrogen therapy have shown that transdermally administered estrogen has little or no effect in elevating prothrombotic substances. It may have beneficial effects on proinflammatory markers, including C-reactive protein, prothrombin activation peptide, and antithrombin activity. It has also been reported that, in contrast to oral use, it may have a suppressive effect on tissue plasminogen activator antigen and plasminogen activator inhibitor activity [29].

Non-oral administration methods of E2 include transdermal patches, gels, sprays, and vaginal rings. Topical vaginal creams and tablets prescribed for the treatment of local urogenital atrophic changes have low levels of systemic absorption with no adverse effects on coagulation proteins or on the incidence of venous thromboembolism [29]. Therefore, transdermal rather than oral use of E2, especially in older ages, is considered to be more advantageous in women with venous thromboembolism, risk of stroke, diabetes mellitus, hypertension, cholecystitis, and other cardiovascular risk factors [24]. A study drawing attention to transdermal estrogen use is the ESTHER study conducted in France in 2007, which investigated the use of HRT in 271 cases of thromboembolism. It was found that oral hormone administration increased the risk by 4.2 times, while transdermal estrogen increased the risk to a lesser extent by 0.9 times. Meanwhile, it was reported that the risk coefficient for natural micronized progesterone use was 0.7, indicating a significant reduction in thromboembolism risk [30].

After the Women's Health Initiative (WHI) study in 2002 disclosed an increased risk of breast cancer, coronary events, stroke, and thromboembolism in women treated for more than 5 years with PremPro®, a combination of conjugated equine estrogen (CEE) and medroxyprogesterone acetate (MPA), the use of HRT in menopause declined sharply. This was due to safety concerns after the halfway termination of the study [31]. In the United States (US), the most widely used brand of CEE for HRT is Premarin® (derived from pregnant mares), which contains about 100 different estrogens, mainly estrone sulfate, equilins, and alpha-estradiol. Following reports from the WHI study, sales of Premarin® also declined by over 30% along with PremPro® [32].

About two thirds of women who use HRT discontinue it, usually within the first 2 years, due to unwanted side effects, mainly weight gain. These side effects include bloating, breast tenderness, and irregular bleeding caused by the synthetic progestin part of HRT [32].

Progesterone was first used in 1934 for HRT in the treatment of women who had undergone oophorectomy. Due to their significant first-pass effect through the liver, progestins were developed in the 1940s as an alternative, initially from progesterone (e.g., medroxyprogesterone acetate: MPA) and then from testosterone (e.g., 19-nortestosterone). Progestins can bind to progesterone, androgen, estrogen, and glucocorticoid receptors with different affinities, which explains the differences in their metabolic effects [32].

Micronized progesterone is approved as an oral capsule by the Food and Drug Administration (FDA) in the United States under the name Prometrium® (Progestan® in Türkiye). It has been reported to prevent endometrial hyperplasia when used with estrogen at a dose of 200 mg/day for 12 days a month. It has also been shown to be more effective than synthetic MPA in improving sleep quality in postmenopausal women when used with estrogen [25]. In an extracorporeal uterine perfusion model, vaginal application of micronized progesterone has been shown to plateau in endometrium and myometrium in approximately 6 h. Considering metabolic pathways and peripheral plasma levels, vaginal use of progesterone HRT may be more advantageous than the oral route [33].

The majority of systemic estrogens prescribed in the United States are in oral form. The most commonly prescribed oral estrogens for the treatment of vasomotor symptoms are E2 and CEE, with standard doses of 1.0 mg and 0.625 mg, respectively [26]. Transdermal patches are commonly used, releasing 0.0375 mg or 0.05 mg of E2 per day, although higher and lower doses are also available. All systemic HRT products have FDA approval for the treatment of vasomotor symptoms. The exception is Menostar®, a transdermal patch that releases 0.014 mg of E2 per day, which is approved for the prevention of osteoporosis. Common side effects associated with estrogen use include breast tenderness, bloating, and uterine bleeding [10].

The most commonly prescribed progestagens in the United States are MPA, available in oral doses of 2.5 mg, 5 mg, and 10 mg; and micronized progesterone, available in oral doses of 100 mg and 200 mg. Progestogen therapy with a dose of 2.5 mg MPA or 100 mg micronized progesterone is sufficient for endometrial protection. There are also treatment regimens with norethindrone acetate, drospirenone, or levonorgestrel serving for the same purpose [10].

As mentioned before, after the publication of the WHI study results, there was a decrease in estrogen and progestagen prescriptions due to women's concerns about their health. This led to an increase in the use of bioidentical hormones based on their more natural structure. However, the FDA did not approve compound preparations of bioidentical hormones for reasons such as lack of standardized dosing, quality monitoring, and adequate controlled studies in terms of safety and efficacy. Bijuva® oral capsules (0.5 mg E2 + 100 mg micronized progesterone or 1 mg E2 + 100 mg micronized progesterone) exceptionally received FDA approval in 2018 for the treatment of moderate to severe vasomotor symptoms associated with menopause [10, 27].

In 2008, a literature review of HRT by the University of Belgium concluded that the safest HRT method is the use of transdermally administered E2 combined with natural progesterone [23].

The United States Preventive Services Task Force statement of November 2022 emphasizes that systemic HRT should not be used for the primary prevention of chronic conditions in postmenopausal women, despite its benefits [26].

In addition to all, undiagnosed abnormal uterine bleeding, breast cancer and other estrogen-dependent neoplasms, history of active or previous deep vein thrombosis, thrombophilia, history of myocardial infarction and transient ischemic attack, liver dysfunction, and uncontrolled hypertension are contraindications for HRT [10].

One of the most important long-term implications of menopausal transition is its negative effect on women's bone health. Bone remodeling is a continuous and dynamic process with simultaneous activities of osteoclast-mediated bone resorption and osteoblast-mediated bone formation. The positive bone balance in favor of bone formation starts to shift to a status in favor of bone resorption between 25 and 35 years of age, leading to a decrease in bone mass of about 0.4% per year. During menopausal transition, in the absence of HRT, this rate increases to 2–5% per year for the first 5–10 years; then, this loss slows down but continues at a pace of 1% per year. This increases the risk of fractures [34]. There are three important components that are involved in osteoclastic and osteoblastic activities in bone formation and destruction: The receptor activator of nuclear factor-kappa B (RANK), the receptor activator of nuclear factor-kappa B ligand (RANKL), and osteoprotegerin (OPG). Increased osteoclast activity in postmenopausal osteoporosis is mediated through the RANKL pathway. RANKL, released by osteoblasts, binds to RANK on the surface of osteoclast precursor cells, activating osteoclast formation and function, leading to bone resorption. To counterbalance this remodeling, OPG secreted by osteoblasts binds to RANKL and blocks RANK activation. In postmenopausal women, decreased estrogen levels provoke greater RANKL expression, and simultaneously, activity of OPG is suppressed. Osteoblasts cannot completely fill the resorption gaps of osteoclastic activity, causing postmenopausal osteoporosis [35]. Therefore, HRT may help to prevent osteoporosis, positively contributing to its standard medical approach by dietary (sufficient calcium and vitamin D, avoidance of alcohol and smoking, etc.) and exercise (regular weight-bearing, etc.) modifications, taking necessary precautions (diminishing the risk of falls, etc.), and pharmacologic treatment (bisphosphonates, denosumab, etc.) [10].

A decrease in estrogen during the menopausal transition lowers the pain threshold, increases substance P release, and decreases opioid peptide and serotonin production and thus causes common muscle and joint pains. These may also benefit from HRT [36].

11.3.1.2 Selective Estrogen Receptor Modulators (SERMs)

SERMs are drugs that can act as estrogen agonists or antagonists upon binding to the estrogen receptor.

Bazedoxifene was FDA approved in 2014 and is available orally in combination with CEE for the treatment of moderate to severe vasomotor symptoms and for the prevention of postmenopausal osteoporosis under the name Duavee® (20 mg Bazedoxifene + 0.45 mg CEE). When used alone, bazedoxifene slows down the loss of bone mineral density but increases the number of hot flushes and the risk of venous thromboembolism. In contrast, when combined with CEE, it does not increase the risk of venous thromboembolism to the same extent as the CEE + MPA combination. Since synthetic progestins of HRT seem to be dicier for breast cancer, it is a suitable choice for women who prefer to use systemic HRT but are concerned about its safety [10].

Ospemifene is a drug in the SERM group approved for oral use in the treatment of menopausal dyspareunia [37]. Once-daily oral use (30, 60, or 90 mg) improves vulvovaginal symptoms similar to local estrogen therapy. However, it is not approved for use in breast cancer and it may increase the risk of venous thromboembolism [34]. It lowers vaginal pH, reduces nocturia and the frequency of urinary tract infections, and improves sexual function but may increase vasomotor symptoms, vaginal discharge, candidiasis, and endometrial thickness [38].

Raloxifene, another drug from the SERM group, is also approved by the FDA to prevent/treat postmenopausal osteoporosis. It selectively activates estrogen receptors only in bone tissue. Raloxifene (60 mg/day) prevents vertebral fractures, but it does not prevent non-vertebral osteoporotic ones [10].

Tibolone is a selective regulator of tissue estrogenic activity used in the treatment of osteoporosis and endometriosis. Similar to estrogen, it improves vaginal dryness, dyspareunia, sudden urges to urinate, and urinary incontinence by maturing the vaginal epithelium. It has estrogenic effects on the vagina but not on the endometrium. It is not FDA approved [38].

11.3.1.3 Local Hormonal Therapy

The genitourinary syndrome of menopause, which includes symptoms such as vaginal dryness, discomfort—dyspareunia, burning—itching, and frequent urination, is common in perimenopausal and postmenopausal periods. The prevalence may be up to 50% in postmenopausal women [38].

Women who do not receive Systemic Hormonal Therapy almost inevitably develop this genitourinary syndrome of menopause. Even women receiving systemic hormone replacement may need additional local estrogen therapy. Local estrogen therapy increases vaginal acidity, allows lactobacilli to dominate the flora, and increases blood flow and thus treats atrophy. It can be applied in various formulations such as vaginal rings, creams, or tablets. These local treatments result in complete improvement within 2–3 months of usage [35].

Topical dehydroepiandrosterone (DHEA) is converted to estrogens and androgens when applied to the vagina. By this mechanism, vaginal estrogen levels are increased, and symptoms of atrophy are relieved. The product approved by the FDA is available in 6.5 mg ovule form (Prasterone®). This has been shown to be effective in the treatment of genitourinary syndrome and can improve dyspareunia and sexual function [38, 39].

Testosterone can also improve objective signs of atrophy, vaginal dryness, and possibly sexual function. When applied topically, it is converted to dihydrotestosterone by 5-alpha reductase. Testosterone in doses of 150–300 μg/day induces the proliferation of vaginal epithelium [38]. However, its oral use has been reported to result in negative effects on lipid profiles [25, 38].

11.3.2 Nonhormonal Drug Therapy

Selective serotonin reuptake inhibitors (SSRIs), serotonin norepinephrine reuptake inhibitors (SNRIs), and gabapentin can be used to treat vasomotor menopausal symptoms. Paroxetine, escitalopram, and venlafaxine, at lower doses than those used for psychiatric conditions, are the most commonly used antidepressants for this purpose. Paroxetine, in particular, is the only drug approved by the FDA. Its therapeutic effect arises starting from the first week of its use at a dose of 7.5 mg/day. However, Paroxetine and Fluoxetine should not be used concomitantly with tamoxifen due to their inhibitory effects on cytochrome P450 phase I enzymes (CYP2D6) [26, 31, 40, 41].

Although not approved by the FDA for the treatment of vasomotor symptoms, gabapentin has also been documented to reduce hot flashes in menopausal women. High-dose gabapentin (900–2400 mg per day) reduces hot flashes to the same extent as estrogen replacement [26, 40].

Clonidine, an α-2 adrenergic agonist, may be moderately effective for mild hot flashes. But it is less effective than SSRIs/SNRIs and gabapentin and therefore is generally not recommended [26, 31, 42].

Neurokinin B, which acts through neurokinin 3 receptors (NK3R) located in the arcuate nucleus of the hypothalamus, has recently been blamed for the hot flashes of menopause. NK3R antagonists have therefore been considered for the treatment of vasomotor symptoms. Initial studies suggest that they may be more effective than SNRIs [30]. Fezolinetant, an NK3R antagonist, is FDA approved for moderate to severe vasomotor symptoms. It is used as a single oral daily dose of 45 mg. Headache is its most common side effect [31, 41, 42].

Oxybutynin, with its anticholinergic properties, may also improve hot flashes and night sweats in a dose-dependent manner up to 15 mg daily. Side effects such as dry mouth, constipation, and urinary retention make patients' adherence to the treatment difficult [24]. It has been demonstrated that oxybutynin is also effective in reducing sleep disturbances in postmenopausal women [31, 40].

11.3.3 Non-drug Treatment

Lifestyle changes such as wearing comfortable and antiperspirant clothing and lowering bed and room temperature seem to be feasible, but these have not been shown to be beneficial in clinical trials [24, 43].

There is limited evidence to support dietary changes in improving vasomotor symptoms of menopause [40]. Alcohol, spicy foods, hot drinks, and foods have been considered triggers of vasomotor symptoms; however, no benefit has been demonstrated by their restriction. Although there are studies suggesting that weight loss may also reduce these symptoms, the mechanism has not been fully explained [43].

Complementary and alternative therapies include phytoestrogens, vitamin E, and omega-3 fatty acids. Vitamin E, milk thistle, and omega-3 fatty acids have been used to treat vasomotor symptoms of menopause. They are generally safe, but studies have shown that they do no better than a placebo. Similarly, cannabinoids, wild potato, dong quai, evening primrose oil, ginseng, chaste berry, and black snakeroot have not been shown to relieve vasomotor symptoms [26, 27].

Relaxation therapy, acupuncture, and paced respiration have not been shown to relieve vasomotor symptoms. More studies are needed to evaluate the positive results of aromatherapy, reflexology, and homeopathy [27, 43].

Exercise and yoga have not been found to be effective as well. However, hypnosis and cognitive behavioral therapy have been shown to improve vasomotor symptoms in some women and are recommended by the North American

Menopause Association as a complementary treatment method in menopause [24, 26, 43].

It has also been shown that vasomotor symptoms decreased in women who applied mindfulness-based stress reduction methods compared to women who did not, but the difference was not statistically significant [43].

Some alternative treatment options have been proposed for the treatment of genitourinary syndrome of menopause. Among these, polycarbophil-based vaginal moisturizers produce a moist film that remains attached to the epithelial cell surface. The resulting hydration of epithelium provides lubrication of the vaginal wall. This also regulates vaginal acidity and is therapeutic for dryness and dyspareunia [26, 38, 39].

Hyaluronic acid is a lubricant with water-retaining ionic properties that can be used to increase tissue volume and epithelial integrity. Similarly, it treats vaginal atrophy and dyspareunia [10, 38, 43].

Fractional carbon dioxide laser therapy has regenerative properties on vaginal epithelium. It seems to improve the symptoms of genitourinary syndrome. However, it is a controversial method since its long-term effects are unknown, and it is costly [10, 38, 43]. More studies are needed before recommending its widespread use [39].

11.4 Conclusion

Menopause is a fundamental transitional stage of a woman's life that all healthcare providers should be informed about. This vital switch of reproductive status is accompanied by many neurologic, cardiovascular, uro-gynecologic, and musculoskeletal symptoms and has a substantial sociopsychological impact. Alleviation of the burden of this transition by a variety of therapy options and preparation of the lady to the new "second chapter" of her life is therefore of utmost importance. Appropriate counseling should target persuading the patient to believe in the fact that menopause is, in reality, a "beginning" rather than an "end."

References

1. Peacock K, Carlson K, Ketvertis KM. Menopause. In: StatPearls [Internet]. Treasure Island: StatPearls Publishing; 2024 [cited 2024 May 26]. Available from: http://www.ncbi.nlm.nih.gov/books/NBK507826/.
2. McNeil MA, Merriam SB. Menopause. Ann Intern Med. 2021;174(7):ITC97–112.
3. US Preventive Services Task Force, Mangione CM, Barry MJ, Nicholson WK, Cabana M, Caughey AB, et al. Hormone therapy for the primary prevention of chronic conditions in postmenopausal persons: US Preventive Services Task Force recommendation statement. JAMA. 2022;328(17):1740–6.
4. Santoro N. Perimenopause: from research to practice. J Womens Health (Larchmt). 2016;25(4):332–9.
5. Harlow SD, Gass M, Hall JE, Lobo R, Maki P, Rebar RW, et al. Executive summary of the Stages of Reproductive Aging Workshop +10: addressing the unfinished agenda of staging reproductive aging. Climacteric. 2012;15(2):105–14.
6. Burkard T, Moser M, Rauch M, Jick SS, Meier CR. Utilization pattern of hormone therapy in UK general practice between 1996 and 2015: a descriptive study. Menopause. 2019;26(7):741–9.
7. Freeman EW, Sammel MD, Gracia CR, Kapoor S, Lin H, Liu L, et al. Follicular phase hormone levels and menstrual bleeding status in the approach to menopause. Fertil Steril. 2005;83(2):383–92.
8. Williams M, Richard-Davis G, Williams PL, Christensen L, Ward E, Schrager S. A review of African American women's experiences in menopause. Menopause. 2022;29(11):1331–7.
9. Finkelstein JS, Lee H, Karlamangla A, Neer RM, Sluss PM, Burnett-Bowie SAM, et al. Antimullerian hormone and impending menopause in late reproductive age: the study of women's health across the nation. J Clin Endocrinol Metab. 2020;105(4):e1862–71.
10. McGraw Hill Medical [İnternet]. [cited 2024 Dec 4]. Menopause and the mature woman. Available from: https://obgyn.mhmedical.com/content.aspx?sectionid=241010835&bookid=2658.
11. Soules MR, Sherman S, Parrott E, Rebar R, Santoro N, Utian W, et al. Executive summary: stages of reproductive aging workshop (STRAW). Fertil Steril. 2001;76(5):874–8.
12. Elting MW, Kwee J, Korsen TJM, Rekers-Mombarg LTM, Schoemaker J. Aging women with polycystic ovary syndrome who achieve regular menstrual cycles have a smaller follicle cohort than those who continue to have irregular cycles. Fertil Steril. 2003;79(5):1154–60.
13. Robert F, Casper MD. Clinical manifestations and diagnosis of menopause [Internet]. Available from: https://www.uptodate.com/contents/clinical-manifestations-and-diagnosis-of-menopause?search=menopoz&source=search_result&selectedTitle=1%7E150&usage_type=default&display_rank=1#H172091386.

14. Black A, Francoeur D, Rowe T, Collins J, Miller D, Brown T, et al. SOGC clinical practice guidelines: Canadian contraception consensus. J Obstet Gynaecol Can. 2004;26(3):219–96.
15. Randolph JF, Zheng H, Sowers MR, Crandall C, Crawford S, Gold EB, et al. Change in follicle-stimulating hormone and estradiol across the menopausal transition: effect of age at the final menstrual period. J Clin Endocrinol Metab. 2011;96(3):746–54.
16. Woods NF, Mitchell ES. Symptoms during the perimenopause: prevalence, severity, trajectory, and significance in women's lives. Am J Med. 2005;118(Suppl 12B):14–24.
17. Hansen KR, Knowlton NS, Thyer AC, Charleston JS, Soules MR, Klein NA. A new model of reproductive aging: the decline in ovarian non-growing follicle number from birth to menopause. Hum Reprod. 2008;23(3):699–708.
18. Greendale GA, Karlamangla AS, Maki PM. The menopause transition and cognition. JAMA. 2020;323(15):1495–6.
19. Szoeke CEI, Cicuttini F, Guthrie J, Dennerstein L. Self-reported arthritis and the menopause. Climacteric. 2005;8(1):49–55.
20. Dennerstein L, Dudley EC, Hopper JL, Guthrie JR, Burger HG. A prospective population-based study of menopausal symptoms. Obstet Gynecol. 2000;96(3):351–8.
21. MacGregor EA. Menstruation, sex hormones, and migraine. Neurol Clin. 1997;15(1):125–41.
22. El Khoudary SR, Greendale G, Crawford SL, Avis NE, Brooks MM, Thurston RC, et al. The menopause transition and women's health at midlife: a progress report from the Study of Women's Health Across the Nation (SWAN). Menopause. 2019;26(10):1213–27.
23. L'hermite M, Simoncini T, Fuller S, Genazzani AR. Could transdermal estradiol + progesterone be a safer postmenopausal HRT? A review. Maturitas. 2008;60(3–4):185–201.
24. L'Hermite M. HRT optimization, using transdermal estradiol plus micronized progesterone, a safer HRT. Climacteric. 2013;16(Suppl 1):44–53.
25. Sites CK. Bioidentical hormones for menopausal therapy. Womens Health (Lond). 2008;4(2):163–71.
26. Practice bulletin no. 141: management of menopausal symptoms. Obstet Gynecol. 2014;123(1):202.
27. Crandall CJ, Mehta JM, Manson JE. Management of menopausal symptoms: a review. JAMA. 2023;329(5):405–20.
28. Davis SR, Baber RJ. Treating menopause—MHT and beyond. Nat Rev Endocrinol. 2022;18(8):490–502.
29. Postmenopausal estrogen therapy route of administration and risk of venous thromboembolism [İnternet]. [cited 2024 Nov 24]. Available from: https://www.acog.org/clinical/clinical-guidance/committee-opinion/articles/2013/04/postmenopausal-estrogen-therapy-route-of-administration-and-risk-of-venous-thromboembolism.
30. Canonico M, Oger E, Plu-Bureau G, Conard J, Meyer G, Lévesque H, et al. Hormone therapy and venous thromboembolism among postmenopausal women: impact of the route of estrogen administration and progestogens: the ESTHER study. Circulation. 2007;115(7):840–5.
31. Levy B, Simon JA. A contemporary view of menopausal hormone therapy. Obstet Gynecol. 2024;144(1):12–23.
32. Moskowitz D. A comprehensive review of the safety and efficacy of bioidentical hormones for the management of menopause and related health risks. Altern Med Rev. 2006;11(3):208–23.
33. Bulletti C, Bulletti FM, Sciorio R, Guido M. Progesterone: the key factor of the beginning of life. Int J Mol Sci. 2022;23(22):14138.
34. Riis BJ, Hansen MA, Jensen AM, Overgaard K, Christiansen C. Low bone mass and fast rate of bone loss at menopause: equal risk factors for future fracture: a 15-year follow-up study. Bone [Internet]. 1996 [cited 2024 Dec 4];19(1). Available from: https://pubmed.ncbi.nlm.nih.gov/8830981/.
35. Sambrook P, Cooper C. Osteoporosis. Lancet (London, England) [Internet]. 2006 [cited 2024 Dec 7];367(9527). Available from: https://pubmed.ncbi.nlm.nih.gov/16782492/.
36. White HD, Robinson TD. A novel use for testosterone to treat central sensitization of chronic pain in fibromyalgia patients. Int Immunopharmacol. 2015;27(2):244–8.
37. Liu JH. Selective estrogen receptor modulators (SERMS): keys to understanding their function. Menopause. 2020;27(10):1171–6.
38. Casiano Evans EA, Hobson DTG, Aschkenazi SO, Alas AN, Balgobin S, Balk EM, et al. Nonestrogen therapies for treatment of genitourinary syndrome of menopause: a systematic review. Obstet Gynecol. 2023;142(3):555.
39. Shifren JL. Genitourinary syndrome of menopause. Clin Obstet Gynecol. 2018;61(3):508–16.
40. "The 2023 Nonhormone Therapy Position Statement of The North American Menopause Society" Advisory Panel. The 2023 nonhormone therapy position statement of The North American Menopause Society. Menopause. 2023;30(6):573–90.
41. Menown SJ, Tello JA. Neurokinin 3 receptor antagonists compared with serotonin norepinephrine reuptake inhibitors for non-hormonal treatment of menopausal hot flushes: a systematic qualitative review. Adv Ther. 2021;38(10):5025–45.
42. Bonga KN, Mishra A, Maiti R, Padhy BM, Meher BR, Srinivasan A. Efficacy and safety of fezolinetant for the treatment of menopause-associated vasomotor symptoms: a meta-analysis. Obstet Gynecol. 2024;143(3):393.
43. Nonhormonal management of menopause-associated vasomotor symptoms: 2015 position statement of The North American Menopause Society. Menopause. 2015;22(11):1155–72; quiz 1173–4.

Diagnosis and Treatment of Andropause

12

Görkem Özenç
and Muhammet Abdurrahim İmamoğlu

12.1 Introduction

Andropause, derived from the Greek words "andras," meaning human male, and "pause," meaning cessation, is characterized as a syndrome linked to diminished sexual satisfaction or a reduction in overall well-being due to reduced testosterone levels in elderly men. This syndrome is also referred to by various names, including male menopause, male climacteric, androclysis, androgen deficit in aging males, aging male syndrome, and late-onset hypogonadism (LOH) [1].

Aging is a gradual physiological process characterized by significant alterations in the release of many hormones. Testosterone synthesis declines with aging. The European Male Aging Study (EMAS) reported a 0.4% per annum (log hormone-age) decrease in total testosterone and a 1.3% per annum decline in free testosterone [2]. The rate of age-related decline in serum testosterone levels varies in different individuals and is affected by chronic disease, such as obesity, new illness, serious emotional stress, and medications [3].

Despite having low levels of testosterone, many men are not symptomatic. This phenomenon is likely attributable to the fact that the testosterone threshold at which symptoms manifest differs among individuals. When these testosterone-deficient patients also demonstrate symptoms of testosterone deficiency, a diagnosis of hypogonadism appears justified. There is a consensus that sexual symptoms and erectile dysfunction (ED), reduced libido, and reduced frequency of nocturnal erections, in particular, are the most important symptoms. Decreased self-confidence, motivation, depression, irritability, trouble concentrating and remembering, sleep disorders or insomnia, and decreased psychomotor activity are all examples of nonspecific symptoms [4–6].

The prevalence of hypogonadism in men aged 30–69 years ranged from 3.1% to 7.0%, while it was 18.4% in men over 70 years [4]. Although it is a common disorder in older men, this disorder is frequently underdiagnosed and often remains untreated. It has been estimated that only 5–35% of hypogonadal men receive treatment for their condition [7].

12.2 Diagnosis

Andropause, commonly known as LOH, is a clinical and biochemical syndrome [8]. Therefore, the mainstay of diagnosis includes signs and symptoms associated with hypogonadism, coupled with biochemical evidence of low morning serum total testosterone levels.

G. Özenç (✉) · M. A. İmamoğlu
Department of Urology, Ministry of Health Ankara Etlik City Hospital, Ankara, Türkiye

T. Akbayrak, E. Üzelpasaci (eds.), *Physiotherapy and Rehabilitation in Pelvic and Women's Health-Related Problems*, https://doi.org/10.1007/978-3-032-28741-0_12

12.2.1 Clinical Diagnosis

The most common symptoms in men with androgen deficiency include low libido, erectile dysfunction, and hot flashes. Other manifestations of hypogonadism encompass reduced muscular mass and strength, increased body fat, decreased morning erections, breast discomfort, gynecomastia, decreased bone mineral density and osteoporosis, and infertility. Although less specific in these patients, personality changes, anger, fatigue, a feeling of exhaustion, depression, decreased memory or other cognitive functions, decreased work performance, and sleep disorders may occur. Depression, hypothyroidism, and chronic alcoholism should be excluded, along with the administration of medications including corticosteroids, cimetidine, spironolactone, digoxin, opioid analgesics, antidepressants, and antifungal drugs. Diagnosis of LOH should never be undertaken during an acute illness, as it may result in temporarily reduced testosterone levels [7].

Because obesity is often associated with hypogonadism, body mass index should be determined and waist circumference should be measured. The dimensions of the testicles and penis and secondary sexual characteristics may provide useful information about overall androgen status. During the physical examination of men with androgen insufficiency, gynecomastia, breast soreness, and diminished muscle strength and mass may be observed. In addition, skin changes such as pale appearance, loss of facial and chest hair, and facial wrinkling, which suggest anemia, may be detected. Finally, before therapy with testosterone, the risk of prostate cancer must be assessed using digital rectal examination (DRE) [9].

The problem is that many of these symptoms and signs are not specific to hypogonadism. But this may raise suspicion of testosterone deficiency, and one or more of these symptoms must be corroborated with a low serum testosterone level [1].

Multiple questionnaires have been developed to assess symptoms and their response to testosterone therapy. These include the Aging Male Symptom Score (AMS) [10] and the Androgen Deficiency in Aging Men (ADAM) [8–11]. However, they are not recommended for the diagnosis of hypogonadism because of low specificity (30% and 39%, respectively) [7].

12.2.2 Laboratory Diagnosis

The diagnosis of LOH should be based on the combination of clinical symptoms and significantly reduced testosterone levels. Serum testosterone levels exhibit diurnal variation, and testosterone levels are also potentially influenced by food intake. Therefore, a serum sample for total testosterone determination should be obtained between 07.00 and 11.00 in a fasting condition. A confirming secondary measurement should always be undertaken in the case of a primary pathological value [12].

No appropriate age-specific reference ranges for testosterone are available. There are no generally accepted lower limits of normal. There are several consensus statements based on existing information and expert opinions on the limits of normal and hypogonadal testosterone levels of aging men. Data from meta-analyses have shown that testosterone therapy is ineffective when baseline levels are >12 nmol/L (350 ng/dL). Similarly, patients with serum total testosterone levels below 8 nmol/l (230 ng/dL) will usually benefit from testosterone treatment. When serum total testosterone levels range from 8 to 12 nmol/l (230–350 ng/dl), it may be advantageous to calculate free testosterone or bioavailable testosterone. Additionally, it is recommended to measure free or bioavailable testosterone levels in some men suspected of having changes in sex hormone binding globulin (SHBG), for example, obesity, diabetes mellitus, chronic illness, use of glucocorticoids, hypothyroidism, hepatic cirrhosis, hepatitis, and hyperthyroidism. Unfortunately, there are no validated thresholds for free testosterone. However, the EMAS study noted that free testosterone improved the diagnosis, especially at borderline levels of total testosterone. If the total testosterone level is between 8 and 11 nmol/L, then free testosterone <220 pmol/L strengthens the diagnosis [13].

The best method for bioavailable testosterone level measurement is sulfate precipitation and for free testosterone level is equilibrium dialysis. Alternatively, free testosterone can be calculated using total testosterone along with serum SHBG and albumin levels [14].

Upon the detection of abnormal total testosterone levels, determination of luteinizing hormone must be performed to distinguish primary from secondary hypogonadism. Unless fertility is an issue, it is usually not necessary to measure follicle-stimulating hormone levels. In cases of diminished sexual desire and secondary hypogonadism, prolactin levels should be measured. Additionally, some studies recommend performing pituitary magnetic resonance imaging (MRI) in cases of severe hypogonadism (<6 nmol/L, 1.75 ng/mL) with inadequate gonadotropin levels [15, 16].

Alterations also occur in other endocrine systems in association with aging. Determinations of estradiol, thyroid hormones, cortisol, dehydroepiandrosterone (DHEA), dehydroepiandrosterone sulfate (DHEA-S), melatonin, growth hormone, and insulin-like growth factor-1 are not indicated unless other endocrine disorders are suspected [17].

12.3 Treatment

The aim of treatment is to increase testosterone levels to physiological limits and correct symptoms of testosterone deficiency. Improving the quality of life, maintaining sexual functions, and reducing disability are the primary objectives [7].

12.3.1 Lifestyle Factors

It is important to consider the general situation of the patient when choosing the most appropriate treatment. LOH is considered functional in the majority of cases, and functional hypogonadism is typically linked to obesity and metabolic problems. Consequently, it would seem most logical to begin treatment with lifestyle modification and weight reduction for all overweight and obese men with hypogonadism. A meta-analysis has shown that lifestyle interventions, including caloric restriction and increased physical activity, may reverse obesity-associated secondary hypogonadism through increases in total and free testosterone levels, although the overall rise in testosterone is relatively modest(1–2 nmol) [18]. There is also evidence that a combination of lifestyle modifications and testosterone therapy in symptomatic hypogonadal men might result in better outcomes [19].

12.3.2 Medical Treatment

Men with symptoms of erectile dysfunction, low libido, and documented testosterone deficiency are candidates for testosterone therapy. Preparations of natural testosterone should be used for substitution therapy. Various pharmacological formulations exist for testosterone replacement therapy, including intramuscular, subdermal, transdermal, oral, and buccal preparations. Patients should be informed by the physician about the pharmacokinetics and advantages and disadvantages of each preparation. The selection of the preparation should be a collaborative decision between the patient and the physician [20]. Short-acting forms should be used at the beginning of treatment. In this way, treatment can be stopped upon the observation of potential side effects. Long-acting forms should be preferred for maintenance treatment [21].

There is inadequate data to determine the optimum serum testosterone level for efficacy and safety. Currently, mid- to lower-young-adult-male serum testosterone levels seem appropriate as the therapeutic goal [22].

There is insufficient data on the therapeutic and side effects of human chorionic gonadotropin treatment in older men; therefore, this treatment cannot be recommended in LOH unless there is a fertility issue. Non-testosterone androgen precursor preparations such as DHEA, DHEA-S, androstenediol, or androstenedione are not recommended. Although antiestrogens and aromatase inhibitors have been shown to increase endogenous testosterone levels, there is insufficient evidence to recommend their use [23].

12.3.2.1 Oral Agents

One of the effective oral androgen formulations, 17-α-alkylated androgen preparations, is obsolete because of their potential liver toxicity. Oral testosterone undecanoate (TU) bypasses first-pass metabolism through its preferential absorption into the lymphatic system. Thus, adverse liver side effects are not observed, and it is safe. But the efficacy of oral TU is limited because of fluctuating serum levels and short half-life, and to improve absorption, take 3–4 40 mg capsules daily with meals [24].

12.3.2.2 Transmucosal Formulations

Buccal administration for testosterone replacement therapy is still available in several countries. Mucoadhesive tablets are applied to the upper gums twice daily. Peak circulating testosterone levels are reached within 10–12 h of initial administration. Testosterone levels decline to baseline 4–6 h after tablet removal [25]. Gum edema, blistering, and gingivitis are the most common side effects [26].

Intranasal administration more closely approximates the normal circadian variation of testosterone. It requires administration two or three times daily using a specific metered-dose pump. Further studies are needed to determine the effect of nasal testosterone administration in hypogonadal men [7, 27].

12.3.2.3 Transdermal Testosterone

Transdermal testosterone is available as a skin patch and gel preparation. This formulation provides continuous transdermal delivery of testosterone for 24 h, producing circulating testosterone levels that approximate the normal levels. The advantage of transdermal patches is that they are non-invasive, painless and easy to apply. But the efficacy of the transdermal patch is often limited by lack of adherence or discontinuation because of skin reactions. Gel preparations have a lower incidence of skin irritation compared with the patch, but testosterone can be transferred from the patient to other people after skin contact [7, 28].

12.3.2.4 Subdermal Testosterone Implants

The implantation of testosterone pellets is the longest-lasting testosterone formulation, enduring from 4 to 7 months. However, the procedure is invasive, requiring skin incision and local anesthesia. The most common side effects are the risk of infection at the implant site and extrusion of the pellets [27, 29].

12.3.2.5 Intramuscular Injection

The intramuscular (IM) preparations approved for the treatment are testosterone cypionate, testosterone enanthate, testosterone propionate, and testosterone undecanoate. Testosterone propionate usually requires administration of 50–100 mg every 2–3 days. This is a significant limitation for its use [9, 27]. Testosterone cypionate and enanthate are short-term formulations, requiring administration every 2–4 weeks. The use of these formulations is associated with wide fluctuations in plasma testosterone concentrations, which can result in mood swings or changes in libido [30]. Testosterone undecanoate shows a longer half-life compared to other IM preparations of testosterone, of about 34 days. Through this long-lasting effect, serum testosterone levels can be maintained for a long time. However, the long washout period may cause problems if complications appear [28].

12.4 Contraindications of Testosterone Replacement Therapy

The primary option for testosterone replacement therapy is the administration of exogenous testosterone. However, exogenous testosterone may impair spermatogenesis by suppressing gonadotropin secretion. Therefore, testosterone therapy is contraindicated in hypogonadal men who desire fertility in the next 6–12 months [31].

Testosterone treatment is contraindicated in men with prostate or breast cancer. But testosterone replacement therapy can be offered to hypogonadal men who have been surgically treated for localized prostate cancer and who are currently without evidence of active disease. Treatment should be restricted to patients with a low risk for recurrent prostatic cancer and should start after at least 1 year of follow-up with a prostate-specific antigen (PSA) level < 0.01 ng/mL. However, the recommendation on this topic is weak in the european association of urology (EAU) guidelines. On the other hand, there is no information on the role of testosterone therapy in patients successfully treated for male breast cancer [32].

There is no data that testosterone therapy increases the severity of lower urinary tract symptoms. The concern is related to patients with severe lower urinary tract symptoms (International Prostate Symptom Score > 19) because of benign prostate hyperplasia, as they are usually excluded from trials. Therefore, testosterone therapy is relatively contraindicated in these patients [9]. This contraindication is no longer applicable after successful treatment of lower urinary tract obstruction [4].

Erythrocytosis is a common adverse effect of testosterone therapy. The elevation in hematocrit above certain levels is weakly associated with an increase in cardiovascular events and mortality [33]. But there are no specific studies in men with testosterone-induced erythrocytosis alone. Periodic hematological assessment is indicated, and while it is not yet clear what critical threshold is desirable, hematocrit should be kept below 52–55% [7, 20].

Men with untreated severe congestive heart failure and untreated obstructive sleep apnea should not be started on treatment with testosterone without prior resolution of the comorbid condition [1].

12.5 Follow-Up

Patients are evaluated for symptomatic improvement, presence of side effects, and compliance with treatment. DRE, serum PSA, voiding function, and sleep-apnea assessment are mandatory before treatment. All patients should be evaluated for prostate cancer and breast cancer. Hematological and cardiological evaluations of patients should be performed.

Testosterone levels should be generally checked at 3, 6, and 12 months and then annually. As testosterone concentrations show large variations related to the formulation used, the timing of measuring testosterone concentration should be guided by the pharmacokinetics of the formulation [28].

Patients at high risk of developing elevated hematocrit should be evaluated every 3 months during the first year of testosterone therapy and at least every 6 months thereafter. If hematocrit levels are elevated, the dose should be reduced, the formulation changed, or phlebotomy performed [32].

The prostate should be monitored with both DRE and PSA levels before and after treatment. The patient should be checked at 3 and 6 months after treatment starts and then annually. PSA increases greater than 1–1.4 ng/mL above baseline, or PSA velocity increases greater than 0.35–0.4 ng/mL per year during sequential PSA measurements, requiring further investigation [28].

Testosterone therapy may be beneficial for hypogonadal men with low or moderate fracture risk [34]; therefore, a dual-energy X-ray absorptiometry (DEXA) bone scan may also be considered at baseline. Bone mineral density should be monitored after 1–2 years of TRT only in men with abnormal BMD at baseline [28, 32].

12.6 Conclusion

LOH is a prevalent syndrome among elderly men. Diagnosis is established by identifying diminished testosterone levels in symptomatic patients. Testosterone replacement therapy is recommended to mitigate the symptoms and signs of androgen deficiency, following the exclusion of pituitary or testicular disorders. The benefits and risks of testosterone therapy should be clearly discussed with the patient, and risk factors should be evaluated prior to initiating treatment. Patients must be monitored for evidence of testosterone-dependent diseases during therapy. If there is no improvement in symptoms and signs, the medication should be terminated, and other possible causes of the symptoms should be explored. Finally, although testosterone replacement therapy is known to be effective in improving symptoms, it should be noted that there is insufficient evidence regarding its safety.

References

1. Singh P. Andropause: current concepts. Indian J Endocrinol Metab. 2013;17(Suppl 3):S621–9. https://doi.org/10.4103/2230-8210.123552. PMID: 24910824; PMCID: PMC4046605.
2. Wu FC, et al. Hypothalamic-pituitary-testicular axis disruptions in older men are differentially linked to age and modifiable risk factors: the European Male Aging Study. J Clin Endocrinol Metab. 2008;93:2737.
3. Morley JE, Kaiser FE, Perry HM, et al. Longitudinal changes in testosterone, luteinizing hormone, and follicle-stimulating hormone in healthy older men. Metabolism. 1997;46:410–3.
4. Araujo AB, Esche GR, Kupelian V, et al. Prevalence of symptomatic androgen deficiency in men. J Clin Endocrinol Metab. 2007;92:4241–7.
5. Kelleher S, Conway AJ, Handelsman DJ. Blood testosterone threshold for androgen deficiency symptoms. J Clin Endocrinol Metab. 2004;89:3813–7.
6. Zitzmann M, Faber S, Nieschlag E. Association of specific symptoms and metabolic risks with serum testosterone in older men. J Clin Endocrinol Metab. 2006;91:4335–43.
7. Bassil N. Late-onset hypogonadism. Med Clin North Am. 2011;95(3):507–23. https://doi.org/10.1016/j.mcna.2011.03.001. PMID: 21549875.
8. Huhtaniemi I. Late-onset hypogonadism: current concepts and controversies of pathogenesis, diagnosis and treatment. Asian J Androl. 2014;16(2):192–202. https://doi.org/10.4103/1008-682X.122336. PMID: 24407185; PMCID: PMC3955328.
9. Rastrelli G, et al. Testosterone and benign prostatic hyperplasia. Sex Med Rev. 2019;7:259.
10. Heinemann LA, Saad F, Heinemann K, Thai DM. Can results of the Aging Males' Symptoms (AMS) scale predict those of screening scales for androgen deficiency? Aging Male. 2004;7:211–8. https://doi.org/10.1080/13685530400004223.
11. Morley JE, Charlton E, Patrick P, Kaiser FE, Cadeau P, et al. Validation of a screening questionnaire for androgen deficiency in aging males. Metabolism. 2000;49:1239–42. https://doi.org/10.1053/meta.2000.8625.
12. Gagliano-Juca T, et al. Oral glucose load and mixed meal feeding lowers testosterone levels in healthy eugonadal men. Endocrine. 2019;63:149.
13. Wu FC, Tajar A, Beynon JM, Pye SR, Silman AJ, et al. EMAS Group. Identification of late-onset hypogonadism in middle-aged and elderly men. N Engl J Med. 2010;363:123–35. https://doi.org/10.1056/NEJMoa0911101.
14. Vermeulen A, et al. A critical evaluation of simple methods for the estimation of free testosterone in serum. J Clin Endocrinol Metab. 1999;84:3666.
15. Dalvi M, et al. The prevalence of structural pituitary abnormalities by MRI scanning in men presenting with isolated hypogonadotrophic hypogonadism. Clin Endocrinol. 2016;84:858.
16. Cipriani S, et al. Biochemical predictors of structural hypothalamus-pituitary abnormalities detected by magnetic resonance imaging in men with secondary hypogonadism. J Endocrinol Investig. 2021;44:2785.
17. Bhasin S, Singh AB, Mac RP, Carter B, Lee MI, Cunningham GR. Managing the risks of prostate disease during testosterone replacement therapy in older men: recommendations for a standardized monitoring plan. J Androl. 2003;24:299–311.
18. Corona G, et al. Body weight loss reverts obesity-associated hypogonadotropic hypogonadism: a systematic review and meta-analysis. Eur J Endocrinol. 2013;168:829.
19. Isidori AM, et al. Outcomes of androgen replacement therapy in adult male hypogonadism: recommendations from the Italian society of endocrinology. J Endocrinol Investig. 2015;38:103.
20. Calof OM, Singh AB, Lee ML, Kenny AM, Urban RJ, Tenover JL, Bhasin S. Adverse events associated with testosterone replacement in middle-aged and older men: a meta-analysis of randomized, placebo-controlled trials. J Gerontol A Biol Sci Med Sci. 2005;60:1451–7. https://doi.org/10.1093/gerona/60.11.1451.
21. Parsons JK, Carter HB, Platz EA, Wright EJ, Landis P, Metter EJ. Serum testosterone and the risk of prostate cancer: potential implications for testosterone therapy. Cancer Epidemiol Biomarkers Prev. 2005;14:2257–60. https://doi.org/10.1158/1055-9965.EPI-04-0715.
22. Zitzmann M, Nieschlag E. Androgen receptor gene CAG repeat length and body mass index modulate the safety of long-term intramuscular testosterone undecanoate therapy in hypogonadal men. J Clin Endocrinol Metab. 2007;92(10):3844–53. https://doi.org/10.1210/jc.2007-0620. Epub 2007 Jul 17. PMID: 17635942.
23. Wang C, Nieschlag E, Swerdloff R, Behre HM, Hellstrom WJ, Gooren LJ, Kaufman JM, Legros JJ, Lunenfeld B, Morales A, Morley JE, Schulman C, Thompson IM, Weidner W, Wu FC. Investigation, treatment and monitoring of late-onset hypogonadism in males: ISA, ISSAM, EAU, EAA and ASA recommendations. Eur J Endocrinol. 2008;159(5):507–14. https://doi.org/10.1530/EJE-08-0601. PMID: 18955511; PMCID: PMC2754376.
24. Bagchus WM, Hust R, Maris F, et al. Important effect of food on the bioavailability of oral testosterone undecanoate. Pharmacotherapy. 2003;23:319–25.
25. Wang C, Cunningham G, Dobs A, et al. Long-term testosterone gel (AndroGel) treatment main-

tains beneficial effects on sexual function and mood, lean and fat mass, and bone mineral density in hypogonadal men. J Clin Endocrinol Metab. 2004;89(5):2085–98.
26. Dinsmore WW, Wyllie MG. The long-term efficacy and safety of a testosterone mucoadhesive buccal tablet in testosterone-deficient men. BJU Int. 2012;110:162–9.
27. Rastrelli G, et al. Pharmacotherapy of male hypogonadism. Curr Opin Pharmacol. 2023;68:102323.
28. Barbonetti A, D'Andrea S, Francavilla S. Testosterone replacement therapy. Andrology. 2020;8(6):1551–66. https://doi.org/10.1111/andr.12774. Epub 2020 Mar 9. PMID: 32068334.
29. Rastrelli G, et al. Pharmacological management of late-onset hypogonadism. Expert Rev Clin Pharmacol. 2018;11:439.
30. Shoskes JJ, Wilson MK, Spinner ML. Pharmacology of testosterone replacement therapy preparations. Transl Androl Urol. 2016;5(6):834–43.
31. Rambhatla A, et al. The role of estrogen modulators in male hypogonadism and infertility. Rev Urol. 2016;18:66.
32. Salonia A, Capogrosso, P, Bettocchi C, et al. EAU guidelines on male hypogonadism; 2024. Accessed from https://uroweb.org/guidelines/sexual-and-reproductive-health/chapter/male-hypogonadism.
33. Gagnon DR, et al. Hematocrit and the risk of cardiovascular disease—the Framingham study: a 34-year follow-up. Am Heart J. 1994;127:674. https://pubmed.ncbi.nlm.nih.gov/8122618.
34. Isidori AM, et al. Effects of testosterone on body composition, bone metabolism and serum lipid profile in middle-aged men: a meta-analysis. Clin Endocrinol. 2005;63:280.

Diagnosis and Treatment of Cancers Specific to Pelvic and Women's Health

13

Nejat Ozgul and Utku Akgor

13.1 Introduction

Pelvic and women's health encompasses cancers unique to or predominantly affecting women, including those of the cervix, ovary, uterus, vagina, and vulva. These malignancies pose significant challenges due to differences in etiology, clinical presentation, and progression, as well as issues in prevention, early detection, and treatment. Although advances in molecular diagnostics, imaging, and targeted therapies have enabled innovative and personalized approaches, the burden of these cancers remains a pressing global concern [1].

Globally, pelvic cancers are among the most common malignancies in women, and some rank within the top ten causes of cancer-related deaths. Despite effective screening programs, such as those for cervical cancer, many pelvic cancers remain undetected until advanced stages, particularly in low-resource settings, underscoring the need for improved diagnostic tools and wider access to screening [1].

N. Ozgul (✉)
Department of Gynecology and Obstetrics, Faculty of Medicine, Başkent University, Ankara, Türkiye
e-mail: nozgul@baskent.edu.tr; nejat.ozgul@hacettepe.edu.tr

U. Akgor
Department of Gynecology and Obstetrics, Faculty of Medicine, Hacettepe University, Ankara, Türkiye
e-mail: utkuakgor@hacettepe.edu.tr

This chapter focuses on the three most common gynecological cancers: cervical, endometrial, and ovarian. Their epidemiology, risk factors, and diagnostic strategies are explored, with special attention to stage-specific management and tailored treatment approaches for each cancer type.

By presenting the latest evidence-based approaches and multidisciplinary care strategies, this chapter aims to provide healthcare providers with the tools to optimize outcomes for these prevalent cancers.

13.2 Cervical Cancer

13.2.1 Epidemiology and Risk Factors

Cervical cancer is the most common gynecological cancer worldwide. However, there has been a significant decline in its incidence in developed countries as a result of the widespread implementation of HPV vaccination and screening programs. In developing countries, cervical cancer remains a major public health problem despite this progress. In particular, with an average age of around 47 years, the average age at diagnosis is younger than for other gynecological cancers [2, 3].

Cervical cancer is strongly associated with persistent human papillomavirus (HPV) infec-

T. Akbayrak, E. Üzelpasaci (eds.), *Physiotherapy and Rehabilitation in Pelvic and Women's Health-Related Problems*, https://doi.org/10.1007/978-3-032-28741-0_13

tion, with almost all cases linked to this viral etiology [4]. Risk factors for HPV-related cervical cancer include early onset of sexual activity, particularly before the age of 18, and having multiple sexual partners, both of which increase the likelihood of HPV exposure [5]. Additional factors include having a high-risk sexual partner, a history of sexually transmitted infections, early age at first childbirth, and high parity. A history of vulvar or vaginal squamous intraepithelial neoplasia or cancer, which are also HPV-driven, further increases the risk. Immunosuppression, such as that caused by HIV infection, significantly amplifies susceptibility to HPV persistence and progression to cervical cancer [5, 6].

Non-HPV-related risk factors include socioeconomic disparities, as individuals from low-income communities often face barriers to healthcare access and regular screening, leading to delayed diagnosis and treatment [7]. Other contributors include prolonged contraceptive use, cigarette smoking, which is thought to act as a cocarcinogen with HPV, and genetic predisposition [8]. Together, these factors underscore the multifaceted nature of cervical cancer risk and the critical importance of prevention strategies, including vaccination and routine screening.

13.2.2 Diagnosis of Cervical Cancer

The most common presenting symptom of cervical cancer is abnormal vaginal bleeding, particularly postcoital bleeding. However, many cases remain asymptomatic in the early stages, highlighting the importance of effective screening programs for early detection. Cervical cancer and cervical intraepithelial neoplasia are primarily detected through two screening methods: HPV DNA testing and cytology (Pap smear) [9, 10]. The combination of both tests, referred to as co-testing, offers enhanced sensitivity and specificity for identifying high-risk cases. While screening methods provide critical insights into cervical pathology, a definitive diagnosis requires a cervical biopsy, often performed during colposcopy. Colposcopy allows for the detailed examination of the cervix under magnification, and the application of acetic acid or Lugol's iodine can help identify suspicious areas for biopsy.

13.2.2.1 The Role of Biopsy and Pathological Assessment

Cervical biopsy remains the gold standard for the diagnosis of cervical cancer. Indications for biopsy include abnormal Pap smear results, visible cervical abnormalities, and symptoms such as postcoital bleeding. During colposcopy, the presence of abnormal findings such as acetowhite areas, punctation, mosaic patterns, and atypical vessels serves as a guide for the selection of biopsy sites. In order to achieve a more comprehensive evaluation, excisional procedures such as the loop electrosurgical excision procedure (LEEP) or conization may be performed, serving both diagnostic and therapeutic purposes [11]. The pathological examination of the biopsy specimen is imperative for the confirmation of the diagnosis and the determination of the histological type of the tumor. Squamous cell carcinoma, the most common histologic type, often shows nuclear polymorphism and tadpole-shaped cells on microscopic examination [12]. Adenocarcinoma, while less prevalent, lacks specific cytological features, necessitating a thorough histopathological evaluation [13]. The histological classification of cervical cancer includes various epithelial tumor subtypes, which influence management strategies.

13.2.2.2 Imaging and Tumor Markers in Staging and Follow-Up

Imaging plays a critical role in staging cervical cancer and guiding treatment decisions. Magnetic resonance imaging (MRI) is considered the gold standard for assessing local disease spread, particularly parametrial invasion. Computed tomography (CT) is frequently utilized for evaluating nodal involvement and detecting distant metastases. Positron emission tomography-computed tomography (PET-CT) offers superior sensitivity in identifying lymph node metastases, making it a valuable tool in advanced disease evaluation. Tumor markers such as CA 125, CA 19-9, CEA, and CA 15-3 are not specific to cervical cancer but may assist in monitoring treatment response and detecting recurrence. Although imaging and tumor markers complement pathological assessment, the combination of comprehensive diagnostic approaches ensures optimal staging and tailored management of cervical cancer [14]. Table 13.1 shows the histological classification of cervical cancer.

13.2.3 Cervical Cancer Staging

Cervical cancer staging plays a critical role in determining the most appropriate treatment approach and predicting patient prognosis. Historically, staging for cervical cancer has been based on clinical evaluation, which includes physical examination and basic diagnostic procedures. However, advancements in radiologic imaging and surgical techniques have influenced staging practices, enabling more accurate assessment of tumor characteristics and extent of disease [15].

In the revised Federation of Gynecology and Obstetrics (FIGO) 2018 staging system, modern diagnostic tools such as CT, MRI, and PET scans, along with pathological findings, are incorporated to enhance the identification of critical prognostic factors like tumor size and lymph node involvement. These updates enable more precise treatment planning while maintaining flexibility for resource-limited settings, where physical examination and basic diagnostic procedures remain the primary staging methods [16]. In Table 13.2, the FIGO 2018 staging system for cervical cancer is demonstrated, providing detailed criteria for each stage [16].

Microinvasive cervical cancer is defined as an invasive carcinoma confined to the cervix with minimal stromal invasion, typically limited to a depth of ≤5 mm, and without lymphovascular space invasion (LVSI) or nodal metastasis. This early-stage disease represents a critical point in cervical cancer management, as precise staging and appropriate treatment can prevent disease progression while preserving fertility in select cases [17].

In the FIGO 2018 cervical cancer staging system, significant revisions have been made to include nodal metastasis assessment as a key component. Retroperitoneal lymph node involvement can now be evaluated using radiologic (r) or pathologic (p) findings, which are explicitly indicated for stage IIIC. This stage is further subdivided into IIIC1, for pelvic node involvement, and IIIC2, for para-aortic node involvement. These changes underline the critical role of

Table 13.1 Histologic subtypes of cervical cancer. Squamous cell carcinoma accounts for 70% and adenocarcinoma for 25% of cases. Other categories include mixed cervical carcinoma, neuroendocrine tumors, and rare types [14]

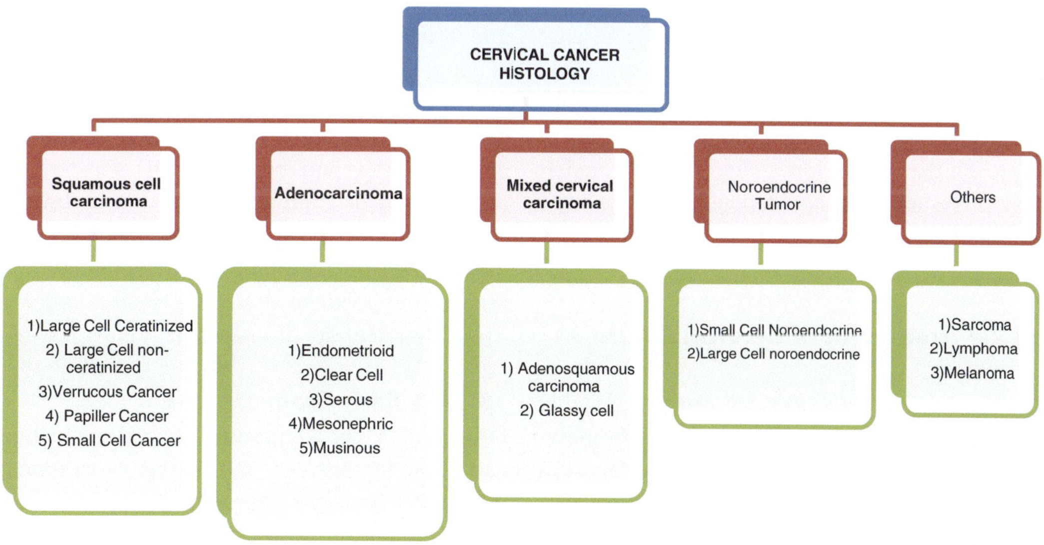

Table 13.2 The FIGO 2018 staging system for cervical cancer is presented, outlining the stages and corresponding descriptions used to classify the extent of disease

FIGO staging system for cervical cancer (2018)	
Stage	Description
I	The carcinoma is strictly confined to the cervix (extension to the uterine corpus should be disregarded)
IA	Invasive carcinoma that can be diagnosed only by microscopy, with a maximum depth of invasion <5 mm
IA1	Measured stromal invasion ≤3 mm in depth
IA2	Measured stromal invasion >3 mm and ≤5 mm in depth
IB	Invasive carcinoma with measured deepest invasion >5 mm (greater than stage IA), lesion limited to the cervix uteri
IB1	Invasive carcinoma >5 mm depth of stromal invasion and ≤2 cm in greatest dimension
IB2	Invasive carcinoma >2 cm and ≤4 cm in greatest dimension
IB3	Invasive carcinoma >4 cm in greatest dimension
II	The carcinoma invades beyond the uterus but has not extended onto the lower third of the vagina or to the pelvic wall
IIA	Involvement limited to the upper two-thirds of the vagina without parametrial involvement
IIA1	Invasive carcinoma ≤4 cm in greatest dimension
IIA2	Invasive carcinoma >4 cm in greatest dimension
IIB	With parametrial involvement but not up to the pelvic wall
III	The carcinoma involves the lower third of the vagina or extends to the pelvic wall and/or causes hydronephrosis or nonfunctioning kidney and/or involves pelvic and/or para-aortic lymph nodes
IIIA	Involvement of the lower third of the vagina, with no extension to the pelvic wall
IIIB	Extension to the pelvic wall and/or hydronephrosis or nonfunctioning kidney (unless known to be due to another cause)
IIIC	Involvement of pelvic and/or para-aortic lymph nodes, irrespective of tumor size and extent (with r and p notations)
IIIC1	Pelvic lymph node metastasis
IIIC2	Para-aortic lymph node metastasis
IV	The carcinoma has extended beyond the true pelvis or has involved (biopsy-proven) the mucosa of the bladder or rectum. Stage IV is subdivided into:
IVA	Spread to adjacent pelvic organs
IVB	Spread to distant organs

This staging system integrates clinical, radiologic, and pathologic findings to optimize treatment planning and prognostic assessment [4]

lymph node assessment in determining disease prognosis and tailoring treatment strategies. Based on this staging system, treatment principles are established, ensuring a multidisciplinary approach that incorporates surgery, chemoradiation, or systemic therapy depending on the stage and individual patient factors [14].

13.2.4 Treatment of Cervical Cancer

The management of cervical cancer is highly dependent on the stage of the disease. For early-stage disease, conservative surgical approaches are the preferred option. For advanced stages, multimodal strategies, including chemoradiation and systemic therapies, are employed. Accurate staging is paramount in determining the most appropriate treatment plan, as it guides decisions on the extent of surgery, the need for radiation or chemotherapy, and considerations for fertility preservation in eligible patients. The following sections will explore treatment modalities in detail based on the FIGO 2018 staging system, highlighting evidence-based approaches tailored to each stage of the disease [14].

13.2.4.1 Early-Stage Disease

Following a comprehensive clinical evaluation and staging process, the primary treatment modality for early-stage cervical cancer generally encompasses either surgical intervention or radiation therapy (RT). Treatment planning is guided by the FIGO staging system, with options tailored to the specific stage and patient characteristics. A fertility-sparing approach may be considered for select patients with stage IA, IB1, and certain cases of IB2 disease. However, fertility-sparing surgery is contraindicated in patients with high-risk histologic subtypes, such as small cell neuroendocrine tumors, gastric-type adenocarcinoma, or adenoma malignum (minimal deviation adenocarcinoma), due to the aggressive nature of these tumors and the limited supporting data available [14].

13.2.4.1.1 Stage IA1 Disease

The management of stage IA1 cervical cancer is contingent on various factors, including the patient's fertility desires, the extent of medical operability, and the presence of lymphovascular space invasion (LVSI). Fertility-sparing options are available for eligible patients, while non-fertility-sparing approaches are preferred for those who do not wish to preserve fertility or have contraindications. The primary objective in all cases is to achieve negative margins and assess nodal involvement to guide further management [18].

For patients desiring fertility preservation, cone biopsy with or without pelvic lymphadenectomy is the primary recommendation. The cone biopsy aims to achieve negative margins for invasive disease and high-grade squamous intraepithelial lesions (HSIL). In the absence of LVSI and with negative margins, observation may be considered. For cases with positive margins, repeat cone biopsy or radical trachelectomy is recommended to evaluate the depth of invasion and rule out stage IA2 or IB disease. If LVSI is present, radical trachelectomy with sentinel lymph node (SLN) mapping or pelvic lymphadenectomy is a reasonable strategy. After childbearing, patients may consider hysterectomy for persistent HPV infection or abnormal cytology [14, 19].

For patients not seeking fertility preservation, extrafascial hysterectomy is the standard recommendation for cases with negative margins and no LVSI. In cases with positive margins for carcinoma or LVSI, a modified radical hysterectomy with SLN mapping or pelvic lymphadenectomy is preferred. For inoperable patients, brachytherapy with or without pelvic external beam radiation therapy (EBRT) is recommended. Observation may be an option for medically inoperable patients with negative margins following cone biopsy [14].

13.2.4.1.2 Stage IA2 Disease

For patients with stage IA2 cervical cancer who do not desire fertility preservation and are medically operable, radical hysterectomy with bilateral pelvic lymph node dissection is the primary treatment recommendation. SLN mapping can be included in the surgical approach, while para-aortic node dissection is advised if pelvic nodal disease is suspected or confirmed. Less radical surgical methods are under investigation but not yet standard practice. For patients who are medically inoperable or refuse surgery, pelvic external beam radiotherapy (EBRT) combined with brachytherapy offers an effective alternative. The radiation dose should be tailored based on tissue tolerance, fractionation, and target volume size, particularly when high-dose-rate brachytherapy is used [20, 21].

For patients desiring fertility preservation, radical trachelectomy with pelvic lymphadenectomy is recommended, with SLN mapping as an alternative. Cone biopsy followed by observation is an option if margins and lymph nodes are negative. In stage IA2–IB1 cases without LVSI, conization with negative margins and pelvic lymphadenectomy or SLN mapping may be performed. For stage IA1–IA2 with LVSI, radical trachelectomy and pelvic lymphadenectomy are preferred. If a cone biopsy shows positive margins, a repeat cone biopsy or trachelectomy is advised [14, 21].

13.2.4.1.3 Stage IB and IIA Disease

For patients with stage IB1 cervical cancer desiring fertility preservation, radical trachelectomy combined with pelvic lymph node dissection, with or without para-aortic node dissection, is an option. This approach is typically reserved for tumors 2 cm or smaller. Tumors between 2 and

4 cm may be considered for fertility-sparing surgery, but these cases require careful selection due to the potential need for adjuvant therapy based on risk factors like positive nodes or Sedlis criteria. SLN mapping may also be performed. Evidence suggests that radical trachelectomy provides comparable oncologic outcomes to radical hysterectomy in selected stage IB1 cases [14, 22].

For stage IB1 and IIA1 patients, radical hysterectomy with bilateral pelvic lymph node dissection is the primary treatment, with para-aortic node dissection optionally included if nodal disease is suspected. SLN mapping is also considered. For stage IB2 and IIA2 tumors, concurrent chemoradiation is the preferred approach, involving external beam radiotherapy (EBRT), brachytherapy, and cisplatin-based chemotherapy. This method has demonstrated significant survival benefits for advanced-stage disease [14, 23].

For patients with positive pelvic lymph node involvement, the recommended course of action involves the immediate initiation of definitive chemoradiation without prior hysterectomy. For individuals who are medically unsuitable for surgery or who elect to decline surgical intervention, the recommended treatment approach incorporates a combination of external beam radiation therapy (EBRT), brachytherapy, and platinum-based chemotherapy [14].

13.2.4.1.4 Advanced-Stage Disease

Advanced cervical cancer encompasses stage IIB to IVA cases, and many clinicians now include stage IB2 and IIA2 in this category. For these patients, treatment planning hinges on precise evaluation of tumor spread and nodal involvement using imaging modalities like PET/CT, which are essential for staging and radiation field determination. MRI aids in assessing local disease extent and optimizing radiation therapy (RT) planning. Needle biopsy may clarify ambiguous imaging findings, while surgical staging via lymph node dissection can uncover microscopic nodal disease undetectable through imaging [14].

For patients without nodal involvement or with disease confined to the pelvis, standard treatment involves pelvic external beam radiotherapy (EBRT) combined with concurrent platinum-based chemotherapy and brachytherapy. Preferred chemotherapy regimens include weekly cisplatin or carboplatin for those intolerant to cisplatin. Research has explored the use of cisplatin/gemcitabine alongside EBRT, followed by additional chemotherapy cycles, showing improved progression-free and overall survival. However, the regimen's high toxicity has limited its adoption [24, 25].

Patients with positive para-aortic or pelvic lymph nodes require an extended imaging workup for metastasis. In these cases, extended-field EBRT, concurrent platinum-based chemotherapy, and brachytherapy are recommended. If distant metastases are detected, systemic chemotherapy, with or without tailored EBRT, becomes the treatment focus [24, 26].

Adjuvant therapy following radical hysterectomy is tailored based on pathological findings. Observation is sufficient for stage IA2, IB1, or IIA1 cases without risk factors (Sedlis criteria: large tumor size, deep stromal invasion, or LVSI). However, patients with intermediate-risk disease benefit from pelvic EBRT, which improves progression-free survival (PFS) and shows a trend toward better overall survival (OS) [14, 27].

For high-risk patients (positive nodes, margins, or parametrial involvement), concurrent chemoradiation using cisplatin or carboplatin with pelvic EBRT and optional brachytherapy is recommended. This approach significantly enhances OS. Imaging and biopsies may guide treatment for suspected metastases, with extended-field RT or systemic chemotherapy indicated for confirmed cases. Neoadjuvant chemotherapy, though sometimes used, has shown limited survival benefit and is not routinely recommended [14, 28].

13.3 Endometrial Cancer

13.3.1 Epidemiology and Risk Factors

Endometrial cancer (EC) is the most common gynecologic malignancy in developed countries, with rising incidence due to aging populations and increasing obesity rates [29]. Most cases are diagnosed in postmenopausal women, with a median age of 60 years. However, approximately 5% occur in women under 40, often linked to hereditary syndromes such as Lynch syndrome [3]. Higher incidence rates are observed in developed countries, primarily attributed to lifestyle factors, while lower rates in developing regions may reflect limited healthcare access and differences in diagnostic practices. Type I cancers, driven by estrogen, constitute the majority of cases and typically have a favorable prognosis, whereas type II cancers, which are non-estrogen-driven, are more aggressive [30, 31].

Hormonal factors play a central role in EC risk, with prolonged unopposed estrogen exposure due to obesity, polycystic ovary syndrome (PCOS), nulliparity, or estrogen-only hormone replacement therapy (HRT) being significant contributors. Obesity, the most modifiable risk factor, increases estrogen production through aromatization in adipose tissue [32]. Other risk factors include diabetes, hypertension, tamoxifen use, and Lynch syndrome, which elevates lifetime EC risk up to 60% [33, 34].

Preventive strategies focus on reducing modifiable risks through weight management, physical activity, and diet. Combined oral contraceptives offer protective benefits by countering estrogen's effects, and high-risk individuals, such as Lynch syndrome carriers, may benefit from endometrial sampling or prophylactic hysterectomy [8].

13.3.2 Diagnosis of Endometrial Cancer

The most significant clinical symptom of endometrial cancer is postmenopausal bleeding, which warrants immediate evaluation. The diagnosis of endometrial cancer primarily relies on histopathologic examination of endometrial tissue obtained via biopsy, curettage, or hysterectomy [35]. Endometrial biopsy is typically the first-line diagnostic procedure due to its high sensitivity and reliability, particularly when a significant portion of the endometrium is involved. Endometrial cancer should be considered and ruled out in the following clinical scenarios: postmenopausal patients with pyometra, detection of endometrial cells—especially atypical cells—on a Pap smear, postmenopausal bleeding, abnormal uterine bleeding or intermenstrual bleeding during perimenopause, premenopausal patients with abnormal bleeding and a history of anovulatory cycles, and postmenopausal patients with an endometrial thickness exceeding 4 mm as assessed by transvaginal ultrasound. Early recognition and evaluation in these cases are crucial for timely diagnosis and management [36, 37].

Pipelle biopsy is one of the diagnostic options for endometrial cancer. Fractional curettage can also be performed for diagnosis. Hysteroscopy is another diagnostic tool; while it is more sensitive for detecting endometrial lesions, it has lower sensitivity for endometrial hyperplasia. Although hysteroscopy may increase the risk of peritoneal contamination, this does not affect prognosis, making it an appropriate method for diagnosing endometrial cancer [38, 39].

Endometrial cancer encompasses a diverse range of histological subtypes, with endometrioid carcinoma being the most common, accounting for approximately 75–80% of cases. These are often low-grade, estrogen-driven tumors with a favorable prognosis [40]. Serous carcinoma, the second most common subtype, is highly aggressive, often associated with p53 abnormalities, and shows extensive myometrial and lymphovascular invasion. Clear cell carcinoma, a rare subtype, shares features with ovarian clear cell carcinoma and exhibits variable behavior based on its molecular profile [41, 42]. Other less common subtypes include carcinosarcoma, undifferentiated carcinoma, and mixed histologies, each characterized by unique pathological and molecular features influencing prognosis and treatment strategies. Molecular classification increasingly aids in stratifying these subtypes to guide personalized therapy [41, 43].

Preoperative imaging is essential in the evaluation and management of endometrial cancer, providing critical information for accurate staging and guiding treatment decisions. Imaging recommendations depend on the disease stage and clinical presentation. A chest X-ray is often utilized to rule out thoracic metastases, while advanced modalities such as CT, MRI, ultrasound, and FDG-PET/CT are employed to evaluate the extent of local and metastatic disease, particularly in the presence of suspicious symptoms, abnormal physical findings, or laboratory abnormalities [44, 45]. In cases of extrauterine disease, serum CA-125 levels can offer additional insight into disease burden and treatment response. However, CA-125 levels must be interpreted with caution, as they can be falsely elevated due to factors such as peritoneal inflammation or infection and may remain normal in cases of isolated vaginal metastases. These limitations underscore the necessity of a multidisciplinary diagnostic approach that incorporates imaging, clinical findings, and laboratory data to ensure comprehensive disease assessment and optimal treatment planning [38].

13.3.3 Molecular Classification and Its Role in Endometrial Cancer

The molecular classification of endometrial cancer (EC) has revolutionized risk stratification and treatment planning by providing a reproducible and objective framework. Based on The Cancer Genome Atlas (TCGA) analysis, EC is categorized into four molecular subtypes: POLE-mutated, mismatch repair-deficient (MMRd), no specific molecular profile (NSMP), and p53-abnormal (p53abn). These subtypes have distinct genomic and clinical features that influence prognosis and guide therapeutic decisions [46]. Molecular testing, which can be performed on diagnostic biopsies or surgical specimens, ensures accurate subtype assignment and has high concordance between biopsy and hysterectomy samples [47, 48].

POLE-mutated EC, characterized by an ultra-mutated genomic profile and a high mutational burden, is associated with favorable outcomes despite aggressive pathological features. Patients with POLE-mutated tumors typically achieve excellent survival rates, prompting discussions about de-escalating adjuvant therapies in clinical trials. MMRd EC, resulting from a mismatch repair deficiency, is associated with a high tumor mutational burden and immune responsiveness. Immune checkpoint inhibitors have shown significant efficacy in metastatic or recurrent MSI-H (microsatellite instability-high) tumors, establishing immunotherapy as a key treatment option [46, 49].

The NSMP subtype, comprising tumors with normal p53 expression and intermediate genomic stability, includes many estrogen-driven endometrioid cancers with favorable outcomes. However, estrogen receptor (ER)-negative NSMP tumors have a worse prognosis. In contrast, p53abn EC, characterized by high genomic instability and frequent p53 mutations, represents the most aggressive subtype [47, 48]. These tumors, often serous or high-grade endometrioid, carry a poor prognosis and require intensive multimodal therapy, including chemotherapy and radiation. Emerging therapies targeting HER2 amplification and homologous recombination deficiency (HRD) in p53abn tumors offer promising avenues for improving outcomes in this high-risk group [38]. Figure 13.1 illustrates the molecular classification of endometrial cancer, highlighting its subtypes—POLE ultramutated, MSI hypermutated, copy-number low, and copy-number high—along with the unclassifiable category [40].

13.3.4 Current Approaches to Staging of Endometrial Cancer

Staging of endometrial cancer is essential for accurate treatment planning and prognostication, requiring a multidisciplinary team skilled in imaging, pathology, and surgery. The extent of surgical staging is guided by preoperative and intraoperative evaluations. For cases apparently confined to the uterus, lymph node evaluation is critical for determining the stage and guiding adjuvant therapy decisions, though it may be unnecessary if final pathology confirms noninvasive endometrioid histology [38].

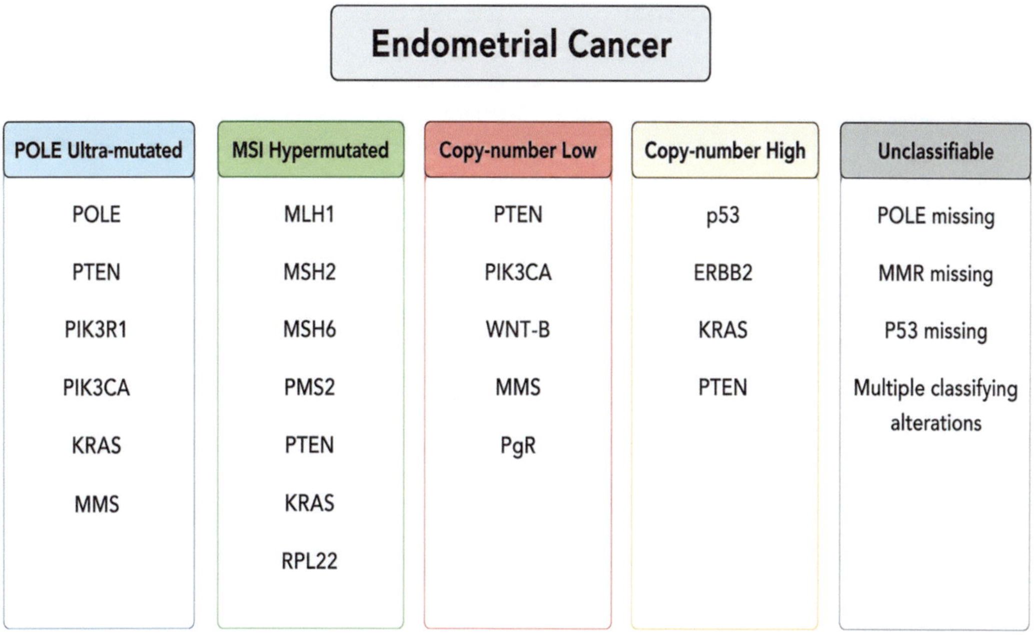

Fig. 13.1 Molecular classification of endometrial cancer depicting its subtypes and associated genetic mutations. The subtypes include POLE ultra-mutated, MSI hypermutated, copy-number low, and copy-number high, along with an unclassifiable category characterized by the absence of defining molecular alterations. This classification provides insights into the genetic heterogeneity and biological behavior of endometrial cancer, aiding in prognostic and therapeutic decision-making [50]

Staging of endometrial cancer is essential for accurate treatment planning and prognostication, particularly with the introduction of the 2023 FIGO staging system [48]. Surgical staging, including total hysterectomy, bilateral salpingo-oophorectomy, and lymphadenectomy, remains the cornerstone of disease evaluation. Lymph node evaluation is crucial for staging and adjuvant therapy decisions, though it may not be necessary for noninvasive endometrioid histology. Advanced imaging modalities such as MRI, CT, and PET/CT are indispensable in assessing extrauterine spread, guiding surgical decisions, and ensuring accurate staging [38].

This updated FIGO staging system integrates molecular classifications, including *p53-abnormal (p53abn)* and *POLE-mutated (POLEmut)* subtypes, alongside traditional pathological parameters. Molecular profiling has significantly enhanced the precision of staging, allowing for reclassification in certain cases. For example, *p53abn tumors*, known for their aggressive behavior, may be upstaged even when confined to the uterus, whereas *POLEmut tumors* with favorable prognoses may be downstaged despite high-grade features. This refined approach underscores the importance of molecular testing in modern endometrial cancer management [48].

Despite these advancements, the integration of molecular classification into clinical practice has highlighted gaps in globally standardized treatment algorithms. While the 2023 FIGO system provides a robust framework, variability in practice and limited long-term data have delayed the development of universally accepted management protocols. This ongoing progression underscores the critical need for a unified international framework to harmonize treatment strategies with molecularly informed staging, paving the way for enhanced patient outcomes and more effective cancer management.

13.3.5 Treatment of Endometrial Cancer

13.3.5.1 Disease Limited to the Uterus

The surgical management of endometrial cancer primarily involves hysterectomy and bilateral salpingo-oophorectomy, which remain the cornerstones of treatment. Over time, surgical approaches have advanced significantly. Traditionally, patients underwent exploratory laparotomy through a midline incision. Today, most patients with presumed early-stage disease are treated with minimally invasive surgery (MIS), such as laparoscopy or robotic surgery, which has become the preferred approach [51]. These changes reflect the broader adoption of advanced surgical techniques and improvements in retroperitoneal lymph node evaluation.

For patients with disease apparently confined to the uterus, as determined by physical examination and/or pelvic imaging, MIS is generally recommended. Randomized controlled trials have demonstrated that laparoscopic hysterectomy is associated with lower morbidity and equivalent oncologic outcomes compared to open hysterectomy [52, 53]. The goals of surgical management are the complete removal of the primary tumor and the identification of prognostic factors to guide decisions regarding adjuvant therapy. MIS techniques effectively achieve these objectives while minimizing surgical morbidity [54].

Robotic surgery has been shown to offer comparable short-term outcomes to conventional laparoscopy, with additional benefits such as shorter operative times and lower conversion rates to laparotomy. In particular, robotic surgery may reduce conversion rates in patients with obesity, who may experience positional intolerance during conventional laparoscopy [55]. However, in experienced hands, conventional laparoscopy is not considered inferior. The higher cost of robotic surgery raises concerns about its cost-effectiveness and highlights the need to identify specific patient populations that would derive the most benefit from this technology [56].

13.3.5.2 Advanced-Stage Disease

The management of advanced-stage endometrial cancer requires a multidisciplinary approach, integrating surgery, systemic therapy, and, in selected cases, radiation therapy. For patients with clinical or radiographic evidence of metastatic disease, surgery plays a pivotal role in establishing a definitive diagnosis, alleviating symptoms, and potentially improving oncologic outcomes. In most cases, surgical procedures are performed via laparotomy through a midline incision to allow comprehensive exploration and maximal surgical control [57].

Cytoreductive surgery, aiming to remove as much visible tumor burden as possible, is often a cornerstone of treatment for advanced disease. The success of cytoreduction is closely associated with improved survival outcomes, mirroring the treatment paradigms observed in advanced ovarian cancer. Indications for cytoreduction in endometrial cancer typically include patients with operable disease, good performance status, and absence of widespread extra-abdominal metastases. The goal of surgery is to achieve no residual disease, as residual tumor burden has been correlated with poorer outcomes [58].

Neoadjuvant chemotherapy followed by interval cytoreduction is emerging as an alternative to primary cytoreduction for selected patients with high tumor burden or poor surgical candidates. Preliminary studies have shown that neoadjuvant chemotherapy may facilitate a higher rate of complete cytoreduction (removal of all visible disease) compared to primary surgery while also reducing operative time and surgical morbidity. These findings suggest that neoadjuvant chemotherapy could play a significant role in optimizing outcomes for patients with advanced endometrial cancer, particularly those with limited operability at initial presentation [57, 58].

The surgical principles of cytoreduction in advanced endometrial cancer are similar to those in ovarian cancer, with an emphasis on removing gross disease from the pelvis, upper abdomen, and other affected regions. Procedures may include omentectomy, bowel resection, and diaphragm stripping or resection, depending on the extent of disease. However, the decision to proceed with extensive cytoreduction must be balanced against potential morbidity, and a tailored approach is essential based on patient-specific factors and disease characteristics [38, 59].

13.3.5.2.1 Adjuvant Therapy in Stage I Disease

There is debate regarding the need for adjuvant therapy in stage I disease. For stage IA, grade 1/2 tumors, observation is often preferred unless risk factors like LVSI or age ≥60 are present, in which case vaginal brachytherapy is recommended. Stage IA, grade 3 patients may also undergo observation if no myometrial invasion exists, but brachytherapy is the preferred option otherwise. For patients with stage IB, grade 1–2 disease, brachytherapy is generally favored unless additional risk factors warrant consideration of external beam radiation therapy (EBRT). For stage IB, grade 3 with adverse factors, systemic therapy may be added to radiation [38].

13.3.5.2.2 Adjuvant Therapy in Stage II Disease

Patients with stage II disease require careful consideration of risk factors such as stromal invasion depth, grade, and LVSI. For those who undergo a radical hysterectomy with negative margins and no extrauterine spread, EBRT is preferred, sometimes combined with vaginal brachytherapy and/or systemic therapy. In contrast, patients undergoing extrafascial hysterectomy are more likely to require adjuvant RT for optimal outcomes. The presence of adverse factors strongly influences the necessity and intensity of adjuvant treatment in stage II cases [38].

13.3.5.2.3 Adjuvant Therapy for Advanced Stage/Extrauterine Endometrial Cancer

Patients with extrauterine endometrial cancer, including nodal or adnexal involvement, face a high risk of recurrence and benefit from adjuvant therapy to improve outcomes. Systemic therapy, often combined with radiotherapy (RT), is the cornerstone of treatment, addressing both local and distant disease. Carboplatin and paclitaxel remain the most commonly utilized chemotherapy regimens due to their proven efficacy in advanced and high-risk cases [38, 60].

Immunotherapy has emerged as a promising option, particularly for tumors exhibiting high microsatellite instability (MSI-H) or deficient mismatch repair (dMMR). Agents such as pembrolizumab and dostarlimab, which target the PD-1 pathway, offer tailored treatment approaches for these molecularly defined subgroups. Additionally, targeted therapies like temsirolimus, which inhibit the mTOR pathway, are being explored in resistant or recurrent cases, broadening the options for personalized treatment [38, 61, 62].

The selection of adjuvant therapy is guided by factors such as histologic subtype, molecular profile, and individual patient characteristics. Multidisciplinary collaboration and ongoing research are essential to refining treatment strategies and improving survival outcomes for patients with advanced-stage endometrial cancer [60].

13.3.5.3 Lymph Node Evaluation in Endometrial Cancer

Lymph node evaluation plays a critical role in the management of endometrial cancer (EC), providing essential information for accurate staging, prognosis, and guiding adjuvant therapy decisions [50]. However, the optimal approach remains a topic of debate, with practices varying across institutions and surgeons. Current strategies for retroperitoneal lymph node management include no lymph node dissection (LND), sentinel lymph node dissection (SLND), systematic LND in all patients, or selective LND based on risk factors for lymph node metastasis [63]. The choice of approach significantly impacts the use and type of adjuvant therapy, emphasizing the need for individualized treatment planning.

Historically, systematic pelvic and para-aortic lymphadenectomy was introduced in the 1980s after studies demonstrated an increased risk of lymph node metastasis associated with higher tumor grade and deeper myometrial invasion. The Gynecologic Oncology Group 33 study highlighted the prognostic value of lymph node dissection, leading to its widespread adoption [64]. However, subsequent randomized trials, including the ASTEC trial and others, failed to show a survival benefit from routine LND. These findings, coupled with the increased morbidity of the procedure, such as lymphedema, have prompted a shift toward less invasive approaches [65].

Sentinel lymph node dissection (SLND) has emerged as an alternative to systematic LND, offering a lower-risk approach while maintaining diagnostic accuracy. Studies have demonstrated the feasibility of SLND, with low false-negative rates and comparable detection of metastatic disease [66]. SLND has been particularly favored for its reduced rates of complications, such as lower-extremity lymphedema, making it a valuable option in the surgical staging of EC [67]. Despite these advantages, the lack of randomized trials directly comparing SLND to other approaches limits definitive conclusions regarding its long-term benefits.

The role of selective LND, guided by preoperative and intraoperative factors, has also gained traction. Criteria such as tumor grade, size, depth of myometrial invasion, and histologic subtype help identify patients at higher risk for lymph node metastasis, allowing for targeted lymphadenectomy. This approach minimizes unnecessary procedures in low-risk patients while maintaining the ability to provide critical staging information for those at higher risk. The Mayo criteria and similar predictive models have been instrumental in stratifying patients for selective LND [63].

While advances in SLND and selective LND have improved the management of lymph nodes in EC, challenges remain. Variability in the use of intraoperative frozen sections and the absence of a universally accepted protocol for lymphatic mapping contribute to inconsistencies in practice. Moreover, the utility of lymph node assessment in guiding adjuvant therapy continues to evolve, underscoring the need for ongoing research and standardization. For now, multidisciplinary collaboration and patient-specific considerations remain paramount in determining the most appropriate approach.

13.3.5.4 Special Considerations in Endometrial Cancer

13.3.5.4.1 Fertility-Sparing Therapy

Fertility-sparing therapy can be considered for select patients with grade 1, stage IA, noninvasive endometrioid cancer. Continuous progestin-based therapy, such as megestrol acetate or a levonorgestrel-releasing intrauterine device, is an option. Patients should undergo regular monitoring with biopsies every 3–6 months. Once childbearing is complete or if treatment fails, hysterectomy with surgical staging is recommended [38].

13.3.5.4.2 Ovarian Preservation

Ovarian preservation is a feasible and safe option for select premenopausal patients with early-stage, low-grade endometrioid endometrial cancer. Research indicates that retaining the ovaries does not significantly increase cancer-related mortality in these cases. This approach is particularly beneficial for younger patients who wish to avoid the adverse effects of premature menopause, such as osteoporosis, cardiovascular disease, and reduced quality of life [68].

Patient selection is critical for this strategy and is typically limited to those without extrauterine disease, adnexal involvement, or high-risk histologic subtypes, such as serous or clear cell carcinoma. Comprehensive imaging and intraoperative assessment are necessary to confirm the absence of metastatic spread before proceeding. Long-term follow-up remains essential to monitor for potential ovarian malignancies, ensuring that this individualized approach aligns with optimal patient outcomes [69].

13.4 Ovarian Cancer

13.4.1 Epidemiology and Risk Factors

Ovarian cancer is a significant gynecologic malignancy, ranking as the second most common gynecologic cancer in resource-rich settings and one of the leading causes of gynecologic cancer-related deaths globally. The average age at diagnosis is typically in the early 60s, although hereditary syndromes, such as those involving BRCA1 or BRCA2 mutations, often lead to an earlier onset. The lifetime risk of developing ovarian cancer is approximately 1.3% [70].

Several factors influence the risk of developing epithelial ovarian cancer (EOC). Increased age, infertility, endometriosis, polycystic ovarian syndrome, and cigarette smoking, particularly for mucinous carcinomas, are associated with a higher risk. Conversely, protective factors include prior pregnancies, breastfeeding, oral contraceptive use, intrauterine device use, and tubal ligation. Genetic predisposition plays a critical role, with BRCA1 and BRCA2 mutations being the most prominent contributors. Other genetic alterations, including those in homologous recombination repair pathways and mismatch repair genes associated with Lynch syndrome, also increase risk. While a family history of breast cancer was traditionally viewed as a risk factor, much of this association is now attributed to underlying BRCA mutations [71].

13.4.2 Diagnostic Evaluation of Ovarian Cancer

Ovarian cancer is a heterogeneous disease comprising several histological subtypes, each with distinct clinical, pathological, and molecular characteristics. The majority of ovarian cancers (approximately 90%) arise from epithelial cells and are classified as epithelial ovarian cancers (EOCs). These include serous (high-grade and low-grade), endometrioid, clear cell, and mucinous carcinomas, as well as rare undifferentiated tumors. High-grade serous carcinoma (HGSC) is the most common and aggressive subtype, often presenting at advanced stages and exhibiting mutations in the *TP53* gene [72]. In contrast, low-grade serous carcinoma typically demonstrates indolent behavior and harbors KRAS and BRAF mutations. Endometrioid and clear cell carcinomas are frequently associated with endometriosis and display distinct molecular profiles, such as ARID1A mutations. Mucinous carcinomas, although less common, require differentiation from metastatic mucinous tumors originating from other organs [73].

Non-epithelial ovarian cancers account for less than 10% of cases and include germ cell and sex cord-stromal tumors. Germ cell tumors, such as dysgerminomas and yolk sac tumors, are more common in younger patients and exhibit rapid growth but are highly sensitive to chemotherapy [74]. Sex cord-stromal tumors, including granulosa cell and Sertoli-Leydig cell tumors, are rare and often produce hormones, leading to clinical presentations such as estrogen or androgen excess [75]. Understanding the histopathological diversity of ovarian cancer is crucial for accurate diagnosis, prognostication, and tailoring treatment strategies, as each subtype responds differently to chemotherapy and targeted therapie. Ovarian tumors are broadly classified according to their cellular origin, as shown in (Fig. 13.2).

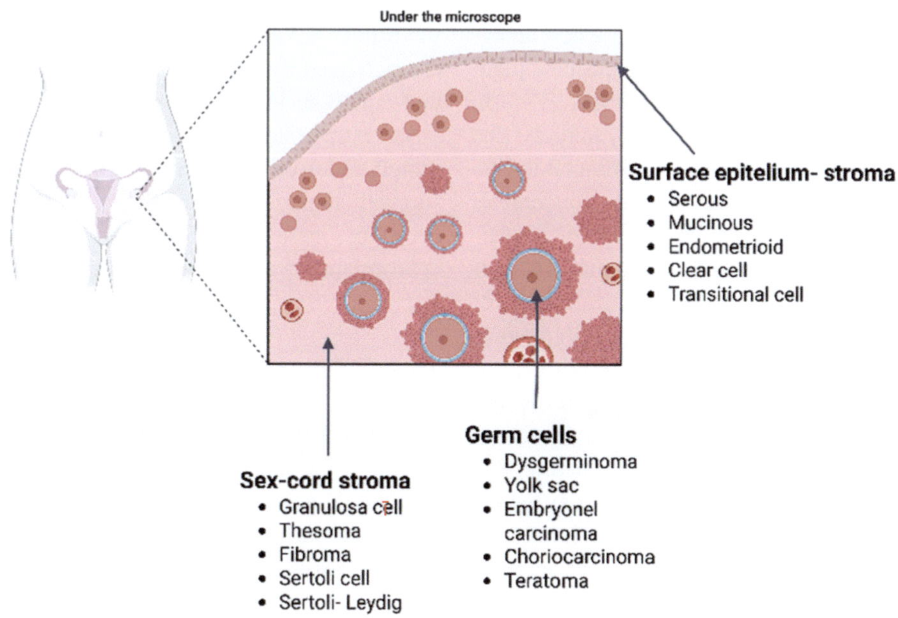

Fig. 13.2 Histological classification of ovarian cancer. (Figure created with biorender)

The most common early symptom of ovarian cancer is abdominal pain, while abdominal distension is more typical in later stages. The most important clinical findings are a palpable pelvic mass and ascites [76].

The diagnosis of ovarian cancer involves a stepwise approach combining clinical evaluation, imaging, laboratory studies, and surgical exploration. The primary objective of the initial evaluation is to determine the likelihood of malignancy and identify patients requiring referral to a gynecologic oncologist. Key components of the initial evaluation include a complete physical examination, pelvic imaging (typically transvaginal ultrasound), and tumor marker assessment [77]. Findings suggestive of malignancy include a complex adnexal mass with solid components, irregular septations, Doppler evidence of vascular flow, and the presence of ascites. Serum cancer antigen 125 (CA-125) is a commonly used tumor marker, elevated in the majority of patients with epithelial ovarian cancer (EOC). However, other biomarkers, such as human epididymis protein 4 (HE4), may be used based on clinical suspicion [78].

For patients with advanced or suspicious findings, further evaluation with computed tomography (CT) or magnetic resonance imaging (MRI) is recommended to assess disease extent, including peritoneal carcinomatosis, lymph node involvement, or distant metastases. Chest imaging, often with CT, is performed to evaluate pleural effusion or pulmonary metastases [79]. In patients unable to undergo primary surgery due to poor performance status or unresectable disease, diagnostic procedures such as paracentesis or image-guided omental biopsies may be performed to confirm malignancy and guide neoadjuvant chemotherapy. Cytologic evaluation of ascitic or pleural fluid may also assist in diagnosis, though sensitivity varies [80].

Definitive diagnosis and staging typically require surgical exploration, including removal of the adnexal mass, histologic confirmation, and staging procedures. Image-guided biopsy of the ovary is avoided due to the risk of cell spillage and potential upstaging of disease. The integration of clinical, radiologic, and pathological findings ensures accurate diagnosis and optimizes individualized treatment planning [81].

13.4.3 Staging System of Ovarian Cancer

Ovarian cancer is surgically staged using the 2017 FIGO Tumor, Node, Metastasis (TNM) classification system. Table 13.3 shows the FIGO 2017 ovarian cancer staging system. This unified system applies to ovarian, fallopian tube, and peritoneal carcinomas, providing a standardized framework for staging. Key distinctions include the inability to classify peritoneal carcinoma as stage I and the categorization of ovarian or fallopian tube surface involvement as an advanced stage. Capsule rupture is a significant determinant of staging: preoperative rupture is categorized as stage IC2, while intraoperative rupture is stage IC1, both of which influence the need for adjuvant therapy. Histologic confirmation of dense adhesions with malignant cells also leads to an upstaging to stage II [76].

The staging system also emphasizes the importance of comprehensive peritoneal evaluation above and below the pelvic brim, as this anatomical landmark differentiates stage II disease (below the brim) from stage III disease (above the brim). Advanced-stage disease (stage IV) is characterized by parenchymal metastases to distant organs such as the liver or spleen, as well as other extra-abdominal metastases like inguinal lymph nodes or umbilical deposits. This precise surgical staging is critical for guiding treatment decisions, assessing prognosis, and ensuring appropriate therapeutic interventions [29].

13.4.4 Treatment

13.4.4.1 Surgical Staging of Ovarian Cancer

Epithelial, germ cell, and stromal cancers of the ovary, fallopian tube, and peritoneum are staged surgically, which remains the corner-

Table 13.3 The FIGO 2017 ovarian cancer staging [82]

FIGO 2017 ovarian cancer staging	
Stage	Definition
I	Tumor confined to ovaries or fallopian tubes
IA	Tumor limited to one ovary or fallopian tube; capsule intact, no tumor on surface, negative washings
IB	Tumor limited to both ovaries or fallopian tubes; capsule intact, no tumor on surface, negative washings
IC	Tumor limited to one or both ovaries or fallopian tubes, with any of the following:
IC1	Intraoperative surgical spill
IC2	Capsule rupture before surgery or tumor on ovarian or fallopian tube surface
IC3	Malignant cells in the ascites or peritoneal washings
II	Tumor involves one or both ovaries or fallopian tubes with pelvic extension (below the pelvic brim) or primary peritoneal cancer
IIA	Extension and/or implants on the uterus and/or fallopian tubes and/or ovaries
IIB	Extension to other pelvic intraperitoneal tissues
III	Tumor involves one or both ovaries or fallopian tubes, or primary peritoneal cancer, with cytologically or histologically confirmed spread to the peritoneum outside the pelvis and/or metastasis to the retroperitoneal lymph nodes
IIIA1	Positive retroperitoneal lymph nodes only (cytologically or histologically confirmed)
IIIA1(i)	Metastasis ≤10 mm in greatest dimension
IIIA1(ii)	Metastasis >10 mm in greatest dimension
IIIA2	Microscopic extrapelvic (above the pelvic brim) peritoneal involvement ± positive retroperitoneal lymph nodes
IIIB	Macroscopic peritoneal metastasis beyond the pelvis ≤2 cm ± positive retroperitoneal lymph nodes
IIIC	Macroscopic peritoneal metastasis beyond the pelvis >2 cm ± positive retroperitoneal lymph nodes (includes extension to the capsule of the liver/spleen without parenchymal involvement)
IV	Distant metastasis (excluding peritoneal metastases)
IVA	Pleural effusion with positive cytology
IVB	Parenchymal metastases and metastases to extra-abdominal organs (including inguinal lymph nodes and lymph nodes outside the abdominal cavity)

stone of diagnosis and management. Comprehensive surgical staging is critical for treatment planning and prognostic counseling. For epithelial ovarian cancer (EOC), most patients are diagnosed at an advanced stage, with 48% presenting with distant metastases, 22% with regional lymph node involvement, and 22% localized at the time of diagnosis, while 8% remain unstaged [83].

Surgical staging aims to accurately determine the extent of the disease, often revealing more advanced disease than initially suspected. Approximately 30% of patients with clinical findings suggestive of stage I EOC are found to have more advanced disease upon thorough surgical staging, such as positive peritoneal cytology, resulting in upstaging and subsequent modification of treatment [84].

Surgical staging is a cornerstone of ovarian cancer management, providing critical information for treatment planning and prognosis. The International Federation of Gynecology and Obstetrics (FIGO) recommends comprehensive surgical staging for all cases of clinically early-stage epithelial ovarian cancer (EOC). This standard procedure includes peritoneal cytology (via washings or ascitic fluid sampling), visual and biopsy assessments of abdominal and pelvic organs, total hysterectomy with bilateral salpingo-oophorectomy, pelvic and para-aortic lymph node dissection, and omentectomy. These steps aim to accurately determine the extent of disease and to identify any occult metastases that may affect the choice of adjuvant therapy [85].

Peritoneal biopsies and cytology play a vital role in staging. Systematic biopsies of the peritoneal surfaces, including the cul-de-sac, bladder, and diaphragmatic peritoneum, help detect occult disease. Positive peritoneal washings or biopsies upstage the disease and influence adjuvant treatment decisions. Accurate documentation of findings in the operative report is essential, as it guides the oncologic management and informs patient prognosis [80].

Minimally invasive surgery (MIS), including traditional and robotic-assisted laparoscopy, has emerged as an alternative to laparotomy for selected early-stage EOC patients. MIS offers advantages such as reduced blood loss, shorter hospital stays, and lower postoperative morbidity. However, concerns remain regarding the risk of tumor rupture, the thoroughness of abdominal inspection, and the potential for port site metastasis. Studies suggest that capsule rupture is more frequent during MIS and may negatively impact prognosis, highlighting the importance of careful surgical technique to prevent spillage of malignant cells [86].

Omentectomy is a critical component of staging, as the omentum is a common site for metastatic disease in ovarian cancer. Infracolic or complete omentectomy allows for both staging and cytoreduction in cases of advanced disease. The procedure involves meticulous dissection of the gastroepiploic vessels and careful mobilization of the hepatic and splenic flexures to ensure complete removal of the omentum. This step not only aids in staging but also reduces tumor burden, which may help decrease postoperative ascites [87].

Debulking surgery remains the cornerstone of treatment for stage II–IV ovarian, fallopian tube, or primary peritoneal cancer. The primary aim is maximal cytoreduction, with the best outcomes achieved when no visible residual disease (R0) is left or when residual disease is reduced to less than 1 cm. These outcomes are associated with improved progression-free and overall survival [88]. For early-stage disease (stage I/II), the focus is on removing all pelvic disease and thoroughly evaluating the upper abdomen and retroperitoneum for occult metastases. In advanced-stage disease (stage III/IV), the surgical objective extends to removing all visible disease throughout the abdomen and pelvis [89].

Additional procedures, including bowel resections, splenectomy, diaphragm stripping, or partial hepatectomy, are often necessary to achieve optimal cytoreduction. Addressing upper abdominal metastases, when feasible, significantly improves survival outcomes [90]. For patients with minimal residual disease in stage II or III, intraperitoneal (IP) catheter placement during surgery can facilitate IP chemotherapy, which has been shown to enhance survival [91]. Comprehensive and strategic debulking surgery thus remains the gold standard in managing advanced ovarian cancer, providing the best possible outcomes through meticulous surgical intervention [88].

13.4.4.2 Lymph Node Evaluation in Ovarian Cancer

Lymph node evaluation plays a critical role in the management of ovarian cancer, particularly for staging and guiding adjuvant therapy. In cases with gross metastatic disease, lymphadenectomy is typically limited to enlarged or suspicious nodes if optimal cytoreduction is feasible [92, 93]. Systematic lymphadenectomy in patients with advanced ovarian cancer has not shown a statistically significant overall survival benefit, emphasizing its selective use in these cases [85].

For patients with apparent early-stage ovarian cancer, bilateral pelvic and para-aortic lymph node sampling is standard practice to detect occult stage III disease, which occurs in approximately one-third of patients with clinical stage I disease. This approach has been associated with improved survival outcomes, as demonstrated in the EORTC ACTION trial [94]. Despite the increased duration of surgery and a risk of lymphocyst formation (approximately 13%), the detection of nodal disease is crucial due to its significant prognostic implications.

Exceptions to routine lymph node sampling include patients with mucinous ovarian tumors that appear confined to the ovary. Studies have shown a low rate (0.7%) of lymph node metastases in these cases, with no survival benefit from lymphadenectomy. In such patients, staging is performed without lymph node sampling [95].

Special attention should be given to para-aortic lymph nodes, particularly those above the inferior mesenteric artery, as these are more likely to harbor metastases. Comprehensive lymph node evaluation remains a vital component of staging, providing critical information for tailoring treatment strategies [88].

13.4.4.3 Fertility-Sparing Options for Ovarian Cancer

Fertility-sparing surgery is an important consideration for young patients with early-stage ovarian cancer who wish to preserve their reproductive potential. This approach is primarily offered to carefully selected individuals with stage IA epithelial ovarian cancer (EOC) or non-epithelial ovarian tumors, where the risk of recurrence is relatively low. The procedure typically involves unilateral salpingo-oophorectomy (USO), preserving the uterus and contralateral ovary, combined with comprehensive surgical staging to ensure accurate assessment and minimize the risk of disease spread [85].

For patients with bilateral stage IB tumors, bilateral salpingo-oophorectomy (BSO) with uterine preservation may be considered as an alternative. While this approach retains the possibility of future fertility through assisted reproductive technologies, such as in vitro fertilization using donor eggs, it requires careful counseling. Patients must be informed of the risks and benefits, as well as the potential impact on their overall prognosis [85].

Fertility-sparing surgery should be performed in a multidisciplinary setting by experienced surgical teams to optimize outcomes. Postoperative follow-up is crucial, involving regular imaging and tumor marker assessments to detect recurrence early and guide further management [69].

13.4.4.4 Adjuvant Therapy of Epithelial Ovarian, Fallopian Tube, or Peritoneal Cancer

Adjuvant chemotherapy plays a critical role in managing early-stage epithelial ovarian cancer (EOC) for patients with high-risk features, including stage IC (tumor confined to the ovary with positive peritoneal washings), stage II (tumor involving the pelvis), clear cell histology, or high-grade (grade 3) tumors [96]. Evidence suggests that these features significantly increase the risk of relapse, with five-year disease-free survival rates ranging from 40% to 80%. Two meta-analyses and the Adjuvant Chemotherapy in Ovarian Neoplasms (ACTION) trial have demonstrated the benefits of platinum-based chemotherapy in reducing recurrence and improving survival, particularly in patients with incomplete surgical staging or residual disease. However, patients with low-risk tumors, such as stage IA or IB grade 1 disease, generally do not benefit from chemotherapy and are managed with observation [81].

The ACTION trial highlighted that the benefit of adjuvant chemotherapy is more pronounced in patients with incomplete surgical staging, showing improved recurrence-free survival and cancer-specific survival compared to observation [81]. Conversely, patients who undergo complete surgical staging may not derive the same benefit, suggesting that thorough surgical staging is critical in tailoring adjuvant therapy decisions. Current guidelines recommend adjuvant chemotherapy for high-risk patients, while observation remains the standard for fully staged, low-risk early EOC [85]. Further research is necessary to refine the criteria for adjuvant therapy, particularly for grade 2 tumors and optimally staged high-risk cases.

The cornerstone of chemotherapy for epithelial ovarian cancer (EOC) is a combination of a platinum agent, typically carboplatin, and a taxane, such as paclitaxel [97]. This regimen is the standard for first-line treatment, offering significant survival benefits. For optimally cytoreduced patients (residual disease <1 cm), options include intravenous (IV) chemotherapy or a combination of IV and intraperitoneal (IP) therapy. IP therapy is associated with better progression-free and overall survival but is limited to those with minimal residual disease due to limited penetration into larger tumors [91].

Studies, such as GOG 172, have demonstrated superior outcomes with IV/IP chemotherapy in patients with optimally reduced disease, showing improved median progression-free survival (PFS) and overall survival (OS) [91]. However, IP therapy often leads to increased toxicity, including abdominal discomfort and neurotoxicity, impacting patients' quality of life (QoL). Subsequent trials, like GOG 252, have explored modifications to the IP regimen, achieving similar survival outcomes with potentially reduced toxicity [98].

Advancements in ovarian cancer management include the integration of targeted therapies. For patients with BRCA mutations or homologous recombination deficiency, maintenance therapy with PARP inhibitors like olaparib has demonstrated prolonged PFS [99, 100]. The addition of angiogenesis inhibitors, such as bevacizumab, to first-line treatment and maintenance therapy has demonstrated survival benefits, particularly in high-risk patients with extensive disease or ascites. Evidence from the GOG-0218 and ICON7 trials supports the inclusion of bevacizumab in the standard chemotherapy regimen of carboplatin and paclitaxel, followed by maintenance therapy with single-agent bevacizumab for patients without disease progression after initial treatment. This approach has shown improved progression-free survival, making it a valuable option in the management of advanced ovarian cancer [101, 102].

Despite advancements, chemotherapy for ovarian cancer remains challenging due to treatment-related toxicities and recurrence risks. Ongoing trials are investigating novel combinations, including immune checkpoint inhibitors and further refinement of IP regimens. Personalized approaches based on molecular profiling, such as BRCA and mismatch repair deficiency testing, are key to optimizing therapy and improving outcomes in ovarian cancer patients.

13.5 Conclusion

Diagnosis and treatment of pelvic and women-specific cancers, such as ovarian, endometrial, and other gynecologic malignancies, have undergone significant advancements. Multidisciplinary approaches integrating surgical, systemic, and targeted therapies, guided by molecular profiling, have greatly improved patient outcomes.

Early detection remains pivotal, with precision diagnostics and individualized treatment strategies ensuring optimal care. Despite these advancements, challenges persist, particularly in resource-limited settings, underscoring the importance of global efforts to enhance accessibility to state-of-the-art diagnostic and therapeutic modalities. Continued research, collaboration, and innovation are essential to address existing gaps and further refine management strategies for these complex malignancies, ultimately improving survival and quality of life for women worldwide.

References

1. Smith RA, Andrews KS, Brooks D, et al. Cancer screening in the United States, 2019: a review of current American Cancer Society guidelines and current issues in cancer screening. CA Cancer J Clin. 2019;69:184–210. https://doi.org/10.3322/caac.21557.
2. Lin S, Gao K, Gu S, et al. Worldwide trends in cervical cancer incidence and mortality, with predictions for the next 15 years. Cancer. 2021;127:4030–9. https://doi.org/10.1002/cncr.33795.
3. Bray F, Laversanne M, Sung H, et al. Global cancer statistics 2022: GLOBOCAN estimates of incidence and mortality worldwide for 36 cancers in 185 countries. CA Cancer J Clin. 2024;74:229–63. https://doi.org/10.3322/caac.21834.
4. Rodríguez AC, Schiffman M, Herrero R, et al. Longitudinal study of human papillomavirus persistence and cervical intraepithelial neoplasia grade 2/3: critical role of duration of infection. J Natl Cancer Inst. 2010;102:315–24. https://doi.org/10.1093/jnci/djq001.
5. International Collaboration of Epidemiological Studies of Cervical Cancer. Comparison of risk factors for invasive squamous cell carcinoma and adenocarcinoma of the cervix: collaborative reanalysis of individual data on 8,097 women with squamous cell carcinoma and 1,374 women with adenocarcinoma from 12 epidemiological studies. Int J Cancer. 2007;120:885–91. https://doi.org/10.1002/ijc.22357.
6. Dugué PA, Rebolj M, Garred P, et al. Immunosuppression and risk of cervical cancer. Expert Rev Anticancer Ther. 2013;13:29–42. https://doi.org/10.1586/era.12.159.
7. Yu L, Sabatino SA, White MC. Rural-urban and racial/ethnic disparities in invasive cervical cancer incidence in the United States,

2010-2014. Prev Chronic Dis. 2019;16:E70. https://doi.org/10.5888/pcd16.180447.
8. Gierisch JM, Coeytaux RR, Urrutia RP, et al. Oral contraceptive use and risk of breast, cervical, colorectal, and endometrial cancers: a systematic review. Cancer Epidemiol Biomarkers Prev. 2013;22:1931–43. https://doi.org/10.1158/1055-9965.Epi-13-0298.
9. Pimple S, Mishra G. Cancer cervix: epidemiology and disease burden. Cytojournal. 2022;19:21. https://doi.org/10.25259/cmas_03_02_2021.
10. Partridge EE, Abu-Rustum NR, Campos SM, et al. Cervical cancer screening. J Natl Compr Cancer Netw. 2010;8:1358–86. https://doi.org/10.6004/jnccn.2010.0103.
11. Sherman ME, Wang SS, Carreon J, et al. Mortality trends for cervical squamous and adenocarcinoma in the United States. Relation to incidence and survival. Cancer. 2005;103:1258–64. https://doi.org/10.1002/cncr.20877.
12. Cooper DB, Dunton CJ. Colposcopy. StatPearls. Treasure Island: StatPearls Publishing. Copyright © 2024, StatPearls Publishing LLC; 2024.
13. Sasieni P, Castanon A, Cuzick J. Screening and adenocarcinoma of the cervix. Int J Cancer. 2009;125:525–9. https://doi.org/10.1002/ijc.24410.
14. Abu-Rustum NR, Yashar CM, Arend R, et al. NCCN guidelines® insights: cervical cancer, version 1.2024. J Natl Compr Cancer Netw. 2023;21:1224–33. https://doi.org/10.6004/jnccn.2023.0062.
15. Bhatla N, Aoki D, Sharma DN, et al. Cancer of the cervix uteri. Int J Gynaecol Obstet. 2018;143(Suppl 2):22–36. https://doi.org/10.1002/ijgo.12611.
16. Corrigendum to "Revised FIGO staging for carcinoma of the cervix uteri" [Int J Gynecol Obstet 145(2019) 129–135]. Int J Gynaecol Obstet. 2019;147:279–80. https://doi.org/10.1002/ijgo.12969.
17. Bhatla N, Berek JS, Cuello Fredes M, et al. Revised FIGO staging for carcinoma of the cervix uteri. Int J Gynaecol Obstet. 2019;145:129–35. https://doi.org/10.1002/ijgo.12749.
18. Marchiole P, Benchaib M, Buenerd A, et al. Oncological safety of laparoscopic-assisted vaginal radical trachelectomy (LARVT or Dargent's operation): a comparative study with laparoscopic-assisted vaginal radical hysterectomy (LARVH). Gynecol Oncol. 2007;106:132–41. https://doi.org/10.1016/j.ygyno.2007.03.009.
19. Plante M, Renaud MC, Hoskins IA, et al. Vaginal radical trachelectomy: a valuable fertility-preserving option in the management of early-stage cervical cancer. A series of 50 pregnancies and review of the literature. Gynecol Oncol. 2005;98:3–10. https://doi.org/10.1016/j.ygyno.2005.04.014.
20. Yoneda JY, Braganca JF, Sarian LO, et al. Surgical treatment of microinvasive cervical cancer: analysis of pathologic features with implications on radicality. Int J Gynecol Cancer. 2015;25:694–8. https://doi.org/10.1097/igc.0000000000000416.
21. Kokka F, Bryant A, Brockbank E, et al. Surgical treatment of stage IA2 cervical cancer. Cochrane Database Syst Rev. 2014;2014:Cd010870. https://doi.org/10.1002/14651858.CD010870.pub2.
22. Li J, Wu X, Li X, et al. Abdominal radical trachelectomy: is it safe for IB1 cervical cancer with tumors ≥ 2 cm? Gynecol Oncol. 2013;131:87–92. https://doi.org/10.1016/j.ygyno.2013.07.079.
23. Keys HM, Bundy BN, Stehman FB, et al. Cisplatin, radiation, and adjuvant hysterectomy compared with radiation and adjuvant hysterectomy for bulky stage IB cervical carcinoma. N Engl J Med. 1999;340:1154–61. https://doi.org/10.1056/nejm199904153401503.
24. Morris M, Eifel PJ, Lu J, et al. Pelvic radiation with concurrent chemotherapy compared with pelvic and para-aortic radiation for high-risk cervical cancer. N Engl J Med. 1999;340:1137–43. https://doi.org/10.1056/nejm199904153401501.
25. Dueñas-González A, Zarbá JJ, Patel F, et al. Phase III, open-label, randomized study comparing concurrent gemcitabine plus cisplatin and radiation followed by adjuvant gemcitabine and cisplatin versus concurrent cisplatin and radiation in patients with stage IIB to IVA carcinoma of the cervix. J Clin Oncol. 2011;29:1678–85. https://doi.org/10.1200/jco.2009.25.9663.
26. Whitney CW, Sause W, Bundy BN, et al. Randomized comparison of fluorouracil plus cisplatin versus hydroxyurea as an adjunct to radiation therapy in stage IIB-IVA carcinoma of the cervix with negative para-aortic lymph nodes: a Gynecologic Oncology Group and Southwest Oncology Group study. J Clin Oncol. 1999;17:1339–48. https://doi.org/10.1200/jco.1999.17.5.1339.
27. Estape RE, Angioli R, Madrigal M, et al. Close vaginal margins as a prognostic factor after radical hysterectomy. Gynecol Oncol. 1998;68:229–32. https://doi.org/10.1006/gyno.1998.4960.
28. Noh JM, Park W, Kim YS, et al. Comparison of clinical outcomes of adenocarcinoma and adenosquamous carcinoma in uterine cervical cancer patients receiving surgical resection followed by radiotherapy: a multicenter retrospective study (KROG 13-10). Gynecol Oncol. 2014;132:618–23. https://doi.org/10.1016/j.ygyno.2014.01.043.
29. Siegel RL, Miller KD, Fuchs HE, et al. Cancer statistics, 2021. CA Cancer J Clin. 2021;71:7–33. https://doi.org/10.3322/caac.21654.
30. American College of Obstericians and Gynecologists. ACOG practice bulletin, clinical management guidelines for obstetrician-gynecologists, number 65, August 2005: management of endometrial cancer. Obstet Gynecol. 2005;106:413–25. https://doi.org/10.1097/00006250-200508000-00050.
31. Bokhman JV. Two pathogenetic types of endometrial carcinoma. Gynecol Oncol. 1983;15:10–7. https://doi.org/10.1016/0090-8258(83)90111-7.
32. Felix AS, Weissfeld JL, Stone RA, et al. Factors associated with Type I and Type II endometrial

cancer. Cancer Causes Control. 2010;21:1851–6. https://doi.org/10.1007/s10552-010-9612-8.
33. Committee Opinion No. 601. Tamoxifen and uterine cancer. Obstet Gynecol. 2014;123:1394–7. https://doi.org/10.1097/01.AOG.0000450757.18294.cf.
34. Ryan NAJ, Glaire MA, Blake D, et al. The proportion of endometrial cancers associated with Lynch syndrome: a systematic review of the literature and meta-analysis. Genet Med. 2019;21:2167–80. https://doi.org/10.1038/s41436-019-0536-8.
35. Clarke MA, Long BJ, Del Mar Morillo A, et al. Association of endometrial cancer risk with postmenopausal bleeding in women: a systematic review and meta-analysis. JAMA Intern Med. 2018;178:1210–22. https://doi.org/10.1001/jamainternmed.2018.2820.
36. Clarke MA, Long BJ, Sherman ME, et al. Risk assessment of endometrial cancer and endometrial intraepithelial neoplasia in women with abnormal bleeding and implications for clinical management algorithms. Am J Obstet Gynecol. 2020;223(549):e541–549.e513. https://doi.org/10.1016/j.ajog.2020.03.032.
37. Purdie DM, Green AC. Epidemiology of endometrial cancer. Best Pract Res Clin Obstet Gynaecol. 2001;15:341–54. https://doi.org/10.1053/beog.2000.0180.
38. Abu-Rustum N, Yashar C, Arend R, et al. Uterine neoplasms, version 1.2023, NCCN clinical practice guidelines in oncology. J Natl Compr Cancer Netw. 2023;21:181–209. https://doi.org/10.6004/jnccn.2023.0006.
39. Cicinelli E, Tinelli R, Colafiglio G, et al. Risk of long-term pelvic recurrences after fluid minihysteroscopy in women with endometrial carcinoma: a controlled randomized study. Menopause. 2010;17:511–5. https://doi.org/10.1097/gme.0b013e3181c8534d.
40. Morice P, Leary A, Creutzberg C, et al. Endometrial cancer. Lancet. 2016;387:1094–108. https://doi.org/10.1016/s0140-6736(15)00130-0.
41. Huang CY, Tang YH, Chiang YC, et al. Impact of management on the prognosis of pure uterine papillary serous cancer—a Taiwanese Gynecologic Oncology Group (TGOG) study. Gynecol Oncol. 2014;133:221–8. https://doi.org/10.1016/j.ygyno.2014.02.010.
42. Murali R, Soslow RA, Weigelt B. Classification of endometrial carcinoma: more than two types. Lancet Oncol. 2014;15:e268–78. https://doi.org/10.1016/s1470-2045(13)70591-6.
43. Hoffman BL, Schorge JO, Halvorson LM, Hamid CA, Corton MM, Schaffer JI. Williams gynecology. 4th ed. New York: McGraw Hill Education; 2020.
44. Ortashi O, Jain S, Emannuel O, et al. Evaluation of the sensitivity, specificity, positive and negative predictive values of preoperative magnetic resonance imaging for staging endometrial cancer. A prospective study of 100 cases at the Dorset Cancer Centre. Eur J Obstet Gynecol Reprod Biol. 2008;137:232–5. https://doi.org/10.1016/j.ejogrb.2007.02.029.
45. Reinhold C, Ueno Y, Akin EA, et al. ACR appropriateness criteria® pretreatment evaluation and follow-up of endometrial cancer. J Am Coll Radiol. 2020;17:S472–s486. https://doi.org/10.1016/j.jacr.2020.09.001.
46. Church DN, Briggs SE, Palles C, et al. DNA polymerase ε and δ exonuclease domain mutations in endometrial cancer. Hum Mol Genet. 2013;22:2820–8. https://doi.org/10.1093/hmg/ddt131.
47. Oaknin A, Bosse TJ, Creutzberg CL, et al. Endometrial cancer: ESMO Clinical Practice Guideline for diagnosis, treatment and follow-up. Ann Oncol. 2022;33:860–77. https://doi.org/10.1016/j.annonc.2022.05.009.
48. Berek JS, Matias-Guiu X, Creutzberg C, et al. FIGO staging of endometrial cancer: 2023. Int J Gynaecol Obstet. 2023;162:383–94. https://doi.org/10.1002/ijgo.14923.
49. Kandoth C, Schultz N, Cherniack AD, et al. Integrated genomic characterization of endometrial carcinoma. Nature. 2013;497:67–73. https://doi.org/10.1038/nature12113.
50. Ben-Shachar I, Pavelka J, Cohn DE, et al. Surgical staging for patients presenting with grade 1 endometrial carcinoma. Obstet Gynecol. 2005;105:487–93. https://doi.org/10.1097/01.AOG.0000149151.74863.c4.
51. Wright JD, Burke WM, Tergas AI, et al. Comparative effectiveness of minimally invasive hysterectomy for endometrial cancer. J Clin Oncol. 2016;34:1087–96. https://doi.org/10.1200/jco.2015.65.3212.
52. Galaal K, Bryant A, Fisher AD, et al. Laparoscopy versus laparotomy for the management of early stage endometrial cancer. Cochrane Database Syst Rev. 2012;9:Cd006655. https://doi.org/10.1002/14651858.CD006655.pub2.
53. Mäenpää MM, Nieminen K, Tomás EI, et al. Robotic-assisted vs traditional laparoscopic surgery for endometrial cancer: a randomized controlled trial. Am J Obstet Gynecol. 2016;215(588):e581–588.e587. https://doi.org/10.1016/j.ajog.2016.06.005.
54. Segarra-Vidal B, Dinoi G, Zorrilla-Vaca A, et al. Minimally invasive compared with open hysterectomy in high-risk endometrial cancer. Obstet Gynecol. 2021;138:828–37. https://doi.org/10.1097/aog.0000000000004606.
55. Wright JD, Burke WM, Wilde ET, et al. Comparative effectiveness of robotic versus laparoscopic hysterectomy for endometrial cancer. J Clin Oncol. 2012;30:783–91. https://doi.org/10.1200/jco.2011.36.7508.
56. Cusimano MC, Simpson AN, Dossa F, et al. Laparoscopic and robotic hysterectomy in endometrial cancer patients with obesity: a systematic review and meta-analysis of conversions and complications. Am J Obstet Gynecol. 2019;221:410–428.e419. https://doi.org/10.1016/j.ajog.2019.05.004.
57. Barlin JN, Puri I, Bristow RE. Cytoreductive surgery for advanced or recurrent endometrial cancer:

a meta-analysis. Gynecol Oncol. 2010;118:14–8. https://doi.org/10.1016/j.ygyno.2010.04.005.
58. Wilkinson-Ryan I, Frolova AI, Liu J, et al. Neoadjuvant chemotherapy versus primary cytoreductive surgery for stage IV uterine serous carcinoma. Int J Gynecol Cancer. 2015;25:63–8. https://doi.org/10.1097/igc.0000000000000321.
59. Landrum LM, Moore KN, Myers TK, et al. Stage IVB endometrial cancer: does applying an ovarian cancer treatment paradigm result in similar outcomes? A case-control analysis. Gynecol Oncol. 2009;112:337–41. https://doi.org/10.1016/j.ygyno.2008.10.009.
60. Burke WM, Orr J, Leitao M, et al. Endometrial cancer: a review and current management strategies: part II. Gynecol Oncol. 2014;134:393–402. https://doi.org/10.1016/j.ygyno.2014.06.003.
61. Jutzi L, Hoskins P, Lim P, et al. The importance of adjuvant chemotherapy and pelvic radiotherapy in high-risk early stage endometrial carcinoma. Gynecol Oncol. 2013;131:581–5. https://doi.org/10.1016/j.ygyno.2013.09.012.
62. Eskander RN, Sill MW, Beffa L, et al. Pembrolizumab plus chemotherapy in advanced endometrial cancer. N Engl J Med. 2023;388:2159–70. https://doi.org/10.1056/NEJMoa2302312.
63. Mariani A, Webb MJ, Keeney GL, et al. Low-risk corpus cancer: is lymphadenectomy or radiotherapy necessary? Am J Obstet Gynecol. 2000;182:1506–19. https://doi.org/10.1067/mob.2000.107335.
64. Creasman WT, Morrow CP, Bundy BN, et al. Surgical pathologic spread patterns of endometrial cancer. A Gynecologic Oncology Group Study. Cancer. 1987;60:2035–41. https://doi.org/10.1002/1097-0142(19901015)60:8+<2035::aid--cncr2820601515>3.0.co;2-8.
65. Kitchener H, Swart AM, Qian Q, et al. Efficacy of systematic pelvic lymphadenectomy in endometrial cancer (MRC ASTEC trial): a randomised study. Lancet. 2009;373:125–36. https://doi.org/10.1016/s0140-6736(08)61766-3.
66. Rossi EC, Kowalski LD, Scalici J, et al. A comparison of sentinel lymph node biopsy to lymphadenectomy for endometrial cancer staging (FIRES trial): a multicentre, prospective, cohort study. Lancet Oncol. 2017;18:384–92. https://doi.org/10.1016/s1470-2045(17)30068-2.
67. Benedetti Panici P, Basile S, Maneschi F, et al. Systematic pelvic lymphadenectomy vs. no lymphadenectomy in early-stage endometrial carcinoma: randomized clinical trial. J Natl Cancer Inst. 2008;100:1707–16. https://doi.org/10.1093/jnci/djn397.
68. Di Donato V, Giannini A, Bogani G. Recent advances in endometrial cancer management. J Clin Med. 2023;12(6):2241. https://doi.org/10.3390/jcm12062241.
69. Matsuo K, Machida H, Shoupe D, et al. Ovarian conservation and overall survival in young women with early-stage low-grade endometrial cancer. Obstet Gynecol. 2016;128:761–70. https://doi.org/10.1097/aog.0000000000001647.
70. La Vecchia C. Ovarian cancer: epidemiology and risk factors. Eur J Cancer Prev. 2017;26:55–62. https://doi.org/10.1097/cej.0000000000000217.
71. Hunn J, Rodriguez GC. Ovarian cancer: etiology, risk factors, and epidemiology. Clin Obstet Gynecol. 2012;55:3–23. https://doi.org/10.1097/GRF.0b013e31824b4611.
72. Kurman RJ, Shih IM. Molecular pathogenesis and extraovarian origin of epithelial ovarian cancer—shifting the paradigm. Hum Pathol. 2011;42:918–31. https://doi.org/10.1016/j.humpath.2011.03.003.
73. Wiegand KC, Shah SP, Al-Agha OM, et al. ARID1A mutations in endometriosis-associated ovarian carcinomas. N Engl J Med. 2010;363:1532–43. https://doi.org/10.1056/NEJMoa1008433.
74. Pectasides D, Pectasides E, Kassanos D. Germ cell tumors of the ovary. Cancer Treat Rev. 2008;34:427–41. https://doi.org/10.1016/j.ctrv.2008.02.002.
75. Young RH. Ovarian sex cord-stromal tumors: reflections on a 40-year experience with a fascinating group of tumors, including comments on the seminal observations of Robert E. Scully, MD. Arch Pathol Lab Med. 2018;142:1459–84. https://doi.org/10.5858/arpa.2018-0291-RA.
76. Doubeni CA, Doubeni AR, Myers AE. Diagnosis and management of ovarian cancer. Am Fam Physician. 2016;93:937–44.
77. Prat J. Staging classification for cancer of the ovary, fallopian tube, and peritoneum. Int J Gynaecol Obstet. 2014;124:1–5. https://doi.org/10.1016/j.ijgo.2013.10.001.
78. Romagnolo C, Leon AE, Fabricio ASC, et al. HE4, CA125 and risk of ovarian malignancy algorithm (ROMA) as diagnostic tools for ovarian cancer in patients with a pelvic mass: an Italian multicenter study. Gynecol Oncol. 2016;141:303–11. https://doi.org/10.1016/j.ygyno.2016.01.016.
79. Musto A, Rampin L, Nanni C, et al. Present and future of PET and PET/CT in gynaecologic malignancies. Eur J Radiol. 2011;78:12–20. https://doi.org/10.1016/j.ejrad.2009.12.035.
80. Naz S, Hashmi AA, Ali R, et al. Role of peritoneal washing cytology in ovarian malignancies: correlation with histopathological parameters. World J Surg Oncol. 2015;13:315. https://doi.org/10.1186/s12957-015-0732-1.
81. Trimbos B, Timmers P, Pecorelli S, et al. Surgical staging and treatment of early ovarian cancer: long-term analysis from a randomized trial. J Natl Cancer Inst. 2010;102:982–7. https://doi.org/10.1093/jnci/djq149.
82. Berek JS, Renz M, Kehoe S, et al. Cancer of the ovary, fallopian tube, and peritoneum: 2021 update. Int J Gynaecol Obstet. 2021;155(Suppl 1):61–85. https://doi.org/10.1002/ijgo.13878.

83. Siegel RL, Giaquinto AN, Jemal A. Cancer statistics, 2024. CA Cancer J Clin. 2024;74:12–49. https://doi.org/10.3322/caac.21820.
84. Hengeveld EM, Zusterzeel PLM, Lajer H, et al. The value of surgical staging in patients with apparent early stage epithelial ovarian carcinoma. Gynecol Oncol. 2019;154:308–13. https://doi.org/10.1016/j.ygyno.2019.06.006.
85. Armstrong DK, Alvarez RD, Backes FJ, et al. NCCN guidelines® insights: ovarian cancer, version 3.2022. J Natl Compr Cancer Netw. 2022;20:972–80. https://doi.org/10.6004/jnccn.2022.0047.
86. Park HJ, Kim DW, Yim GW, et al. Staging laparoscopy for the management of early-stage ovarian cancer: a metaanalysis. Am J Obstet Gynecol. 2013;209(58):e51–8. https://doi.org/10.1016/j.ajog.2013.04.013.
87. Chi DS, Musa F, Dao F, et al. An analysis of patients with bulky advanced stage ovarian, tubal, and peritoneal carcinoma treated with primary debulking surgery (PDS) during an identical time period as the randomized EORTC-NCIC trial of PDS vs neoadjuvant chemotherapy (NACT). Gynecol Oncol. 2012;124:10–4. https://doi.org/10.1016/j.ygyno.2011.08.014.
88. du Bois A, Reuss A, Pujade-Lauraine E, et al. Role of surgical outcome as prognostic factor in advanced epithelial ovarian cancer: a combined exploratory analysis of 3 prospectively randomized phase 3 multicenter trials: by the Arbeitsgemeinschaft Gynaekologische Onkologie Studiengruppe Ovarialkarzinom (AGO-OVAR) and the Groupe d'Investigateurs Nationaux Pour les Etudes des Cancers de l'Ovaire (GINECO). Cancer. 2009;115:1234–44. https://doi.org/10.1002/cncr.24149.
89. Vergote I, Tropé CG, Amant F, et al. Neoadjuvant chemotherapy or primary surgery in stage IIIC or IV ovarian cancer. N Engl J Med. 2010;363:943–53. https://doi.org/10.1056/NEJMoa0908806.
90. Eisenkop SM, Spirtos NM, Friedman RL, et al. Relative influences of tumor volume before surgery and the cytoreductive outcome on survival for patients with advanced ovarian cancer: a prospective study. Gynecol Oncol. 2003;90:390–6. https://doi.org/10.1016/s0090-8258(03)00278-6.
91. Armstrong DK, Bundy B, Wenzel L, et al. Intraperitoneal cisplatin and paclitaxel in ovarian cancer. N Engl J Med. 2006;354:34–43. https://doi.org/10.1056/NEJMoa052985.
92. Morice P, Joulie F, Camatte S, et al. Lymph node involvement in epithelial ovarian cancer: analysis of 276 pelvic and paraaortic lymphadenectomies and surgical implications. J Am Coll Surg. 2003;197:198–205. https://doi.org/10.1016/s1072-7515(03)00234-5.
93. Marpeau O, Schilder J, Zafrani Y, et al. Prognosis of patients who relapse after fertility-sparing surgery in epithelial ovarian cancer. Ann Surg Oncol. 2008;15:478–83. https://doi.org/10.1245/s10434-007-9651-x.
94. Timmers PJ, Zwinderman K, Coens C, et al. Lymph node sampling and taking of blind biopsies are important elements of the surgical staging of early ovarian cancer. Int J Gynecol Cancer. 2010;20:1142–7. https://doi.org/10.1111/igc.0b013e3181ef8e03.
95. Hoogendam JP, Vlek CA, Witteveen PO, et al. Surgical lymph node assessment in mucinous ovarian carcinoma staging: a systematic review and meta-analysis. BJOG. 2017;124:370–8. https://doi.org/10.1111/1471-0528.14226.
96. Young RC, Walton LA, Ellenberg SS, et al. Adjuvant therapy in stage I and stage II epithelial ovarian cancer. Results of two prospective randomized trials. N Engl J Med. 1990;322:1021–7. https://doi.org/10.1056/nejm199004123221501.
97. Kyrgiou M, Salanti G, Pavlidis N, et al. Survival benefits with diverse chemotherapy regimens for ovarian cancer: meta-analysis of multiple treatments. J Natl Cancer Inst. 2006;98:1655–63. https://doi.org/10.1093/jnci/djj443.
98. Walker JL, Brady MF, Wenzel L, et al. Randomized trial of intravenous versus intraperitoneal chemotherapy plus bevacizumab in advanced ovarian carcinoma: an NRG Oncology/Gynecologic Oncology Group study. J Clin Oncol. 2019;37:1380–90. https://doi.org/10.1200/jco.18.01568.
99. Tew WP, Lacchetti C, Ellis A, et al. PARP inhibitors in the management of ovarian cancer: ASCO guideline. J Clin Oncol. 2020;38:3468–93. https://doi.org/10.1200/jco.20.01924.
100. González-Martín A, Pothuri B, Vergote I, et al. Niraparib in patients with newly diagnosed advanced ovarian cancer. N Engl J Med. 2019;381:2391–402. https://doi.org/10.1056/NEJMoa1910962.
101. Burger RA, Brady MF, Bookman MA, et al. Incorporation of bevacizumab in the primary treatment of ovarian cancer. N Engl J Med. 2011;365:2473–83. https://doi.org/10.1056/NEJMoa1104390.
102. Perren TJ, Swart AM, Pfisterer J, et al. A phase 3 trial of bevacizumab in ovarian cancer. N Engl J Med. 2011;365:2484–96. https://doi.org/10.1056/NEJMoa1103799.

Part III

Physiotherapy and Rehabilitation for Pelvic and Women's Health

Physiotherapy and Rehabilitation in Lower Urinary Tract Disorders

14

Demet Öztürk and Emine Baran

14.1 Introduction

Upon examining the terminology studies of the International Continence Society (ICS) and the International Children's Continence Society (ICCS), lower urinary tract dysfunction (LUTD) is defined as the presence of multiple subcategories of functional disorders within the lower urinary tract [1, 2]. LUTD is a broad term encompassing a wide range of lower urinary tract symptoms (LUTS). LUTD significantly affects patients' quality of life, contributing to psychological distress, social embarrassment, and limitations in physical activities. These impacts highlight the necessity for comprehensive assessment and treatment strategies. Physiotherapists play a vital role as part of the multidisciplinary team in the evaluation and management of LUTD.

A large-scale prevalence study from 2017, which included 8284 individuals, reported LUTS prevalence rates of 62.8% in men and 59.6% in women. The study also noted that LUTS become more common with advancing age [3, 4]. The 2023 study, which included data from 36 countries, highlighted that the prevalence of any LUTS was 63.2% [5]. According to the results of another study published by Kim et al. in 2023, which examined the prevalence of LUTD, the prevalence of LUTD in men in the age groups 60–69, 70–79, and ≥80 years in 2018 was 26.7%, 28.9%, and 16.0%, respectively. In women, the prevalence in the same age groups was 19.3%, 20.5%, and 18.1%. Furthermore, a significant increase in the prevalence of LUTD was observed over the past decade (from 2009 to 2018) [6].

While LUTD is prevalent in adults, it also affects specific populations, such as children and individuals with neurological conditions. It has been identified as a condition affecting 15% of school-age children [7]. Particularly, although more common in male children, nocturnal incontinence (enuresis) is observed in 10% of 7-year-old children, 3.1% of 11–12-year-olds, and 0.5–1.7% of 16–17-year-olds [8]. This condition, which is commonly observed among healthy individuals without any diagnosis, is even more prevalent in individuals with a diagnosis [9, 10]. Neurological conditions (such as multiple sclerosis and Parkinson's disease) often affect bladder control by disrupting the nerves that innervate the lower urinary tract. According to the results of a meta-analysis published in 2020 investigating the prevalence of LUTS in individuals with multiple sclerosis, the presence of LUTS was reported in 68.41% of patients based on self-reported outcomes and in 63.95% based on urodynamic measurement results [11]. A meta-analysis conducted

D. Öztürk (✉)
Department of Physiotherapy and Rehabilitation, Faculty of Health Sciences, Lokman Hekim University, Ankara, Türkiye

E. Baran
Faculty of Physical Therapy and Rehabilitation, Hacettepe University, Ankara, Türkiye

T. Akbayrak, E. Üzelpasaci (eds.), *Physiotherapy and Rehabilitation in Pelvic and Women's Health-Related Problems*, https://doi.org/10.1007/978-3-032-28741-0_14

in 2022 examining the prevalence of LUTS in Parkinson's disease highlighted the presence of LUTS in 61% of individuals with Parkinson's disease. Besides, the prevalence of storage symptoms was calculated to be 59%, while the prevalence of voiding symptoms was 24% in this population [12]. According to a study investigating LUTS in neuromuscular diseases, LUTD was found in 44.44% of children with Duchenne muscular dystrophy [13]. Moreover, at least one lower urinary tract symptom was detected in 86.66% of the children with Duchenne muscular dystrophy [14].

The pathophysiology of LUTD is heterogeneous due to underlying disorders, and no single cause can be solely attributed [4]. It is more advantageous to examine the etiology of each symptom separately. For example, the causes of stress urinary incontinence include insufficiency in the closure pressure of the internal urethral sphincter, deficiencies in external support mechanisms, and urethral hypermobility [15]. The presence of urgency has been identified as an indicator of overactive bladder. Pain at the onset of urination suggests a urethral-related problem, while pain that emerges after urination may indicate a problem originating from the bladder [2]. The feeling of incomplete emptying and increased residual urine volume has been suggested to be etiologically related to the frequent use of holding maneuvers [16]. It has also been emphasized that constipation is a significant risk factor in the presence of bladder- and bowel-related symptoms [17, 18]. Therefore, conducting a separate analysis for each symptom and focusing specifically on the etiology and risk factors would be beneficial. Physiotherapy and rehabilitation are an integral part of the management of LUTD, providing targeted interventions to alleviate symptoms, enhance bladder function, and improve patients' quality of life.

14.2 Classification of Lower Urinary Tract Disorders

Normal micturition function is a cycle that involves the storage of urine in the bladder and its emptying in a timely and appropriate manner under voluntary control. This cycle is referred to as the micturition cycle. Symptoms are categorized based on which phase of the micturition cycle is affected. LUTS can be categorized into three groups: storage symptoms, voiding symptoms, and other symptoms. Storage symptoms include increased or decreased voiding frequency, urgency, nocturia, and incontinence. Voiding symptoms include hesitancy, straining, weak urine stream, intermittent urination, and dysuria. Other symptoms, aside from storage and voiding symptoms, include holding maneuvers, the sensation of incomplete emptying, post-micturition dribbling, and painful conditions [2, 19]. According to some sources, symptoms are also categorized into three groups: storage, voiding, and post-micturition symptoms [4, 20]. However, painful conditions can occur not only after urination but also before and/or during urination. Similarly, holding maneuvers can occur at any stage of the storage phase. Therefore, it would be more accurate to classify these symptoms under the "other symptoms" category [2]. Detailed descriptions of these symptoms are presented in Table 14.1 [1].

In addition to classification based on the physiological functions of the bladder, LUTS is also divided into neurogenic and non-neurogenic types. Non-neurogenic lower urinary tract dysfunction refers to a disorder caused by structural and functional changes in the lower urinary system without an obvious neurological diagnosis. Neurogenic lower urinary tract dysfunction (NLUTD), on the other hand, results from central or peripheral nerve disorders that impair the function of the lower urinary system, affecting lower urinary tract function [4].

NLUTD is further categorized both anatomically and physiologically. Anatomical classification is based on the lesion's location (supraspinal, suprasacral, and infrasacral), while physiological classification considers the specific functional impairment of the bladder (storage disorders or voiding disorders) [21, 22]. According to the findings of Gierup et al. the effects of upper motor neuron lesions and lower motor neuron lesions on the bladder differ [23]. If the cause of neurogenic bladder is related to upper motor neuron lesions, it is expected to cause detrusor and

Table 14.1 Lower urinary tract symptoms (LUTS) and definitions

LUTS	Definitions
Storage symptoms	
Increased voiding frequency	The need to urinate more than 7 times a day
Decreased voiding frequency	Urinating less than 4 times a day
Incontinence	Involuntary urinary incontinence that causes social or hygienic problems and can be objectively demonstrated
Urgency	The sudden and urgent feeling of needing to urinate unexpectedly
Nocturia	Waking up one or more times at night to urinate
Voiding symptoms	
Hesitancy	Difficulty initiating urination despite being ready to void
Straining	The need to increase intra-abdominal pressure to initiate, maintain, and/or complete urination
Weak stream	Weak urine flow observed during urination
Intermittency	Urination characterized by multiple start and stop phases
Dysuria	Burning sensation or discomfort experienced during urination
Other symptoms	
Holding maneuvers	Strategies used by children to postpone urination or suppress the feeling of urgency (e.g., crossing legs, making dance-like movements, applying pressure to the genital area)
Feeling of incomplete emptying	The sensation of incomplete bladder emptying after urination
Post-micturition dribble	Involuntary leakage of urine immediately after completing urination
Pain	Pain experienced during and/or after urination

Table 14.2 Anatomical and physiological classification of neurogenic bladder

Classification type	Classification title	Possible characteristics of lesion/disorder
Anatomical classification	*Supraspinal lesion*	Hyperactive detrusor, low bladder capacity, involuntary detrusor contractions, sensory impairment, high intravesical pressure, increased voiding frequency, urgency and urge incontinence, etc.
	Suprasacral lesion	Hyperactive detrusor, detrusor-external sphincter dyssynergia, sensory impairment, risk of vesicoureteral reflux, etc.
	Infrasacral lesion	Acontractile detrusor (weak or absent contractions), sensory impairment, increased bladder capacity, difficulty initiating voiding, etc.
Physiological classification	*Storage disorders*	Hyperactive detrusor, denervated external sphincter, denervated pelvic diaphragm, bladder neck insufficiency
	Voiding disorders	Acontractile or hypocontractile detrusor, detrusor-sphincter dyssynergia, spastic external sphincter, mechanical obstruction

sphincter hyperactivity, as well as urethral sphincter dyssynergia. This is due to the loss of the inhibitory effect of higher centers on the lower centers. On the other hand, if the cause of neurogenic bladder is related to lower motor neuron lesions, reduced detrusor activity, detrusor areflexia, sphincter denervation, and sphincter insufficiency may occur [22, 23]. The condition resulting from NLUTD is referred to as neurogenic bladder. The anatomical and physiological classification of neurogenic bladder is summarized in Table 14.2 [21].

14.3 Assessment Methods

Individuals diagnosed with LUTD, which results in bladder and bowel symptoms, may experience a wide range of symptoms. These symptoms can negatively affect individuals physically, psychologically, socially, and sexually. Therefore, a detailed assessment is crucial for ensuring the optimal management of patients and for developing a rehabilitation program tailored to the patient's clinical findings. A multidisciplinary approach is essential for the holistic evaluation of patients with LUTD. Chapter 4 of this book will discuss the medical assessments and treatments related to LUTD. Therefore, this section will present the assessments within the scope of physiotherapists' expertise in a structured manner. Physiotherapist evaluations are summarized in Table 14.3.

Table 14.3 Physiotherapist evaluations and detailed assessment methods

Assessment title	Details
Comprehensive history-taking	During history-taking, various factors should be assessed, including age, body mass index, occupation, other relevant medical conditions (neurological conditions, diabetes mellitus, irritable bowel syndrome, previous pelvic injury, oncological diseases, and cognitive impairment, etc.), past urological surgeries (hysterectomy, episiotomy, prostatectomy, etc.), and urinary tract infections [24–27]. Urinary symptoms, including frequency, urgency, incontinence (presence, type, and severity), and nocturia, should be thoroughly explored. For female patients, gynecological history should include menstrual regularity, menopausal status, and any associated symptoms, while obstetric history should evaluate the number of pregnancies, types of deliveries (vaginal, cesarean, or assisted), birth weights, and complications such as perineal trauma. To better understand lifestyle modifications and identify which changes may be necessary for treatment, the individual's daily routines should also be examined in detail, such as daily fluid intake and types of fluids consumed, dietary habits, whether daily energy and protein requirements are met, and sleep quality [28, 29]. Additionally, pelvic pain assessment can be conducted during history-taking. The type, location, and intensity of the pain, as well as all factors that alleviate or exacerbate it, should be thoroughly evaluated [30]
Physical examination	Physical examination primarily begins with inspection and palpation of the perineum. During inspection, various aspects are assessed, including discoloration in the pelvic floor, the presence of edema, cystic structures, scar tissue, asymmetry, and atrophic changes [31]. Through palpation, valuable information can be obtained regarding pelvic floor muscle tone, voluntary contraction capability, voluntary relaxation ability, coordination, muscle strength, endurance, elasticity, tension, painful points, and reflexes such as the anal reflex and bulbocavernosus reflex. Additionally, when necessary, detailed motor, sensory, and reflex assessments of lumbosacral dermatomes (L1-S5) should be performed. Furthermore, the presence and severity of pelvic organ prolapse can be evaluated [32]. Physical examination should include an abdominal examination to detect any abdominal or pelvic mass, presence of tense tissue, trigger points, diastasis recti abdominis, and herniations [32]. In male patients, prostate size, prostate nodules, smoothness of the prostate wall, prostate density, and penile and scrotal evaluation are important [24, 33]
LUTS assessments	Evaluation should identify the types (e.g., stress, urge, mixed), the timing, and the severity of incontinence. The most bothersome symptom should be determined [24]. The use of validated patient questionnaires (King's Health Questionnaire, International Incontinence Questionnaire, Incontinence Impact Questionnaire, The Dysfunctional Voiding and Incontinence Scoring System, etc.) is recommended by guidelines [2, 27, 34]
Pelvic floor assessments	Pelvic floor muscle strength, endurance, tone, spasticity, and function can be assessed using clinical methods such as digital evaluation with scales like the Modified Oxford Scale and the PERFECT Scale (Fig. 14.1). For more detailed assessments, tools such as manometers, perineometers, dynamometers, electromyography, and biofeedback may be utilized. In complex cases, advanced imaging techniques such as ultrasound, computed tomography, or magnetic resonance imaging can provide comprehensive insights into pelvic floor function [31, 35–37]
Diaries	In the assessment of LUTD, commonly used diaries include bladder diaries (frequency-volume charts) and bowel diaries [2]. These diaries are reproducible, practical, reliable, valid, and even have therapeutic benefits. Therefore, their use is recommended by clinical guidelines. The recommended duration for completing a bladder diary is 3–7 days, while for a bowel diary, it is 7–14 days [2, 18, 27]

(continued)

Table 14.3 (continued)

Assessment title	Details
Pad test	It is used to determine the presence of urinary incontinence, measure its severity if present, and evaluate treatment effectiveness. It has high diagnostic accuracy. While some protocols are standardized, others involve tests where standardizing activity levels can be challenging. These assessments can be conducted in various formats, such as 1-hour, 8-hour, 24-hour, 48-hour, or 72-hour tests [27, 38]
Q-tip test	The Q-tip test is performed to evaluate urethral hypermobility [39]. A change of at least 30° between the angle of the Q-tip and the transverse plane during straining or coughing is defined as the clinically significant threshold for urethral hypermobility [40]
Laboratory tests	LUTD symptoms frequently lead to urinary tract infections [41]. Therefore, during patient evaluation, questions related to urinary tract infections should be asked, and a urinalysis should be conducted if necessary. According to a guideline published by McKibben et al. in 2015, if the urinalysis result is negative, no further testing is needed. However, if it is positive, a culture test should be performed. A negative culture test indicates the absence of infection, while a positive result suggests that further assessment of additional symptoms is warranted. In cases of asymptomatic bacteriuria, no treatment (e.g., antibiotics) is recommended; however, if symptoms such as fever, pain, or changes in vital signs are present, a 1–2 week course of antibiotics is advised [42]. Among the duties, authorities, and responsibilities of physiotherapists, performing tests for urinary tract infections, collecting cultures, prescribing medications, or monitoring these processes are not included. However, the presence of a urinary tract infection may influence the physiotherapist's assessment findings and rehabilitation sessions. Therefore, physiotherapists should have general knowledge of laboratory tests, be able to review and interpret findings obtained by other healthcare professionals, and refer patients to a specialist when deemed necessary
Functional assessment of voiding parameters	Uroflowmetry provides important data regarding urination symptoms that may be associated with pelvic floor dysfunction. It is an objective tool for noninvasive and/or non-pharmacological data collection and therefore falls within the scope of physiotherapists' practice (Fig. 14.2). Uroflowmetry provides key data such as voided volume, voiding time, maximum flow rate, voiding curve patterns, and flow rate [43]. Uroflow curve patterns are crucial for diagnosis [2]
Post-void residual measurement	The volume of urine remaining in the bladder after voiding is measured to assess bladder emptying efficiency. Ultrasound, catheterization, and portable dedicated bladder scanner methods are commonly used for this evaluation, aiding in the diagnosis of incomplete emptying or urinary retention [44]
Urodynamic studies	Since urodynamic assessment is an invasive procedure, physiotherapists are not authorized to perform urodynamic evaluations. However, to enhance the quality and effectiveness of rehabilitation, physiotherapists should also be knowledgeable about urodynamic interventional assessments and, when necessary, be able to interpret the results of these evaluations. Urodynamics is a diagnostic method used to evaluate the storage and voiding functions of the lower urinary tract. These methods provide detailed information about the bladder's capacity, compliance, and contraction. The goal of these techniques is to elicit clinical symptoms, perform relevant measurements during the procedure, and identify underlying pathology [18]
Core stabilization assessments	Core stabilization assessments focus on evaluating the strength, endurance, and coordination of muscles responsible for trunk stability, such as the transversus abdominis, multifidus, pelvic floor, and diaphragm. These evaluations include functional tests (e.g., abdominal drawing-in maneuver) and endurance tests (e.g., side plank, Sorensen test), providing insight into core muscle performance and imbalances
Quality-of-life assessments	The presence of LUTS negatively impacts individuals' participation in daily life activities and social roles. In children and adolescents, it can adversely affect academic performance [8]. In geriatric individuals, LUTS can lead to the rejection of caregiving roles by family members and may even prevent the elderly person from receiving institutional care [45]. All of these effects negatively influence quality of life. Therefore, reliable and valid questionnaires (e.g., Incontinence Quality of Life Questionnaire, King's Health Questionnaire, the Dysfunctional Voiding Symptom Score, and the Pediatric Urinary Incontinence Quality of Life Score) that assess quality of life should be used. In addition, the patient's expectations from treatment should be questioned [24]

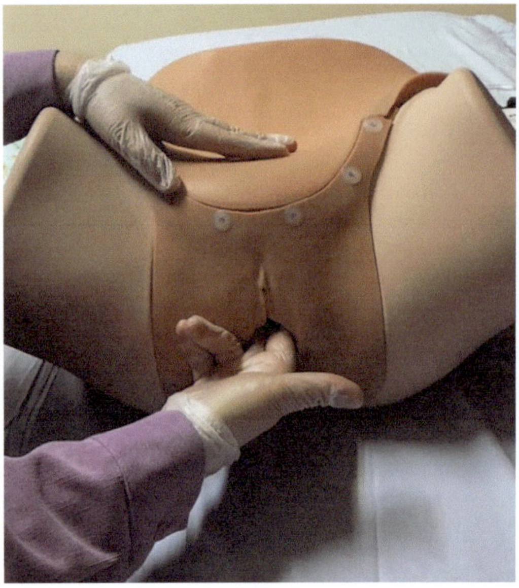

Fig. 14.1 Digital assessment of the pelvic floor

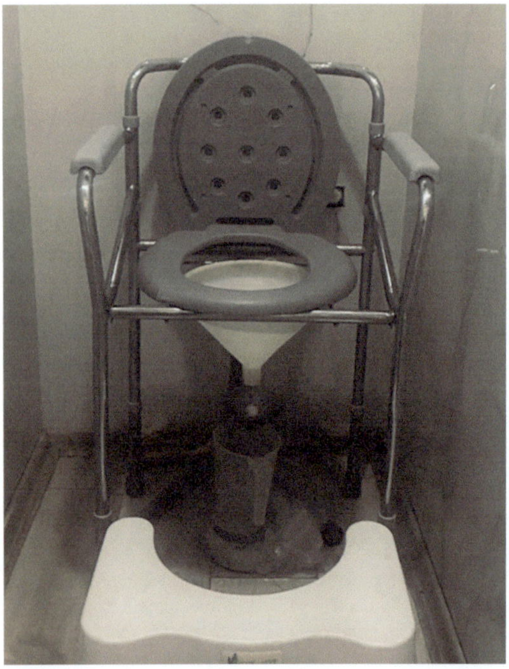

Fig. 14.2 Uroflowmetry assessment

14.4 Treatment Modalities

In the literature, numerous modalities have been presented for the treatment of LUTD. These modalities can be listed as follows [46, 47]: Lifestyle modifications, dietary changes, bladder training, exercise modalities (especially pelvic floor muscle exercises), catheterization, catheter-free bladder emptying techniques, pharmacological treatments, minimally invasive procedures, surgical interventions, emerging and experimental treatments, etc. In this section of the book, only physiotherapy and rehabilitation practices will be discussed. Treatment topics will be classified based on neurological and non-neurological conditions.

14.5 Physiotherapy and Rehabilitation in Non-neurological Conditions

Evidence-based practices used in the management of non-neurological LUTD have been outlined under specific headings:

14.5.1 Lifestyle Changes and Patient Education (Urotherapy)

Urotherapy is the first-line treatment for bladder and bowel dysfunction, encompassing non-surgical and non-pharmacological lifestyle modifications [17]. It reduces the severity of LUTS and has therapeutic effects on existing symptoms. Urotherapy improves uroflowmetry parameters, decreases post-void residual urine volume, enhances pelvic floor muscle awareness and functionality, facilitates pelvic floor relaxation, alleviates constipation symptoms, and protects against upper urinary tract complications [18, 48].

According to the most recent guideline published by the ICCS in 2021, urotherapy is categorized into two main types: standard urotherapy and specific urotherapy [49]. Standard urotherapy includes providing information about lower urinary tract function, educating the patient and their family, offering recommendations for addressing specific LUTS, implementing behavioral changes (e.g., regular bowel and voiding habits, proper toilet posture), promoting lifestyle modifications (e.g., adequate fluid intake, caffeine reduction, high-fiber diet), scheduling voiding, recording voiding symptoms and habits, enhancing pelvic floor muscle awareness, and ensuring regular clinical follow-ups. Specific urotherapy, on the other hand, encompasses pelvic floor training, the use of biofeedback, alarm therapy, electrical stimulation, and clean intermittent catheterization. Besides, the guidelines highlight psychotherapy and cognitive-behavioral therapy as potential interventions that can complement urotherapy [17, 48, 49].

Urotherapy primarily involves patient education, focusing on enhancing individuals' knowledge and awareness. This educational component includes a simplified explanation of the anatomy and physiology of the pelvic floor, urinary system, and bowel system. Patients are informed about LUTS, their pathophysiology, potential risk factors, prognosis, and possible complications. To facilitate understanding and visualization, the use of pelvic floor-related images, videos, models, and metaphors is recommended. Additionally, sufficient time should be allocated for the educational sessions, which can be conducted individually or in group settings [18, 50].

The details of necessary lifestyle changes should be thoroughly explained. Adjustments should be made to water intake, voiding frequency, bowel movement schedules, voiding and defecation postures, consumption of bladder irritants, dietary routines, and sleep habits. Furthermore, information should be provided on physical activity levels, genital hygiene, weight management strategies, and the consequences of exposure to smoking and alcohol [48, 49].

14.5.2 Pelvic Floor Muscle Training

Pelvic floor muscle training is a conservative approach recommended as a first-line treatment for preventing and treating many issues related to pelvic floor dysfunction and LUTD [32, 51]. Due to its low-risk nature and noninvasive characteristics, it is safely recommended for all populations. It is a treatment modality with high-level evidence supporting its positive outcomes in the management of LUTS and pelvic floor dysfunction [32]. The goal of pelvic floor muscle training is to improve the strength, endurance, power, relaxation, or a combination of these parameters [33]. According to a study by Sheng et al. in 2022 explaining the mechanism of pelvic floor muscle training, there are three main effects of pelvic floor muscle exercises: enhanced pelvic floor muscle strength, maximized awareness of timing, and strengthened core muscles [52]:

1. *Enhanced Pelvic Floor Muscle Strength:* This mechanism focuses on the levator ani muscles and involves repetitive contractions to strengthen the levator ani muscle group.
2. *Maximized Awareness of Timing:* This mechanism targets the urethral striated muscles. It aims to ensure continence by increasing the urethral closing pressure when needed. The Knack maneuver is examined under this theory.
3. *Strengthened Core Muscles:* This mechanism targets the transversus abdominus muscle. It focuses on eliciting a contraction in the transversus abdominus muscle through pelvic floor muscle contraction.

The individual can perform pelvic floor exercises in any position. As long as the exercises are performed correctly, they can be done in all static positions, such as prone, supine, side-lying, lithotomy, sitting, standing, and squatting positions. Moreover, it is recommended to perform the exercises in dynamic positions like walking and climbing stairs. It is crucial that the movements are done correctly. Therefore, the physiotherapist should teach the patient to perform isolated pelvic floor muscle contractions without triggering compensation mechanisms or accessory muscle contractions [53]. The selection of commands given to achieve the correct movement is also very important. A systematic review conducted in 2022 demonstrated the effects of verbal instructions on pelvic floor contraction skills and strengthening of the pelvic floor muscles [53, 54].

The 5F rule should be followed in pelvic floor muscle training: find, feel, force, follow-through, and functional training of pelvic floor muscles [55]. Additionally, it is recommended that pelvic floor muscle exercises be performed intensively [27]. However, it should be noted that the number of daily contractions should not exceed 200 repetitions. It has been shown that significant changes in urinary incontinence can be achieved with short sessions (10–45 min) performed 3–7 days a week [56]. Furthermore, it has been demonstrated that performing pelvic floor muscle exercises for 12 months significantly improves pelvic floor function. This result underscores the importance of prolonged exercise in the recovery of pelvic floor health [57].

14.5.3 Biofeedback

Biofeedback is a process in which an individual's performed activity is transformed into perceivable auditory or visual signals, enabling the person to become aware of activities typically carried out unconsciously by the body. Feedback can be provided through internal (self-awareness by the individual) or external (feedback from clinicians, devices, or other external stimuli) [35].

Its application in the pelvic floor involves a video game format that allows patients to move objects on a screen, helping them learn how to relax their pelvic floor muscles effectively [58]. In some devices, the sound intensity increases as muscle contraction strengthens, or brighter lights are displayed as the contraction force grows. Theoretically, these feedback mechanisms help patients develop better awareness of performing correct and strong contractions. This, in turn, effectively enhances the strength of the pelvic floor muscles [59]. Biofeedback devices can be utilized through intravaginal, intraanal, and transperineal applications. Moreover, feedback can also be provided using the individual's finger or the therapist's finger, which is considered a form of biofeedback application [60].

Biofeedback not only helps enhance concentric contraction of the muscles but also facilitates relaxation of the pelvic floor muscles. When combined with pelvic floor muscle training, biofeedback allows patients to visualize the muscle's movement during contraction, the strength of the contraction, the degree of relaxation, and the overall effectiveness of the treatment [17].

Biofeedback is effective in the treatment of LUTD due to its benefits for symptoms; however, it is not superior to standard urotherapy or pelvic floor muscle training when used alone [17, 61]. Therefore, biofeedback is not considered a standalone treatment modality. Its use is recommended only in combination with other modalities [62].

14.5.4 Electrical Stimulation

Electrical stimulation is presented as a passive method for strengthening pelvic floor muscles [35]. Through the use of electrical stimulation, isolated contractions of the pelvic floor muscles can be achieved without involving auxiliary or compensatory muscle contractions. These isolated contractions are believed to strengthen the pelvic floor. Additionally, they are thought to enhance motor learning by increasing awareness of the pelvic floor muscles [56]. Electrical stimulation applied to the pelvic floor induces a form of neuromodulation. Neuromodulation has been shown to increase bladder capacity, reduce the sense of urgency, improve continence, and decrease the frequency of urinary tract infections [17]. Furthermore, it is hypothesized that electrotherapy agents may stimulate angiogenesis, cellular proliferation, and regeneration, thereby contributing to symptom improvement [62].

The primary mechanism of action involves activating motor units by innervating the pudendal nerve originating from the S2 to S4 levels, thereby inducing repetitive pelvic floor muscle contractions. In addition to muscle contraction, stimulation of the pudendal nerve is thought to activate the sacral segments, facilitating autonomic and somatic modulation in the pelvic organs [63]. Specifically, electrical stimulation of S3 activates the pelvic floor muscles and coordinates sacral reflexes by regulating the innervation of the bladder, external urethral sphincter, and pelvic floor [17].

Electrical stimulation can be applied in various forms (e.g., intravaginal, intrarectal, transperineal, posterior tibial nerve stimulation, sacral neuromodulation) and using different types of currents (e.g., transcutaneous electrical nerve stimulation, interferential current, faradic currents, extracorporeal magnetic stimulation, ultrasound, low-intensity laser) [60, 64]. Applications such as parasacral transcutaneous electrical nerve stimulation, posterior tibial nerve stimulation, and interferential stimulation have been identified as distinct neuromodulation modalities that can be employed in the treatment of LUTD [65] (Fig. 14.3).

Electrical stimulation of the pelvic floor has been proposed as an option for patients who are unable to perform voluntary contractions of the pelvic floor muscles [66]. It is particularly recommended for individuals with low treatment adherence as a means to enhance their motivation to participate in therapy. However, similar to biofeedback applications, studies have shown that despite its benefits, electrical stimulation alone is not sufficient for the treatment of LUTS. It must be incorporated into a combined program with pelvic floor muscle exercises and/or another therapeutic modality [62].

14.5.5 Manual Therapy

Manual therapy is a general term for noninvasive interventions that involve various techniques and principles applied through hands-on methods. Being a noninvasive and non-pharmacological treatment, it has been presented as an alternative therapeutic approach [67]. In LUTD, various noninvasive manual therapy techniques can be applied. These techniques are gentle, non-damaging methods that affect different tissues in the body, including fascia, nerves, joints, bones, organs, and the vascular system [68].

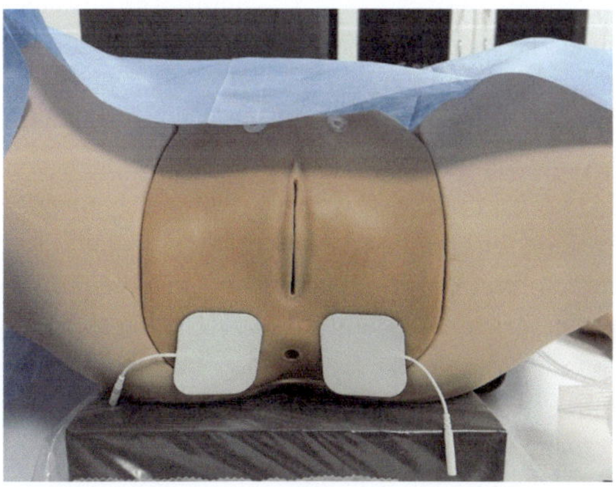

Fig. 14.3 Superficial electrotherapy application to pelvic floor muscles

Experienced and trained physiotherapists can apply various direct and indirect techniques targeting the pelvic floor, abdomen (diaphragm, ileocecal valve, duodenojejunal flexure), skull, spine, and sacrum. These techniques may include articular, visceral, vascular, muscular, and myofascial approaches. It is noted that these techniques help normalize neurovegetative functions as well as muscle and joint functions [69].

Manual interventions applied in the treatment of LUTD include classical massage, connective tissue massage, myofascial releases, diaphragm mobilization, Wurn technique, transvaginal applications, trigger point therapy, Thiele massage, compression maneuvers, transverse friction, skin rolling, joint manipulations, visceral mobilization, and proprioceptive neuromuscular facilitation techniques. These methods aim to address various musculoskeletal, visceral, and neurophysiological dysfunctions, contributing to the improvement of pelvic floor and overall lower urinary tract health [35, 70, 71].

14.5.6 Breathing Exercises

The diaphragm works in coordination with the pelvic floor and core muscles, performing co-contractions that contribute to the generation and regulation of intra-abdominal pressure [72]. Due to this synergy, dysfunction in any of these muscle groups can negatively impact the others. Similarly, including one muscle group in a rehabilitation program can positively influence the others [73]. Therefore, incorporating breathing exercises is considered crucial in the treatment of LUTD symptoms associated with the pelvic floor.

Breathing exercises aim to achieve a proper breathing pattern, induce pelvic floor muscle contractions, enhance pelvic floor muscle awareness, establish a consistent abdominal breathing model, improve blood circulation in the mesenteric region to influence pelvic organs, enhance colonic transit, and strengthen and relax the abdominal muscles

[72, 74]. Moreover, during breathing exercises, the diaphragm moves caudally during inspiration, the thoracic cavity expands, and the abdominal wall displaces anteriorly. These movements and displacements have been shown to reduce urethral pressure, thereby facilitating urination and defecation [75]. Most children with LUTD exhibit an overactive abdominal wall, which prevents the relaxation of the pelvic floor muscles [76]. Consequently, diaphragmatic breathing exercises can be employed in their treatment to promote relaxation of the abdominal muscles [72].

14.5.7 Trunk Stabilization Exercises

Core stabilization exercises can be implemented in individuals diagnosed with LUTS to enhance coordination among core muscles, support the regulation of intra-abdominal pressure, improve stabilization, and enhance pelvic floor muscle function [77]. These exercises are noninvasive, carry no side effects, and are particularly utilized in the treatment of LUTS symptoms, especially incontinence [76]. Core stabilization exercises are not limited to a strictly defined or fixed set of movements. Instead, they represent a versatile pool of exercises that can be performed in various positions and across different populations. These exercises can be carried out in positions such as supine hook-lying, crawling, prone, sitting, and standing. Furthermore, concept-based therapies targeting core stabilization, such as Pilates, can also be utilized [78]. Combining core stabilization exercises with breathing exercises can provide an integrated treatment approach. Moreover, Pilates balls may be incorporated into the exercises to further enhance their effectiveness [79].

14.6 Physiotherapy and Rehabilitation in Neurological Conditions (NLUTD)

Neurogenic bladder is a bladder dysfunction caused by diseases or traumas affecting the central nervous system centers or peripheral nerves responsible for controlling urination [80]. It is most commonly associated with neurological disorders [81]. In the etiology of neurogenic bladder in the young population, the most frequently reported diagnosis is neurospinal dysraphism. Neural tube defects (e.g., spina bifida) account for 90% of neurogenic bladder cases in infancy and childhood. The remaining 10% includes conditions such as sacral agenesis, tethered cord syndrome, spinal cord-associated masses, cerebral palsy, and central nervous system pathologies [82].

In adults and geriatric individuals, the most common cause of neurogenic bladder is spinal cord lesions. These include compressive lesions, spinal cord injuries, cauda equina syndrome, spinal fractures, intervertebral disc herniations, and tumors. In addition to spinal lesions, conditions affecting the spinal cord, such as vascular problems (e.g., infarctions, vascular malformations), inflammation (e.g., myelitis, meningitis), widespread infections (e.g., herpes virus, varicella-zoster virus), and medication use, can also lead to neurogenic bladder. Furthermore, cerebrovascular events, multiple sclerosis, Parkinson's disease, peripheral neuropathy, dementia, and Alzheimer's disease are among the etiologies of neurogenic bladder in adults [21].

Neurogenic bladder pathology is associated with a wide range of symptoms. The most common among these are urinary incontinence, increased post-void residual urine, and the inability to initiate micturition. The presence of these symptoms alone imposes a significant physical, financial, and emotional burden on individuals' lives. Additionally, patients with NLUTD often experience advanced complications, frequently reported in parallel with the disease's progression [41]. Complications of neurogenic bladder include recurrent urinary tract infections, vesicoureteral reflux, hydronephrosis, pyelonephritis, prostatitis, urinary stones, bladder tumors, autonomic dysreflexia, and kidney failure [41, 83, 84]. Beyond physical findings, psychosocial impacts such as reduced participation in daily activities, social isolation, and depression have also been reported [83]. Consequently, untreated NLUTD, a lower urinary tract pathology, can lead to upper urinary tract pathologies and psychosocial problems. If additional neurological symptoms such as spasticity, rigidity, or autonomic dysfunction are present, the severity of LUTS tends to increase. The presence of these issues significantly reduces individuals' quality of life and may even result in mortality [41]. Therefore, treatment of NLUTD is of critical importance.

Due to the multifaceted impacts experienced by individuals with NLUTD, a multidisciplinary approach has been recommended for the evaluation and treatment of bladder and bowel dysfunctions [85]. Moreover, to reduce healthcare costs and facilitate adherence to the disease management process, all assessments should be tailored to the individual [86]. In the management of NLUTD, all comprehensive assessments used for non-neurogenic LUTD management can be applied. Furthermore, additional evaluations such as cystoscopy, neurophysiological assessments, and glomerular filtration rate calculations are suggested [21]. In addition, urodynamic assessments hold greater significance in NLUTD. However, current evidence indicates that due to their invasive nature and potential complications, urodynamic assessments are not recommended for routine evaluation [27]. They are emphasized in cases of persistent LUTS, treatment-resistant overactive bladder, and neurogenic conditions [87]. Early treatment based on urodynamic findings has been shown to reduce both upper and lower urinary tract dysfunctions in NLUTD management [88]. Although procedures such as cystoscopy, urodynamic assessments, and evaluations of blood and kidney markers fall outside the scope of the physiotherapist's duties, responsibilities, and authority, it is crucial for physiotherapists to be proficient in interpreting these findings to effectively manage the patient's treatment process.

In the evaluation of NLUTD, conducting a neurological assessment—including sensory, motor, and reflex evaluations—is more critical compared to LUTD evaluation [25]. Sensory assessment should primarily focus on the S2–S4 segments, responsible for the sensory innervation of the pelvic floor, as well as other potentially related regions [89]. Additionally, assessments tailored to the patient should include gait analysis, evaluation of hand dexterity, vital signs, autonomic dysfunction, muscle tone, and cognitive level [21, 90]. Furthermore, evaluating transfer activities, mobility, functional level, and wheelchair usability, if applicable, is also essential.

In addition to general neurological assessments, disease-specific evaluation tools should also be included in the assessment process. Tools such as the ASIA scoring system for spinal cord injuries, the Expanded Disability Status Scale for Multiple Sclerosis, and the Hoehn and Yahr scale for Parkinson's disease are crucial for understanding disease-specific impacts. Awareness of disease symptoms and potential complications helps prevent issues that may arise during rehabilitation. Furthermore, considering the biopsychosocial model, a comprehensive evaluation of the individual's intellectual capacity and available social support systems is as important as the other assessments [91].

To enhance the efficiency of rehabilitation and ensure patient participation in the treatment program, a personalized rehabilitation plan should be developed. The primary goals of NLUTD treatment include protecting the upper urinary tract, maintaining adequate bladder compliance and capacity, treating incontinence if present, preventing bladder distension, reducing the risk of urinary tract infections, and achieving an acceptable quality of life [92]. In line with these objectives, interventions addressing the symptoms caused by neurological impairments should be incorporated into the rehabilitation program. These may include implementing follow-up programs for clean intermittent catheterization if required, teaching patients the use of urinary collecting systems, employing neurophysiological approaches (e.g., Bobath concept, proprioceptive neuromuscular facilitation, Brunnstrom, Johnstone therapy, Todd-Davies), and providing orthotic supports when necessary. These measures can effectively support the overall rehabilitation process.

Two of the treatment methods (bladder training and catheterization) that are important in the treatment of NLUTD are explained under the following headings:

14.6.1 Bladder Training

Bladder training is applied differently in patients with storage symptoms compared to those with voiding symptoms. In patients with storage symptoms, the goal is to increase bladder capacity and reduce urinary frequency by alleviating urgency. As part of bladder retraining, patients are taught pelvic floor muscle contractions, relaxation techniques, and distraction methods. The ICS recommends adjusting voiding intervals based on the patient's baseline frequency [35]. To determine this, patients are asked to maintain a bladder diary to identify their longest voiding interval. Based on this interval, an additional 15–30 min is added, and the patient is instructed to maintain this extended interval between voids for 1 week. If successful, the interval is increased by another 15–30 min each subsequent week. If the patient is unable to achieve the interval, the same duration is maintained until they succeed. This process is typically continued for 6–12 weeks, progressively increasing the time between voiding episodes and restoring control over bladder function [93].

For patients with voiding dysfunction associated with neurological conditions who are unable to completely empty their bladder, the goal is to achieve catheter-free bladder emptying. Before initiating training, video-urodynamic studies should be conducted to assess the upper and lower urinary tracts during both filling and voiding phases. Additionally, routine ultrasound evaluations of post-void residual urine volume are recommended. Patients are instructed to void upon waking, 1–1.5 h after consuming large amounts of fluid (e.g., during meals or excessive fluid intake), every 3–4 h during the day, and before bedtime. During bladder training, the bladder should ideally hold 300–600 mL of urine. Post-void residual volume should not exceed 20% of the voided volume or remain below 100 mL, and detrusor pressure must stay under 80 cm H_2O to prevent overdistension. A daily fluid intake of approximately 1800 mL is recommended. With voiding intervals of 4–6 h, the bladder volume can be maintained between 300 and 450 mL, thus preventing excessive bladder stretching [94].

There are four primary techniques for achieving catheter-free voiding by reflexively stimulating detrusor muscle contractions. These include triggered voiding, which uses sensory stimuli to initiate the voiding reflex; straining voiding, which engages abdominal muscles to assist in voiding; the Credé maneuver, which involves applying suprapubic pressure to aid bladder emptying; and anal sphincter stretching to stimulate detrusor contractions. If residual urine remains in the bladder after voiding, catheterization is required. It is crucial to note that certain techniques are contraindicated in specific conditions. For instance, straining voiding is contraindicated in patients with overactive bladder or detrusor-sphincter dyssynergia, while the Credé maneuver is contraindicated in cases of hyperreflexive sphincter or detrusor-sphincter dyssynergia [95, 96].

14.6.2 Catheterization

14.6.2.1 Permanent Catheterization

Permanent catheterization is used as a bladder emptying method in patients with little or no bladder control, severe cognitive impairments, poor motor skills, or unstable medical conditions. Since these patients have a higher risk of urinary tract infections, daily fluid intake should be approximately 3000 mL. Long-term use of permanent catheters may lead to reduced bladder compliance and capacity, increased intravesical pressure, and a negative impact on body image. Therefore, transitioning to intermittent catheterization or catheter-free voiding methods is recommended as soon as possible [97].

14.6.2.2 Intermittent Catheterization

For patients experiencing difficulty emptying their bladder, residual urine retention, or inability to void, the International Continence Society and the European Association of Urology (EAU) recommend clean intermittent catheterization (CIC) with an A-level evidence rating. If residual urine after catheter-free voiding exceeds 100 mL or is greater than 20% of the voided urine volume, CIC should be used to remove the residual urine [98].

CIC is a technique that patients can perform independently or with assistance. Before initiating CIC, fluid intake should be restricted to approximately 1800–2000 mL per day. The procedure should be performed every 4–6 h, with 400–500 mL of urine emptied during each session. Excessive urine accumulation in the bladder may lead to complications affecting the upper urinary tract. Overdistension of the bladder can cause autonomic hyperreflexia, making it essential to monitor urine output and prevent overfilling of the bladder. Compared to permanent catheterization, CIC carries a lower risk of infection and preserves bladder storage function. Furthermore, CIC allows for a more social lifestyle and has a lesser negative impact on body image and sexuality [97].

14.6.2.3 External Catheters (Condom Catheter—Drip Collector)

If urinary incontinence is mild and involves dribbling, these products can be used. Proper attention should be given to the cleaning and maintenance of the products, as well as hand hygiene and hygiene of the application site. They need to be changed at regular intervals. Prolonged use can lead to skin damage and urinary tract infections. If the patient has a latex allergy, latex-free products should be preferred [99].

14.7 Conclusion

Lower urinary tract dysfunction is quite common among individuals in the community and must be treated due to its potentially life-threatening complications. To design a personalized rehabilitation program, a comprehensive assessment by a specialized physiotherapist is essential. Given its wide range of symptoms, a holistic evaluation plan should be implemented. Based on the findings of this assessment and the clinical decision-making processes of the therapist, a symptomatic and biopsychosocial treatment program should be developed.

References

1. Abrams P, Cardozo L, Fall M, Griffiths D, Rosier P, Ulmsten U, et al. The standardisation of terminology in lower urinary tract function: report from the standardisation sub-committee of the International Continence Society. Urology. 2003;61(1):37–49.
2. Austin PF, Bauer SB, Bower W, Chase J, Franco I, Hoebeke P, et al. The standardization of terminology of lower urinary tract function in children and adolescents: update report from the standardization committee of the International Children's Continence Society. Neurourol Urodyn. 2016;35(4):471–81.
3. Chapple C, Castro-Diaz D, Chuang Y-C, Lee K-S, Liao L, Liu S-P, et al. Prevalence of lower urinary tract symptoms in China, Taiwan, and South Korea: results from a cross-sectional, population-based study. Adv Ther. 2017;34:1953–65.
4. Kamei J, Fujimura T. Urinary tract infection in patients with lower urinary tract dysfunction. J Infect Chemother. 2023;29(8):744–8.
5. Huang J, Chan C-K, Yee S, Deng Y, Bai Y, Chan SC, et al. Global burden and temporal trends of lower urinary tract symptoms: a systematic review and meta-analysis. Prostate Cancer Prostatic Dis. 2023;26(2):421–8.
6. Kim YH, Hong SH, Kang TW, Chung HC, Kim TH, Kim SC, et al. Trends in age-specific prevalence of lower urinary tract dysfunction: a nationwide population-based cohort study. Urogenit Tract Infect. 2023;18(3):101–6.
7. Argibay S, Beloy C. Urinary incontinence and lower urinary tract dysfunction prevalence in schoolchildren: risk factors. Cir Pediatr. 2019;32(3):145–9.
8. Kuwertz-Bröking E, von Gontard A. Clinical management of nocturnal enuresis. Pediatr Nephrol. 2018;33(7):1145–54.
9. Chao TC, Yang SSD, Chang SJ, Tsai LP. High prevalence of lower urinary tract dysfunction in patients with Prader–Willi syndrome. Neurourol Urodyn. 2021;40(4):1063–8.
10. Moussa M, Papatsoris A, Abou Chakra M, Fares Y, Dellis A. Lower urinary tract dysfunction in common neurological diseases. Turk J Urol. 2020;46(Suppl 1):S70.
11. Al Dandan HB, Coote S, McClurg D. Prevalence of lower urinary tract symptoms in people with multiple sclerosis: a systematic review and meta-analysis. Int J MS Care. 2020;22(2):91–9.
12. Li F-F, Cui Y-S, Yan R, Cao S-S, Feng T. Prevalence of lower urinary tract symptoms, urinary incontinence and retention in Parkinson's disease: a systematic

review and meta-analysis. Front Aging Neurosci. 2022;14:977572.
13. Öztürk D, Karaduman AA, Akbayrak T. Lower urinary tract symptoms in children with Duchenne muscular dystrophy: an evaluation in terms of functional level, posture, and muscle strength. Neurourol Urodyn. 2024;43(8):2130–9.
14. Öztürk D, Karaduman AA, Akbayrak T. The relationship between lower urinary system symptoms and the level of independence and quality of life in children with Duchenne muscular dystrophy. Pediatr Nephrol. 2024;39(10):3005–12.
15. Yang X, Wang X, Gao Z, Li L, Lin H, Wang H, et al. The anatomical pathogenesis of stress urinary incontinence in women. Medicina (Kaunas). 2022;59(1):5.
16. van den Heijkant M, Bogaert G. Lower urinary tract terminology in daytime lower urinary tract symptoms in children: a view of the pediatric urologist. Eur Urol Focus. 2017;3(2–3):189–97.
17. Chang SJ, Van Laecke E, Bauer SB, von Gontard A, Bagli D, Bower WF, et al. Treatment of daytime urinary incontinence: a standardization document from the International Children's Continence Society. Neurourol Urodyn. 2017;36(1):43–50.
18. Santos JD, Lopes RI, Koyle MA. Bladder and bowel dysfunction in children: an update on the diagnosis and treatment of a common, but underdiagnosed pediatric problem. Can Urol Assoc J. 2017;11(1–2Suppl1):S64–72.
19. D'Ancona C, Haylen B, Oelke M, Abranches-Monteiro L, Arnold E, Goldman H, et al. The International Continence Society (ICS) report on the terminology for adult male lower urinary tract and pelvic floor symptoms and dysfunction. Neurourol Urodyn. 2019;38(2):433–77.
20. Drake MJ. Fundamentals of terminology in lower urinary tract function. Neurourol Urodyn. 2018;37(S6):S13–S9.
21. Panicker JN. Neurogenic bladder: epidemiology, diagnosis, and management. Semin Neurol. 2020;40(5):569–79.
22. Ersöz M. Pediyatrik medulla spinalis yaralanmalarında nörojen mesane ve nörojen barsak. Turk J Phys Med Rehab. 2008;54(Suppl 2):75–80.
23. Gierup J. Micturition studies in infants and children. Intravesical pressure, urinary flow and urethral resistance in boys without infravesical obstruction. Scand J Urol Nephrol. 1970;4(3):217–30.
24. Chung E, Katz DJ, Love C. Adult male stress and urge urinary incontinence—a review of pathophysiology and treatment strategies for voiding dysfunction in men. Aust Fam Physician. 2017;46(9):661–6.
25. Mahoney C, Smith A, Marshall A, Reid F. Pelvic floor dysfunction and sensory impairment: current evidence. Neurourol Urodyn. 2017;36(3):550–6.
26. Peinado-Molina RA, Hernández-Martínez A, Martínez-Vázquez S, Rodríguez-Almagro J, Martínez-Galiano JM. Pelvic floor dysfunction: prevalence and associated factors. BMC Public Health. 2023;23(1):2005.
27. Nambiar AK, Arlandis S, Bø K, Cobussen-Boekhorst H, Costantini E, de Heide M, et al. European association of urology guidelines on the diagnosis and management of female non-neurogenic lower urinary tract symptoms. Part 1: diagnostics, overactive bladder, stress urinary incontinence, and mixed urinary incontinence. Eur Urol. 2022;82(1):49–59.
28. Maeda K, Yamana T, Takao Y, Mimura T, Katsuno H, Seki M, et al. Japanese practice guidelines for fecal incontinence part 1-definition, epidemiology, etiology, pathophysiology and causes, risk factors, clinical evaluations, and symptomatic scores and qol questionnaire for clinical evaluations-English version. J Anus Rectum Colon. 2021;5(1):52–66.
29. Everaert K, Hervé F, Bosch R, Dmochowski R, Drake M, Hashim H, et al. International Continence Society consensus on the diagnosis and treatment of nocturia. Neurourol Urodyn. 2019;38(2):478–98.
30. Louis-Charles K, Biggie K, Wolfinbarger A, Wilcox B, Kienstra CM. Pelvic floor dysfunction in the female athlete. Curr Sports Med Rep. 2019;18(2):49–52.
31. Haylen BT, de Ridder D, Freeman RM, Swift SE, Berghmans B, Lee J, et al. An International Urogynecological Association (IUGA)/International Continence Society (ICS) joint report on the terminology for female pelvic floor dysfunction. Int Urogynecol J. 2010;21(1):5–26.
32. Wallace SL, Miller LD, Mishra K. Pelvic floor physical therapy in the treatment of pelvic floor dysfunction in women. Curr Opin Obstet Gynecol. 2019;31(6):485–93.
33. Kocjancic E, Chung E, Garzon JA, Haylen B, Iacovelli V, Jaunarena J, et al. International Continence Society (ICS) report on the terminology for sexual health in men with lower urinary tract (LUT) and pelvic floor (PF) dysfunction. Neurourol Urodyn. 2022;41(1):140–65.
34. Rodrigues MP, Paiva LL, Ramos JGL, Ferla L. Vibratory perineal stimulation for the treatment of female stress urinary incontinence: a systematic review. Int Urogynecol J. 2018;29(4):555–62.
35. Bo K, Frawley HC, Haylen BT, Abramov Y, Almeida FG, Berghmans B, et al. An International Urogynecological Association (IUGA)/International Continence Society (ICS) joint report on the terminology for the conservative and nonpharmacological management of female pelvic floor dysfunction. Int Urogynecol J. 2017;28(2):191–213.
36. Volløyhaug I, Mørkved S, Salvesen Ø, Salvesen K. Assessment of pelvic floor muscle contraction with palpation, perineometry and transperineal ultrasound: a cross-sectional study. Ultrasound Obstet Gynecol. 2016;47(6):768–73.
37. Faubion SS, Shuster LT, Bharucha AE. Recognition and management of nonrelaxing pelvic floor dysfunction. Mayo Clin Proc. 2012;87(2):187–93.
38. Milios JE, Ackland TR, Green DJ. Pelvic floor muscle training in radical prostatectomy: a randomized controlled trial of the impacts on pelvic floor mus-

cle function and urinary incontinence. BMC Urol. 2019;19(1):116.
39. Meyer I, Szychowski JM, Illston JD, Parden AM, Richter HE. Vaginal swab test compared with the urethral Q-tip test for urethral mobility measurement: a randomized controlled trial. Obstet Gynecol. 2016;127(2):348–52.
40. Robinson BL, Geller EJ, Parnell BA, Crane AK, Jannelli ML, Wells EC, et al. Diagnostic accuracy of visual urethral mobility exam versus Q-Tip test: a randomized crossover trial. Am J Obstet Gynecol. 2012;206(6):528.e1-6.
41. Amarenco G, Sheikh Ismaël S, Chesnel C, Charlanes A, Frederique LEB. Diagnosis and clinical evaluation of neurogenic bladder. Eur J Phys Rehabil Med. 2017;53(6):975–80.
42. McKibben MJ, Seed P, Ross SS, Borawski KM. Urinary tract infection and neurogenic bladder. Urol Clin North Am. 2015;42(4):527–36.
43. Burgers RE, Mugie SM, Chase J, Cooper CS, von Gontard A, Rittig CS, et al. Management of functional constipation in children with lower urinary tract symptoms: report from the Standardization Committee of the International Children's Continence Society. J Urol. 2013;190(1):29–36.
44. Ballstaedt L, Leslie SW, Woodbury B. Bladder post void residual volume. StatPearls. Treasure Island: StatPearls Publishing LLC; 2024.
45. Milsom I, Gyhagen M. The prevalence of urinary incontinence. Climacteric. 2019;22(3):217–22.
46. Ginsberg DA, Boone TB, Cameron AP, Gousse A, Kaufman MR, Keays E, et al. The AUA/SUFU guideline on adult neurogenic lower urinary tract dysfunction: treatment and follow-up. Urol J. 2021;206(5):1106–13.
47. Kakizaki H, Kita M, Watanabe M, Wada N. Pathophysiological and therapeutic considerations for non-neurogenic lower urinary tract dysfunction in children. LUTS. 2016;8(2):75–85.
48. Assis GM, Silva C, Martins G. Urotherapy in the treatment of children and adolescents with bladder and bowel dysfunction: a systematic review. J Pediatr. 2019;95(6):628–41.
49. Nieuwhof-Leppink AJ, Hussong J, Chase J, Larsson J, Renson C, Hoebeke P, et al. Definitions, indications and practice of urotherapy in children and adolescents: a standardization document of the International Children's Continence Society (ICCS). J Pediatr Urol. 2021;17(2):172–81.
50. Braga LH, Rickard M, Farrokhyar F, Jegatheeswaran K, Brownrigg N, Li C, et al. Bladder training video versus standard urotherapy for bladder and bowel dysfunction: a noninferiority randomized, controlled trial. Urol J. 2017;197(3):877–84.
51. Alouini S, Memic S, Couillandre A. Pelvic floor muscle training for urinary incontinence with or without biofeedback or electrostimulation in women: a systematic review. Int J Environ Res Public Health. 2022;19(5):2789.
52. Sheng Y, Carpenter JS, Ashton-Miller JA, Miller JM. Mechanisms of pelvic floor muscle training for managing urinary incontinence in women: a scoping review. BMC Womens Health. 2022;22(1):161.
53. Carvalho AAA, de Oliveira Rocha AC, da Silva Viana JK, Dias SFL. Assessment of the pelvic floor in young women in the presence and absence of verbal instruction from a physical therapist. Man Ther Posturol Rehabil J. 2024;22:1328.
54. Díaz-Álvarez L, Lorenzo-Gallego L, Romay-Barrero H, Prieto-Gómez V, Torres-Lacomba M, Navarro-Brazález B. Does the contractile capability of pelvic floor muscles improve with knowledge acquisition and verbal instructions in healthy women? A systematic review. Int J Environ Res Public Health. 2022;19(15):9308.
55. Berghmans B, Seleme M. The '5 F's concept for pelvic floor muscle training: from finding the pelvic floor to functional use. J Womens Health Dev. 2020;3(2):131–4.
56. García-Sánchez E, Ávila-Gandía V, López-Román J, Martínez-Rodríguez A, Rubio-Arias JÁ. What pelvic floor muscle training load is optimal in minimizing urine loss in women with stress urinary incontinence? A systematic review and meta-analysis. Int J Environ Res Public Health. 2019;16(22):4358.
57. Schütze S, Heinloth M, Uhde M, Schütze J, Hüner B, Janni W, et al. The effect of pelvic floor muscle training on pelvic floor function and sexuality postpartum. A randomized study including 300 primiparous. Arch Gynecol Obstet. 2022;306(3):785–93.
58. Altunkol A, Abat D, Sener NC, Gulum M, Ciftci H, Savas M, et al. Is urotherapy alone as effective as a combination of urotherapy and biofeedback in children with dysfunctional voiding? Int Braz J Urol. 2018;44(5):987–95.
59. Lasak AM, Jean-Michel M, Le PU, Durgam R, Harroche J. The role of pelvic floor muscle training in the conservative and surgical management of female stress urinary incontinence: does the strength of the pelvic floor muscles matter? PM&R. 2018;10(11):1198–210.
60. Harvey MA. Pelvic floor exercises during and after pregnancy: a systematic review of their role in preventing pelvic floor dysfunction. J Obstet Gynaecol Can. 2003;25(6):487–98.
61. Tremback-Ball A, Gherghel E, Hegge A, Kindig K, Marsico H, Scanlon R. The effectiveness of biofeedback therapy in managing Bladder Bowel Dysfunction in children: a systematic review. JPRM. 2018;11(3):161–73.
62. Nunes EFC, Sampaio LMM, Biasotto-Gonzalez DA, Nagano R, Lucareli PRG, Politti F. Biofeedback for pelvic floor muscle training in women with stress urinary incontinence: a systematic review with meta-analysis. Physiotherapy. 2019;105(1):10–23.
63. Lukanović D, Kunič T, Batkoska M, Matjašič M, Barbič M. Effectiveness of magnetic stimulation in the treatment of urinary incontinence: a system-

atic review and results of our study. J Clin Med. 2021;10(21):5210.
64. Moroni RM, Magnani PS, Haddad JM, Castro RA, Brito LGO. Conservative treatment of stress urinary incontinence: a systematic review with meta-analysis of randomized controlled trials. Rev Bras Ginecol Obstet. 2016;38:97–111.
65. Fuentes M, Magalhães J, Barroso U Jr. Diagnosis and management of bladder dysfunction in neurologically normal children. Front Pediatr. 2019;7:298.
66. Hu JS, Pierre EF. Urinary incontinence in women: evaluation and management. Am Fam Physician. 2019;100(6):339–48.
67. Abrams P, Cardozo L, Fall M, Griffiths D, Rosier P, Ulmsten U, et al. The standardization of terminology of lower urinary tract function: report from the standardization sub-committee of International Continence Society. In: Textbook of female urology and urogynecology. CRC Press; 2010. p. 1098–108.
68. Zollars JA, Armstrong M, Whisler S, Williamson S. Visceral and neural manipulation in children with cerebral palsy and chronic constipation: five case reports. Explore (NY). 2019;15(1):47–54.
69. Blanco Díaz M, Bousoño García C, Segura Ramírez DK, Rodríguez Rodriguez ÁM. Manual physical therapy in the treatment of functional constipation in children: a pilot randomized controlled trial. J Altern Complement Med. 2020;26(7):620–7.
70. Deodato M, Grosso G, Drago A, Martini M, Dudine E, Murena L, et al. Efficacy of manual therapy and pelvic floor exercises for pain reduction in primary dysmenorrhea: a prospective observational study. J Bodyw Mov Ther. 2023;36:185–91.
71. Trahan J, Leger E, Allen M, Koebele R, Yoffe MB, Simon C, et al. The efficacy of manual therapy for treatment of dyspareunia in females: a systematic review. JWPHPT. 2019;43(1):28–35.
72. Zivkovic VD, Stankovic I, Dimitrijevic L, Kocic M, Colovic H, Vlajkovic M, et al. Are interferential electrical stimulation and diaphragmatic breathing exercises beneficial in children with bladder and bowel dysfunction? Urology. 2017;102:207–12.
73. Korkmaz Dayican D, Keser I, Celiker Tosun O, Yavuz O, Tosun G, Kurt S, et al. Exercise position to improve synergy between the diaphragm and pelvic floor muscles in women with pelvic floor dysfunction: a cross sectional study. J Manip Physiol Ther. 2024;46:201–11.
74. Yuksel H, Cayir Y, Kosan Z, Tastan K. Effectiveness of breathing exercises during the second stage of labor on labor pain and duration: a randomized controlled trial. J Integr Med. 2017;15(6):456–61.
75. Zivkovic V, Lazovic M, Vlajkovic M, Slavkovic A, Dimitrijevic L, Stankovic I, et al. Diaphragmatic breathing exercises and pelvic floor retraining in children with dysfunctional voiding. Eur J Phys Rehabil Med. 2012;48(3):413–21.
76. Sapsford R. Rehabilitation of pelvic floor muscles utilizing trunk stabilization. Man Ther. 2004;9(1):3–12.
77. Almousa S, Lamprianidou E, Kitsoulis G. The effectiveness of stabilising exercises in pelvic girdle pain during pregnancy and after delivery: a systematic review. Physiother Res Int. 2018;23(1):e1699.
78. Ladi Seyedian SS, Sharifi-Rad L, Ebadi M, Kajbafzadeh AM. Combined functional pelvic floor muscle exercises with Swiss ball and urotherapy for management of dysfunctional voiding in children: a randomized clinical trial. Eur J Pediatr. 2014;173(10):1347–53.
79. Ghaderi F, Mohammadi K, Amir Sasan R, Niko Kheslat S, Oskouei AE. Effects of stabilization exercises focusing on pelvic floor muscles on low back pain and urinary incontinence in women. Urology. 2016;93:50–4.
80. Lee JK. Neurogenic bladder management. Radiol Technol. 2021;92(3):281–95.
81. Hogue LL, Kennelly M. The ideal neurogenic bladder management team. Urol Clin North Am. 2024;51(2):297–303.
82. Yücel S. Çocuklarda nörojen mesaneye genel yaklaşım. Turk J Urol. 2010;36:160–6.
83. Erden E, Ersöz M, Erden E, Tiftik T. Urodynamic findings and therapeutic approaches for neurogenic lower urinary tract dysfunction in patients with thoracic spinal cord injury. Ir J Med Sci. 2023;192(5):2513–20.
84. Taweel WA, Seyam R. Neurogenic bladder in spinal cord injury patients. Res Rep Urol. 2015;7:85–99.
85. Riaz H, Nadeem H, Rathore FA. Recent advances in the pelvic floor assessment and rehabilitation of women with pelvic floor dysfunction. J Pak Med Assoc. 2022;72(7):1456–9.
86. Andretta E, Pagliacci MC, Zuliani C, Filocamo MT, Losavio E, Krassioukov A. A survey of clinical practice concerning long-term follow-up of neurogenic lower urinary tract dysfunction due to spinal cord injury in Italy. J Spinal Cord Med. 2022;45(6):907–15.
87. Birkhäuser V, Anderson CE, Kozomara M, Bywater M, Gross O, Kiss S, et al. Urodynamics are essential to predict the risk for upper urinary tract damage after acute spinal cord injury. Biomedicine. 2023;11(6):1748.
88. Kozomara M, Birkhäuser V, Anderson CE, Bywater M, Gross O, Kiss S, et al. Neurogenic lower urinary tract dysfunction in the first year after spinal cord injury: a descriptive study of urodynamic findings. Urol J. 2023;209(1):225–32.
89. Doumouchtsis SK, de Tayrac R, Lee J, Daly O, Melendez-Munoz J, Lindo FM, et al. An International Continence Society (ICS)/ International Urogynecological Association (IUGA) joint report on the terminology for the assessment and management of obstetric pelvic floor disorders. Int Urogynecol J. 2023;34(1):1–42.
90. Sripathi V, Mitra A. Management of neurogenic bladder. Indian J Pediatr. 2017;84(7):545–54.
91. DeWitt-Foy ME, Elliott SP. Neurogenic bladder: Assessment and operative management. Urol Clin North Am. 2022;49(3):519–32.

92. Kurpad R, Kennelly MJ. The evaluation and management of refractory neurogenic overactive bladder. Curr Urol Rep. 2014;15:1–7.
93. Kaya S, Akbayrak T, Gursen C, Beksac S. Short-term effect of adding pelvic floor muscle training to bladder training for female urinary incontinence: a randomized controlled trial. IUJ. 2015;26:285–93.
94. Dorsher PT, McIntosh PM. Neurogenic bladder. Adv Urol. 2012;2012(1):816274.
95. Erden E, Ersöz M, Tiftik T, Erden E. The neurogenic bladder characteristics and treatment approaches in the patients with multiple sclerosis. Mult Scler Relat Disord. 2022;58:103439.
96. Andrews AW, Thomas MW, Bohannon RW. Normative values for isometric muscle force measurements obtained with hand-held dynamometers. Phys Ther. 1996;76(3):248–59.
97. Corcos J, Ginsberg DD, Karsenty G. Textbook of the neurogenic bladder. Boca Raton: CRC Press; 2015.
98. Stöhrer M, Blok B, Castro-Diaz D, Chartier-Kastler E, Del Popolo G, Kramer G, et al. EAU guidelines on neurogenic lower urinary tract dysfunction. Eur Urol. 2009;56(1):81–8.
99. Jamison J, Maguire S, McCann J. Catheter policies for management of long term voiding problems in adults with neurogenic bladder disorders. Cochrane Database Syst Rev. 2013;2013(11):CD004375.

15 Physiotherapy and Rehabilitation in Pelvic Organ Prolapse

Zehra Korkut and Seyda Toprak Celenay

15.1 Introduction

Pelvic organ prolapse (POP) is a major problem for patients and the healthcare system that affects millions of women worldwide. POP, which can be asymptomatic and symptomatic, is observed in almost half of women who have given birth [34]. In addition, the incidence of its symptoms increases with age, and it has been reported that the risk rate of POP increases by 10% with each new age [16]. Although the pathophysiology of POP is multifactorial, the primary factor is the weakness of the pelvic floor muscles (PFM) and associated connective tissues, which play a crucial role in maintaining normal pelvic organ support [42, 68]. It represents a nonthreatening disorder that leads to bladder, bowel, and sexual dysfunctions; thus, POP negatively affects the physical, social, and psychological conditions of the individual. The diagnosis of POP is based on a combination of the patient-reported symptoms and details of the clinical evaluations [3]. A multidisciplinary approach is important in the treatment of POP. POP treatment options are generally classified as conservative and surgical approaches [15]. Physiotherapy and rehabilitation approaches, which are among the conservative treatments, are recommended to be used in mild and moderate POP cases [34]. Within the scope of physiotherapy and rehabilitation approaches, different treatment methods such as pelvic floor muscle training (PFMT), electrical stimulation (ES), biofeedback, different exercise approaches, and kinesio taping can be applied [41].

15.2 Pelvic Organ Prolapse

POP is defined in the report of the International Urogynecological Association (IUGA)/International Continence Society (ICS) on the terminology of female POP as the descent and anatomical change of one or more of the anterior vaginal wall, posterior vaginal wall, uterus (cervix), or vaginal apex (vaginal vault or vaginal cuff after hysterectomy) downward from the vagina (Fig. 15.1) [41]. *Anterior vaginal wall (compartment) prolapse* is the descent of the anterior vaginal compartment from the vagina due to weakness of the anterior vaginal wall and ligaments. The descent of the bladder down the anterior vaginal wall is called cystocele, and the descent of the urethra down the vagina is called urethrocele [41]. *Posterior vaginal wall (compartment) prolapse* is the descent

Z. Korkut (✉)
Department of Physiotherapy and Rehabilitation, Faculty of Health Sciences, Selcuk University, Konya, Türkiye
e-mail: zehra.korkut@selcuk.edu.tr

S. Toprak Celenay
Department of Physiotherapy and Rehabilitation, Faculty of Health Sciences, Ankara Yildirim Beyazit University, Ankara, Türkiye

T. Akbayrak, E. Üzelpasaci (eds.), *Physiotherapy and Rehabilitation in Pelvic and Women's Health-Related Problems*, https://doi.org/10.1007/978-3-032-28741-0_15

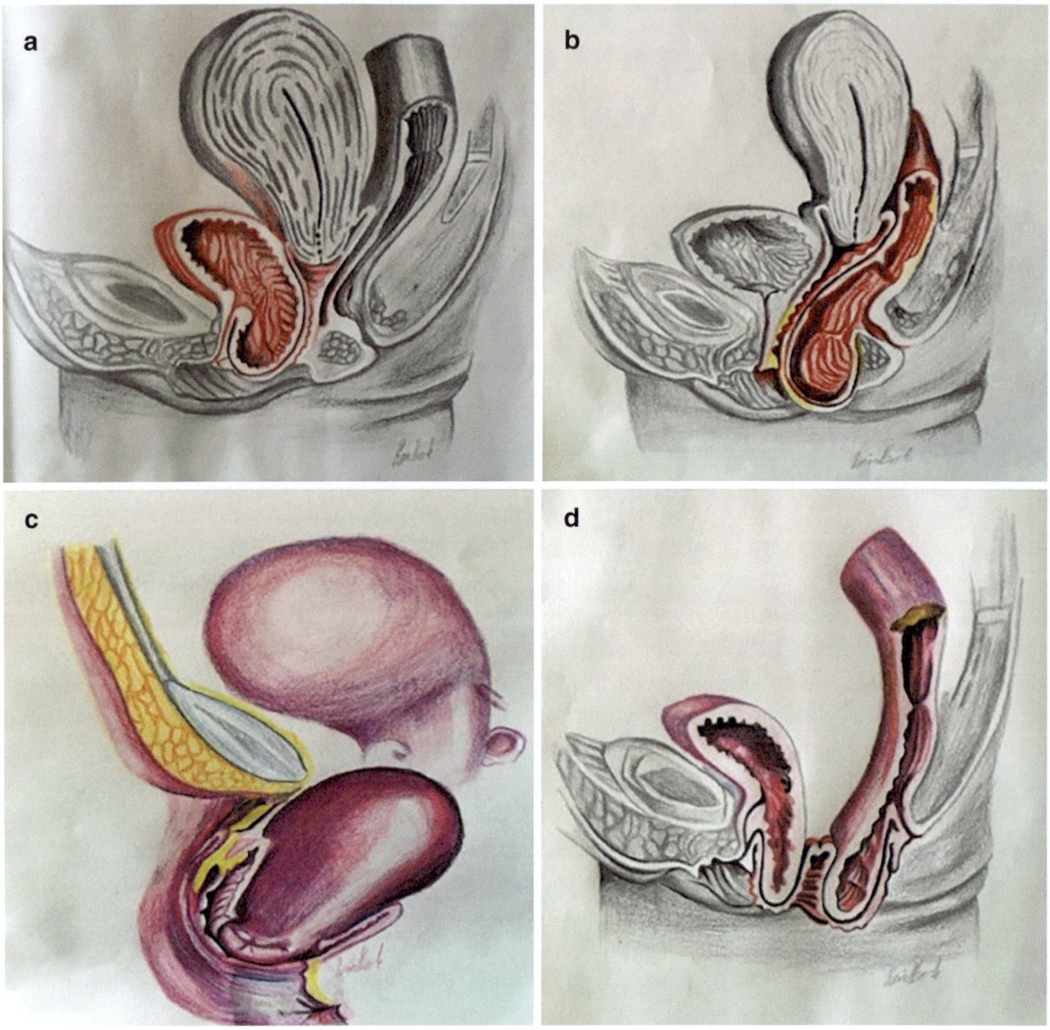

Fig. 15.1 Types of POP. (**a**) Cystocele, (**b**) rectocele, (**c**) uterine prolapse, (**d**) vaginal cuff prolapse

of the posterior vaginal compartment downward from the vagina. Rectocele, a bulge in the posterior vaginal wall related to herniation of the anterior wall of the rectum, is often seen. Enterocele, which is the displacement of the vaginal cuff and the small intestine and peritoneum into the vagina, often accompanies advanced posterior vaginal wall prolapse after hysterectomy [65]. *Uterine/cervical prolapse* is defined as the descent of the uterus or uterine cervix downward from the vagina due to apical weakness of the cardinal or uterosacral ligament [65]. *Vaginal cuff prolapse* is the downward descent of the vaginal vault (after hysterectomy) [65].

Women with symptomatic POP may experience pelvic, bladder, bowel, and sexual symptoms associated with pelvic floor dysfunctions (PFD) (Table 15.1). The most prominent symptom of POP is seeing or feeling a bulge at the opening of the vagina [50]. It has been reported that there is a strong association between POP and lower urinary tract symptoms (LUTS) [50]. LUTS are commonly seen in patients with POP, especially obstructive voiding, which is one of the most common symptoms associated with POP [39]. Studies have reported that overactive bladder

Table 15.1 Common symptoms in pelvic organ prolapse (POP) [34, 41]

Pelvic symptoms	*Bladder symptoms*
Feeling of pressure/heaviness in the vagina Feeling/seeing a bulge in/coming out of vagina Vaginal/perineal pain Vaginal dryness Vaginal bleeding Feeling of heaviness in lower abdomen/pelvis Lumbopelvic pain	Urinary incontinence Sensation of urinary urgency Increased urinary frequency Delay in initiating micturition Urinary slow stream Intermittency of urine flow/straining to void Feeling of incomplete bladder emptying Manual fixation of the prolapse for urination
Bowel symptoms	*Sexual symptoms*
Fecal and/or flatal incontinence Constipation Inability to delay defecation Feeling of incomplete bowel emptying Manual fixation of the prolapse for defecation Difficulty in defecation Rectal protrusion during or after defecation	Dyspareunia Obstructed intercourse Orgasm disorder Dissatisfaction with the coitus Urinary incontinence during coitus Vaginal laxity

(OAB) symptoms were observed as a result of bladder outlet obstruction caused by POP [24]. In a study conducted in 237 women with POP, it was reported that 73% of women had urinary incontinence (UI), 86% had urinary urgency and urinary frequency, 34–62% had voiding dysfunction, and 31% had fecal incontinence [30].

15.2.1 Prevalence and Risk Factors

Studies examining the prevalence of POP have reported prevalence rates ranging up to 50% [69]. In the literature, it has been reported that the prevalence of POP is observed at different rates according to the symptomatic and asymptomatic course of the disease. While the prevalence of POP determined during gynecological examination reaches up to 50%, the rate determined according to the symptoms reported by the patient remains in the range of 3–6% [7, 54]. This difference in prevalence rates may be explained by the asymptomatic course of POP in some women. It has been observed that older women are more likely to experience symptoms of POP [72]. According to a recent narrative review, it was reported that POP prevalence rates range between 1% and 65% according to geographical regions, with the highest rates observed in the United States [17]. A study in the United States reported that the number of women suffering from symptomatic POP will increase to 46% in 2050 [71].

Several risk factors associated with POP have been identified. Advanced age increases the risk of developing POP by 10% each year. Vaginal delivery, especially the first delivery, has been reported to be a strong risk factor for POP [27]. Other risk factors identified for POP include pregnancy, genetics, connective tissue problems, menopause, obesity, and hysterectomy [69]. According to the results of a recent meta-analysis study investigating risk factors related to POP, body mass index (BMI) > 30 kg/m^2, large waist circumference, dyslipidemia, hypertension, constipation, persistent cough, and varicose veins were reported to be determinant risk factors for POP [31].

15.2.2 Pathophysiology

The pathophysiology of POP is complex and multifactorial, involving various mechanisms that contribute to the weakening of pelvic support structures, including muscle, ligament, and fascia. Normal pelvic organ support is provided by the PFM and connective tissue connections (endopelvic fascia, ligaments). Damage or weakening of these muscles, due to various reasons such as neuropathic and/or mechanical muscular damage, causes the endopelvic fascia and ligaments to be under long-term and excessive stress and lose their normal anatomical structure by stretching, thinning, and tearing over time. This loss is accompanied by alterations in the vectorial forces acting on the organs, which ultimately can lead to the development of POP [4, 69].

Two major theories have been proposed to explain the pathophysiology of POP. According to the Integral Theory by Petros, the relationship between the pelvic floor muscles (PFMs), fascia, and supportive ligaments is crucial. Weakening, damage, or laxity of any of these structures can lead to POP in the anterior, middle, or posterior compartments [59]. In recent years, scientists have started to investigate collagen tissue in women with POP, with the knowledge that the main component of pelvic floor fascia and ligaments is collagen. In patients with POP, there have been findings of different metabolic issues related to collagen types I, III, and V. In the literature, it was reported that there was an increased incidence of collagen tissue problems, such as varicose veins and joint hypermobility, in women with POP [23]. In addition, a decrease in the amount of total collagen and an increase in the amount of collagen-degrading proteinases were found in the pelvic floor tissues of women with POP [23].

The other prominent theory in the pathophysiology of POP was proposed by DeLancey. According to this theory, pelvic organ support is provided at three critical levels. At *level I,* weakening of the cardinal and uterosacral ligaments leads to apical prolapse, such as uterine or vaginal vault prolapse, and enterocele. At *level II,* loss of paravaginal support can result in cystocele or rectocele. Finally, *level III* consists of the fibromuscular connective tissue and muscles surrounding the perineum and distal vagina. Damage at this level may lead to anterior and posterior vaginal wall prolapse and perineal body defects [25]. The levator ani muscle integrity has a critical role in maintaining pelvic organ support [26]. Levator muscle damage has been reported in approximately half of women with prolapse. In a study by Dietz et al., it was found that levator ani muscle strength decreased in women with POP in the 6th month postpartum compared to antepartum, and also muscle strength decreased significantly compared to women without POP [28]. According to the results of various studies conducted in women with POP in recent years, it has been found that the length, thickness, strength, and stiffness of the PFM decreased and the genital hiatus area enlarged [38, 55, 66].

15.3 Assessment

15.3.1 History

A comprehensive medical history taken from patients with POP provides valuable insights into the etiology of POP as well as associated pathological conditions. Obstetric history should include gravidity, parity, type of delivery, episiotomy, and use of forceps, and gynecologic history should include menstrual cycle, presence of menopause, hormone replacement therapy, and surgical history. In addition, medical history (presence of cancer, constipation, chronic cough, neurological disease, etc.), medications, previous treatments, and habits (smoking, alcohol, and exercise habits) should be recorded. It is important to conduct a comprehensive evaluation of the discomfort levels and symptoms related to the vagina, bladder, bowel, and sexual function in patients with POP. According to current clinical guidelines, the use of validated pelvic floor symptom scales is recommended as a crucial tool for accurate assessment and treatment planning (NICE [53]). Some of these scales are the Pelvic Floor Distress Inventory, Pelvic Floor Distress Inventory-20 (PFDI-20), Global Pelvic Floor Discomfort Scale (GPFDS), and Pelvic Organ Prolapse Symptom Score (POP-SS) [6, 8, 35]. The presence of pain accompanying POP should also be questioned. Therefore, pain localization, intensity, duration, type, and factors that increase and decrease pain can be recorded.

15.3.2 Physical Assessment

Observations of any abdominal masses or bulges, bladder retention or fullness, and the existence of incisions or scars should be recorded [40].

Electromyography (EMG), stabilizer pressure biofeedback units, and core stability tests can also be used for abdominal muscle function [57, 58, 64]. A comprehensive pelvic examination should also focus on external genitalia observation (lesions, rash, etc.), anatomy of the pelvic organs, the presence and severity of POP, and PFM functions.

The Pelvic Organ Prolapse-Quantification (POP-Q) system, a gold standard method officially accepted by the American College of Obstetricians and Gynecologists (ACOG), is used in the evaluation of POP [18]. Before the evaluation, the patient is asked to empty the urine and lie down in the lithotomy position. At this stage, the patient is asked to strain or cough with maximum force. Six points are measured on the anterior (Aa, Ba), posterior (Ap, Bp), and upper parts of the vagina (C, D) using a speculum and ruler according to the hymen reference points. In addition, the genital hiatus, perineal body, and vaginal length are assessed. The proximal part of the hymen is recorded in centimeters with negative values and the distal part with positive values. Genital hiatus (gh) is the length between the external urethral meatus and the posterior remnant of the hymen (Fig. 15.2) [18]. Perineal body (pb) is the length between the posterior aspect of the hymen and the middle of the anal opening. Total vaginal length (TVL) is the vaginal length between the posterior fornix and the hymen. The measurements are recorded, and the POP type and stages are determined. Prolapse stage is graded from stage 0 (no prolapse) to stage 4 (complete eversion of the lower genital tract) (Table 15.2).

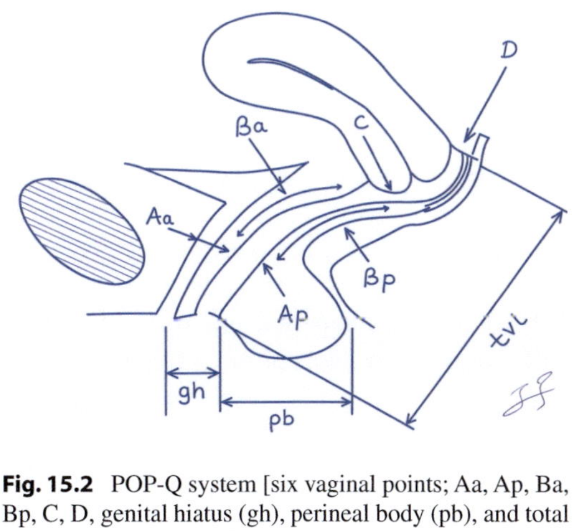

Fig. 15.2 POP-Q system [six vaginal points; Aa, Ap, Ba, Bp, C, D, genital hiatus (gh), perineal body (pb), and total vaginal length (tvl)] [18]

Although the POP-Q system is accepted as the gold standard for evaluation, it is less frequently used in the clinic due to its time-consuming nature. Therefore, the system was modified over time, and the simplified POP-Q system was developed. In this system, four points (C, D, Ba, and Bp) are measured by taking the reference point as hymen, so it takes less time to apply in the clinic [56].

15.3.3 Pelvic Floor Muscle Function Assessment

The assessment of PFMs involves techniques such as observation, digital palpation, dynamometry, myotonometry, manometry, electromyography, and various imaging methods. During observational evaluation of the perineum at rest, the presence of scars, lesions, trophic changes/atrophy, discoloration, erythema, etc. that may affect PFM function is noted. Moreover, the length of the perineum, position of the perineum at rest, introital, and anal openings should be evaluated. Movement of the perineum (perineal ascent, absence of perineal movement, perineal descent) should be observed during different intra-abdominal pressure increases (e.g., Valsalva maneuver, straining, coughing) [32, 41]. In the resting state, vaginal and rectal digital palpation can provide information about scar tissue, sensation, tone, tenderness, the presence of tender

Table 15.2 Pelvic organ prolapse (POP) staging

Stage	Description
0	No prolapse
I	The most distal part of the prolapse is more than 1 cm above the hymen
II	The most distal part of the prolapse is between 1 cm above and 1 cm below the hymen
III	The most distal part of the prolapse protrudes more than 1 cm below the hymen
IV	Complete eversion of the lower genital tract

points, the elasticity of the vaginal opening, levator muscle injury, and the integrity of the anal sphincter. In addition, PFM contraction can be examined by palpation of the superficial perineal muscles [15, 32]. PFM strength can be assessed using digital muscle tests. The modified Oxford grading scale is frequently used in the assessment of PFM strength [11]. PFM endurance (duration or number of contractions) and number of rapid contractions (usually the maximum number of rapid contractions in 10 s) are also recorded. PFM coordination (present or absent) and co-contractions (synergistic or counterproductive to normal function) can be evaluated [15].

Dynamometers are devices that measure muscle strength during PFM contraction. Researchers have developed specialized intravaginal dynamometers to evaluate PFM function in women. These devices measure the resting and contractile strength of the PFM with strain gauges attached to a speculum inserted into the vagina [32]. Manometers have been developed in intravaginal, intraanal, and intraurethral formats. The perineometer, a type of manometer, can be used to measure PFM strength and endurance [14] (Fig. 15.3).

Electromyography is the recording of electrical potentials generated by depolarization of muscle fiber membranes. These recordings allow symmetrical assessment of the activation pattern/behavior of a particular muscle during a defined activity [32, 61]. Ultrasound is one of the imaging methods that provides detailed information about PFM morphology and mechanical properties (thickness, cross-sectional area, stiffness, etc.), anatomical location, genital hiatus, and PFM displacement due to contraction/relaxation [32]. Magnetic resonance imaging (MRI) provides direct information about the damage and morphology of PFMs and the position of the involved organs and PFMs [40].

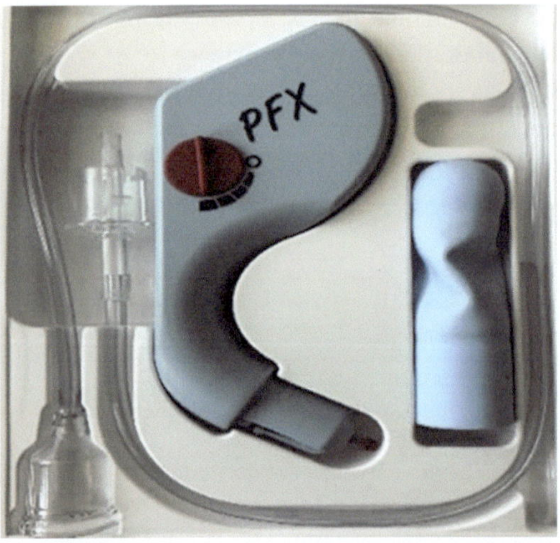

Fig. 15.3 Perineometer device. (Cardio Design Pty Ltd., Australia)

15.3.4 Neurological Assessment

It includes sensory, motor, and reflex examinations of the lumbosacral level, which is responsible for the innervation of the pelvic floor, perineum, and pelvic organs. In the presence of neurological disease, pelvic surgery, trauma, or neuropathy that may accompany POP, and before different physiotherapy applications (electrotherapy, heat modalities, etc.), sensory assessment should be performed. In motor assessment, myotomes, including the nerve roots of the lumbosacral region, are examined. PFM (S2-S4) strength should also be evaluated in detail in terms of motor function. The integrity of the pudendal nerve can be evaluated by the bulbocavernous reflex and anal reflex [46].

15.3.5 Posture Assessment

The pelvic floor can be adversely affected by changes in posture in the spine and pelvic plane due to several factors such as obesity, aging, osteoporosis, and menopause. In addition, the connections between the pelvic floor and other body parts (muscles, fascia, ligaments, etc.) are very important in maintaining the correct posture [62]. It has been reported that a healthy spine with normal curvatures allows optimal contraction of the PFMs and protects the pelvic floor from the negative effects of intra-abdominal pressure [9]. It has been reported that women with POP have less lumbar lordosis and increased thoracic kyphosis compared to women without POP

[47, 52]. A detailed posture analysis, especially focusing on the spine and pelvis, will help determine the treatment protocol to be followed. Some techniques that can be used in posture analysis are observation, posture mirrors, inclinometers, goniometry, mobile applications, and computer-based analysis systems [70].

15.3.6 Hypermobility Assessment

In the literature, it is reported that the prevalence of joint hypermobility increases in women with POP, and the relationship between hypermobility and POP may be clinically significant [67]. Beighton or Brighton diagnostic criteria are used in the evaluation of hypermobility [33, 37].

15.3.7 Sexual Function Assessment

POP negatively affects sexual function. Medical and psychosocial history in POP patients with active sexual lives should be questioned in detail to understand the sexual function cycle and to define where the problem is in the cycle, and it is important for the partner to participate in the evaluation. In the joint report of the IUGA and ICS on the assessment of sexual health in POP, general and PFD-specific sexual function scales (Female Sexual Function Index, Pelvic Organ Prolapse/Urinary Incontinence Sexual Questionnaire, etc.) were determined according to the level of evidence, and their use was recommended [63]. In addition, a detailed pelvic evaluation and pain assessment should be performed.

15.3.8 Quality of Life Assessment

POP affects the individual physically, socially, and psychologically and causes deterioration in quality of life. General or disease-specific quality of life scales (Short Form-36, Prolapse Quality of Life Scale, etc.) can be used to evaluate the impact of POP symptoms on quality of life and to determine the effects of the treatment program.

15.4 Physiotherapy and Rehabilitation

15.4.1 Patient Education and Lifestyle Recommendations

The patient education should include patient-specific information on the anatomy and functions of the pelvic floor, pelvic organs, POP pathophysiology, POP symptoms, risk factors, recommendations, and treatment options [36]. Lifestyle recommendations for POP have an important role in managing the prolapse process and preventing its progression. Lifestyle recommendations include the management of modifiable risk factors such as chronic cough, constipation, and obesity, which may increase the symptoms and severity of POP due to increased intra-abdominal pressure (NICE [53]). Patients should be taught the Knack maneuver during activities such as weight lifting, pushing, pulling, and jumping. Patients should increase physical activity levels and participate in an individually planned regular exercise program to ensure weight control and improve well-being. The International Urogynecology Consultation reported that lifestyle changes (weight loss, constipation treatment, activity restriction, etc.) have a positive impact on the prevention and treatment of POP [43]. In the literature, it has been reported that lifestyle recommendations given to women with POP are more effective in reducing POP symptoms when given in combination with PFMT rather than alone [19, 29].

15.4.2 Pelvic Floor Muscle Training

Pelvic floor muscle training (PFMT) is defined as a treatment method aimed at improving pelvic floor muscle strength, endurance, power, relaxation, or a combination of these parameters [2]. During PFM contraction, the levator hiatus narrows, urethral and anal closure pressure increases, and the pelvic organs are elevated. PFMT is one of the clinically evidence-based physiotherapy techniques that manage and prevent POP [12]. Regular follow-up of PFMT is important in terms of providing optimal exercise training and exercise habits. PFMT can be used alone or in combination with electrical stimulation (ES), biofeedback, and vaginal cone/tampon training. PFMT varies in intensity, frequency, and duration, and there is no standardized treatment protocol. PFMT is known to be effective in the treatment management of POP at the level of evidence 1, grade of recommendation A. A recent guideline for the management of POP suggests supervised PFMT for at least 16 weeks as the first-line treatment option for women with symptomatic stage 1 or 2 POP [53]. The International Urogynecology Consultation published a recent report that PFMT is effective in reducing POP symptoms and/or improving POP stage (by one stage) in women with POP-Q stages I, II, and III [12]. In the same report, it was reported that PFMT is effective in alleviating specific prolapse symptoms such as vaginal bulge by a level of evidence rated at 1 and a grade of recommendation at B [12].

Biofeedback can be used to teach how to contract and relax the PFMs correctly, to increase the patient's motivation to do PFM exercises, and to ensure continuity in the exercise [73]. Biofeedback is not a therapy on its own but supports the existing structure of the therapy. Relaxation training can be provided with biofeedback for increased PFM tone, and awareness-raising and strengthening training can be provided with biofeedback for decreased PFM tone. Electromyographic devices, manometers, intravaginal vibration devices, and real-time ultrasound devices can be used as biofeedback types in pelvic floor rehabilitation [5].

Vaginal cones are small weights that are placed inside the vagina above the level of the levator muscle. Their purpose is to provide sensory biofeedback and to progressively load the PFMs to strengthen them [60]. Vaginal tampons are disposable, cheap, and hygienic and can be used to perform resistant PFMT.

15.4.3 Alternative Exercise Approaches

PFM is known to work synergistically with trunk muscle groups (abdominal, paraspinal, diaphragm, etc.) to stabilize the spine. In addition to PFMT, spinal stabilization exercises can be used to provide dynamic stability of the spine and intra-abdominal pressure balance, to improve trunk muscle and PFM function, and to decrease POP symptoms [1, 10, 22, 44]. And also, hypopressive exercises can be preferred to reduce intra-abdominal pressure, regulate pelvic floor and abdominal wall tone, and reduce muscle stiffness of the antagonists of aponeurotic structures (diaphragm, quadratus lumborum, and hamstring) [21]. In the literature, it was reported that adding hypopressive exercise to PFMT had no additional effect, and PFMT was more effective than hypopressive exercise alone. There was no evidence that other exercises such as hypopressive, yoga, breathing, and hip exercises in an inverted position were more effective than PFMT for POP [13].

15.4.4 Electrical Stimulation

The main purpose of ES in the treatment of POP is to provide awareness of PFM, improve its strength and endurance, and thus increase pelvic organ support. ES applications for POP can be performed with superficial external electrodes (perineal, sacral, etc.) or intravaginal or intraanal probes. ES applications are not used in pregnant women, patients with malignancy and infection, pacemaker users, and patients with sensory impairment [48]. It has been reported that ES may reduce the POP stage in patients [45, 49]. ES applications can be applied alone or as combined treatments.

15.4.5 Mechanical Support

Mechanical support, or a pessary, is a device designed to support the prolapsed organ in women with POP that is placed in the vagina. It is generally used for patients who are contraindicated for surgery or who do not want surgery in order to prevent an increase in the severity of POP and to reduce symptom severity. Complications that may frequently occur from the use of pessaries are vaginal discharge, odor, irritation, dislocation of the pessary, ulceration, pain, and bleeding [51]. To prevent these complications, pessaries should be changed at least every 6 months. Pessaries are produced in many shapes and sizes in accordance with individual needs. The 7th International Consultation on Incontinence recommends the combined use of a vaginal pessary plus PFMT instead of PFMT alone for the treatment of prolapse with a recommendation grade of B [20].

15.5 Conclusion

POP, which negatively affects the quality of life, is a PFD with a high prevalence in society. Treatment should be planned individually for each patient. Conservative treatment and surgical applications are included in the management of POP. Physiotherapy and rehabilitation, as conservative treatment approaches, are very important for reducing and preventing POP symptoms, improving the PFM strength, and enhancing the quality of life.

References

1. Abdel-Aziem AA, Abdelraouf OR, El-Basatiny HMY, Draz AH. The effects of stabilization exercises combined with pelvic floor exercise in women with nonspecific low back pain: a randomized clinical study. J Chiropr Med. 2021;20(4):229–38. https://doi.org/10.1016/j.jcm.2021.12.008.
2. Abrams P, Cardozo L, Fall M, Griffiths D, Rosier P, Ulmsten U, et al. The standardisation of terminology in lower urinary tract function: report from the standardisation sub-committee of the International Continence Society. Urology. 2003;61(1):37–49. https://doi.org/10.1016/s0090-4295(02)02243-4.
3. American College of Obstetricians and Gynecologists and the American Urogynecologic Society. Pelvic organ prolapse. Female Pelvic Med Reconstr Surg. 2019;25(6):397–408. https://doi.org/10.1097/SPV.0000000000000794.
4. Ashton-Miller JA, DeLancey JOL. Functional anatomy of the female pelvic floor. Ann N Y Acad Sci. 2007;1101:266–96. https://doi.org/10.1196/annals.1389.034.
5. Barber MD. Pelvic organ prolpase. In: Bø K, Berghmans B, Morkved S, van Kampen M, editors. Evidence based physical therapy for the pelvic floor: bridging science and clinical practice. 2nd ed. Toronto: Elsevier; 2015. p. 226–7.
6. Barber MD, Kuchibhatla MN, Pieper CF, Bump RC. Psychometric evaluation of 2 comprehensive condition-specific quality of life instruments for women with pelvic floor disorders. Am J Obstet Gynecol. 2001;185(6):1388–95. https://doi.org/10.1067/mob.2001.118659.
7. Barber MD, Maher C. Epidemiology and outcome assessment of pelvic organ prolapse. Int Urogynecol J. 2013;24:1783–90. https://doi.org/10.1007/s00192-013-2169-9.
8. Barber MD, Walters MD, Bump RC. Short forms of two condition-specific quality-of-life questionnaires for women with pelvic floor disorders (PFDI-20 and PFIQ-7). Am J Obstet Gynecol. 2005;193(1):103–13. https://doi.org/10.1016/j.ajog.2004.12.025.
9. Bassani T, Casaroli G, Galbusera F. Dependence of lumbar loads on spinopelvic sagittal alignment: an evaluation based on musculoskeletal modeling. PLoS One. 2019;14:0. https://doi.org/10.1371/journal.pone.0207997.
10. Bayramoğlu Demirdöğen E, Ulcay T, Bağbanci MŞ, Toprak Çelenay Ş. A comparison of pelvic floor muscle exercises and spinal stabilization exercises in women with stress urinary incontinence. Int Urogynecol J. 2024;19 https://doi.org/10.1007/s00192-024-05978-y.
11. Bø K, Sherburn M. Evaluation of female pelvic-floor muscle function and strength. Phys Ther. 2005;85(3):269–82.
12. Bø K, Anglès-Acedo S, Batra A, Brækken IH, Chan YL, Jorge CH, Kruger J, Yadav M, Dumoulin C. International urogynecology consultation chapter 3 committee 2; conservative treatment of patient with pelvic organ prolapse: pelvic floor muscle training. Int Urogynecol J. 2022;33(10):2633–67. https://doi.org/10.1007/s00192-022-05324-0.
13. Bø K, Anglès-Acedo S, Batra A, Brækken IH, Chan YL, Jorge CH, Kruger J, Yadav M, Dumoulin C. Are hypopressive and other exercise programs effective for the treatment of pelvic organ prolapse? Int Urogynecol J. 2023;34(1):43–52. https://doi.org/10.1007/s00192-022-05407-y.
14. Bo K, Frawley HC, Haylen BT, Abramov Y, Almeida FG, Berghmans, et al. An International Urogynecological Association (IUGA)/International Continence Society (ICS) joint report on the terminology for the conservative and nonpharmacological management of female pelvic floor dysfunction. Neurourol Urodyn. 2017;36(2):221–44. https://doi.org/10.1002/nau.23107.
15. Bø K, Frawley HC, Haylen BT, Abramov Y, Almeida FG, Berghmans B, et al. An International

Urogynecological Association (IUGA)/International Continence Society (ICS) joint report on the terminology for the conservative and nonpharmacological management of female pelvic floor dysfunction. Int Urogynecol J. 2017;28(2):191–213. https://doi.org/10.1007/s00192-016-3123-4.
16. Brito LGO, Pereira GMV, Moalli P, Shynlova O, Manonai J, Weintraub AY, Deprest J, Bortolini MAT. Age and/or postmenopausal status as risk factors for pelvic organ prolapse development: systematic review with meta-analysis. Int Urogynecol J. 2022;33(1):15–29. https://doi.org/10.1007/s00192-021-04953-1.
17. Brown HW, Hegde A, Huebner M, et al. International urogynecology consultation chapter 1 committee 2: epidemiology of pelvic organ prolapse: prevalence, incidence, natural history, and service needs. Int Urogynecol J. 2022;33:173–87. https://doi.org/10.1007/s00192-021-05018-z.
18. Bump RC, Mattiasson A, Bø K, Brubaker LP, DeLancey JO, Klarskov P, et al. The standardization of terminology of female pelvic organ prolapse and pelvic floor dysfunction. Am J Obstet Gynecol. 1996;175(1):10–7. https://doi.org/10.1016/s0002-9378(96)70243-0.
19. Caagbay D, Raynes-Greenow C, Dangal G, Mc Geechan K, Black KI. Impact of an informational flipchart on lifestyle advice for Nepali women with a pelvic organ prolapse: a randomized controlled trial. Int Urogynecol J. 2020;31(6):1223–30. https://doi.org/10.1007/s00192-020-04228-1.
20. Cardozo L, Rovner E, Wagg A, Wein A, Abrams P, editors. Incontinence. 7th ed. Bristol: ICI-ICS. International Continence Society; 2023. ISBN: 978-0-9569607-4-0
21. Caufriez M. Gymnastique abdominale hypopressive. Brussels: Ed. Bruxelles; 1997. p. 8–10.
22. Celenay ST, Korkut Z, Bulbul SB, Altay H, Oskay K. Effects of spinal stabilization exercises focusing on the pelvic floor in women with overactive bladder. Int Urogynecol J. 2023;34(12):2959–67. https://doi.org/10.1007/s00192-023-05638-7.
23. Chen B, Yeh J. Alterations in connective tissue metabolism in stress incontinence and prolapse. J Urol. 2011;186:1768–72. https://doi.org/10.1016/j.juro.2011.06.054.
24. De Boer TA, Salvatore S, Cardozo L, Chapple C, Kelleher C, Van Kerrebroeck P, et al. Pelvic organ prolapse and overactive bladder. Neurourol Urodyn. 2010;29(1):30–9. https://doi.org/10.1002/nau.20858.
25. DeLancey JO. Anatomy and biomechanics of genital prolapse. Clin Obstet Gynecol. 1993;36:897–909. https://doi.org/10.1097/00003081-199312000-00015.
26. DeLancey JO, Morgan DM, Fenner DE, Kearney R, Guire K, Miller JM, et al. Comparison of levator ani muscle defects and function in women with and without pelvic organ prolapse. Obstet Gynecol. 2007;109(2):295–302. https://doi.org/10.1097/01.AOG.0000250901.57095.ba.
27. Deprest JA, Cartwright R, Dietz HP, et al. International Urogynecological Consultation (IUC): pathophysiology of pelvic organ prolapse (POP). Int Urogynecol J. 2022;33:1699–710. https://doi.org/10.1007/s00192-022-05081-0.
28. Dietz HP, Simpson JM. Levator trauma is associated with pelvic organ prolapse. BJOG. 2008;115(8):979–84. https://doi.org/10.1111/j.1471-0528.2008.01751.x.
29. Dwyer LKR. Conservative management of pelvic organ prolapse. Obstet Gynaecol Reprod Med. 2020;31(2):35–41.
30. Ellerkmann RM, Cundiff GW, Melick CF, Nihira MA, Leffler K, Bent AE. Correlation of symptoms with location and severity of pelvic organ prolapse. Am J Obstet Gynecol. 2001;185(6):1332–8. https://doi.org/10.1067/mob.2001.119078.
31. Fitz FF, Bortolini MAT, Pereira GMV, Salerno GRF, Castro RA. PEOPLE: lifestyle and comorbidities as risk factors for pelvic organ prolapse-a systematic review and meta-analysis PEOPLE: PElvic Organ Prolapse Lifestyle comorbiditiEs. Int Urogynecol J. 2023;34(9):2007–32. https://doi.org/10.1007/s00192-023-05569-3.
32. Frawley H, Shelly B, Morin M, Bernard S, Bø K, Digesu GA, Dickinson T, Goonewardene S, McClurg D, Rahnama'i MS, Schizas A, Slieker-Ten Hove M, Takahashi S, Voelkl Guevara J. An International Continence Society (ICS) report on the terminology for pelvic floor muscle assessment. Neurourol Urodyn. 2021;40(5):1217–60. https://doi.org/10.1002/nau.24658.
33. Grahame R, Bird HA, Child A. The revised (Brighton 1998) criteria for the diagnosis of benign joint hypermobility syndrome (BJHS). J Rheumatol. 2000;27(7):1777–9.
34. Hagen S, Stark D. Conservative prevention and management of pelvic organ prolapse in women. Cochrane Database Syst Rev. 2011;12:CD003882. https://doi.org/10.1002/14651858.
35. Hagen S, Glazener C, Sinclair L, Stark D, Bugge C. Psychometric properties of the pelvic organ prolapse symptom score. BJOG. 2009;116(1):25–31. https://doi.org/10.1111/j.1471-0528.2008.01903.x.
36. Hagen S, Stark D, Glazener C, Dickson S, Barry S, Elders A, et al. Individualised pelvic floor muscle training in women with pelvic organ prolapse (POPPY): a multicentre randomized controlled trial. Lancet. 2014;383(9919):796–806. https://doi.org/10.1016/S0140-6736(13)61977-7.
37. Hakim A, Grahame R. Joint hypermobility. Best Pract Res Clin Rheumatol. 2003;17(6):989–1004. https://doi.org/10.1016/j.berh.2003.08.001.
38. Handa VL, Roem J, Blomquist JL, Dietz HP, Muñoz A. Pelvic organ prolapse as a function of levator ani avulsion, hiatus size, and strength. Am J Obstet Gynecol. 2019;221(1):41. https://doi.org/10.1016/j.ajog.2019.03.004.
39. Harvey MA, Chih HJ, Geoffrion R, Amir B, Bhide A, Miotla P, et al. International Urogynecology Consultation Chapter 1 Committee 5: relation-

ship of pelvic organ prolapse to associated pelvic floor dysfunction symptoms: lower urinary tract, bowel, sexual dysfunction and abdominopelvic pain. Int Urogynecol J. 2021;32(10):2575–94. https://doi.org/10.1007/s00192-021-04941-5.
40. Haylen BT, De Ridder D, Freeman RM, Swift SE, Berghmans B, Lee J, et al. An International Urogynecological Association (IUGA)/International Continence Society (ICS) joint report on the terminology for female pelvic floor dysfunction. Neurourol Urodyn. 2010;29(1):4–20. https://doi.org/10.1002/nau.20798.
41. Haylen BT, Maher CF, Barber MD, Camargo S, Dandolu V, Digesu A, et al. An International Urogynecological Association (IUGA)/International Continence Society (ICS) joint report on the terminology for female pelvic organ prolapse (POP). Int Urogynecol J. 2016;27(2):165–94. https://doi.org/10.1007/s00192-015-2932-1.
42. Iglesia CB, Smithling KR. Pelvic organ prolapse. Am Fam Physician. 2017;96(3):179–85.
43. Jeppson PC, Balgobin S, Wheeler T, Forner L, Caagbay D, Thompson J, Muffly TM, Meyer I, Beestrum M, Collins S, Sung V. Impact of lifestyle modifications on the prevention and treatment of pelvic organ prolapse. Int Urogynecol J. 2024; https://doi.org/10.1007/s00192-024-05992-0.
44. Kisner C, Colby LA, Borstad J. Therapeutic exercise: foundations and techniques. Fa Davis; 2017.
45. Korkut Z, Demir ET, Celenay ST. Effects of interferential current stimulation in women with pelvic organ prolapse: a prospective randomized sham-controlled study. Int Urogynecol J. 2023;34(1):279–89. https://doi.org/10.1007/s00192-022-05402-3.
46. LeBlond RF, DeGowin RL. The neurologic examination. In: Shanahan JEK, editor. DeGowin's diagnostic examination. 9th ed. New York: McGraw-Hill Medical; 2009. p. 683–763.
47. Lind LR, Lucente V, Kohn N. Thoracic kyphosis and the prevalence of advanced uterine prolapse. Obstet Gynecol. 1996;87(4):605–9. https://doi.org/10.1016/0029-7844(95)00477-7.
48. Martellucci J. Electrotherapy for pelvic floor disorders: historical background. In: Electrical stimulation for pelvic floor disorders. Cham: Springer; 2015. p. 1–18.
49. Min L, Chunxue Y, Qiubo L, Xudong D, Yan Z, Guifang Z, Kejia H, Tianzi G, Qing F. Effectiveness of intravaginal electrical stimulation combined with electromyography biofeedback-mediated pelvic floor muscle training for postpartum symptomatic pelvic organ prolapse: protocol for the PROSPECT randomized trial. Trials. 2022;23(1):131. https://doi.org/10.1186/s13063-022-06051-z.
50. Munno GM, La Verde M, Lettieri D, Nicoletti R, Nunziata M, Fasulo DD, Vastarella MG, Pennacchio M, Scalzone G, Pieretti G, et al. Pelvic organ prolapse syndrome and lower urinary tract symptom update: what's new? Healthcare. 2023;11(10):1513. https://doi.org/10.3390/healthcare11101513.
51. Neumann P. Use of pessaries to prevent and treat pelvic organ prolapse. In: Bø K, Berghmans B, Morkved S, van Kampen M, editors. Evidence based physical therapy for the pelvic floor: bridging science and clinical practice. 2nd ed. Toronto: Elsevier; 2015. p. 230–3.
52. Nguyen JK, Lind LR, Choe JY, McKindsey F, Sinow R, Bhatia NN. Lumbosacral spine and pelvic inlet changes associated with pelvic organ prolapse. Obstet Gynecol. 2000;95(3):332–6. https://doi.org/10.1016/s0029-7844(99)00561-x.
53. NICE Guidance. Urinary incontinence and pelvic organ prolapse in women: management: © NICE (2019) Urinary incontinence and pelvic organ prolapse in women: management. BJU Int. 2019;123(5):777–803. https://doi.org/10.1111/bju.14763.
54. Nygaard I, Barber MD, Burgio KL, Kenton K, Meikle S, Schaffer J, et al. Pelvic Floor Disorders Network. Prevalence of symptomatic pelvic floor disorders in US women. JAMA. 2008;300:1311–6. https://doi.org/10.1001/jama.300.11.1311.
55. Oversand SH, Atan IK, Shek KL, Dietz HP. The association between different measures of pelvic floor muscle function and female pelvic organ prolapse. Int Urogynecol J. 2015;26(12):1777–81. https://doi.org/10.1007/s00192-015-2793-7.
56. Parekh M, Swift S, Lemos N, Iskander M, Freeman B, Arunkalaivanan AS, et al. Multicenter inter-examiner agreement trial for the validation of simplified POPQ system. Int Urogynecol J. 2011;22(6):645–50. https://doi.org/10.1007/s00192-011-1395-2.
57. Park DJ, Lee SK. What is a suitable pressure for the abdominal drawing-in maneuver in the supine position using a pressure biofeedback unit? J Phys Ther Sci. 2013;25(5):527–30. https://doi.org/10.1589/jpts.25.527.
58. Park DJ, Park SY. Which trunk exercise most effectively activates abdominal muscles? A comparative study of plank and isometric bilateral leg raise exercises. J Back Musculoskelet Rehabil. 2019;32(5):797–802. https://doi.org/10.3233/BMR-181122.
59. Petros PE, Woodman PJ. The integral theory of continence. Int Urogynecol J Pelvic Floor Dysfunct. 2008;19:35–40. https://doi.org/10.1007/s00192-007-0475-9.
60. Plevnik S. New methods for testing and strengthening the pelvic floor muscles. In: Proceedings of the 15th annual meeting of the international continence society. London: LCS; 1985. p. 267–8.
61. Podnar S, Vodušek DB. Protocol for clinical neurophysiologic examination of the pelvic floor. Neurourol Urodyn. 2001;20(6):669–82. https://doi.org/10.1002/nau.1018.
62. Rocca Rossetti S. Functional anatomy of pelvic floor. Arch Ital Urol Androl. 2016;88:28. https://doi.org/10.4081/aiua.2016.1.28.

63. Rogers RG, Pauls RN, Thakar R, Morin M, Kuhn A, Petri E, et al. An International Urogynecological Association (IUGA)/International Continence Society (ICS) joint report on the terminology for the assessment of sexual health of women with pelvic floor dysfunction. Neurourol Urodyn. 2018;37:1220–40. https://doi.org/10.1002/nau.23508.
64. Stanton R, Reaburn PR, Humphries B. The effect of short-term Swiss ball training on core stability and running economy. J Strength Cond Res. 2004;18(3):522–8. https://doi.org/10.1519/1533-4287(2004)18<522:TEOSSB>2.0.CO;2.
65. Sultan AH, Monga A, Lee J, Emmanuel A, Norton C, Santoro G, et al. An International Urogynecological Association (IUGA)/International Continence Society (ICS) joint report on the terminology for female anorectal dysfunction. Int Urogynecol J. 2017;28(1):5–31. https://doi.org/10.1007/s00192-016-3140-3.
66. Tang JH, Zhong C, Wen W, Wu R, Liu Y, Du LF. Quantifying levator ani muscle elasticity under normal and prolapse conditions by shear wave elastography: a preliminary study. J Ultrasound Med. 2020;39(7):1379–88. https://doi.org/10.1002/jum.15232.
67. Veit-Rubin N, Cartwright R, Singh AU, Digesu GA, Fernando R, Khullar V. Association between joint hypermobility and pelvic organ prolapse in women: a systematic review and meta-analysis. Int Urogynecol J. 2016;27(10):1469–78. https://doi.org/10.1007/s00192-015-2896-1.
68. Wang CN, Chung DE. Etiology, diagnosis, and management of pelvic organ prolapse: overview. In: Martins FE, Holm HV, Sandhu JS, McCammon KA, editors. Female genitourinary and pelvic floor reconstruction. Cham: Springer; 2023.
69. Weintraub AY, Glinter H, Marcus-Braun N. Narrative review of the epidemiology, diagnosis and pathophysiology of pelvic organ prolapse. Int Braz J Urol. 2020;46(1):5–14. https://doi.org/10.1590/S1677-5538.
70. Wong WY, Wong MS, Lo KH. Clinical applications of sensors for human posture and movement analysis: a review. Prosthetics Orthot Int. 2007;31(1):62–75. https://doi.org/10.1080/03093640600983949.
71. Wu JM, Hundley AF, Fulton RG, Myers ER. Forecasting the prevalence of pelvic floor disorders in U.S. Women: 2010 to 2050. Obstet Gynecol. 2009;114(6):1278–83. https://doi.org/10.1097/AOG.0b013e3181c2ce96.
72. Wu JM, Vaughan CP, Goode PS, Redden DT, Burgio KL, Richter HE, et al. Prevalence and trends of symptomatic pelvic floor disorders in U.S. women. Obstet Gynecol. 2014;123:141–8. https://doi.org/10.1097/AOG.0000000000000057.
73. Yıldız N. Pelvik Taban Disfonksiyonunda Elektriksel Stimulasyon Tedavisi. In: Karan A, editor. Ürojinekolojide Fizik Tedavi ve Rehabilitasyon. İstanbul: Nobel Tıp Kitabevi; 2016. p. 71–80.

16 Physiotherapy and Rehabilitation in Menstrual Disorders

Gamze Nalan Çinar and Türkan Akbayrak

16.1 Introduction

Menstrual disorders are frequently observed during adolescence, especially during the initial 2–3 years after menarche as a result of the incomplete maturation of the hypothalamic-pituitary-ovarian axis [1]. These disorders include amenorrhea (primary or secondary), menstrual bleeding disorders (oligomenorrhea, dysfunctional uterine bleeding), conditions associated with menstruation (dysmenorrhea), and polyendocrine metabolic ovarian syndrome. To study menstrual disorders comprehensively, it is essential to first review normal pubertal development and menarche.

16.2 Menstrual Cycle

For reproductive functions to proceed normally, various changes are expected throughout the body, particularly in the reproductive system. The entirety of the changes that occur every month in the female reproductive system, from menarche (the first menstrual bleeding during puberty) to menopause, allowing fertilization and pregnancy, is called the menstrual cycle [2]. The cycle duration, defined from the first day of menstruation to the day before the onset of the next menstruation, is approximately 28 days (28 ± 7 days) [3]. Menstruation occurs in the endometrium and ovaries under the influence of reproductive hormones. Therefore, the menstrual cycle is studied under two main headings:

- **Ovarian cycle**
- **Endometrial cycle**

The ovarian cycle, as illustrated in Fig 16.1, is characterized by fluctuations in ovarian hormones and is divided into three phases: the follicular phase, ovulation phase, and luteal phase. During the follicular phase, ovarian follicles containing oocytes mature. This phase begins with menstruation, marked by the shedding of the proliferative endometrium, and continues through ovulation (release of the oocyte from the dominant follicle), predominantly under the influence of follicle-stimulating hormone (FSH). During this stage, progesterone levels remain consistently low, while estrogen levels begin to rise during the mid-follicular phase, peaking just before ovulation. The ovulation phase occurs on days 12–14 of the menstrual cycle, during which the mature follicle releases the oocyte from the ovary. This phase is characterized by the highest estro-

G. N. Çinar (✉)
Department of Physiotherapy and Rehabilitation, Faculty of Health Sciences, Gazi University, Ankara, Türkiye
e-mail: gamzenalancinar@gazi.edu.tr

T. Akbayrak
Faculty of Physical Therapy and Rehabilitation, Hacettepe University, Ankara, Türkiye
e-mail: takbayra@hacettepe.edu.tr

T. Akbayrak, E. Üzelpasaci (eds.), *Physiotherapy and Rehabilitation in Pelvic and Women's Health-Related Problems*, https://doi.org/10.1007/978-3-032-28741-0_16

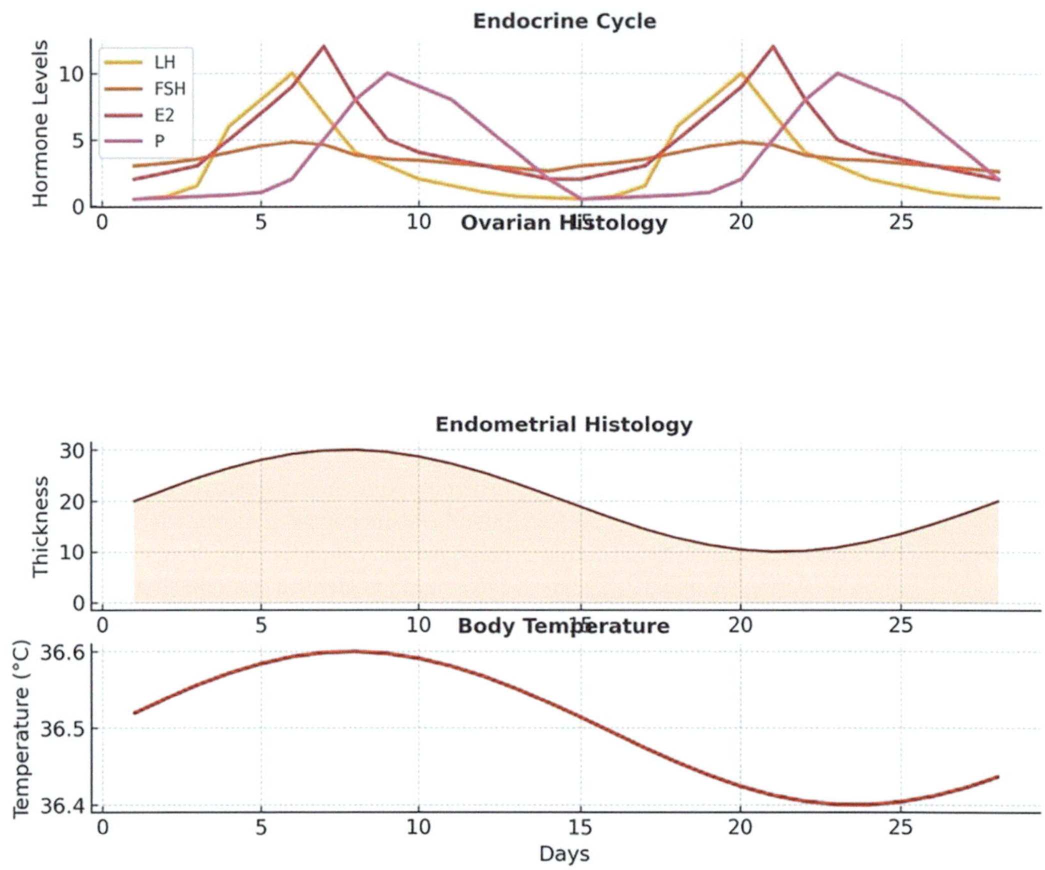

Fig. 16.1 Menstrual cycle phases and hormone levels. *LH* luteinizing hormone, *FSH* follicle-stimulating hormone, *E2* estrogen, *P* progesterone

gen levels in the bloodstream. In the luteal phase, following ovulation, the remaining follicular cells accumulate cholesterol, acquiring a yellow hue, and form the corpus luteum. Following ovulation, the corpus luteum secretes a substantial amount of progesterone alongside lower levels of estrogen. In the absence of fertilization, the corpus luteum starts to regress approximately one week prior to menstruation. The subsequent decline in estrogen and progesterone levels triggers menstruation [4].

The endometrial cycle occurs within the endometrium, which prepares for the implantation of a fertilized ovum. Like the ovarian cycle, the endometrial cycle is divided into three phases: Proliferative phase spans from the end of menstruation (approximately the sixth day of the menstrual cycle) to around the 12th or 13th day of the cycle. Following menstruation, the functional layer of the endometrium regenerates from the basal layer, a process driven by estrogen. Proliferation continues until ovulation (days 12–14 of the cycle). The secretory phase includes the time from ovulation to the onset of menstruation (days 13–28 of the cycle); this phase is marked by a significant increase in progesterone, which limits endometrial thickness, causing the endometrium to thicken. Spiral arterioles become coiled, and vasoconstriction increases. Endometrial glands begin to secrete mucus to support the fertilized ovum, hence the name "secretory phase." This phase is governed by the luteal phase of the ovarian cycle. If fertilization does not occur within 24–48 h post-ovulation, the corpus luteum regresses, and estrogen and progesterone levels in the blood drop. The functional layer of the endometrium deteriorates, leading to ischemia. This phase, lasting 14 days post-ovulation, is also referred to as the premenstrual phase. During the menstrual phase, if the ovum is not fertilized, the corpus luteum degenerates, leading to a decline in estrogen and progesterone levels. The withdrawal of progesterone triggers menstruation (progesterone withdrawal bleeding). The resulting decrease in hormone levels induces ischemia and stasis in the endometrial arteries, leading to the shedding of the endometrial layer over approximately 4–7 days.

In the first year after menarche, the menstrual cycle typically ranges between 21 and 45 days, with an average duration of 32.2 days. Normal menstruation typically lasts 2–7 days, with a monthly blood loss of 10–80 ml (average 35 ml) [5]. Early menstrual cycles are often characterized by anovulatory cycles. Ovulation frequency correlates with the time elapsed since menarche and the age at which menarche occurs. For girls who experience menarche before the age of 12, approximately 50% of cycles in the first gynecological year are ovulatory. Conversely, in women with later menarche, achieving regular ovulatory cycles may take 8–12 years. Menstrual cycles tend to be longer in the first three gynecological years, becoming shorter and more regular with age. A World Health Organization study involving 3073 girls reported an average cycle length of 34 days after the first menarche, with 38% of cycles exceeding 40 days. By the third year, 60–80% of cycles align with the adult range of 21–34 days, with regular cycles typically established by the sixth gynecological year, around the ages of 19–20 [6].

16.3 Menstrual Disorders

As per the definition provided by the World Health Organization, "health" refers to "a condition of overall physical, mental, and social wellness, rather than simply the absence of illness or impairment. For women, menstrual health is an integral component of overall health, significantly impacting physical, mental, and social well-being from menarche to menopause. Normal menstruation is defined as the cyclical bleeding originating from the uterine corpus between menarche and menopause. Four basic questions outline its characteristics: the frequency, regularity or predictability, duration, and volume of menstruation.

Menstrual problems are common gynecological issues, affecting approximately 50% of women and particularly adolescent girls, requiring medical treatment [7]. The American College of Obstetricians and Gynecologists (ACOG) outlined the causes of menstrual disorders in its 2020 guidelines [8]. The underlying causes can be classified into four primary groups: pregnancy; endocrine-related conditions such as diabetes mellitus, polyendocrine metabolic ovarian syndrome (PMOS), Cushing's syndrome, thyroid irregularities, premature ovarian failure, and late-onset congenital adrenal hyperplasia; acquired factors including stress-induced hypothalamic dysfunction, medication effects, amenorrhea caused by excessive exercise, and eating disorders like anorexia or bulimia; and various tumors, including those affecting the ovaries, adrenal glands, and prolactin-secreting glands. Common menstrual disorders include amenorrhea, dysmenorrhea, and PMOS, especially in adolescent girls, who are frequently affected by acute gynecological issues such as dysfunctional and abnormal uterine bleeding.

16.3.1 Dysfunctional Uterine Bleeding (DUB): Abnormal Uterine Bleeding (AUB)

Dysfunctional uterine bleeding (DUB) and abnormal uterine bleeding (AUB) are widespread problems affecting 10–30% of women of reproductive age, significantly impacting quality of life and fertility [9]. DUB refers to prolonged, excessive, or irregular endometrial bleeding without any underlying structural or systemic cause. Bleeding occurring at intervals shorter than 21 days due to organic causes, such as pregnancy complications, coagulation disorders, systemic diseases, reproductive system pathologies, endocrine disorders, or iatrogenic factors, is classified as AUB [10]. The European Society of Human Reproduction and Embryology (ESHRE) defines DUB as excessive uterine bleeding (in terms of severity, duration, or frequency) not associated with pelvic disease, pregnancy complications, or systemic disorders. DUB can be ovulatory or anovulatory in origin. AUB etiologies are categorized under the PALM-COEIN classification:

- **PALM Group (Structural Causes):** Polyps, adenomyosis, leiomyomas, malignancy (diagnosed via imaging or biopsy)
- **COEIN Group (Non-structural Causes):** Coagulopathy, ovulatory dysfunction, endometrial dysfunction, iatrogenic causes (e.g., implants, intrauterine devices, oral contraceptives), and non-iatrogenic uterine bleeding [11]

The ACOG report establishes normal menstrual parameters for adolescents as follows: menarche occurring between 11 and 14 years, cycle intervals of 21–45 days, and average menstrual blood loss of approximately 35 ml (usually not exceeding 60 ml) per cycle [12]. Deviations from these norms result in uterine bleeding classified as AUB or DUB, further subdivided into:

- **Menorrhagia (Hypermenorrhea):** Regular but heavy (>80 ml) and/or prolonged bleeding (>7 days)
- **Hypomenorrhea:** Regular but scant bleeding (<30 ml)
- **Menometrorrhagia:** Irregular, heavy bleeding (>80 ml) with prolonged duration (>7 days)
- **Metrorrhagia:** Intermenstrual spotting or light bleeding
- **Oligomenorrhea:** Irregular bleeding occurring at intervals longer than 45 days, common in early post-menarche, premenopausal, or lactational phases
- **Polymenorrhea:** Frequent bleeding at intervals shorter than 21 days [13]

16.3.1.1 Evaluation

The approach to patients presenting with AUB and DUB involves hemodynamic assessment, particularly anemia parameters, identification of the bleeding source, pregnancy testing, and comprehensive differential diagnosis to exclude pathological conditions such as endometrial carcinoma. This requires a detailed history and physical examination.

Key aspects include obtaining information on the patient's menstrual history, particularly the age of menarche and menstrual cycle length. Additionally, the duration of menstruation, volume of bleeding, presence of clots, and any associated pain or cramps should be evaluated. A systems review should investigate other unusual or abnormal bleeding. Psychosocial factors, recent weight fluctuations, dietary and exercise habits, substance or alcohol use, and signs of hyperandrogenism (acne, hirsutism) should also be considered. Family history should be evaluated for endocrine disorders, thyroid dysfunctions, functional ovarian hyperandrogenism, and hematological conditions like von Willebrand disease. Sexual activity, contraceptive use, and history of infections spread through sexual contact should be thoroughly reviewed [14].

16.3.1.2 Treatment

AUB and DUB are among the most urgent gynecological issues in adolescence. The initial goal in treating DUB is to control bleeding and regulate menstruation. The secondary aim is correcting anemia and replenishing iron stores. Hormonal therapy is the cornerstone for most patients, with the type and route of administration tailored to the severity of DUB [5]. In mild cases, menstruation may be slightly prolonged or irregular, but hemoglobin levels remain above 12 g/dl. Hormonal therapy is rarely needed; instead, patient education and monitoring through a menstrual calendar are typically sufficient [15]. In moderate DUB, characterized by prolonged menstrual periods, short intervals, and heavy bleeding, symptoms interfere with daily activities, often accompanied by mild anemia (hemoglobin $\geq$10 g/dl). Treatment primarily involves pharmacological interventions such as low-dose oral contraceptives or cyclic (10-day) oral progesterone. Oral iron supplements may be added in cases of iron-deficiency anemia. Nonsteroidal anti-inflammatory drugs (NSAIDs) can reduce bleeding by approximately 50% through the inhibition of prostaglandin synthesis. Oral contraceptives should be continued for at least 3–6 months [5]. In severe DUB, where hemoglobin levels fall below 10 g/dl, treatment requires close monitoring, particularly if hypovolemia is present. Rapid control is often achieved using combined oral contraceptives. In more severe cases, surgical interventions such as dilation and curettage may be necessary [16].

16.3.2 Amenorrhea

For menstruation to occur, certain physiological conditions must be met: the uterus and genital tract must be intact, the endometrium and ovaries must function properly, and the pituitary and hypothalamus must maintain normal functions, all working in harmony. Amenorrhea is defined as the absence or abnormal cessation of menstruation during the reproductive years [16]. The prevalence of amenorrhea, excluding causes such as pregnancy, lactation, or menopause, is approximately 3–4% [17]. Clinically, amenorrhea is classified as primary or secondary. Primary amenorrhea refers to the lack of menstrual cycles by the age of 16 when secondary sexual features, such as breast development, the growth of pubic and underarm hair, and voice changes, are present, or by the age of 14 if these characteristics are absent [18]. Primary amenorrhea causes include endocrine abnormalities (40% of cases) and developmental anomalies (60%) [19]. Secondary amenorrhea refers to the cessation of menstruation for more than 3 months in women who previously had regular cycles or for more than 9 months in those with prior oligomenorrhea [20]. The causes of primary and secondary amenorrhea often overlap and are examined together (Table 16.1).

Excessive exercise level is among the causes of amenorrhea, particularly in adolescents, as it can suppress pubertal development. Menstrual dysfunction associated with amenorrhea, low energy availability, and decreased bone mineral density constitutes the "Female Athlete Triad," observed in many female athletes, although its exact prevalence is unknown. Athletes with amenorrhea face an increased risk of bone loss

Table 16.1 Causes of amenorrhea [22]

Genital anomalies	Hypothalamic/pituitary anomalies	Endocrine abnormalities
Acquired	Autoimmune diseases	Adrenal insufficiency
Cervical stenosis	Brain exposure to radiation	Androgen-secreting tumor
Intrauterine adhesions	Functional disorders	Cushing syndrome
Congenital	Eating disorders	Diabetes mellitus, uncontrolled
Closed hymen	Excessive weight loss	Late-onset congenital adrenal
Transverse vaginal	Intense exercise	hyperplasia
septum	Stress disorders Gonadotropin deficiency	Polycystic ovary syndrome
Vaginal agenesis	(Kallmann syndrome)	Thyroid disease
Primary ovarian failure	Hyperprolactinemia	Hyperthyroidism
Acquired	Adenoma	Hyperthyroidism
Autoimmune	Chronic kidney disease	Amenorrhea due to chronic
Chemotherapy and	Medications or illicit	disease
radiotherapy	Drugs	Celiac disease
Congenital	Pregnancy	Inflammatory bowel disease
Gonadal dysgenesis	Infarction (e.g., Sheehan syndrome)	Other chronic diseases
Turner syndrome	Infiltrative disease (e.g., sarcoidosis)	Physiologic or induced
	Infection (e.g., meningitis, tuberculosis)	Breastfeeding
	Trauma or surgery	Birth control
	Tumor (primary or metastatic)	Exogenous androgens
		Menopause
		Pregnancy

and osteoporosis, which is often irreversible and occurs during peak bone mass development. In such cases, increasing caloric intake and reducing training intensity by about 10% is often sufficient to resume menstruation. Additionally, resistance exercises can provide partial protection against bone loss, but continued medical intervention is typically necessary [21].

One of the earliest signs of eating disorders is menstrual dysfunction, particularly amenorrhea. The American Psychiatric Association recommends using the Diagnostic and Statistical Manual of Mental Disorders (DSM-IV) to identify severe metabolic disturbances that may affect eating habits and physiological systems in individuals with amenorrhea.

DSM-IV Criteria for Anorexia Nervosa:

- Failure to sustain body weight at or above a minimally normal level for age and height (body weight <85% of expected)
- Intense fear of increasing body weight
- Distorted body image (denial of the seriousness of low body weight)
- Amenorrhea for three consecutive cycles in postmenarchal females

DSM-IV Criteria for Bulimia Nervosa:

- Recurrent episodes of binge eating accompanied by a sense of loss of control
- Compensatory behaviors to prevent weight gain (self-induced vomiting, misuse of laxatives, diuretics, excessive exercise, fasting)
- Dissatisfaction with body shape and weight [23]

Studies on anorexia nervosa and bulimia nervosa indicate that menarche can occur when body fat constitutes approximately 17% of total body weight. Secondary amenorrhea can arise when body fat falls below 22% [24].

16.3.2.1 Evaluation

The assessment of amenorrhea begins with a thorough history and physical examination to exclude pregnancy. For individuals at extremes of body weight (cachexia or obesity), ovulatory dysfunction, insulin resistance, and diabetes mellitus should be considered. Calculating the body mass index (BMI) is crucial for determining an individual's weight category. A detailed inquiry into the patient's medical history, including concurrent illnesses, symptoms, family history, and the usage of medication, is essential. The menstrual history should encompass age at menarche, cycle length, intermenstrual intervals, and the date of the last menstrual period. In addition, clinical signs such as hirsutism or acne may suggest polycystic ovary syndrome (PCOS). Symptoms like fatigue, temperature intolerance, or galactorrhea warrant investigation for hyperprolactinemia or thyroid disorders. In such cases, referral to a physician is advised.

Since amenorrhea can also be seen in premenopausal women, vasomotor symptoms other than irregular menstrual bleeding occurring during this period should be questioned in detail. Women diagnosed with functional hypothalamic amenorrhea require detailed evaluation of stress, exercise, and dietary habits, as obsessive behavior in these areas may lead to menstrual dysfunction. Recent stressors should also be documented, as they can indicate a higher likelihood of hypothalamic disruption. Psychological factors, including stress, anxiety, depressive symptoms, sleep quality, and activity levels, should be evaluated.

Routine pelvic examination is not necessary for every case but should be performed if indicated. Key areas to assess include:

- Vaginal orifice size (to evaluate for outlet obstruction; average depth in postpubertal females is 7–8 cm)
- Vaginal moisture (indicates adequate estrogenization of genital tissues)
- Presence of nodules or masses upon palpation
- Perineal sensitivity
- Skin assessment (rash, ulcers) [25]

If anatomical abnormalities are detected, pelvic ultrasonography should be conducted [26].

16.3.2.2 Treatment

The treatment of amenorrhea varies depending on its etiology. For functional hypothalamic amenorrhea, management often begins with weight restoration to regulate menstruation. A 5-year retrospective study involving 373 university women reported that 20% experienced oligo-amenorrhea and 18% achieved complete remission within 15 months through improved diet and adjusted energy expenditure [27]. There is a lack of literature on physiotherapy and rehabilitation interventions for amenorrhea, though physiotherapy approaches for PCOS are discussed in a separate section.

Addressing factors such as stress, anxiety disorders, dietary changes, and sleep disturbances is critical, as these can influence menstruation. Techniques like cognitive-behavioral therapy, meditation, mindfulness, and yoga (asana, pranayama, and meditation) help manage stress and promote relaxation.

While the Female Athlete Triad—characterized by menstrual irregularities, low energy availability, and decreased bone mineral density—is recognized as a significant public health issue, it should not be viewed as an inevitable consequence of regular exercise or sports participation. The overall health benefits of physical activity outweigh the risk of developing the triad. Return-to-play criteria for athletes depend on clinical and psychosocial evaluations. Athletes who restrict their diets more than four times per week or have a BMI below 16 kg/m^2 should have their training restricted. The increasing number of women engaging in professional sports underscores the need for education and intervention strategies to prevent and treat the triad effectively [21].

Successful management and prevention of the triad require a multidisciplinary team approach. Although the prevalence of athletes exhibiting all three components simultaneously is low, many physically active women may have one or two components and are at risk of developing the triad [28]. Regular screening and monitoring of at-risk athletes are crucial. Early detection and awareness of triggering factors are vital for implementing treatment strategies. Physiotherapists play an essential role in the treatment and prevention of the Female Athlete Triad as part of a multidisciplinary team [29]. According to the American College of Sports Medicine, the primary goal for athletes exhibiting triad symptoms is to increase energy intake and decrease energy expenditure. This improves menstrual health and bone mineral density while guiding athletes toward appropriate dietary and exercise practices [30].

16.3.3 Premenstrual Syndrome

Premenstrual syndrome (PMS) is a health problem characterized by the cyclical onset of physical, behavioral, and psychological symptoms, typically starting about a week before menstruation, peaking at the onset of menstruation, and resolving within a few days thereafter (occurring during the luteal phase of the menstrual cycle). Most women experience physical and emotional changes (molimina) related to menstruation each month. The most commonly reported physical issues include abdominal pain, acne on the skin/face, and breast pain/tenderness, while psychological issues include mood sensitivity and irritability [31]. However, for a diagnosis of PMS to be made, there must be a significant disruption in occupational, familial, and personal functioning [32]. Prevalence studies suggest that between 30% and 80% of women experience some symptoms before menstruation, though determining the true prevalence of PMS is difficult due to factors such as medical care, diagnostic criteria, tendencies for self-treatment, and cultural differences. When strict diagnostic criteria are applied, it is estimated that the prevalence of severe PMS in women of reproductive age is approximately 2.5% [33].

Although the specific etiology of PMS is not fully understood, proposed causes include genetic factors, hormonal imbalances, sodium retention, nutritional deficiencies, abnormal neurotransmitter effects on ovarian function, insulin resistance, abnormal changes in glucose metabolism, and abnormal hypothalamic-pituitary-adrenal axis function [34].

16.3.3.1 Evaluation

Accurate diagnosis of PMS requires a comprehensive history, physical examination, and ongoing symptom assessment. PMS refers to the presence of multiple symptoms not associated with a serious disorder (Table 16.2). To definitively diagnose PMS, patients are asked to complete a form over two menstrual cycles. For symptoms to be classified as PMS, the following criteria must be met:

- Symptoms must become prominent in the final week of the luteal phase, diminish during menstruation, and resolve in the follicular phase.
- Symptoms should be severe enough to interfere with the patient's usual activities or daily life.
- Finally, symptoms must not be caused by another medical or psychiatric disorder or be confused with the effects of the use of a drug or any substance.

Quality of life, anxiety and depressive symptom levels, sleep quality, and physical activity levels of individuals must be assessed using questionnaires specific to the individual and situation [36]. In their study, Bosman et al. listed various questionnaires and diaries used in the literature to assess PMS severity. These include:

- Cyclicity Diagnoser (CD)
- Premenstrual Tension Syndrome Self-Rating Scales (PMTS-SR)
- Calendar of Premenstrual Experiences (COPE)
- Prospective Record of the Impact and Severity of Menstrual Symptomatology (PRISM)
- Daily Rating Form (DRF), Daily Assessment Form (DAF), Daily Record of Severity of Problems (DRSP), and Daily Symptom Report [37]

Table 16.2 PMS diagnostic criteria [35]

Premenstrual syndrome can be diagnosed if the patient reports at least one of the following affective and somatic symptoms on the 5 days before menstruation in each of the three menstrual cycles	
Affective symptoms	Somatic symptoms
Outbursts of anger	Abdominal bloating
Anxiety	Breast tenderness or edema
Confusion	Headache
Depression	Joint or muscle pain
Irritability	Extremity edema
Social isolation	Weight gain

16.3.3.2 Treatment

The main goal of studies in the literature has been to alleviate symptoms of PMS and reduce the negative impact on individuals' daily lives. Pharmacotherapy (antidepressants, diuretics, progesterone and estrogen implants, combined contraceptives, pyridoxine, and gonadotropin-releasing hormone agonists) is commonly used as a first-line treatment for PMS; however, since no medication completely halts all symptoms, women often seek traditional and alternative methods [38]. Recent clinical studies suggest the use of cognitive and behavioral therapies, aerobic exercises, manual therapies, dietary and nutritional changes, and complementary treatments like acupuncture and reflexology in the management of PMS [39, 40]. Additionally, a 3-month aerobic training program applied to sedentary women has been found to reduce premenstrual symptoms, leading the American College of Obstetricians and Gynecologists to recommend regular physical exercise as a non-pharmacological treatment for PMS [41].

Exercise increases the release of various neurotransmitters, including endorphins (natural painkillers), estrogen, dopamine, and endogenous opiate peptides; suppresses prostaglandin release; and increases the estrone-estradiol ratio, reducing endometrial proliferation (thickening). This increases uterine blood flow and reduces the intensity of pain perceived by individuals. Furthermore, exercise can reduce stress, anxiety, and depression by clearing negative thoughts and promoting positive thinking, thereby improving mood and behavior. Studies show that women who regularly engage in aerobic exercise experience improved psychological well-being. Furthermore, increasing the frequency of physical activity is noted to reduce PMS [42].

A study investigating the effectiveness of yoga in PMS found that regular yoga practice positively affects the menstrual cycle and psychological health by regulating the neuroendocrine axis. The mechanism of this effect is attributed to yoga's ability to adjust the amount and synthesis of immunoglobulin A, which protects the immune system. In this way, yoga reduces harmful inflammatory secretions and alleviates stress-induced negative effects, providing relaxation for women with PMS [43]. Research comparing the effects of aerobic exercise and yoga on PMS indicates that 1 month of consistent practice in either form can alleviate pain intensity and PMS symptoms. However, yoga was found to be more beneficial than aerobic exercise in alleviating PMS symptoms [44]. Swimming is also noted as an effective treatment for PMS symptoms [44].

Another treatment option for PMS is lifestyle changes (diet, participation in activities, smoking cessation, etc.). Literature suggests that lifestyle modifications can alleviate mild and moderate PMS symptoms without the need for pharmacological treatment. Relaxation exercises are essential for managing both stress levels and PMS symptoms. Therefore, breathing exercises, relaxation techniques, meditation, and classical massage therapy using various herbal oils, performed by specialized physiotherapists, are important in the treatment of PMS [45].

16.3.4 Dysmenorrhea

The word dysmenorrhea, originating from Greek (dys–difficult, mens–month, and rhoia–flow), describes painful menstrual cramps and is the most prevalent gynecological symptom experienced by women [46]. The prevalence of dysmenorrhea worldwide varies between 28% and 71% [47]. Dysmenorrhea is classified into primary or secondary forms based on its pathophysiology. In both cases, the perception of pain can lead to not only physical discomfort but also psychological and emotional disturbances. It is known that this condition affects daily life activities and social relationships and causes a high rate of social isolation (school/work absenteeism) [48]. One study reports that 12% of adolescent girls and young women aged 14–20 miss school or work every month due to dysmenorrhea [49].

Primary dysmenorrhea (PD) refers to chronic, cyclical menstrual pain beginning 6–12 months after menarche without any underlying pelvic pathology [50]. In PD, pain usually lasts 48–72 h and is felt just before and/or during menstruation. The pain is typically colicky and is primarily felt in the suprapubic area, radiating to both lower abdominal quadrants, the lower back, or the thighs. In women with PD, along with pain, many systemic menstrual symptoms may occur, such as back pain, headaches, abdominal bloating, breast pain/tenderness/tightness, fatigue, nausea/vomiting, diarrhea, constipation, irritability, and depression. All these symptoms interfere with women's participation in daily life activities and lead to school/work absenteeism [50]. Additionally, PD causes psychological symptoms like anxiety, depressive signs, and increased stress levels, negatively impacting quality of life. However, most individuals consider PD to be a normal physiological condition rather than a disorder. As a result, approximately one-third of women with PD seek medical attention for this condition [51]. In PD, excessive production and release of endometrial prostaglandins (PGs) during menstruation cause uterine hypercontractility, which is a key factor in reducing uterine blood flow, leading to uterine hypoxia and the sensitization of pain fibers [52]. Women with PD exhibit high Doppler indices throughout the cycle, creating high impedance against uterine blood flow and reducing uterine artery blood flow [53].

Secondary dysmenorrhea (SD) is more common, particularly in women aged 25–29, and is associated with pathological conditions [54]. Severe menstrual pain that occurs 3 years after menarche is considered pathological. SD is characterized by chronic pain felt in the pelvic or lower abdominal region, typically 1–2 days before menstruation, and may also be accompanied by irregular and heavy menstruation, dyspareunia, and irritable bowel symptoms. This condition is associated with underlying organic pathology [16]. The most common causes of SD in adolescents include endometriosis, pelvic inflammatory disease, and Müllerian duct malformations. Other less common causes in women include uterine retroversion, cervical canal stenosis, inappropriate intrauterine devices, uterine fibroids, endometrial or endocervical polyps, adenomyosis, and pelvic venous congestion [55]. Studies have shown that women with SD and endometriosis have a relationship between dyspareunia, low back pain, pain during ovulation, rectal pain, dysuria, and chronic pelvic pain [56, 57].

Studies show that many factors are associated with menstrual pain, influencing the frequency and severity of dysmenorrhea. These factors include younger age, low body mass index (BMI), early menarche, smoking and alcohol use, perimenstrual somatic complaints, pelvic infections, and psychological disorders [58, 59].

16.3.4.1 Evaluation

In PD, the diagnosis requires excluding the possibility of underlying pelvic pathology and confirming that the pain is periodic. Therefore, for individuals with dysmenorrhea, pregnancy tests, routine smear tests, cancer screening, and abdominal and pelvic mass screenings should be performed to eliminate the possibility of pregnancy. A detailed history should be taken, and usage of medication and previous surgeries should be questioned. Family history and parental modeling play an important role not only in how a young patient perceives and reports pain but also in their experience of pain. Therefore, a detailed family history should be obtained. Additionally, family history in the evaluation of dysmenorrhea is often used to distinguish SD from PD [60].

The symptoms accompanying menstrual pain and the attitudes and behaviors of individuals also need to be evaluated. Common methods used in clinics include self-developed forms, the menstrual symptom scale, the menstruation attitude scale, and the menstrual distress scale. Besides menstrual symptoms and attitudes, it is extremely important to assess cultural differences that might influence an individual's behavior. Especially in individuals with dysphoric disorder or underlying psychiatric conditions, premenstrual symptoms and pain exacerbation can lead to significant changes in emotional, cognitive, and behavioral functioning [61]. This situation reduces individuals' quality of life and affects various physical, mental, and social dimensions of overall well-being, including sleep efficiency, concentration, work/school attendance, and social relationships. Therefore, in the evaluation of dysmenorrhea, it is important to thoroughly assess individuals' quality of life, sleep quality, stress and anxiety levels, and psychological impact.

The therapeutic mechanism of physical activity on dysmenorrhea is well known in the literature. According to the guidelines of the American College of Obstetricians and Gynecologists, moderate physical activity is particularly noted for its therapeutic role in dysmenorrhea. Therefore, the level of physical activity in individuals should be evaluated using subjective or objective methods. In addition, factors identified as risk factors for dysmenorrhea, such as smoking and alcohol use, fluid intake, and nutritional knowledge, should be thoroughly assessed.

In individuals with dysmenorrhea, the peripheral nociceptive input resulting from uterine activity throughout the menstrual cycle is reported to be greater than in individuals without dysmenorrhea. However, there are gaps in the literature regarding the relationship between dysmenorrhea and chronic pain, which highlights the need to determine whether dysmenorrhea directly contributes to the development of chronic pain [62]. Therefore, in the assessment of dysmenorrhea, the characteristic features of the pain (onset, location, duration, type, intensity, and whether it is acute or chronic) should be carefully evaluated. Some commonly used scales and tests in clinics for this purpose include:

- Visual Analog Scale
- Numeric Pain Rating Scale
- Verbal Pain Scale
- McGill Pain Questionnaire
- Algometer—Pain threshold assessment
- Central Sensitization Scale
- Sensory tests

Another commonly used method in dysmenorrhea evaluation (for SD differential diagnosis) is pelvic examination. If the patient's history suggests organic disease or congenital malformations of the genital system, and if the patient does not respond to conventional PD treatments, a pelvic examination is indicated. However, this method may cause mild to moderate tenderness in individuals. Uterosacral nodules and pelvic masses are rare findings in adolescent patients with endometriosis, but it has been found that patients with a family history of endometriosis are more likely to have SD [63]. Another aspect of physical examination in dysmenorrhea is trigger point palpation. Literature suggests that individuals with dysmenorrhea may have myofascial trigger points in the abdominal wall [64].

16.3.4.2 Treatment

Studies examining treatment approaches for dysmenorrhea indicate that individuals often view this condition as something they can resolve on their own, with low rates of seeking help from doctors or healthcare facilities (ranging from 8.9% to 32.6%) [65], while over-the-counter or non-prescribed medication use is quite high (70–82%) [66]. Treatment approaches for dysmenorrhea can be categorized into pharmacological methods, alternative treatments, physiotherapy and rehabilitation, and surgical methods. The primary aim of treatment is to regulate myometrial tone and reduce prostaglandin production. The choice of treatment depends on the characteristics of the menstrual cycle, the need for contraception, the individual's age, and the severity of the symptoms.

16.3.4.2.1 Pharmacological Methods

Pharmacological treatments for dysmenorrhea are classified into hormonal and nonhormonal approaches. Hormonal medical treatments include combined oral contraceptives (COCs) and progestin derivatives, while nonhormonal treatments include analgesics, anticholinergics, muscle relaxants, nonsteroidal anti-inflammatory drugs (NSAIDs), beta-adrenergic agents, transdermal glyceryl trinitrate, and calcium channel blockers [67].

The most commonly used drug group for primary dysmenorrhea (PD) treatment is prostaglandin synthesis inhibitors (e.g., ibuprofen, naproxen, NSAIDs). These drugs bind to prostaglandin receptors and reduce the effects of prostaglandins. NSAIDs decrease endometrial prostaglandin levels, reducing the intensity of uterine contractions. In individuals who can predict the start of menstruation, taking these medications 1–2 days before the onset of menstruation has been shown to have a positive effect ranging from 67% to 95% [63]. However, NSAIDs or COCs are less likely to respond to chronic pelvic pain associated with endometriosis, a common cause of secondary dysmenorrhea (SD). If there is a lack of response to NSAIDs and COCs for at least 3 months, laparoscopy becomes indicated. In SD, it is crucial to address both pain management and the treatment of the underlying organic pathology [16].

Calcium channel blockers, COCs, and transdermal nitroglycerin are also frequently used in dysmenorrhea treatment. Calcium channel blockers work by affecting the uterine smooth muscles, inhibiting PGF2a and vasopressin, thus reducing pain. COCs are widely used for PD and work by inhibiting the development of estrogen and progesterone during the ovulatory phase of the menstrual cycle, reducing menstrual pain. Thus, oral contraceptives are effective not only for preventing pregnancy but also for managing menstrual pain. Transdermal nitroglycerin is thought to create vasodilation, improving blood circulation in smooth muscles and reducing myometrial contractions, thus alleviating menstrual pain [68].

16.3.4.2.2 Alternative Treatments

- Acupuncture and Acupressure

Among the oldest forms of alternative medicine and traditional Chinese therapies, acupuncture and acupressure have been found effective in treating dysmenorrhea by blocking pain impulses through the release of serotonin and endorphins. It is believed that these therapies reduce dysmenorrhea intensity by increasing estradiol release. In acupuncture, analgesia can be achieved by applying pressure between T5 and L4 levels [68], while acupressure involves applying pressure on the medial malleolus with three fingers to provide pain relief [69]. Studies in the literature suggest that pain decreases following acupuncture and acupressure, but the effect is short-term [70, 71]. Additionally, a review suggests that, based on placebo-controlled studies in PD, the effects of acupuncture and acupressure could be placebos [72].

- Herbal Products and Dietary Supplements

Herbal products and dietary supplements are popular treatment modalities in dysmenorrhea management as they are easily accessible to patients at supermarkets, pharmacies, or various health stores. While this easy accessibility may seem beneficial, it can pose problems due to insufficient control over the dosage, quality, and interactions with other medications. Systematic reviews and randomized controlled trials in the literature have indicated that thiamine, pyridoxine, magnesium, and fish oil can be effective in relieving pain. However, when consumed without proper dosage or supervision from healthcare professionals, they may cause side effects such as syncope, dizziness, and acne [73]. Foods rich in arachidonic acid, a fatty acid involved in prostaglandin production, are known to increase the severity of dysmenorrhea. Therefore, the excessive consumption of foods rich in arachidonic acid, such as butter, corn, dates, coconut, soybean oil, turkey, and chicken, is believed to increase the severity of dysmenorrhea [74, 75]. Moreover, excessive sugar intake can lead to an increase in the absorption of certain vitamins and minerals, potentially causing nutritional imbalances that can result in muscle spasms and pain. In such cases, increasing the intake of fiber-rich foods (such as whole-grain bread, dry legumes, apples, and oranges) can reduce the absorption of fats and sugars, regulate bowel movements, and effectively reduce dysmenorrhea severity [76].

Certain vitamins (B and E vitamins) and minerals (magnesium, calcium, zinc) have also been shown to be effective in the treatment of dysmenorrhea. In a randomized controlled trial, daily intake of 100 mg of vitamin B1 was found to reduce menstrual pain by over 90%. Vitamin E, used in dysmenorrhea treatment, inhibits protein kinase C, preventing the conversion of arachidonic acid and phospholipids in the cell membrane into prostaglandins, thus reducing dysmenorrhea severity [77]. Similarly, magnesium, with its muscle-relaxant and vasodilatory effects, is used in dysmenorrhea treatment by inhibiting prostaglandin synthesis [78]. The literature also suggests that adequate calcium intake can maintain normal muscle tone and prevent menstrual cramps. Insufficient calcium intake, however, may increase fluid retention, making menstrual pain more severe [75]. Additionally, fish oil, zinc, and herbal products such as black cohosh, rose tea, and fennel tea have been shown to be effective in managing dysmenorrhea, although further research is needed for stronger evidence [79].

- Psychotherapy and Mind–Body Techniques

Dysmenorrhea develops as a result of increased uterine muscle contractions under the influence of the sympathetic nervous system. Therefore, high stress levels can activate the sympathetic nervous system, potentially exacerbating dysmenorrhea. Behavioral treatments used in dysmenorrhea management include biofeedback, desensitization training, relaxation exercises, hypnotherapy, psychotherapy, and behavioral therapy. Studies have shown that menstrual pain is often learned from family members, particularly that girls lack sufficient information before menarche, leading to emotional issues related to academic and social problems. Behavioral changes addressing such issues can be effective in treating dysmenorrhea. Techniques such as deep breathing, meditation, and imagining pleasant scenarios can redirect attention away from pain, reduce anxiety, and result in less menstrual pain. A Cochrane review that compiled five randomized studies comparing behavioral therapies to placebo or other treatments indicated that behavioral therapies are somewhat effective in reducing dysmenorrhea severity [80].

- Reflexology

Foot reflexology is a noninvasive treatment method that involves the application of direct topical pressure to specific points and areas on the feet, believed to correspond to certain somatic organs. The underlying theory of reflexology suggests that during damage to any part of the body, the accumulation of uric acid or calcium crystals may occur, which then affects the nerve endings in the feet and impedes lymphatic flow. By applying pressure to these areas, it is thought that crystal deposits are broken down, and the damage is alleviated. Although the physiological mechanisms are not fully understood, the treatment is believed to work by inducing peripheral vasodilation and subsequently activating A-delta fibers, delaying or eliminating pain perception [81]. In studies examining the effectiveness of reflexology in dysmenorrhea, where its effects were compared with connective tissue manipulation (CTM) and ibuprofen, reflexology was found to reduce dysmenorrhea severity and symptoms. It was noted as an effective, side-effect-free approach, particularly as an alternative to pharmacological methods [82].

16.3.4.2.3 Physiotherapy and Rehabilitation

- Exercise

The effectiveness of various exercises, such as aerobic, stretching, flexibility, relaxation, strengthening, and isometric exercises, in the treatment of dysmenorrhea has been widely researched in the literature. Studies also exist on the effectiveness of specific exercise approaches like Pilates and yoga [72]. Exercise is thought to reduce menstrual pain through a range of mechanisms affecting opioid and non-opioid systems [83]. Research has shown that aerobic exercise, particularly, influences beta-endorphin production, which is linked to changes in pain perception [84]. Intense aerobic exercises have been reported to stimulate beta-endorphin concentrations more significantly [85]. Beta-endorphins work by inhibiting the release of substance P, a key protein involved in pain transmission, and gamma-aminobutyric acid, a neurotransmitter that inhibits pain control structures [86]. Therefore, exercise approaches are considered a cost-effective, low-side-effect treatment option for dysmenorrhea.

Literature suggests that a general stretching program, specific stretching, Kegel exercises, jogging, and relaxation exercises effectively reduce dysmenorrhea symptoms [87]. Strength exercises have been shown to reduce inflammatory cytokines like tumor necrosis factor (TNF-a) and interleukin-6, which increase in the presence of inflammatory reactions in the body, thus reducing pain transmission and suggesting their use in dysmenorrhea treatment [88]. A study examining the effectiveness of strength exercises in dysmenorrhea found that they were effective in reducing dysmenorrhea severity and associated symptoms, as well as reducing school/work absenteeism due to dysmenorrhea [89].

Yoga is another commonly used exercise type in dysmenorrhea treatment. Yoga is an ancient mind–body discipline originating from India, designed to enhance physical, mental, and emotional balance, thereby promoting overall health. Traditionally, yoga integrates a structured philosophy with meditation (dhyana), physical postures (asanas), breathing techniques (pranayama), and deep relaxation (Yoga Nidra). Yoga helps calm the body and mind through controlled breathing exercises, enhances muscle strength, flexibility, and balance through physical postures and warm-up exercises, and promotes mindfulness through relaxation techniques. These properties positively impact quality of life [90]. According to literature, when practiced under the guidance of a trained instructor, yoga is considered a safe complementary and alternative treatment for PD, reducing menstrual pain by reducing prostaglandin production and myometrial ischemia through "hypothalamic-pituitary-adrenal axis and sympathetic nervous system downregulation" [91].

Other approaches examined for their effectiveness in dysmenorrhea include oriental dance and Zumba. Zumba, an aerobics-based form of oriental dance that incorporates Latin rhythms and coordinated full-body movements, has the advantage of being less formal and involving simpler choreography compared to other group exercises [92]. In a study examining Zumba's effectiveness in dysmenorrhea, it was found that Zumba exercises were effective in reducing menstrual pain and related symptoms [93].

- Electrotherapy

The most commonly used electrotherapy modality in dysmenorrhea treatment is TENS (Transcutaneous Electrical Nerve Stimulation), which is widely used for treating acute and chronic pain conditions. TENS is a noninvasive, non-pharmacological, inexpensive, and easy-to-use treatment method. The analgesic effect in primary dysmenorrhea (PD) is based on the activation of opioid receptors in the central nervous system and the stimulation of A-beta fibers, which block pain input through the dorsal horn and reduce pain via a reflex mechanism. Additionally, the electrical stimulation of the skin leads to local axonal reflex vasodilation, increasing blood flow to the area and reducing uterine muscle ischemia. Studies have shown that high-frequency TENS (100–120 Hz) is more effective in reducing PD severity compared to low-frequency TENS (<10 Hz) and placebo groups [94].

Another electrotherapy method used in dysmenorrhea treatment is interferential current. Interferential current directly affects muscle, nerve, and cellular metabolism, increasing permeability in both intracellular and extracellular spaces, stimulating the lymphatic system, facilitating the removal of toxic metabolic waste, reducing edema, and providing analgesic effects, thus preventing tissue anoxia [95]. Literature reports that interferential current set to the same frequency (90–100 Hz) as high-frequency TENS provides similar effects in dysmenorrhea treatment [96, 97].

Although there is limited evidence in the literature, another preferred method in dysmenorrhea treatment is biofeedback. A study found that thermal biofeedback was effective in treating dysmenorrhea symptoms, especially when initiated before menstruation, and was more effective in alleviating symptoms [98]. Another study indicated that EMG biofeedback was more effective in improving symptoms in dysmenorrhea patients compared to those receiving only relaxation training [99].

- Thermotherapy

Thermotherapy approaches, which are traditional methods in dysmenorrhea treatment, include superficial and deep applications of heat and cold. Physiological changes in the body depend on various factors, such as the duration of heat application, the rate of energy transfer to tissues, and the volume of the tissue being treated.

Superficial thermotherapy (such as hot packs, infrared applications, hot towels, whirlpools, and heating pads) is commonly used in clinical practice to stimulate tissues up to 1 cm deep with a temperature range of 40–45 °C. Its effectiveness in reducing pain is comparable to or even superior to anti-inflammatories, analgesics, and exercise approaches. Deep thermotherapy methods, such as microwave diathermy and shortwave diathermy, stimulate tissues up to 2–5 cm deep by inducing local vasodilation, affecting the transmission of painful stimuli, reducing nociceptive stimulation, and decreasing prostaglandin production to alleviate muscle spasms and local ischemia due to hypoxia. Microwave diathermy, which reaches deeper tissues, directly affects the uterus and is believed to provide a stronger analgesic effect compared to superficial thermotherapy [94]. However, studies have also reported that applying superficial heat to the back and abdomen can reduce menstrual cramps and treat dysmenorrhea [100]. Akın et al. found that low-dose local heat application to the lower abdominal area was as effective as ibuprofen in relieving menstrual pain in dysmenorrhea [101].

Another thermotherapy approach studied for PD effectiveness is cold application. The literature indicates that low temperatures lead to the release of endorphins and enkephalins. As skin temperature decreases, the body's heat production mechanisms intensify, which can reduce the severity of dysmenorrhea [102].

- Kinesiotaping

Kinesiotape, a latex-free cotton-based treatment tool that mimics the properties of human skin, works by providing positional stimulus on the skin, which then stimulates cutaneous receptors. Additionally, the taping technique lifts the fascia and soft tissues in the application area, increasing the distance between the skin, muscles, and interstitial space, thus improving blood and lymphatic circulation. This effect facilitates lymphatic drainage, stimulates muscle activity, supports weak muscles, increases joint position and kinesthetic awareness, and reduces pain and tension through improved circulation [103]. In a study by Toprak Çelenay et al., kinesiotaping was found to be effective in reducing menstrual pain severity, anxiety levels, and menstrual symptoms in PD patients. They suggested that kinesiotaping could be an effective, easy, and complementary approach for alleviating pain severity and symptoms in PD treatment [104, 105].

- Manual Therapy

Connective tissue manipulation (CTM) is a manual therapy approach that can be employed in the treatment of PD. CTM is a reflexive treatment with local, segmental, and general effects where manual traction is applied to the connective tissue interfaces in the skin, stimulating the autonomic nerve endings. The goal of this treatment is to regulate the balance between the sympathetic and parasympathetic nervous systems by stimulating segmental and suprasegmental autonomic cutaneous-visceral reflexes and reducing visceral dysfunction. In this context, CTM is believed to increase uterine circulation through reflex stimulation [106]. Additionally, the mechanical stimuli applied to the skin through CTM release opioids such as enkephalins from the dorsal horn of the spinal cord, inhibiting the transmission of nociceptive signals to higher centers [107]. Studies investigating the effectiveness of CTM in dysmenorrhea have shown that it is effective in reducing menstrual pain severity and discomfort from menstrual symptoms and improving quality of life while being a noninvasive, easy-to-apply treatment widely used in clinical practice [108–110].

Classical massage is a soft tissue manipulation technique applied to promote mental relaxation, overall body relaxation, and tissue healing. Classical massage increases blood flow in the treated area, reduces muscle tension, and increases endorphin release, raising the pain threshold [111]. Aromatherapy massage, used in dysmenorrhea treatment, is a therapeutic method where essential oils are applied to the abdominal area to induce general sedation and analgesic effects. A meta-analysis examining the effects of aromatherapy massage with lavender oil on the abdomen found it to be effective in relieving menstrual pain [112].

Another manual therapy method used in dysmenorrhea treatment is musculoskeletal manipulation. The parasympathetic and sympathetic pelvic nerve pathways, particularly the spinal vertebrae related to S2–S4 and T10–L2 segments, are closely connected. Literature suggests that mechanical dysfunctions in the spinal column may contribute to the underlying causes of dysmenorrhea. This dysfunction, by increasing sympathetic stimulation, can cause vasoconstriction in the blood vessels feeding the pelvic organs, resulting in increased dysmenorrhea severity. Therefore, manipulating the levels where dysfunction occurs is thought to enhance spinal mobility and pelvic blood flow. Another theory is that referred pain from the lumbar spine, pelvis, and hips may cause pelvic pain and dysmenorrhea-related symptoms. Despite these theories, a Cochrane systematic review evaluating spinal manipulation in dysmenorrhea found no significant difference between spinal manipulation and placebo manipulation [113].

16.3.4.2.4 Surgical Treatment

Surgical methods are considered the last option for treating dysmenorrhea and are used in cases of persistent menstrual pain despite medical and other treatments. Surgical methods, such as laparoscopy, hysterectomy, presacral neurectomy, and laparoscopic uterosacral nerve ablation (LUNA), are used in appropriate cases [67]. Observational data shows that 1 year after surgery, 82% of women who underwent presacral neurectomy and 51% of women who underwent LUNA reported continued relief from menstrual pain [114].

16.3.5 Polyendocrine Metabolic Ovarian Syndrome (PMOS)

Polyendocrine metabolic ovarian syndrome (PMOS) is a heterogeneous disorder characterized by ovarian cysts, anovulation, androgen excess (hirsutism and/or hyperandrogenemia), and ovarian dysfunction, which can severely affect a woman's life. PMOS, formerly known as polycystic ovary syndrome (PCOS), was recently renamed flooring an international consensus to better reflect its multi system endocrine and metabolic nature. PMOS is the most common endocrine disorder among women of reproductive age, with an overall prevalence ranging from 6% to 20% [115]. Hormonal imbalances in LH, FSH, estrogen, and testosterone can disrupt the normal menstrual cycle, leading to menstrual irregularities such as oligomenorrhea and amenorrhea. PMOS is diagnosed by the presence of hyperandrogenism, menstrual irregularities, and varying sizes of cysts in the ovaries, although there are significant individual differences. This multifactorial condition is more likely to occur in individuals with comorbidities such as obesity, type II diabetes, infertility, endometrial dysplasia, cardiovascular disorders, and psychotic disorders [116].

Polycystic ovaries are defined as ovaries containing 12 or more follicles (ranging from 2 to 9 mm in diameter) or ovaries with a volume greater than 10 mL, as seen in ultrasonography. To diagnose polycystic ovaries, at least one of the criteria mentioned in the above consensus must be met. However, polycystic ovaries, which meet these criteria, can be found in 62% of patients with normal ovulation, and the prevalence of PMOS decreases with age [117].

Although there is no complete consensus on the diagnostic criteria for PMOS, previously referred to as PCOS in earlier international guidelines, three consensus reports have been published to date: the National Institute of Health (NIH) 1990, the Rotterdam Consensus 2003, and the AE-PCOS Definition 2006 [118]. In addition to these criteria, anti-Müllerian hormone (AMH) is also an important hormonal indicator in the diagnosis of PMOS and plays a crucial role in the maturation and development of ovarian follicles. Overproduction of AMH leads to ovarian dysfunction by inhibiting follicular development [119]. The exact etiology of PMOS is not fully understood, but it is believed to result from a complex interaction of genetic and environmental factors. One study suggests a strong correlation between familial factors and the presence of PMOS. The pathogenesis involves persistent hyperandrogenism, insulin resistance, hypothalamic-pituitary feedback dysfunction, LH hypersecretion, abnormal oocyte maturation, and the cessation of activated primary follicle secretion [118]. Among the clinical features of PMOS are short-term symptoms such as hirsutism (excessive hair growth), acne, obesity, metabolic disorders (dyslipidemia, impaired glucose tolerance), irregular menstruation, chronic anovulation (amenorrhea), and infertility. Long-term symptoms include diabetes mellitus, cardiovascular diseases, metabolic syndrome, and endometrial cancer [120].

16.3.5.1 Evaluation

In the evaluation of PMOS, the process should begin with a comprehensive history and physical examination, followed by a general cancer screening. The patient's medical history, family history, medications, previous surgeries, menstrual history, and physical findings should be recorded, and skin signs should be observed. Laboratory test results should then be reviewed, and if necessary, ultrasound or other imaging results should be considered. The evaluation should include a thorough inquiry about the individual's pregnancy status, including delivery type, baby weight, gravida, parity, history of abortion, and curettage for those who have given birth.

Since obesity is a risk factor in PMOS, the individual's dietary habits, smoking and alcohol consumption, physical activity levels, and quality of life (including sleep, anxiety, and stress levels) should be thoroughly assessed. Additionally, body fat analysis, especially abdominal fat percentage, and anthropometric measurements should be taken [115].

16.3.5.2 Treatment

PMOS is a multifaceted syndrome that affects multiple organ systems, with significant impacts on both metabolic and reproductive systems. As the etiology of PMOS is not fully understood, treatment methods are typically symptomatic. Therefore, treatment should be individualized and adapted to the patient's specific needs. Mild cases (e.g., those with mild oligomenorrhea) may not require treatment. Additionally, there are no drugs approved specifically for the treatment of PMOS. Pharmacological treatments commonly include combined oral contraceptives (COCs), anti-androgens, insulin regulators, and ovulation-inducing medications. Lifestyle changes, such as preventing or treating obesity, are also commonly recommended [118].

Treatment for PMOS should begin by educating the patient about the syndrome, associated factors, and symptoms. In the education process, visual aids may be used if necessary. Following the assessment, therapeutic methods should be explained, with discussions on lifestyle and psychological factors that can influence treatment and the disease's progression. Training should include information about the role and benefits of physical activity and exercise in PCOS, as well as potential barriers to exercise and strategies to overcome them.

Given the beneficial effects of exercise on insulin resistance-related complications, moderate-intensity exercise is thought to have a positive impact on treating PMOS. Moderate- to high-intensity aerobic exercise, defined as an intensity of 50–85% of maximum oxygen uptake (VO_2max) or 60–90% of maximum heart rate, has been shown to increase glucose disposal in the body and improve insulin sensitivity in skeletal muscles in the short term. Furthermore, moderate-intensity exercise performed three to five times a week has been shown to reduce the risk of type 2 diabetes and improve cardiovascular risk factors in high-risk groups. Studies have also demonstrated that combined aerobic exercise with resistance or weight-bearing training improves health outcomes in high-risk groups. In line with this, studies exploring treatment approaches for PMOS have found that moderate- to high-intensity exercise effectively improves PCOS symptoms [121, 122].

Mood disorders, particularly depression, are common in women with PMOS. Current guidelines recommend addressing mood and health-related quality of life during diagnosis and treatment using general and/or specific questionnaires like the PMOS scale. However, there is limited evidence in the literature supporting that treatment methods for PMOS directly improve individuals' mood and psychological well-being [123]. Yoga exercises have been frequently used as a complementary and alternative therapy in PMOS treatment due to their ability to aid weight loss, relax the body and mind, reduce stress, and enhance metabolism by improving blood circulation [124].

Another approach in PMOS treatment is lifestyle change strategies, which include reducing or eliminating smoking and alcohol consumption, restricting calorie intake or modifying the diet, and increasing physical activity levels. The aim is to promote weight loss, increase insulin sensitivity, and improve ovulation rates. However, there is no evidence in the literature that specific dietary behaviors (e.g., high-protein/low-carbohydrate diets) lead to long-term improvements in the treatment of women with PMOS. Studies indicate that for improvement in PMOS, weight loss must be sustained long-term and be maintainable [122].

16.4 Conclusion

Menstrual disorders are multifaceted conditions with significant implications for women's health and quality of life. Early and accurate diagnosis, coupled with individualized treatment plans, is essential in managing these disorders effectively. Physiotherapy and rehabilitation play a pivotal role in addressing the physical and psychological impacts of menstrual dysfunctions, offering holistic care. By integrating physiotherapeutic interventions with conventional medical treatments, healthcare professionals can enhance the overall well-being and functional capacity of affected individuals, underscoring the importance of a multidisciplinary approach in managing menstrual health.

Competing Interests The authors declare no conflict of interest.

References

1. Golden NH, Carlson JL. The pathophysiology of amenorrhea in the adolescent. Ann N Y Acad Sci. 2008;1135(1):163–78.
2. Karanisoğlu H, Dinç H. Üreme organ yapı ve fonksiyon bozuklukları. İçinde: Coşkun A editör Kadın sağlığı ve hastalıkları hemsireliği el kitabı. 2012;1:435.
3. Clark VL, Kruse JA. Clinical methods: the history, physical, and laboratory examinations. JAMA. 1990;264(21):2808–9.
4. Akbayrak T, Kaya S. Kadın sağlığında fizyoterapi ve rehabilitasyon. Baskı, Ankara, Kalkan Matbaacılık; 2016, pp. 141–166
5. Deligeoroglou E, Tsimaris P, Deliveliotou A, Christopoulos P, Creatsas G. Menstrual disorders during adolescence. Pediatr Endocrinol Rev. 2006;3:150–9.
6. Organization WH. Multicenter study on menstrual and ovulatory patterns in adolescent girls II. Longitudinal study of menstrual patterns in the early postmenarcheal period, duration of bleeding episodes and menstrual cycles. J Adolesc Health. 1986;7:236–44.
7. Caufriez A. Menstrual disorders in adolescence: pathophysiology and treatment. Horm Res Paediatr. 1991;36(3–4):156–9.
8. Critchley HO, Babayev E, Bulun SE, Clark S, Garcia-Grau I, Gregersen PK, Kilcoyne A, Kim JJ, Lavender M, Marsh EE. Menstruation: science and society. Am J Obstet Gynecol. 2020;
9. Dean BB, Gerner D, Gerner RH. A systematic review evaluating health-related quality of life, work impairment, and healthcare costs and utilization in bipolar disorder. Curr Med Res Opin. 2004;20(2):139–54.
10. Fraser IS, Bonnar J, Peyvandi F. Requirements for research investigations to clarify the relationships and management of menstrual abnormalities in women with hemostatic disorders. Fertil Steril. 2005;84(5):1360–5.
11. Munro MG, Critchley HO, Broder MS, Fraser IS. FIGO classification system (PALM-COEIN) for causes of abnormal uterine bleeding in nongravid women of reproductive age. Int J Gynecol Obstet. 2011;113(1):3–13.
12. Care ACoAH. Menstruation in girls and adolescents: using the menstrual cycle as a vital sign. Obstet Gynecol. 2006;108(5):1323–8.
13. Foster C, Al-Zubeidi H. Menstrual irregularities. Pediatr Ann. 2018;47(1):e23–8.
14. Gülbala NAKİP TrA. Vajinismus Tedavisinde Fizyoterapi ve Rehabilitasyon. In: Karaduman PDA, Ülger DDÖ, Yağlı DDNV, Kılınç YDDM, ARSLAN DFSS (eds) Fizyoterapi Seminerleri, vol 1; 2017. p 57.
15. Deligeoroglou E. Dysfunctional uterine bleeding. Ann N Y Acad Sci. 1997;816:158–64.
16. Deligeoroglou E, Creatsas G. Menstrual disorders. Pediatr Adolesc Gynecol. 2012;22:160–70.
17. Bachmann GA, Kemmann E. Prevalence of oligomenorrhea and amenorrhea in a college population. Am J Obstet Gynecol. 1982;144(1):98–102.
18. Breech L. Menstruation in girls and adolescents: using the menstrual cycle as a vital sign. ACOG Committee opinion. Obstet Gynecol. 2006:1323–8.
19. Hickey M, Balen A. Menstrual disorders in adolescence: investigation and management. Hum Reprod Update. 2003;9(5):493–504.
20. Medicine PCotASfR. Current evaluation of amenorrhea. Fertil Steril. 2006;86(5):S148–55.
21. Chamberlain R. The female athlete triad: recommendations for management. Am Fam Physician. 2018;97(8):499–502.
22. Klein DA, Poth MA. Amenorrhea: an approach to diagnosis and management. Am Fam Physician. 2013;87(11):781–8.
23. American Psychiatric Association. Diagnostic and statistical manual of mental disorders, vol. 3. Washington: American Psychiatric Association; 1980.
24. Frisch RE, McArthur JW. Menstrual cycles: fatness as a determinant of minimum weight for height necessary for their maintenance or onset. Science. 1974;185(4155):949–51.
25. Miller PB. Infrequent menstrual bleeding and amenorrhea during the reproductive years. In: Disorders of menstruation; 2011. p. 124–38.
26. Gray SH, Emans SJ. Abnormal vaginal bleeding in adolescents. Pediatr Rev. 2007;28(5):175.
27. Arends JC, Cheung M-YC, Barrack MT, Nattiv A. Restoration of menses with nonpharmacologic therapy in college athletes with menstrual disturbances: a 5-year retrospective study. Int J Sport Nutr Exerc Metab. 2012;22(2):98–108.
28. Nichols JF, Rauh MJ, Lawson MJ, Ji M, Barkai H-S. Prevalence of the female athlete triad syndrome among high school athletes. Arch Pediatr Adolesc Med. 2006;160(2):137–42.
29. Pantano KJ. Strategies used by physical therapists in the US for treatment and prevention of the female athlete triad. Phys Ther Sport. 2009;10(1):3–11.
30. Nattiv A, Loucks AB, Manore MM, Sanborn C, Sundgot-Borgen J, Warren M. The female athlete triad. American College of Sports Medicine position stand. Med Sci Sports Exerc. 2007;39(10):1867–82.
31. Kırcan N, Ergin F, Adana F, Arslantaş H Hemşirelik öğrencilerinde premenstrüel sendrom prevalansı ve yaşam kalitesi ile ilişkisi; 2012
32. Stevinson C, Ernst E. Complementary/alternative therapies for premenstrual syndrome: a systematic review of randomized controlled trials. Am J Obstet Gynecol. 2001;185(1):227–35.

33. Mortola JF. Premenstrual syndrome – pathophysiologic considerations. Mass Medical Soc. 1998;338:256.
34. Chrousos GP, Torpy DJ, Gold PW. Interactions between the hypothalamic-pituitary-adrenal axis and the female reproductive system: clinical implications. Ann Intern Med. 1998;129(3):229–40.
35. Hofmeister S, Bodden S. Premenstrual syndrome and premenstrual dysphoric disorder. Am Fam Physician. 2016;94(3):236–40.
36. Tsai S-Y. Effect of yoga exercise on premenstrual symptoms among female employees in Taiwan. Int J Environ Res Public Health. 2016;13(7):721.
37. Bosman RC, Jung SE, Miloserdov K, Schoevers RA. Daily symptom ratings for studying premenstrual dysphoric disorder: a review. J Affect Disord. 2016;189:43–53.
38. Kloss BA, Marcom LA, Odom AM, Tuggle CL. PMS treatment through the use of CAM. Int J Childbirth Educ. 2012;27(3):60.
39. Taavoni S, Barkhordari F, Goushegir A, Haghani H. Effect of Royal Jelly on premenstrual syndrome among Iranian medical sciences students: a randomized, triple-blind, placebo-controlled study. Complement Ther Med. 2014;22(4):601–6.
40. Tolossa FW, Bekele ML. Prevalence, impacts and medical managements of premenstrual syndrome among female students: cross-sectional study in college of health sciences, Mekelle University, Mekelle, Northern Ethiopia. BMC Womens Health. 2014;14(1):1–9.
41. Dehghani M, Emami M, Ghamkhar L. The effects of 3 months of regular aerobic exercise on premenstrual syndrome symptoms. J Med Sci Rafsanjan. 2008;7:89–98.
42. Craft LL, Perna FM. The benefits of exercise for the clinically depressed. Primary care Compan J Clin Psychiatry. 2004;6(3):104.
43. Kamalifard M, Yavari A, Asghari-Jafarabadi M, Ghaffarilaleh G, Kasb-Khah A. The effect of yoga on women's premenstrual syndrome: a randomized controlled clinical trial. Int J Women's Health Reproduc Sci. 2017;5(3):205–11.
44. Vaghela N, Mishra D, Sheth M, Dani VB. To compare the effects of aerobic exercise and yoga on premenstrual syndrome. J Educ Health Promotion. 2019;8:199.
45. Taylor D. Perimenstrual symptoms and syndromes: guidelines for symptom management and self-care. Adv Stud Med. 2005;5(5):228–41.
46. Carroquino-Garcia P, Jiménez-Rejano JJ, Medrano-Sanchez E, De La Casa-Almeida M, Diaz-Mohedo E, Suarez-Serrano C. Therapeutic exercise in the treatment of primary dysmenorrhea: a systematic review and meta-analysis. Phys Ther. 2019;99(10):1371–80.
47. Unsal A, Ayranci U, Tozun M, Arslan G, Calik E. Prevalence of dysmenorrhea and its effect on quality of life among a group of female university students. Ups J Med Sci. 2010;115(2):138–45.
48. Obstetricians ACo, Gynecologists. Dysmenorrhea and endometriosis in the adolescent. ACOG Committee opinion no. 760. Obstet Gynecol. 2018;132(6):e249–58.
49. Zannoni L, Giorgi M, Spagnolo E, Montanari G, Villa G, Seracchioli R. Dysmenorrhea, absenteeism from school, and symptoms suspicious for endometriosis in adolescents. J Pediatr Adolesc Gynecol. 2014;27(5):258–65.
50. Ferries-Rowe E, Corey E, Archer JS. Primary dysmenorrhea: diagnosis and therapy. Obstet Gynecol. 2020;136(5):1047–58.
51. Wong LP. Attitudes towards dysmenorrhoea, impact and treatment seeking among adolescent girls: a rural school-based survey. Aust J Rural Health. 2011;19(4):218–23.
52. Pulkkinen M. Prostaglandins and the non-pregnant uterus the pathophysiology of primary dysmenorrhea. Acta Obstet Gynecol Scand. 1983;62(sup113):63–7.
53. Dmitrović R. Transvaginal color Doppler study of uterine blood flow in primary dysmenorrhea. Acta Obstetricia et Gynecologica Scandinavica: ORIGINAL ARTICLE. 2000;79(12):1112–6.
54. Banikarim C, Geffner M, Blake D, Hoppin A. Primary dysmenorrhea in adolescents. UpToDate; 2015
55. Deligeoroglou E. Dysmenorrhea. Ann N Y Acad Sci. 2000;900(1):237–44.
56. Porpora M, Koninckx P, Piazze J, Natili M, Colagrande S, Cosmi E. Correlation between endometriosis and pelvic pain. J Am Assoc Gynecol Laparosc. 1999;6(4):429–34.
57. Silva GPOG, Nascimento AL, Michelazzo D, et al. High prevalence of chronic pelvic pain in women in Ribeirão Preto, Brazil and direct association with abdominal surgery. Clinics. 2011;66(8):1307–12.
58. Çinar GN, Akbayrak T, Gürşen C, Baran E, Üzelpasacı E, Nakip G, Bozdağ G, Beksaç MS, Özgül S. Factors related to primary dysmenorrhea in Turkish women: a multiple multinomial logistic regression analysis. Reprod Sci. 2021;28(2):381–92.
59. Latthe P, Mignini L, Gray R, Hills R, Khan K. Factors predisposing women to chronic pelvic pain: systematic review. BMJ. 2006;332(7544):749–55.
60. Boerner KE, Chambers CT, McGrath PJ, LoLordo V, Uher R. The effect of parental modeling on child pain responses: the role of parent and child sex. J Pain. 2017;18(6):702–15.
61. Wei S-M, Schiller CE, Schmidt PJ, Rubinow DR. The role of ovarian steroids in affective disorders. Curr Opin Behav Sci. 2018;23:103–12.
62. Li R, Li B, Kreher DA, Benjamin AR, Gubbels A, Smith SM. Association between dysmenorrhea and chronic pain: a systematic review and meta-analysis of population-based studies. Am J Obstet Gynecol. 2020;223:350.
63. Proctor M, Farquhar C. Diagnosis and management of dysmenorrhoea. BMJ. 2006;332(7550):1134–8.
64. Huang Q-M, Liu L. Wet needling of myofascial trigger points in abdominal muscles for treat-

ment of primary dysmenorrhoea. Acupunct Med. 2014;32(4):346–9.
65. Burnett MA, Antao V, Black A, Feldman K, Grenville A, Lea R, Lefebvre G, Pinsonneault O, Robert M. Prevalence of primary dysmenorrhea in Canada. J Obstet Gynaecol Can. 2005;27(8):765–70.
66. Campbell MA, McGrath PJ. Use of medication by adolescents for the management of menstrual discomfort. Arch Pediatr Adolesc Med. 1997;151(9):905–13.
67. Burnett M, Lemyre M. No. 345-primary dysmenorrhea consensus guideline. J Obstet Gynaecol Can. 2017;39(7):585–95.
68. Harel Z. Dysmenorrhea in adolescents and young adults: etiology and management. J Pediatr Adolesc Gynecol. 2006;19(6):363–71.
69. Jun E-M, Chang S, Kang D-H, Kim S. Effects of acupressure on dysmenorrhea and skin temperature changes in college students: a non-randomized controlled trial. Int J Nurs Stud. 2007;44(6):973–81.
70. Chen M-N, Chien L-W, Liu C-F. Acupuncture or acupressure at the Sanyinjiao (SP6) acupoint for the treatment of primary dysmenorrhea: a meta-analysis. Evid Based Complement Alternat Med. 2013;
71. Mirbagher-Ajorpaz N, Adib-Hajbaghery M, Mosaebi F. The effects of acupressure on primary dysmenorrhea: a randomized controlled trial. Complement Ther Clin Pract. 2011;17(1):33–6.
72. Kannan P, Claydon LS. Some physiotherapy treatments may relieve menstrual pain in women with primary dysmenorrhea: a systematic review. J Physiother. 2014;60(1):13–21.
73. Proctor M, Murphy PA. Herbal and dietary therapies for primary and secondary dysmenorrhoea. Cochrane Database Syst Rev. 2001;2
74. Demirturk F, Gungor T, Demirturk F, Akbayrak T, Aker EM. Relief of primary dysmenorrhea by supplementation with omega-3 fatty acids. Pain Clinic. 2002;14(1):81–4.
75. Hudson T. Using nutrition to relieve primary dysmenorrhea. Altern Complement Ther. 2007;13(3):125–8.
76. Ozerdogan N, Sayiner D, Ayranci U, Unsal A, Giray S. Prevalence and predictors of dysmenorrhea among students at a university in Turkey. Int J Gynecol Obstet. 2009;107(1):39–43.
77. Ziaei S, Zakeri M, Kazemnejad A. A randomised controlled trial of vitamin E in the treatment of primary dysmenorrhoea. BJOG Int J Obstet Gynaecol. 2005;112(4):466–9.
78. Fontana-Klaiber H, Hogg B. Therapeutic effects of magnesium in dysmenorrhea. Schweizerische Rundschau fur Medizin Praxis. 1990;79(16):491–4.
79. Tseng Y-F, Chen C-H, Yang Y-H. Rose tea for relief of primary dysmenorrhea in adolescents: a randomized controlled trial in Taiwan. J Midwifery Womens Health. 2005;50(5):e51–7.
80. Wilson M, Murphy PA, Pattison HM, Farquhar CM. Behavioural interventions for primary and secondary dysmenorrhoea. Cochrane Database Syst Rev. 2000;3
81. Ernst E, Posadzki P, Lee M. Reflexology: an update of a systematic review of randomised clinical trials. Maturitas. 2011;68(2):116–20.
82. Valiani M, Babaei E, Heshmat R, Zare Z. Comparing the effects of reflexology methods and ibuprofen administration on dysmenorrhea in female students of Isfahan University of Medical Sciences. Iran J Nurs Midwifery Res. 2010;15(Suppl1):371.
83. Koltyn KF, Brellenthin AG, Cook DB, Sehgal N, Hillard C. Mechanisms of exercise-induced hypoalgesia. J Pain. 2014;15(12):1294–304.
84. Naugle KM, Fillingim RB, Riley JL III. A meta-analytic review of the hypoalgesic effects of exercise. J Pain. 2012;13(12):1139–50.
85. Schwarz L, Kindermann W. Changes in β-endorphin levels in response to aerobic and anaerobic exercise. Sports Med. 1992;13(1):25–36.
86. Sprouse-Blum AS, Smith G, Sugai D, Parsa FD. Understanding endorphins and their importance in pain management. Hawaii Med J. 2010;69(3):70.
87. Ortiz MI, Cortés-Márquez SK, Romero-Quezada LC, Murguía-Cánovas G, Jaramillo-Díaz AP. Effect of a physiotherapy program in women with primary dysmenorrhea. Eur J Obstet Gynecol Reprod Biol. 2015;194:24–9.
88. Brown J, Brown S. WITHDRAWN: exercise for dysmenorrhoea. Cochrane Database Syst Rev. 2017;2:CD004142-CD004142.
89. Abbaspour Z, Rostami M, Najjar S. The effect of exercise on primary dysmenorrhea. J Res Health Sci. 2006;6(1):26–31.
90. McGovern CE, Cheung C. Yoga and quality of life in women with primary dysmenorrhea: a systematic review. J Midwifery Womens Health. 2018;63(4):470–82.
91. Kanojia S, Sharma VK, Gandhi A, Kapoor R, Kukreja A, Subramanian SK. Effect of yoga on autonomic functions and psychological status during both phases of menstrual cycle in young healthy females. J Clin Diagn Res. 2013;7(10):2133.
92. Luettgen M, Foster C, Doberstein S, Mikat R, Porcari J. ZUMBA®: is the "fitness-party" a good workout? J Sports Sci Med. 2012;11(2):357.
93. Samy A, Zaki SS, Metwally AA, Mahmoud DSE, Elzahaby IM, Amin AH, Eissa AI, Abbas AM, Hussein AH, Talaat B. The effect of zumba exercise on reducing menstrual pain in young women with primary dysmenorrhea: a randomized controlled trial. J Pediatr Adolesc Gynecol. 2019;32(5):541–5.
94. Machado AFP, Perracini MR, Rampazo ÉP, Driusso P, Liebano RE. Effects of thermotherapy and transcutaneous electrical nerve stimulation on patients with primary dysmenorrhea: a randomized, placebo-controlled, double-blind clinical trial. Complement Ther Med. 2019;47:102188.
95. Kitchen S, Bazin S, Bellis E (2002) Electrotherapy: evidence-based practice.
96. Tugay N, Akbayrak T, Demirtürk F, Karakaya İIÇ, Kocaacar Ö, Tugay U, Karakaya MG, Demirtürk F. Effectiveness of transcutaneous electrical nerve

stimulation and interferential current in primary dysmenorrhea. Pain Med. 2007;8(4):295–300.
97. Ziaei S, Faghihzadeh S, Sohrabvand F, Lamyian M, Emamgholy T. A randomised placebo-controlled trial to determine the effect of vitamin E in treatment of primary dysmenorrhoea. BJOG Int J Obstet Gynaecol. 2001;108(11):1181–3.
98. Balick L, Elfner L, May J, Moore JD. Biofeedback treatment of dysmenorrhea. Biofeedback Self Regul. 1982;7(4):499–520.
99. Bennink CD, Hulst LL, Benthem JA. The effects of EMG biofeedback and relaxation training on primary dysmenorrhea. J Behav Med. 1982;5(3):329–41.
100. Polden M. Pain relief in obstetrics and gynaecology. In: Pain management by physiotherapy. London: Butterworth Heineman; 1994.
101. Akin MD, Weingand KW, Hengehold DA, Goodale MB, Hinkle RT, Smith RP. Continuous low-level topical heat in the treatment of dysmenorrhea. Obstet Gynecol. 2001;97(3):343–9.
102. Gerzson LR, Padilha JF, Braz MM, Gasparetto A. Physiotherapy in primary dysmenorrhea: literature review. Revista Dor. 2014;15(4):290–5.
103. Wallis J, Kase T, Kase K (2003) Clinical therapeutic applications of the kinesio taping method.
104. Celenay ST, Kavalci B, Karakus A, Alkan A. Effects of kinesio tape application on pain, anxiety, and menstrual complaints in women with primary dysmenorrhea: a randomized sham-controlled trial. Complement Ther Clin Pract. 2020;39:101148.
105. Doğan H, Eroğlu S, Akbayrak T. The effect of kinesio taping and lifestyle changes on pain, body awareness and quality of life in primary dysmenorrhea. Complement Ther Clin Pract. 2020;39:101120.
106. Jamieson DJ, Steege JF. The prevalence of dysmenorrhea, dyspareunia, pelvic pain, and irritable bowel syndrome in primary care practices. Obstet Gynecol. 1996;87(1):55–8.
107. Melzack R, Wall PD. On the nature of cutaneous sensory mechanisms. Brain. 1962;85(2):331–56.
108. Demirtürk F, Yilar Erkek Z, Alparslan Ö, Demirtürk F, Demir O, Inanir A. Comparison of reflexology and connective tissue manipulation in participants with primary dysmenorrhea. J Altern Complement Med. 2016;22(1):38–44.
109. Özgül S, Üzelpasaci E, Orhan C, Baran E, Beksaç MS, Akbayrak T. Short-term effects of connective tissue manipulation in women with primary dysmenorrhea: a randomized controlled trial. Complement Ther Clin Pract. 2018;33:1–6.
110. Reis CAAS, Hardy E, Sousa MH. The effectiveness of connective tissue massage in the treatment of primary dysmenorrhea among young women. Revista Brasileira de Saúde Materno Infantil. 2010;10:247–56.
111. Apay SE, Arslan S, Akpinar RB, Celebioglu A. Effect of aromatherapy massage on dysmenorrhea in Turkish students. Pain Manag Nurs. 2012;13(4):236–40.
112. Sut N, Kahyaoglu-Sut H. Effect of aromatherapy massage on pain in primary dysmenorrhea: a meta-analysis. Complement Ther Clin Pract. 2017;27:5–10.
113. Proctor M, Hing W, Johnson TC, Murphy PA. Spinal manipulation for primary and secondary dysmenorrhoea. Cochrane Database Syst Rev. 2001;4
114. Proctor M, Latthe P, Farquhar C, Khan K, Johnson N. Surgical interruption of pelvic nerve pathways for primary and secondary dysmenorrhoea. Cochrane Database Syst Rev. 2005;4
115. Escobar-Morreale HF. Polycystic ovary syndrome: definition, aetiology, diagnosis and treatment. Nat Rev Endocrinol. 2018;14(5):270–84.
116. Kite C, Lahart IM, Afzal I, Broom DR, Randeva H, Kyrou I, Brown JE. Exercise, or exercise and diet for the management of polycystic ovary syndrome: a systematic review and meta-analysis. Syst Rev. 2019;8(1):1–28.
117. Johnstone EB, Rosen MP, Neril R, Trevithick D, Sternfeld B, Murphy R, Addauan-Andersen C, McConnell D, Pera RR, Cedars MI. The polycystic ovary post-Rotterdam: a common, age-dependent finding in ovulatory women without metabolic significance. J Clin Endocrinol Metabol. 2010;95(11):4965–72.
118. Williams T, Mortada R, Porter S. Diagnosis and treatment of polycystic ovary syndrome. Am Fam Physician. 2016;94(2):106–13.
119. Bulsara JP, Patel P, Soni A, Acharya S. A review on brief insight into polycystic ovarian syndrome. Endocrine Metabolic Sci. 2021:100085.
120. Palomba S, Daolio J, La Sala GB. Oocyte competence in women with polycystic ovary syndrome. Trends Endocrinol Metabol. 2017;28(3):186–98.
121. Dos Santos IK, Ashe MC, Cobucci RN, Soares GM, de Oliveira Maranhão TM, Dantas PMS. The effect of exercise as an intervention for women with polycystic ovary syndrome: a systematic review and meta-analysis. Medicine. 2020;99(16)
122. Harrison CL, Lombard CB, Moran LJ, Teede HJ. Exercise therapy in polycystic ovary syndrome: a systematic review. Hum Reprod Update. 2011;17(2):171–83.
123. Conway G, Dewailly D, Diamanti-Kandarakis E, Escobar-Morreale HF, Franks S, Gambineri A, Kelestimur F, Macut D, Micic D, Pasquali R. The polycystic ovary syndrome; a position statement from the European Society of Endocrinology. Eur J Endocrinol. 2014;171(4):P1–P29.
124. Thakur D, Singh SS, Tripathi M. Effect of yoga on polycystic ovarian syndrome: a systematic review. J Bodyw Mov Ther. 2021;

17 Physiotherapy and Rehabilitation in Sexual Dysfunctions

Hanife Doğan and Hanife Abakay

17.1 Introduction

Sexual function is a multifaceted process including various anatomical, physiological, psychological, emotional, and interpersonal components [1, 2]. Sexuality includes the functions of sexual organs, perception of sexual functions, sexual expressions, and preferences [3]. Sexual dysfunction (SD) is a problem in any of the physiological processes in the desire, arousal, and orgasm phases of the sexual response cycle in humans" [4, 5]. Physiotherapists specialized in the field of women's/men's health are included in the multidisciplinary team that provides training related to sexual function, plans and teaches pelvic floor rehabilitation combined with cognitive behavioral therapy, and provides adequate functionality for sexual function [6].

H. Doğan (✉)
Department of Physiotherapy and Rehabilitation, Faculty of Health Sciences, Necmettin Erbakan University, Konya, Türkiye

H. Abakay
Incesu Ayşe and Saffet Arslan Health Services Vocational School, Kayseri University, Kayseri, Türkiye

17.2 Sexual Dysfunction in Women

17.2.1 Normal Sexual Response Cycle in Women

Sexual response phases in women consist of four phases, including arousal, plateau, orgasm, and resolution [7]:

17.2.1.1 Arousal Phase

The arousal phase, which is the first phase of the sexual response process in women, may occur as a result of any somatogenic and psychogenic stimulation [8]. It is basically characterized by the emergence of erotic feelings and thoughts, the emergence of vaginal lubrication in the woman, and pelvic vasocongestion and myotonia in the body. Increases in sympathetic activity cause increased vascular blood flow to the genitals, leading to physical swelling of the vulva, clitoris, and vagina; increased temperature and secretions; and relaxation of the pelvic floor, resulting in increased pudendal and genitofemoral nerve conduction [9].

17.2.1.2 Plato Phase

The plateau phase is a continuation of the arousal phase. With the continuation of effective sexual stimulation and the increase in sexual excitement, the woman enters the plateau phase, the second phase. With increasing congestion, dilata-

T. Akbayrak, E. Üzelpasaci (eds.), *Physiotherapy and Rehabilitation in Pelvic and Women's Health-Related Problems*, https://doi.org/10.1007/978-3-032-28741-0_17

tion of the clitoris occurs with the contraction of the ischiocavernous and bulbocavernous muscles. In this phase, areolae become darker, and vaginal dilatation and lubrication levels increase more with the activation of Bartholin glands [10].

17.2.1.3 Orgasm Phase

It is the third phase in which sexual tension is released. Involuntary rhythmic contractions of the pelvic floor muscles release tension and positive emotions with the reduction of vasocongestion. In orgasm, three to five contractions may occur, or more contractions may occur [10]. Women can reach orgasm by various methods, most commonly direct clitoral and vaginal stimulation, but it is also included in the literature that they may rarely experience orgasm through breast/nipple stimulation, mental imaging, fantasy, and hypnosis [11].

17.2.1.4 Thawing Phase

A few seconds after the orgasm phase, vasocongestion and contractions begin to decrease rapidly. Whole-body responses such as muscle tension, heart rate, blood pressure, and respiratory rate are the last phase, rapidly returning to pre-orgasmic levels unless there is further sexual stimulation [2, 10].

17.2.2 Sexual Dysfunctions in Women

The International Association for the Study of Women's Sexual Health has categorized sexual dysfunctions into four categories: sexual desire disorders, sexual arousal disorders, orgasm disorders, and sexual pain disorders [5, 12, 13].

17.2.2.1 Sexual Desire Disorders

17.2.2.1.1 Hypoactive Sexual Desire Disorder

It is defined as a permanent or recurrent loss of sexual thoughts or fantasies and/or an inability to initiate, participate in, or respond to a sexual activity in a way that causes personal distress [14]. Spontaneous menopause, surgical menopause, or disruption in hormonal balance caused by endocrine disorders may also lead to inhibition of sexual desire [13].

17.2.2.1.2 Sexual Aversion Disorder

It is the state of feeling phobic disgust and avoidance of sexual intercourse with a partner permanently or repetitively, and this state causes personal distress [10]. In DSM-IV, it is defined as feeling extreme disgust for having genital sexual intercourse with a sexual partner continuously or repetitively and avoiding it completely [14].

17.2.2.1.3 Sexual Arousal Disorders

It is a permanent or repetitive condition characterized by the absence of subjective excitement, genital (lubrication/swelling) or other somatic responses, and the inability to reach or maintain adequate sexual excitement, and this condition causes personal problems [15]. Sexual arousal disorders may cause individuals to experience distress and have difficulty in interpersonal relationships [16]. Natural menopause, surgical menopause, medical menopause, and endocrine disorders may cause arousal disorders. Arousal problems can be seen at any age, and it has been shown in the literature that they increase with age [17].

17.2.2.1.4 Orgasm Disorders

It is the state of continuous or recurrent difficulty, delay, or absence of orgasm following an adequate sexual stimulation and arousal phase, and this situation causes personal distress. According to DSM-IV, orgasm disorder is defined as a persistent or recurrent delay or absence of orgasm following the normal sexual arousal phase. This condition may occur after surgeries, trauma, or hormonal failure [15].

17.2.2.1.5 Sexual Pain Disorders

- *Dyspareunia*

It is defined as recurrent or persistent genital pain during sexual intercourse. Dyspareunia includes genital pain disorders and is commonly observed in the premenopausal population [18].

Postpartum episiotomy scars, adhesions following urogenital surgical procedures, neuropathic changes, genetic or immune factors, chronic pelvic pain, hypertonus of the pelvic floor, postmenopausal vaginal atrophy and dryness, and urinary system infections such as cystitis may cause dyspareunia [19, 20].

- *Vaginismus*

It is a state of involuntary contraction of the muscles of the distal one third part of the vagina in a way that prevents vaginal penetration and this causes personal distress [15]. In DSM-IV, vaginismus is classified as a sexual dysfunction and included in the subcategory of sexual pain disorders. Sexual trauma, sexually transmitted diseases, endometriosis, hymenal and congenital abnormalities, traumas after genital surgery or radiotherapy, vaginal atrophy, endometriosis, urinary incontinence, pelvic organ prolapse, pelvic inflammatory diseases, hypertonic pelvic floor, chronic pelvic pain, and vaginal lesions may cause vaginismus [21].

17.2.3 Etiology of Sexual Dysfunction in Women

17.2.3.1 Age and Menopause

With advancing age and menopause, atrophy in the smooth muscles of the vaginal wall and estrogen deficiency in the vaginal tissues may lead to deterioration of the erection of the clitoris and enlargement of the vagina; decrease in vaginal secretions and vaginal dryness; and desire, arousal, orgasm, and vaginal lubrication disorders in women. In addition, a decrease in vaginal and rectal contractions, pain during sexual intercourse, and bleeding afterwards may be observed [22].

17.2.3.2 Vascular Causes

Atherosclerosis of the iliohypogastric and pudendal arteries, impaired genital blood flow due to trauma or hormonal causes, and clitoral and vaginal vascular insufficiency can be seen. Hypertension, hypercholesterolemia, smoking, pelvic surgery, trauma, iliohypogastric pudendal artery injury, myocardial infarction, and diabetes, which are considered among the vascular causes of sexual dysfunction, may cause fibrosis in the smooth muscle tissue of the vaginal wall and clitoris. Accordingly, sexual dysfunctions such as dryness in sexual intercourse, pain, inability to orgasm, sexual arousal disorder, and sexual reluctance may be observed [23, 24].

17.2.3.3 Neurological Causes

In studies, it has been reported that spinal cord injuries, multiple sclerosis, and central and peripheral nervous system diseases, which are among the causes of sexual dysfunction, negatively affect sexual desire, arousal, orgasm, and lubrication. Psychosocial problems such as deterioration in body image, performance anxiety, and fear of rejection that develop with these diseases are also reported to affect sexual life negatively [25].

17.2.3.4 Hormonal Causes

Estrogen, androgens, and progesterone are hormones that have a direct effect on sexual function in women by causing changes in nerve transmission and sensory perception, peripheral blood flow, muscle tone, and capacity. Decreased levels of these hormones in the blood, long-term use of contraceptives that cause hormonal changes, a decrease in the level of estrogen seen with menopause, and atrophy of vaginal smooth muscles cause negative effects at various stages of sexual activity [22, 26].

17.2.3.5 Pregnancy and Labor

Sexual activity in pregnancy is affected by physical and emotional changes as well as sexual beliefs [27]. Studies on sexual function in pregnancy have shown that there is a slight decrease in sexual desire and sexual activity in the first trimester and a steep decrease in the third trimester, but there is a great variability in the second trimester. In the first year after birth, coital frequency decreases in most couples [15]. During the 6–8 weeks after birth and during breastfeeding, sexual arousability decreases due to low estrogen levels, the vaginal wall becomes thinner, and a decrease in the frequency and intensity of orgasm may be observed. This condition is reported to persist for 12 months and longer after birth [28].

17.2.3.6 Pelvic Floor Dysfunctions

The pelvic floor, levator ani, bulbocavernous, and ischiocavernous muscles, which have a direct effect on sexual function, regulate the motor response during coitus and orgasm, and the strength of these muscles increases lubrication, arousal, and orgasm. While excessive tonus increase in these muscles causes genito-pelvic pain/penetration disorders, hypotonia in these muscles may lead to vaginal sensitivity, a decrease in orgasm intensity, and coital incontinence [18].

Coital incontinence may be a result of decreased frequency of sexual activity, experiencing fear of leakage, wearing pads during the night, or feeling unattractive [29]. Symptomatic POP has been reported to negatively affect personal hygiene, sexual function, quality of life, and psychological status [30].

17.2.3.7 Psychological Causes

Studies have shown that some drugs used for anxiety, depression, decreased sense of self, body image, general relationship quality between partners, benzodiazepines, and selective serotonin receptor inhibitors affect sexual life [26, 31, 32].

17.2.3.8 Surgical Interventions

The negative effects of surgical interventions such as mastectomy, hysterectomy, and vulvectomy on women's body image and self-esteem, causing many physiological, hormonal, and structural changes, may lead to sexual dysfunction [33–36].

17.2.4 Evaluation of Female Sexual Dysfunction

The first step in the evaluation of female sexual dysfunction is to take a comprehensive physical, demographic, obstetric, gynecological, medical, and sexual activity history [24]. The presence of vulvovaginal or pelvic pain, itching, dryness, or discharge; urinary or fecal incontinence; and pelvic organ prolapse should be questioned in terms of sexual function. In addition, obstetric characteristics such as number of births, mode of delivery, and birth weight should also be questioned [11].

17.2.4.1 Sexual Function Questionnaires

Scales with Turkish validity and reliability can be used to evaluate the effect of subjective sexual function and sexual function on the quality of life. The Female Sexual Function Index (FSFI), Female Sexual Distress Scale, Pelvic Organ Prolapse/Incontinence Sexual Questionnaire (Pelvic Organ Prolapse/Incontinence Sexual Questionnaire-12, PISQ-12), McCoy's Female Sexual Function Questionnaire in menopausal women, and Pregnancy Sexual Response Inventory (PSRI) in pregnancy are among the questionnaires that can be used in the clinic [15, 37–41].

17.2.4.2 Musculoskeletal Assessment

Generally, anxious body language and frequent breathing patterns, decreased thoracic and diaphragmatic movements, decreased pelvic joint mobility, and shortening of the hip and pelvic muscles can be observed in patients with SD [22]. Evaluation of the strength and flexibility of the iliopsoas, gluteal muscles, quadratus lumborum, obturator internus, and piriformis muscles associated with pelvic floor dysfunction is especially important in pelvic pain/penetration disorder [19, 20].

17.2.4.3 Evaluation of the Pelvic Floor

After the evaluation of the musculoskeletal system and connective tissue is completed, a specific pelvic evaluation should be performed. Especially women with severe vaginismus are prone to fear, anxiety, and behavioral escape behaviors during pelvic evaluations [42].

In women, mucosal integrity, atrophy, and the presence of a birth-related scar or episiotomy-related incision should be considered. It is recommended to observe the pelvic floor with straining to determine paradoxical contractions, perineal edema, and prolapse [43].

Pelvic floor muscle strength can be evaluated by vaginal palpation, the force of contraction felt around the therapist's finger, whether there is a palpable elevation of the finger, the number of contractions, and the duration of the contraction with the modified Oxford grading system [43].

17.2.5 Physiotherapy and Rehabilitation Approaches in Female Sexual Dysfunction

The treatment aims to correct the factors that cause sexual dysfunction specific to each individual. Physiotherapists usually create a multimodal treatment plan including manual therapy techniques, relaxation training, pain management, pelvic floor rehabilitation, and physical modalities, as well as patient education [44].

17.2.5.1 Patient Education

In patient education, pelvic models are preferred to teach the location of the genitals and pelvic floor muscles, the physiology of the sexual cycle, and pelvic floor contraction and relaxation. After the training given with models and visual materials, it can be ensured that the patient examines the anatomical position of the genital organs, especially the clitoris and vaginal introitus, with the help of a mirror and desensitizes the painful or anxious areas by touching [18]. Lifestyle modifications include behavioral changes related to factors such as physical inactivity, unhealthy diet, weight gain, smoking, and alcohol addiction, which may contribute to SD [44, 45].

17.2.5.2 Posture Training and Treatment of Musculoskeletal Problems

Musculoskeletal problems such as excessive increase in lumbar lordosis, increase in anterior pelvic tilt of the pelvis, decreased hip internal rotation, shortened iliopsoas, and hypertonic pelvic floor may be observed in patients with a psychologically affected sexual pain disorder [19, 20]. The aim of posture training is to have spinal curves in a neutral position, body awareness, balanced posture, and controlled movement by reducing the strain on elongated tissues and joints as much as possible [46]. High-voltage galvanic stimulation, perineal intermittent ultrasound, transcutaneous electrical nerve stimulation (TENS), and extracorporeal shock wave therapy (ESWT) can be applied in individuals with levator ani syndrome and hypertonus of the pelvic floor [47]. Manual techniques for the pelvic floor muscles and related muscle groups are applied to increase awareness of the pelvic floor muscles, relax trigger and tender points, and increase the strength of the pelvic floor muscles [18, 48]. In patients with sexual pain disorders, perineal massage is an effective manual therapy technique that can be performed both by the physiotherapist in the clinic and by the patient himself as a home program [48].

17.2.5.3 Cognitive Behavioral Therapy

Cognitive behavioral therapy, which focuses on reducing anxiety-provoking thoughts and cognitions that cause sexual difficulties, includes sensory focusing, pelvic floor exercises, progressive desensitization techniques, communication skills training, and direct clitoral stimulation training aimed at increasing intimacy and trust between partners [49]. It is important to explain the protective role of voluntary muscle contraction in response to pain or anxiety in sexual pain disorders. In the patient education session, treatment components that help muscle relaxation despite pain or fear of pain are applied. The patient's partner should be encouraged to attend treatment sessions and to include the partner in exercises in the home program [11]. Women who experience pain and sexual dysfunction due to overactive pelvic floor muscles may benefit from the use of dilators. Dilators help to eliminate myofascial trigger points and elongate shortened muscle fibers [18].

It is important to add diaphragmatic breathing and progressive relaxation techniques to the treatment program in all sexual dysfunctions, especially in genito-pelvic pain disorders. Desensitization training is given first to decrease the level of anxiety, and then progressive relaxation techniques are taught to the patient. In addition to this technique, maximal contraction and maximal relaxation of the pelvic floor muscles should be added to the relaxation exercises [18, 49].

17.2.5.4 Pelvic Floor Rehabilitation

An exercise prescription consisting of strengthening, relaxation, coordination, and endurance exercises should be prepared for the pelvic floor muscles of the patients (depending on whether they are hypotonic or hypertonic) [18]. EMG biofeedback, which is used to increase the patient's awareness, is an important aid in teaching the patient how to perform normal activity of the pelvic floor muscles [50]. Biofeedback used in combination with digital palpation will contribute to the better development of pelvic floor muscles. In the literature, digital biofeedback has been reported to be effective in teaching the patient to control the activity of the pelvic floor muscles, especially during sexual intercourse [18]. In addition, it has been shown that strong pelvic floor muscle strength in women improves vaginal sensitivity and increases the ability to reach orgasm [11].

17.3 Sexual Dysfunction Disorders in Men

17.3.1 Sexual Function Cycle in Men

Sexual function cycle consists of arousal, plateau, orgasm, and resolution phases in men. Stages of the sexual function cycle (arousal, plato, orgasm, and dissolution phases):

- Arousal (Libido) Phase: In addition to psychological factors such as erotic thoughts or fantasies, physical contact can affect arousal. These stimuli cause erection in men. If there is not enough stimulation or the person has a low response, the next cycle cannot be started.
- Plato Phase: It is the process in which sexual stimulation intensifies and continues. After sexual pleasure increases and reaches its peak level, the orgasm phase begins.
- Orgasm Phase: It is the climax of the sexual response cycle, providing the most intense pleasure and relaxation. The sensation of orgasm intensifies in the penis and prostate, and ejaculation occurs with reflex clonic muscle contractions.
- Dissolution Phase: It is the recovery of the genital area and other parts of the body after the orgasm phase or in case there is no orgasm. The hardness of the sexual organ, breathing rate, heart rate, and blood pressure decrease and return to normal [51–54].

17.3.2 Sexual Function Disorders in Men

According to the DSM-V guide by the American Psychiatric Association, sexual dysfunction in men is classified as follows [55]:

I. Sexual Desire Disorders (Hypoactive Sexual Desire): It is the decrease or absence of sexual desire, desires, and fantasies. It can decrease neural activation in the medial orbitofrontal region and periaqueductal gray matter, which provides sexual arousal or inadequate stimulation of the centers in the cognitive process. These reasons can include some medical drugs, relationship problems, depression, anxiety, feelings and attraction toward the partner, conflicts, and sexual satisfaction [56].
II. Sexual Arousal Disorder (Erectile Dysfunction): The most common erectile dysfunction is the inability to achieve and maintain an erection of the penis during sexual intercourse that has lasted for at least 3 months.
III. Orgasm Disorders (Premature Ejaculation, Delayed Ejaculation): A man with premature ejaculation has difficulty in controlling ejaculation and ejaculates before the desired time. Delayed ejaculation is defined as a significant delay in ejaculation and the inability to ejaculate. While the minimum duration of ejaculation is between 8 and 12 min, exceed-

ing 20–25 min indicates delayed ejaculation. The duration of delaying ejaculation in men is between 4 and 10 min [57].

IV. Sexual Pain Disorders: It is reported that sexual pain is not due to infection and is generally caused by pelvic pain and testicular pain of myofascial origin. Sexual pain disorders can cause sexual anxiety, decreased interest in sexuality, and impaired orgasm and erectile function [19, 20].

V. Other Sexual Dysfunctions (those that develop due to organic causes).

17.3.3 Evaluation of Sexual Dysfunction in Men

Evaluation of sexual dysfunction in men, detailed physical and sexual history, neurological, orthopedic, and musculoskeletal evaluation of the pelvic area, evaluation of bladder-bowel symptoms and sexual function, and creation of the individual's psychosocial profile are very important for planning the treatment [19, 20, 53].

17.3.3.1 Detailed Physical and Sexual History

The time of onset of sexual problems, partner relationship, arousal, orgasm experience, pain associated with sexual activity, morning erection, nocturnal erection, duration of ejaculation, presence of painful ejaculation, and endocrine tests should be questioned. General health status (existing diseases), body mass index, hormone profile, insulin level, blood lipid level, and radiological results should be examined [19, 20, 58].

Note: Lack of erection during sexual intercourse, while having a morning erection, may suggest psychogenic erectile dysfunction. However, if there is no erection both in the morning and during sexual intercourse, this indicates an organic problem.

Note: It has been shown that metabolic problems such as obesity reduce erection by disrupting penile hemodynamics [59].

17.3.3.2 Observational, Neurological, and Musculoskeletal Evaluation of the Pelvic Region

The anatomical structure and posture of the pelvic structure should be examined while the patient is in the lithotomy position. The structure of the penis and testicles, color change, contraction, and relaxation ability of the pelvic floor muscles should be observed, and the presence of pain while performing this should be questioned. Additionally, the range of motion and mobility of the pelvic skeleton, the presence of trigger points (whether there is pain with compression), and tissue mobility should be examined [60].

Note: When the pelvic floor muscles contract, the tissue in the anus wrinkles, elevation of the testicles, and retraction of the radix penis are observed [59].

EMG biofeedback (with internal or superficial electrodes), ultrasound (anorectal angle, urethrovesical angle, urethra position, and bladder neck mobility can be evaluated), and digital rectal evaluation (anal contraction, muscle strength) to evaluate the activation, strength, and tone of the pelvic floor muscles can be done [60–62].

Orthopedic and neurological tests for the lumbosacral and hip joint regions (straight leg lift, Lasegue test, slump test, Faber test, compression distraction tests, Thomas test, sensory test, evaluation of dermatomes and myotomes) and static and dynamic evaluation of posture should be performed [63].

17.3.3.3 Evaluation of Bladder, Bowel Symptoms, and Sexual Function

Bladder and bowel functions, micturition, and defecation habits can also affect sexuality. To evaluate bladder functions, micturition times, volumes, feelings of urgency, and the presence of painful urination can be evaluated with a bladder diary. In addition, the presence of urinary symptoms, their severity, and their impact on quality of life can be evaluated with the International Incontinence Questionnaire Form (ICIQ-SF), King Health Questionnaire (KSA), and Urinary Incontinence Awareness Scale [64].

To evaluate bowel symptoms, defecation times, feelings of urgency, pain during evacuation, and stool type can be questioned through a bowel diary. Stool type can be evaluated with the Bristol Stool Scale [65].

17.3.3.4 Evaluation of Sexual Function

Scales can be used to determine the type and severity of sexual dysfunction.

- International Erectile Function Index (IEFI): Evaluates erectile function, orgasmic function, sexual desire, sexual intercourse satisfaction, and general satisfaction. IEFI consists of 15 questions and is scored in five different sexual function areas according to the answers received. A higher score indicates better function [66].
- Premature ejaculation evaluation questionnaire: It shows the presence of premature ejaculation. It consists of five questions and is scored between 0 and 5. As the score increases, the risk of PE increases. A score of 8 points or less from the questionnaire indicates that the risk of PE is very low. A score of 9–10 points indicates possible PE, and a score of 11 points or more indicates the presence of PE [67].

Apart from these scales, Premature Ejaculation Profile (Male), Male Sexual Health Form, and Gloombok-Rust Sexual Satisfaction Scale-Male Form evaluate sexual function [66, 67].

17.3.4 Physiotherapy and Rehabilitation Approaches in Male Sexual Dysfunction

Planning individual, gradual, and biopsychosocial approaches in the physiotherapy and rehabilitation program for sexual dysfunction in men will be more effective. Physiotherapy and rehabilitation approaches that can be applied in sexual dysfunction include sexual education, development of pelvic floor awareness, myofascial techniques, exercise approaches, and relaxation techniques [54].

17.3.4.1 Sexual Education

Individuals who experience decreased sexual interest, ejaculation, and erectile problems should be told about false beliefs and behaviors regarding sexuality and should be given information about anatomical and physiological processes. Some examples of training are sensory focus, penis squeezing, stop–start training, and couple training [54, 68].

- Sensate Focus: It is a sexual therapy technique used to improve sexual intimacy between couples, reduce sexual anxiety, and strengthen their bond. Partners explore their bodies and pleasure points by touching their bodies. This technique only aims to focus partners on sexuality [69].
- Penile Squeezing Technique: In this technique, the individual increases his bulbocavernous reflex and orgasm ability to control ejaculation. When the individual is approaching orgasm while masturbating, the penis is squeezed with the thumb and index finger (between the head and the body), and they wait for approximately 30 s until ejaculation is controlled. This is repeated several times in a row [54, 68, 69].
- Stop–Start Technique: It stimulates the penis until the individual reaches orgasm and aims to delay ejaculation before it begins. It is useful for controlling orgasm and ejaculation and directing the bulbocavernous reflex and ejaculation [69].
- Couple Education: It includes ensuring individual satisfaction, informing about sexual behavior, and analyzing problems and aims to increase partner sharing [54, 69].

17.3.4.2 Improving Pelvic Floor Awareness

Pelvic floor muscle training, EMG biofeedback, and electrical stimulation can be applied to improve pelvic floor awareness [54].

17.3.4.3 Pelvic Floor Muscle Training

Pelvic floor muscle training involves improving the perception, contraction, relaxation, and endurance of the pelvic floor muscles in different body positions specific to the individual (supine, crawling, lithotomy, standing, etc.). In this training, while the individual is in the side-lying position or lithotomy position, the individual is first helped to perceive and recognize the pelvic floor muscles with directives such as "shorten the length of the penis," "try to hold in urine and feces," and "tighten the muscles at the root of the penis." While doing this, they should be informed not to squeeze their legs, hips, and abdominal area and not to hold their breath. The movement of the tissue during contraction and relaxation should be demonstrated by using a single finger or by placing your hand in the perineal area. In this training, the person can learn through visual imagery, such as "drawing water with a straw, jellyfish movement, elevator movement, or tap on–off movements."

- For fast-twitch fibers (type II fibers), it can be taught in an on–off manner with maximal voluntary contraction and relaxation.
- For slow-twitch fibers (type I fibers- fatigue-resistant fibers), muscle awareness and strength can be increased by explaining the example of the elevator slowly going up in 5 s, waiting there for 5 s, and coming down again in 5 s [68, 69].

Note: To increase muscular strength, maximal contractions for both type I and type II fibers should be given with eight to ten repetitions in a set, and to improve muscular endurance, submaximal contractions should be given in a higher number of repetitions (15 to 30 repetitions on average).

Erectile dysfunction may develop in patients who have undergone radical prostatectomy. Some investigations showed that pelvic floor training can improve erectile function. However, more comprehensive protocols need to be created, including the content of exercise protocols, compliance with exercise, and activation of basic muscles in erection and ejaculation, and randomized controlled studies need to be planned in this context [54, 70, 71].

17.3.4.4 EMG Biofeedback

In men, EMG biofeedback is applied using internal sensors (inter-rectal) or superficial electrodes. Visual and auditory signals are used in this application. It helps or improves the individual's ability to perceive the pelvic floor muscles in isolation and to perform muscle contraction and relaxation. In order to apply EMG biofeedback, the individual must have minimal muscle contraction ability. This practice requires the active participation of the person in order to increase the strength and endurance of the voluntary muscles and develop the ability to relax in isolation [72].

In the effect of EMG biofeedback application on sexual dysfunction, strengthening especially the bulbocavernosus and ischiocavernosus muscles increases the intracavernosus pressure in the penis and improves erectile function by reducing venous return [73].

Systematic review and meta-analysis studies conducted in recent years show that EMG biofeedback training applied in addition to pelvic floor training after prostate surgery improves sexual function more than pelvic floor muscle training alone [74, 75]. Additionally, EMG biofeedback application (rectally) applied to male patients with chronic pelvic pain has been shown to reduce sexual function symptoms by providing relaxation in pelvic muscle tone [76].

17.3.4.5 Electrical Stimulation

Electrical stimulation is especially preferred in individuals who cannot make active pelvic floor muscle contractions. In this method, electrodes can be applied superficially or inter-anally. With the help of electrodes, the motor fibers of the pudendal nerve are stimulated, and the superficial and deep muscles of the pelvic floor are stimulated. Stimulation both strengthens the pelvic floor muscles and increases the urethral closure pressure. Additionally, when the pudendal nerve is stimulated, parasympathetic activity and detrusor overactivity can be reduced [77].

Transcutaneous electrical stimulation (TENS) applied to individuals with premature ejaculation has been found effective in prolonging and controlling ejaculation time. It is also reported that perineal electrical stimulation applied before sexual activity increases the inhibition of the bulbocavernosus reflex and the control of ejaculation by providing rhythmic contraction in the m. bulbocavernosus and m. isciocavernosus muscles [78].

17.3.4.6 Myofascial Treatments

Myofascial trigger points cause pelvic pain and hyperalgesia in the pelvic floor muscles. Pain areas may be in the penis, perineum, urethra, pelvic floor muscles, lumbar, abdomen, or legs. After detecting myofascial trigger points and taut bands (by skin rolling, digital algometer, and palpation method), massage, myofascial release, fascial mobilization, internal and external soft tissue mobilization, self-myofascial techniques, and ischemic compression techniques can be applied to increase fascial mobility [79]. The literature showed that myofascial techniques and manual applications reduce sexual dysfunction by providing relaxation in the pelvic floor muscles [80].

17.3.4.7 Physical Activity and Exercise

Regular physical activity and exercise contribute to erection by positively affecting vascular endothelial responses. In addition, exercise stimulates systemic nitric oxide production and provides vasodilation in vascular structures. Insulin is also released more during regular exercise, is used more in the muscle, and stimulates the release of nitric oxide. Exercise will improve sexual function by both improving the vascular response and removing pro-inflammatory cytokines. In the literature, physical activity prescription for erectile dysfunction developing due to organic reasons (such as obesity, metabolic syndrome, hypertension) requires an average energy expenditure of 50–1000 kcal for a total of 160 min at least 4 days a week and moderate-intensity (4 to 6 METs) physical activity for 6 months or more. Activities or exercises starting from 40 to 60% of maximum heart rate are recommended. Since high-intensity exercise may damage the vascular endothelium, aerobic, moderate-intensity, resistive, and personalized exercises should be planned [81, 82].

17.3.4.8 Relaxation Methods

Mindfulness, breathing techniques, progressive relaxation exercises, and meditation provide both emotional and physical (pelvic floor muscles) relaxation. Relaxation exercises reduce negative sexual thoughts and can increase erection and controlled ejaculation by increasing sexual desire, focus, and performance [83].

In a study conducted in the treatment of erectile dysfunction, mindfulness techniques, goal-oriented sex, and psychoeducation about the physiology of erectile function and sexual response models were given, and an increase in sexual function and satisfaction was achieved. More randomized controlled studies are needed on the effect of relaxation techniques on sexual dysfunction [80].

17.4 Conclusion

Physiotherapists play an active role in the management of sexual dysfunction. The aim of physiotherapists is to regulate the musculoskeletal system and pelvic floor dysfunctions that cause sexual dysfunction and to restore a painless and normal sexual function cycle. Following a comprehensive evaluation of physiotherapy and rehabilitation approaches that can be applied in this field, a biopsychosocial, multidisciplinary, and multifaceted treatment approach should be planned. The literature is limited, and comparative and multidisciplinary studies with large samples are needed.

References

1. Crooks R, Baur K. Our sexuality: sexual coercion. Belmont: Cengage Learning Wadsworth; 2011. p. 515–48.
2. Demirezen E, Erdoğan S, Önem K. Birinci Basamak Sağlık Merkezine Başvuran Kirk Yaşın Altındaki Kadınlarda Cinsel Fonksiyon Değerlendirmesi. Androloji Bülteni. 2006;25:177–80.
3. Doğan O. Sağlık Alanında Davranış Bilimleri. Sivas Dilek matbaacılık; 1995.
4. American Psychiatric Association A. Diagnostic and statistical manual of mental disorders. Washington, DC: American Psychiatric Association; 1980.

5. Edition F. Diagnostic and statistical manual of mental disorders, vol. 21. Am Psychiatric Assoc; 2013.
6. Gulliford AL, Haslam JM, Lewis RDH, Sidney JRL, Todd J, Vits K, et al. Physiotherapy in women's health. In: Tidy's Physiotherapy E-Book; 2008. p. 113.
7. World Health Organization. Education and treatment in human sexuality: the training of health professionals: report of a WHO meeting. Geneva: World Health Organization; 1975. (WHO Technical Report Series No. 572).
8. Yeni E. Menopoz ve Cinsellik. In: Kadıoğlu A, Başar M, Semerci İ, Orhan İ, Aşçı R, Yaman MÖ, Çayan S, Usta MF, Kendirci M, editors. Erkek ve Kadın Cinsel Sağlığı. İstanbul: Türk Androloji Derneği Yayınları; 2004. p. 652–66.
9. Basson R. Human sex-response cycles. Journal of Sex &Marital Therapy. 2001;27(1):33–43.
10. İncesu C. Cinsel işlevler ve cinsel işlev bozuklukları. Derg Klin Psikiyatri. 2004;7(Suppl 3):3–13.
11. Berman JR, Goldstein I. Female sexual dysfunction. Urol Clin. 2001;28(2):405–16.
12. Guze SB. Diagnostic and statistical manual of mental disorders, (DSM-ıv). Am J Psychiatry. 1995;152(8):1228.
13. McCool-Myers M, Theurich M, zuelke A, Knuettel H, Apfelbacher C. Predictors of female sexual dysfunction: a systematic review and qualitative analysisthrough gender inequality paradigms. BMC Womens Health. 2018;18(1):1–15.
14. Brotto LA. The DSM diagnostic criteria for hypoactive sexual desire disorder in women. Arch Sex Behav. 2010;39(2):221–39.
15. Basson R, Berman J, Burnett A, Derogatis L, Ferguson D, Fourcroy J, et al. Report of the nternational consensus development conference on female sexual dysfunction: definitions and classifications. J Urol. 2000;163:888–93.
16. Basson R, Weijmar Shultz WCM. Bölüm 22, Kadınlarda Cinsel İstek ve Uyarılma Bozuklukları ve Cinsel Ağrı. In: Seksüel Tıp; 2004. p. 860.
17. Laumann ED, Paik A, Rosen RC. Sexual dysfunction in the United States, Prevalance and Predictors. JAMA. 1999;281(6):5537–44.
18. Rosenbaum TY. The role of physical therapy in female sexual dysfunction. Curr Sex Health Rep. 2008;5(2):97–101.
19. Stein A, Sauder SK, Reale J. The role of physical therapy in sexual health in men and women: evaluation and treatment. Sexual medicine reviews. 2019a;7(1):46–56.
20. Stein A, Sauder SK, Reale J. The role of physical therapy in sexual health in men and women: evaluations and treatments. Sex Med Rev. 2019b;7(1):46–56.
21. Van Lankveld JJ, Granot M, Schultz WCW, Binik YM, Wesselmann U, Pukall CF, et al. Women's sexual pain disorders. J Sex Med. 2010;7(1):615–31.
22. Qureshi S, Ara Z, Qureshi VF, Al-Rejaie S, Aleisa A, Bakheet S, et al. Sexual dysfunction in women: an overview of psychological/psychosocial, pathophysiological, etiological aspects and treatment strategies. Pharmacognosy Rev. 2007;1:41–8.
23. Anastasiadis AG, Davis AR, Ghafar MA, Burchardt M, Shabsigh R. The epidemiology and definition of female sexual disorders. World J Urol. 2002;20(2):74–8.
24. Berman JR, Berman L, Goldstein I. Female sexual dysfunction: incidence, pathophysiology, evaluation, and treatment options. Urology. 1999;54(3):385–91.
25. Rees PM, Fowler CJ, Maas CP. Sexual function in men and women with neurological disorders. Lancet. 2007;369(9560):512–25.
26. Berman JR, Bassuk J. Physiology and pathophysiology of female sexual function and dysfunction. World J Urol. 2002;20(2):111–8.
27. Erol B, Sanli O, Korkmaz D, Seyhan A, Akman T, Kadioglu A. A cross-sectional study of female sexual function and dysfunction during pregnancy. J Sex Med. 2007;4(5):1381–7.
28. Brtnicka H, Weiss P, Zverina J. Human sexuality during pregnancy and the postpartum period. Bratisl Lek Listy. 2009;110(7):427–31.
29. El-Azab AS, Yousef HA, Seifeldein GS. Coital incontinence: relation to detrusor overactivity and stress incontinence. Neurourol Urodyn. 2011;30(4):520–4.
30. Özengin N, Çankaya H, Duygu E, Uysal MF, Bakar Y. The effect of pelvic organ prolapse type on sexual function, muscle strength, and pelvic floor symptoms in women: a retrospective study. Turk J Obstet Gynecol. 2017;14(2):121.
31. Nurnberg HG. Biologic basis of serotonin reuptake inhibitor antidepressantassociated female sexual dysfunction: a novel signaling perspective. Curr Sex Health Rep. 2005;2(2):85–92.
32. Stephenson KR, Meston CM. Why is impaired sexual function distressing to women? The primacy of pleasure in female sexual dysfunction. J Sex Med. 2015;12(3):728–37.
33. Kammerer-Doak D. Assessment of sexual function in women with pelvic floor dysfunction. Int Urogynecol J. 2009;20(1):45–50.
34. Kuscu NK, Oruc S, Ceylan E, Eskicioglu F, Goker A, Caglar H. Sexual life following total abdominal hysterectomy. Arch Gynecol Obstet. 2005;271(3):218–21.
35. Lee D, Zimmern PE. Female sexual dysfunction management after Pubovaginal/Midurethral sling surgery. Curr Sex Health Rep. 2014;6(3):184–91.
36. Önen Sertöz Ö, Elbi Mete H, Noyan A, Alper M, Kapkaç M. Meme kanserinde ameliyat tipinin beden algısı, cinsel işlevler, benlik saygısı ve eş uyumuna etkileri: kontrollü bir çalışma. Turk Psikiyatri Derg. 2004;15(4):264–75.
37. Aydın S, onaran OI, Topalan K, Aydın CA, Dansuk R. Development and validation of Turkish version of the female sexual distress scale-revised. Sexual medicine. 2016;4(1):e43–50.
38. Celik DB, Beji NK, Yalcin O. Turkish adaptation of the short form of the pelvic organ prolapse/urinary incontinence sexual function questionnaire (PıSQ-

12): a validation and reliability study. Neurourol Urodyn. 2013;32(8):1068–73.
39. Efe H, Bozkurt M, Sahin l, Mutlu MF, Api M, Cetin A. The effects of pregnancy on the sexual life of Turkish women. Proceedings in obstetrics and Gynecology. 2014;4(1):1–11.
40. Nakip G, Gursen C, Baran E, Uzelpasaci E, Çinar GN, Ozgul S, Beksac MS, Akbayrak T. Psychometric properties of the Turkish version of the pregnancy sexual response inventory in pregnant women. archives of Obstet Gynecol. 2021;304:101–7. https://doi.org/10.1007/s00404-020-05933-4.
41. Sonbahar AE, Culha MG, Jannini E. The validity and reliability of the Turkish version of the 6-item female sexual function index (FSFı-6) and the relationship between climacturia and female sexual dysfunction. Int J Impot Res. 2021;1–4:610–613.
42. Saadat SH. Vaginismus: a review of literature and recent updated treatments. J Med Rev. 2014;1(3):97–100.
43. FitzGerald M, Kotarinos R. Rehabilitation of the short pelvic floor: background and patient evaluation. ınternational urogynecology Journal. 2013;14(4):261–8.
44. Stanten N, Yeager S. Four workouts to improve your love life. Prevention. 2003;55:76–8.
45. Dąbrowska J, Drosdzol A, Skrzypulec v, Plinta R. Physical activity and sexuality in perimenopausal women. Eur J Contracept Reprod Health Care. 2010;15(6):423–32.
46. Nakip GAT. Vajinismus Tedavisinde Fizyoterapi ve Rehabilitasyon. Fizyoterapi Seminerleri. Ankara: H.Ü.S.B.F; 2017. p. 57–62.
47. Rosenbaum TY, Owens A. The role of pelvic floor physical therapy in the treatment of pelvic and genital pain-related sexual dysfunction. Erratum. 2008;5(6):1513.
48. Karakaya İC. Gebelerde, Bebeklerde ve Çocuklarda Masaj. Yüksel i, editör. Masaj Teknikleri. Ankara: Asil Yayın; 2013. p. 197–232.
49. Graziottin A. Female sexual dysfunction. In: Evidence based physical therapy for the pelvic Xoor: bridging science and clinical practice. Churchill Livingstone: Elsevier; 2007. p. 266–87.
50. Ghaderi F, Bastani P, Hajebrahimi S, Jafarabadi MA, Berghmans B. Pelvic floor rehabilitation in the treatment of women with dyspareunia: a randomized controlled clinical trial. Int Urogynecol J. 2019;30(11):1849–55.
51. Argiolas A, Melis MR. The neurophysiology of the sexual cycle. J Endocrinol Investig. 2003;26(3):20–2.
52. Kandell FR, Koussa VKT, Swerdloff RS. Male sexual function and its disorders: physiology, pathophysiology, clinic investigation, and treatments. Endocr Rev. 2001;22(3):342–88.
53. Nicol A, Chung E. Male sexual dysfunction: clinical diagnosis and management strategies for common sexual problems. AJGP. 2023;52(1):41–5.
54. Ozgül S, Dericioğlu B. Erkeklerde Cinsel İşlev Bozukluğunda Fizyoterapi ve Rehabilitasyon. In: Akbayrak T, Özgül S, Gürşen C, editors. Multidisipliner Bakış Temeli ile Pelvik Sağlıkta Fizyoterapi ve Rehabilitasyon. Hedef CS Basın Yayın, vol. Cilt 2. 2023; 2023. p. 415–49.
55. MP MC, et al. Definitions of sexual dysfunctions in women and men: a consensus statement from the fourth international consultation on sexual medicine. J Sex Med. 2016;13(2):135–43.
56. Althof SE, et al. An update of the international Society of Sexual Medicine's guidelines for the diagnosis and treatments of premature ejaculation (PE). J Sex Med. 2014;11(6):1392–422.
57. Abdel-Hamid IA, Ali OI. Delayed ejaculation: pathophysiology, diagnosis, and treatments. World J Men's Health. 2018;36(1):22–40.
58. Brookmeyer KA, et al. Sexual history taking in clinical settings: narrative review. Sex Transm Dis. 2021;48(6):393–40.
59. Polackwich AS, Shoskes DA. Chronic prostatitis/chronic pelvic pain syndrome: a review of evaluations and therapy. Prostate Cancer Prostatic Dis. 2016;19(2):132–8.
60. Koh CE, et al. Systematic review of randomized controlled trials of the effectiveness of biofeedback for pelvic floor dysfunction. Br J Surg. 2008;95(9):1079–87.
61. Martin HD, Shears SA, Palmer IJ. Evaluation of the hip. Sports Med Arthrosc Rev. 2010;18(2):63–75.
62. Rosenbaum TY. Reviews: pelvic floor involvement in male and female sexual dysfunction and the role of pelvic floor rehabilitation in treatments: a literatüre review. J Sex Med. 2007;4(1):4–13.
63. Ouchi M, Kitta T, Takahashi Y, Chiba H, Higuchi M, Togo M, et al. Reliability of manometry for assessing pelvic floor muscle function in healthy men. Neurourol Urodyn. 2020;39:1464–71.
64. Bordeianou LG, et al. Measuring pelvic floor disorder symptoms using patient-reported instruments: proceedings of the consensus meeting of the pelvic floor consortium of the American Society of Colon and Rectal Surgeons, the international continence society, the American Urogynecologic Society, and the Society of Urodynamics, female pelvic medicine and urogenital reconstruction. Female Pelvic Med Reconstr Surg. 2020;26(1):1–15.
65. Blake MR, Raker JM, Whelan K. Validity and reliability of the Bristol stool form scale in healthy adults snd patients with diarrhoea-predominant irritable bowel syndrome. Aliment Pharmacol Ther. 2016;44(7):693–703.
66. Bayraktar Z. The reability of the Turkish version of the international index of erectile function (IIEF): literatüre review. Yeni Üroloji Dergisi. 2017;12(1):63–70.
67. Doğantekin E, Dağgüllü M, Söylemez H. Prematür ejakülasyon sıklığı ve tedavi oranı; kesitsel bir anket çalışması. Yeni üroloji dergisi. 2014;9(1):63–6.
68. Brotto L, et al. Physiological and interpersonal dimensions of sexual function and dysfunction. J Sex Med. 2016;13(4):538–71.
69. Pupupo V, Puppo G. Comprehensive review of the anatomy and physiology of male ejaculation: pre-

mature ejaculation is not as a disease. Clin Anat. 2016;29(1):111–9.
70. Gomes CS, et al. The effects of Pilates method on pelvic floor muscle strength in patients with post-prostatectomy urinary incontinence: a randomized clinical trial. Neurol Urodyn. 2018;37(1):346–53.
71. Wong C, Louie DR, Beach C. A systematic review of pelvic floor muscle training for erectile dysfunction after prostatectomy and recommendations to guide further research. J Sex Med. 2020;17(4):737–48.
72. Messelink B, Benson T, Berghmans B, Bø K, Corcos J, Fowler C, et al. Standartdization of terminology of pelvic floor muscle function and dysfunction: report from the pelvic floor clinical assessment group of the international continence society. Neurourol Urodyn. 2005;24(4):374–80.
73. Colpi GM, et al. Perineal floor efficiency in sexually potent and impotent men. Int J Impot Res. 1999;11(3):153–7.
74. Hsu LF, Liao YM, Lai FC, Tsai PS. Beneficial effects of biofeedback assisted pelvic floor muscle training in patients with urinary incontinence after radical prostatectomy: systematic review and metaanalysis. Int J Nurs Stud. 2016;60(1):99–111.
75. Kurne HG, Akbayrak T. The validity and reliability of the Postmenopause sexuality questionnaire. Int J Gynecol Obstet. 2024;165(1):188–93. https://doi.org/10.1002/ijgo.15293.
76. Clemens JQ, Mullins C, Ackerman AL, Bavendam T, Bokhoven AV, Ellingson BM, et al. Urologic chronic pelvic pain syndrome insight from the MAPP research network. Nat Rev Urol. 2019;16(3):187–200.
77. Berghmans B, Hendriks E, Bernards A, Bie R, Omar MI. Electrical stimulation with non-implanted electrodes for urinary incontinence in men. Cochrane Database Syst Rev. 2013;6:CD001202.
78. Shecter A, Serefoglu EC, Gollan T, Springer S, Gideon M, Appel B, et al. Transcuteneous functional elecrical stimulation-a novel therapy for premature ejaculation:results of a proof of concept study. Int J Impot Rec. 2019;32(4):440–5.
79. Masterson TA, Masterson JM, Azzinaro J, Manderson L, Swain S, Ramasamy R. Comprehensive pelvic floor physical therapy program for men with idiopathic chronic pelvic pain syndrome: a prospective study. Transl Androl Urol. 2017;6(5):910–5.
80. Fuentez-Marquez P, Cabrera-Martos I. Physiotherapy Interventations for patients with chronic pelvic pain: systematic review of the literature. Physiother Theory Pract. 2019;35(12):1131–8.
81. Meldrum DR, Gambone JC, Morris MA, Esposito K, Giugliano D, Ignarro LJ. Lifestyle and metabolic approaches to maximizing erectile and vascular health. Int J Impot Res. 2012;24(2):61–8.
82. Silva AB, Sousa N, Azevedo LF, Martins C. Physical activity and exercise for erectile dysfunction: systematic review and meta-analysis. Br J Sports Med. 2017;51(19):1419–24.
83. Jaderek I, Lew-Starowicz M. A systematic review on mindfulness meditation-based interventions for sexual dysfunctions. J Sex Med. 2019;16:1581–96.

Physiotherapy and Rehabilitation in Colorectoanal Dysfunctions

18

Gülbala Gülören and Ceren Gürşen

18.1 Introduction

The storage and defecation of intestinal contents occur through the coordinated functioning of the colon, rectum, and anus. The anal canal has functions such as sensation of rectal content, realization of defecation at the appropriate place and time, and maintenance of resting tonus for continence in the absence of appropriate conditions [1]. Colorectoanal dysfunctions are complex conditions that include anal incontinence, functional constipation, defecatory disorders, hemorrhoids, and functional anorectal pain disorders, and they negatively affect the quality of life [2]. Due to its complex nature, assessment and treatment should be individualized based on a multidisciplinary approach. Specialized physiotherapists should be part of a multidisciplinary team in the management of colorectal dysfunction. Patient reluctance to seek medical help due to embarrassment and limited effective treatment options is a barrier to the assessment and management of these disorders [3]. Despite these limitations, many patients benefit greatly from physiotherapy applications [2, 3].

G. Gülören (✉)
Department of Physiotherapy and Rehabilitation, Hamidiye Faculty of Health Sciences, University of Health Sciences, İstanbul, Türkiye

C. Gürşen
Faculty of Physical Therapy and Rehabilitation, Hacettepe University, Ankara, Türkiye

18.2 Colorectoanal Dysfunctions

Coordination of bowel function requires the colon, rectum, and anus in order to work in harmony. Anorectal continence is controlled by the delivery of colonic contents to the rectum, sensation of rectal contents, rectal capacity and compliance, nocturnal control, internal and external anal sphincter mechanisms, pelvic floor muscles, and nerves. In addition, the anatomy and functional integrity of the pelvic floor muscles and anorectum contribute to continence and defecation. The structures that are functionally important for anal continence and defecation are the rectum, m. levator ani, m. puborectalis, external and internal anal sphincters, anal canal mucosa, and the nerves that innervate these structures [1].

The anal sphincter mechanism consists of two muscle structures, the internal anal sphincter (IAS), which has a smooth muscle structure that forms the inner layer of the sphincter, and the external anal sphincter (EAS), which has a striated muscle structure that forms the outer layer of the sphincter, which contracts voluntarily to prevent feces from escaping from the anus [4]. The levator ani and anal sphincter muscles contribute to continence by maintaining continuous tonic activity with spinal reflexes. The puborectalis muscle, which surrounds the anal sphincter, acts like a muscular sling, pulling the anorectal junction toward the pubic bone to form the anorectal angle. The anorectal angle is the main mecha-

T. Akbayrak, E. Üzelpasaci (eds.), *Physiotherapy and Rehabilitation in Pelvic and Women's Health-Related Problems*, https://doi.org/10.1007/978-3-032-28741-0_18

nism of anorectal constancy and is normally between 60 and 105^0, exceeding this value reduces its effectiveness [1, 4]. Fecal material in the rectum can cause the angle to increase. The anal sphincters close the anal canal to retain gas and liquid feces.

The anal sphincters are responsible for closing the anal canal to retain gas and liquid feces, while the puborectalis muscle and the anorectal angle are responsible for maintaining fecal continence in relation to solid material [5]. If the environment and conditions are not suitable for defecation, repeated contractions of the EAS will delay defecation. The EAS can provide this delay by voluntarily contracting with the puborectalis muscle [4, 5].

Defecation is initiated by the colon's ileocolic reflex contraction and voluntary contraction of the abdominal muscles and gastrocolic reflex filling of the rectum with feces. Increased intrarectal pressure stimulates distension receptors in the puborectalis muscle and associated tissues, and a conscious desire to defecate is felt. At the same time, a reflex relaxation of the IAS occurs. The reflex relaxation of the IAS increases the sensitivity of the mucosa of the anal canal. This allows discrimination between gas, liquid, and solid feces. During defecation, the anorectal angle increases and the pelvic floor moves downwards [1, 4].

Structural and functional disorders of this system, which plays a role in continence and defecation, cause colorectal anal dysfunction such as anal incontinence, functional constipation, bowel dysfunction, anorectal pain, and hemorrhoids [4].

18.2.1 Anal Incontinence

Anal incontinence (AI) is a general condition defined as involuntary leakage of feces and/or gas that causes social or hygienic problems. Fecal incontinence (FI) is the involuntary loss of solid or liquid feces. Flatus incontinence is defined as the involuntary leakage of gas [2]. FI is analyzed in four groups: solid, liquid, passive (involuntary leakage without sensation), and coital (involuntary leakage during vaginal intercourse). According to the guidelines published by the International Classification of Diseases (ICD-10), FI is divided into two sections: passive and urge incontinence according to etiology and symptoms. The Rome III criteria state that incontinence should have occurred at least once in the previous 3 months for FI to be diagnosed. In the Rome IV diagnostic criteria, this criterion has been updated, and it is reported that at least two episodes of incontinence should have occurred in the previous 4 weeks for the diagnosis of FI [6].

The continence mechanism should have more control over liquid feces than over solid feces. The presence of solid feces may indicate severe sphincter weakness. Patients with passive incontinence are unaware of the need to void prior to the incontinence episode. Passive incontinence is usually associated with pudendal nerve injury [7]. Patients with urge incontinence have the need to void but are unable to reach the toilet in time. In these patients, there is a decrease in anal sphincter contraction pressure or time and/or a decrease in rectal capacity leading to rectal hypersensitivity, whereas in patients with passive incontinence, the resting pressure of the anal sphincter is lower [8].

Trauma, anorectal surgery (hemorrhoidectomy, fistulotomy, sphincterotomy), coloanal or ileoanal reconstruction, neurological disease, diabetes mellitus, diarrhea, irritable bowel syndrome, gluten intolerance, constipation, obstetric injury, and overflow incontinence are risk factors for FI [7, 9]. There is some evidence that the prevalence of FI also varies according to socioeconomic status and ethnicity. In one systematic review, the prevalence of FI was reported to vary between 11% and 18.9% [10, 11].

18.2.2 Chronic Constipation

Constipation is a condition defined by symptoms such as straining during more than 25% of bowel movements, fewer than three bowel movements per week, hard stools, abdominal pain and bloating, a sensation of incomplete evacuation, and the need for manual maneuvers. It is common at all ages and negatively affects all sub-dimensions of quality of life [12]. According to the Rome IV criteria, chronic constipation should last for at least 3 months, and there should be at least 6 months between the onset of symptoms and the diagnosis (Table 18.1) [13]. The prevalence of constipation is reported to be between 3% and 27% worldwide and between 22% and 40% in Türkiye [14, 15]. Risk factors for constipation include older age, Black race, low socioeconomic and educational status, physical inactivity, obesity, pregnancy, smoking and alcohol consumption, low-fiber diets, adverse effects of medication, and genetic predisposition [14].

Chronic constipation is divided into two groups according to its etiology: primary (functional) and secondary. Secondary constipation develops due to an underlying cause such as a neurological or metabolic disease that affects bowel motility (Parkinson's disease, hypothyroidism, diabetes mellitus, hypercalcemia, scleroderma, spinal cord injury, multiple sclerosis), leading to a mechanical obstruction in the bowel [16]. Treatment approaches for secondary constipation aim to improve these underlying factors. Primary (functional) constipation is divided into three groups according to the American Gastroenterological Association: normal transit time constipation, slow transit time constipation, and defecation disorders [17]. In normal transit time constipation, stool passes through the colon at a normal rate and the frequency of bowel movements is normal. Patients complain of hard stools, difficult defecation, abdominal distension, and pain. Slow transit constipation, slowing of bowel motility with reduced neuromuscular function in the colon. Normally, the frequency of bowel movements ranges from a maximum of three times a day to at least 3 days a week, but in slow-onset constipation, the frequency of bowel movements is usually less than once a week. It is often associated with pelvic floor dysfunction and has been reported to occur during pregnancy, after childbirth, or following hysterectomy [18]. Defecation dysfunction is the inability to empty the rectum as a result of poor coordination of the abdominal, pelvic floor, and anorectal muscles. It is also known as pelvic floor dysfunction or defecation and evacuation disorders. About half of these patients have slow transit constipation [2, 18].

Table 18.1 Diagnosis of chronic constipation according to Rome IV criteria [13]

Exclusion of irritable bowel syndrome
Rare occurrence of soft stools without the use of laxatives
Defecation frequency <3/week
At least 2 or more of the following symptoms must be present in at least 25% of defecations: Excessive straining during defecation Lumpy or hard stools Feeling of incomplete emptying Sensation of anorectal obstruction Manual maneuvers used to assist evacuation

18.2.3 Functional Defecation Disorders

Functional defecation disorders are caused by an inability to evacuate the contents of the rectum due to incoordination of the abdominal muscles and pelvic floor muscles, particularly the puborectalis muscle and external anal sphincter [19]. Dyssynergic defecatory disorders and inadequate defecatory propulsion are the most common defecatory disorders [20]. In inadequate defecator propulsion, colonic transit time is normal, and there is a slowing of rectal movements. In abdominal straining, the internal pressure of the rectum does not increase sufficiently to expel stool. There is abnormal contraction of the pelvic floor muscles during fecal impaction and defecation [12].

In dyssynergic defecation, paradoxical anal contraction during defecation and inadequate relaxation of the pelvic floor muscles, particularly the puborectalis muscle and external anal sphincter, result in incomplete evacuation of the rectal contents. It has been reported to occur after acquired incorrect toilet training or incorrect toilet habits such as prolonged delay and sexual abuse [21]. Symptoms include difficult straining during defecation, decreased frequency of defecation, sensation of urgency to defecate, sensation of incomplete evacuation, sensation of abdominal fullness, and use of digital maneuvers to evacuate.

In the dyssynergic pattern, there is a relaxation of less than 20% of the resting anal sphincter pressure and insufficient abdominal muscle pushing. The disorder is diagnosed by a balloon expulsion test and anorectal manometry [22].

18.2.4 Functional Anorectal Pain Disorders

Functional anorectal pain disorders are divided into three groups: proctalgia fugax, levator ani syndrome, and unspecified anorectal pain disorders. These are mainly distinguished by the duration of the pain and the presence of anorectal tenderness [2]. Proctalgia fugax is a severe pain in the rectum and anus that lasts for a few minutes. Chronic proctalgia, according to the Rome IV criteria, is continuous or recurrent pain in the perineal region that started at least 6 months ago, has lasted for 3 months, and occurs in cycles of at least 20 min. There is a sensation of pressure, itching, and tenderness in the rectal area. Patients with chronic proctalgia symptoms have no abnormalities in the pelvic and anorectal region [2, 23]. Levator ani syndrome is usually defined as a vague, dull pain with a sensation of pressure in the upper part of the rectum. There is a spasm of the levator ani muscles and hypersensitivity to palpation, usually on the left side, or tenderness of the pelvic floor and vaginal wall. Studies have reported the incidence of anorectal pain to be between 6.6% and 11.6% [2, 24]. Levator ani syndrome has been reported to be caused by spasm of the pelvic floor muscles and high anal resting pressures. In one randomized controlled trial, 85% of patients with dyssynergic defecation had levator ani muscle tenderness [25].

18.2.5 Hemorrhoids

Hemorrhoids are veins that bulge in or around the anus. They are cushions filled with blood at rest and act as buffers during periods of increased intra-abdominal pressure, such as when you cough or sneeze. In this way, they prevent involuntary leakage of feces and gas without contraction of the anal sphincter. During defecation, hemorrhoids compress and drain, making it easier to empty the rectum. If the structure is damaged, the normal function of hemorrhoids is disrupted, and they prolapse and become symptomatic [4]. Hemorrhoids are divided into two groups, internal and external. Internal hemorrhoids can be seen by endoscopic examination of the anal canal, while external hemorrhoids are easily seen by anal examination. Hemorrhoids can cause mild discomfort in the perianal region, while severe hemorrhoids can cause severe discomfort when walking, sitting, and defecating, limiting the patient's daily activities [2]. The most common anorectal symptoms associated with hemorrhoids are bleeding, pain, prolapse, thrombosis, fissures, discharge, itching and irritation, hygiene problems, discomfort, and perianal pain [26, 27]. Since hemorrhoids are innervated by somatic nerves, they cause severe pain [28].

18.3 Assessment of Colorectoanal Dysfunctions

The assessment of colorectoanal dysfunctions for physiotherapy and rehabilitation should include a detailed history, physiological and special tests, physical examination, and pelvic examination. The interpretation of physiological assessments and radiological imaging is very important in the correct clinical evaluation of colorectoanal dysfunction. In addition, since colorectoanal dysfunction is a topic that is avoided and the disclosure of which is embarrassing, care should be taken to ensure that the treatment room is closed and soundproofed to ensure privacy during evaluation and treatment. Annual cancer screening and gynecological check-ups for female patients should be recommended before patients are included in the assessment and treatment program [29].

18.3.1 Medical History

General information such as the patient's age, height, weight, employment status, primary complaint, and the family's approach to the problem should be recorded. Female patients should be asked about their obstetric and gynecological history, including the number of births, birth weight, duration of the second stage of labor, interventions during labor (episiotomy, forceps, vacuum, etc.), anal sphincter injury, and perineal trauma. In addition, the presence of inflammatory, neurological, and metabolic diseases such as diabetes mellitus, which may cause colorectoanal dysfunction, should be recorded. In addition, any colorectal, bowel, abdominal, obstetric/gynecological surgery, or trauma should be assessed. It is important to ask about medication, use of fiber or laxatives, dietary habits, and how the symptoms affect social, sexual, and family relationships [18].

The presence of anorectal symptoms such as difficulty passing stools, sensation of incomplete emptying, sensation of constipation, use of the toilet less than 3 days a week, presence of hard stools, use of digital maneuvers, abdominal distension, abdominal pain or discomfort, and rectal pain or bleeding; the onset, severity, duration, frequency, and impact on life should be assessed. The number of failed defecations, time spent in the toilet, and previous conservative treatment should also be questioned [30].

The most important symptom when taking the history of a patient with FI is whether the patient has a strong urgency associated with incontinence or passive incontinence. Fecal urgency is associated with a violent and sudden sensation of defecation, resulting in leakage of liquid feces before it reaches the toilet. Passive incontinence is more likely to indicate advanced sphincter weakness, inadequate rectal sensation, or structural changes [31]. The Modified Cleveland Score, Wexner Score, and Vaizey Score can be used to assess the severity of incontinence and the effectiveness of treatment [32, 33].

Patients' dietary habits and physical activity levels should be questioned in detail. The number of daily meals, energy intake, fiber intake, and fluid intake should be recorded in diaries. The defecation diary, which is an effective and reliable method, can be used to assess bowel habits, defecation frequency, and incontinence severity. This diary records the frequency and intensity of defecation, the type of incontinence and the presence of urgency, the severity of pain experienced, and the use of medications that cause changes in stool type [34]. Stool consistency and type are assessed using the Bristol Stool Scale (BSS). The BSS, which classifies stool type from 1 to 7, is a quick indicator of colonic transit time. Type 1–2 indicates constipation; type 3 and especially type 4 indicate ideal stool type; types 5–7 indicate the presence of diarrhea [35].

A detailed evaluation of pain is very important in patients with functional anorectal pain. The predominant type of pain is nociceptive (inflammatory), neuropathic, or nociplastic (central sensitization) [36]. In addition, the McGill Pain Questionnaire—Short Form can be used to assess whether the pain is compatible with nociceptive input [37]. The Pain Body Diagram can be used to identify painful areas [38]. However, if there is insufficient evidence of injury, objective findings, or pathology in the patient and sensory hypersensitivity is suspected, the Central Sensitization Inventory and the Pain Catastrophizing Scale should be used at this stage [39, 40]. In addition to these assessments, factors that decrease or increase pain; its relationship to the menstrual cycle, bowel, urinary, and sexual function; its effect on activities of daily living; and quality of life should be explored. In addition to the medical history, a psychosocial assessment is important [38]. Traumatic conditions such as sexual harassment and physical abuse and psychological symptoms such as stress, anxiety, and depression should be assessed. Finally, patients' quality of life can be assessed using disease-specific scales. The Gastrointestinal Quality of Life Index, or the Fecal Incontinence Quality of Life Questionnaire, can be used to assess the impact of anal incontinence on quality of life [41, 42]. The Constipation Quality of Life Scale can be used to assess the impact of constipation on quality of life [43].

18.3.2 Physiological Tests

Specific tests used in colorectoanal dysfunctions are preferred in patients who do not respond to routine treatment, whose symptoms are refractory, and whose underlying pathological mechanism cannot be fully determined. Methods such as anal endosonography, defecography, neurophysiological tests, and magnetic resonance imaging can be used in the evaluation of anal incontinence [44]. Tests such as defecography, colonic transit tests, anorectal manometry, and colonoscopy can be used to assess chronic constipation. In patients with dyssynergic defecation, anorectal manometry provides important information in diagnosing the condition. The anorectal manometer can be used to assess internal anal sphincter pressure, the amount of pressure generated by voluntary contraction and relaxation of the external anal sphincter and puborectal muscle, rectal sensation, and the length of the anal canal. The study and interpretation of all the physiological tests carried out in colorectoanal dysfunction by physiotherapists specialized in this field will provide information in terms of determining the severity of the disease, the choice, and the effectiveness of physiotherapy applications [45].

18.3.3 Physical Evaluation

Physical evaluation in patients with colorectoanal dysfunction includes inspection and palpation of the abdominal and anorectal regions.

Inspection

The abdominal examination begins with the identification of surgical incisions and abdominal masses in the pelvic examination room with the patient in the supine position. The best position for anorectal examination is left lateral decubitus with thighs and knees flexed and buttocks slightly outside the table edges [46]. The skin should be examined for scarring, contamination around the anus, external hemorrhoids, skin blemishes, redness, hematoma, fistula, fissure, structural abnormality, and rash. Check whether the anus is completely closed at rest or during contractions, or whether it opens during straining. In defecation disorders, it is very important to assess the degree of descent of the perineum at rest and during straining [47]. In female patients, the anterior vaginal wall, urethra, and perineum should also be assessed. The presence of an episiotomy and scarring associated with labor should be noted. The presence of feces in the vagina in patients with FI may suggest an anovaginal or rectovaginal fistula, possibly due to obstetric trauma [48].

Palpation

Assessment of trigger points and adherent scar tissue in the abdominal region, the rolling test, light touch, and deep touch can be applied to painful areas. The physiotherapist places the index finger with sufficient gel in the anterocephalic direction while the patient is asked to exhale. The therapist then assesses the puborectalis muscle by rolling the distal phalanx of the finger over the puborectalis muscle [7]. Anal sphincter tone, intrarectal scars, fissures, fistulae, and internal hemorrhoids are assessed. Anal sphincter tone and pressure at rest and during voluntary compression are assessed. Patients with anorectal pain may have tenderness or pain on palpation of the posterior wall of the rectum and tightness of the puborectal muscle and should therefore be treated very gently and carefully [49]. The degree of descent of the perineum during the Valsalva maneuver should also be assessed. Normally, this movement is expected to be between 1 and 3.5 cm, but a decrease in the downward movement of the perineum would be a sign of inadequate relaxation of the pelvic floor muscles during defecation. An excessive downward movement of the perineum of more than 3.5 cm indicates perineal relaxation [47]. Finally, the integrity of the pudendal nerve should be assessed using the anal and bulbocavernosus reflexes. For sensory assessment, the ability to discriminate between light touch, pinprick, and cold sensation should be tested over the lumbosacral dermatomes (S2-S4) [50].

18.3.4 Assessment of the Pelvic Floor

Pelvic floor muscle strength and endurance can be assessed by vaginal/anal palpation, electromyography (EMG), vaginal impingement pressure measurement, urethral pressure measurement, pelvic floor dynamometer, ultrasound, and magnetic resonance imaging [51]. If there is no voluntary contraction and relaxation of the pelvic floor muscles, and if it contracts when it should relax, it is classified as a hypertonic pelvic floor; if voluntary contraction is reduced, it is classified as a hypotonic pelvic floor. For example, in patients with anorectal pain, the ability of the pelvic floor to relax should be assessed, as the tone of the pelvic floor muscles may be high and the muscle fibers may be tight and stiff. In addition to hypertonus, especially in patients with levator ani syndrome, there is hypersensitivity of the pelvic floor, decreased strength, endurance, speed, and coordination [25].

The most practical way to rate pelvic floor muscle strength is to use the Modified Oxford Scale (MOS), which ranges from 0 to 5. The MOS is the internationally accepted and most commonly used grading system for muscle strength and is applied by digital palpation. The assessment of strength, endurance, and maximum strength allows the appropriate exercise program to be prescribed [52]. According to the MOS, patients with AI with a strength grade of 0, 1, or 2 are more suitable for rectal balloon training or electrical stimulation than for pelvic floor exercises [53]. A perineometer is widely used for the objective assessment of anal compression pressure. A perineometer is widely used to objectively assess anal squeezing pressure. The patient is asked to squeeze the anal sphincter as hard as she can (maximum force), to hold the contraction (endurance), or to repeat the contractions as often as she can (endurance) [50].

Physiotherapists can also use superficial EMG measurements to assess muscle activation of the pelvic floor. To assess pelvic floor muscle activation, and in particular the EAS, an anal sensor is inserted to obtain an extracellular recording of bioelectrical activity. During the assessment, this information is presented to the patient via visual and auditory signals on the screen of the device or computer [51].

18.4 Physiotherapy and Rehabilitation in Colorectoanal Dysfunctions

Physiotherapy and rehabilitation approaches for colorectoanal dysfunction are inexpensive and noninvasive, do not require complex equipment, have almost no side effects, and are therefore generally used as first-line treatment. Physiotherapy and rehabilitation methods include patient education, bowel and defecation training, pelvic floor rehabilitation (PFR), exercise training, and manual therapy techniques. Pelvic floor rehabilitation in patients with colorectoanal dysfunction should be carried out by physiotherapists specializing in pelvic floor dysfunction [7].

18.4.1 Patient Education

In patient education, the pelvic physiotherapist should explain the function of the rectum and anus, the formation of feces, the relationship between the rectum, anus, and pelvic floor, the relationship between the pelvic floor and abdominal muscles, possible causes of colorectoanal disorders, and the function of the pelvic floor using visual materials such as pelvic models, presentations, and pictures (Fig. 18.1). Dietary education and physical activity modification as lifestyle changes should be included in patient education.

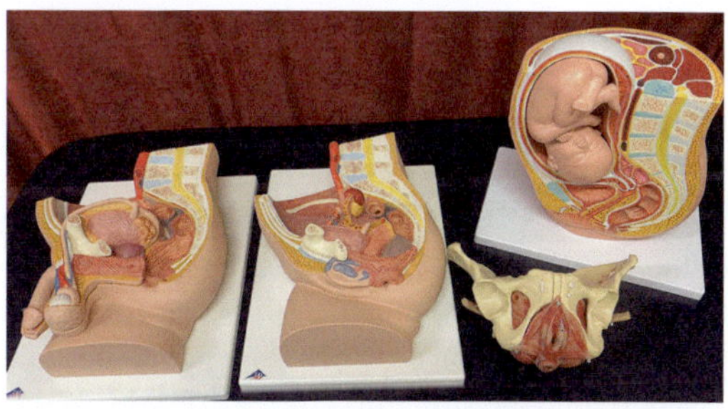

Fig. 18.1 Some models used in patient education

They are often used as first-line treatment strategies, especially for anorectal disorders. This is because these disorders are also associated with various lifestyle factors such as low dietary fiber intake, low fluid intake, and physical inactivity [54]. A high-fiber diet is recommended for people with constipation, and the recommended fiber intake is at least 25–30 g per day [55]. As there is an association between foods containing indigestible complex carbohydrates (fructose, lactose) and caffeine and the incidence of bowel dysfunction, patients should be informed about these foods/drinks. Dietary restrictions are important in regulating stool frequency and size in patients with FI [56]. The patient should be asked to complete a bowel diary along with the dietary diary, and the patient should be referred to a specialist dietitian if necessary. In addition, the patient should be informed about the negative effects of caffeine, alcohol, carbonated/sugary drinks, and smoking on bowel structure [7].

Physical activity is known to increase colonic motility, and hormones that change with exercise also contribute to this motility [57]. After determining the patient's physical activity level using objective or subjective tests, advice on physical activity should be given at this stage.

18.4.2 Bowel and Defecation Education

Patients with anal incontinence should be given toilet training to teach them the habit of regular bowel movements. As the peristaltic movement of the colon increases after waking and after meals (especially after breakfast), these are ideal times for bowel movements. As part of bowel training, patients are advised to sit on the toilet and hold the stool as long as they can for about 5 min. If they are successful at this stage, they are asked to hold the stool for a further 10 min. In the next stage, they are asked to hold the stool for 5 min while standing in the bathroom. In the final stage, patients are asked to hold the stool outside the washbasin for 10 min. The aim is to improve the patient's ability to voluntarily delay the need to defecate [7, 18].

Patients should be taught behavioral changes to reduce incontinence episodes, including regular bowel movements, timing of defecation according to activity, techniques to reduce straining, appropriate bowel movements while sitting on the toilet, and techniques to delay defecation. The positions used for optimal defecation are sitting and squatting, which widen the anorectal angle. The use of the squatting position for defecation has been reported to be a preventive factor, particularly in the development of hemorrhoids and constipation [58]. In the optimal defecation position, the knees should be apart and above the hip joint. Knees above the hip joint can be achieved with the help of a step. In addition, the trunk should be flexed forward and supported with the forearms, and, if possible, the heels should be raised [18]. Particularly in patients with dyssynergic defecation, if there is a compulsive habit of straining, it should be explained that this puts stress on the pelvic floor, and they should be asked to take deep breaths and push the pelvic floor downwards during defecation. The following information should be given to the patient in the patient education session and then practiced in the examination room, in order of importance [47]:

- Take a deep breath and expand your abdomen.
- Expand your abdomen by saying the sound "MMM."
- Say "OOO" by pushing your abdomen forward. This will relax the surrounding muscles and open your anal sphincter. This will make it easier for your stool to come out.
- Release your pelvic floor muscles when you have finished defecating.

18.4.3 Pelvic Floor Rehabilitation

The aim of pelvic floor rehabilitation is to increase the strength, effective contraction and relaxation, tone, endurance, and coordination of the pelvic floor and anal sphincter in order to reduce anorectal symptoms and improve function. It also aims to increase the patient's awareness of the pelvic floor and sphincter, the ability to defecate effectively, and to improve rectal sensation [59]. The literature reports success rates of 49–72% for pelvic floor rehabilitation approaches used in conjunction with bowel and hygiene education, dietary counseling, and bowel management education as patient education [53].

Pelvic Floor Muscle and Anal Sphincter Training

Pelvic floor muscle education (PFME) is an approach to increasing the strength, endurance, and coordination of the pelvic floor and anal sphincters. The standard form of PFME involves pelvic floor and anal sphincter contractions with verbal instruction from a physiotherapist. Patients can be taught to contract and relax their pelvic floor in different positions [60]. Pelvic floor exercises include endurance and strength exercises for both slow-twitch and fast-twitch fibers. Pelvic physiotherapists aim to be able to teach the patient the correct technique of exercise by perineal/vaginal or anal palpation [61]. The prescription of pelvic floor exercises for FI should be individualized, as the type, number, and intensity of exercises will vary from patient to patient [62]. In a systematic review, Visser et al. [63] suggested that PFME should be considered as the first step in functional rehabilitation after low anterior resection. Lin et al. [64] reported that a regular PFME program within the first 6 months after discharge from low anterior resection is a preventive intervention for FI.

Pelvic Floor Training with Biofeedback and Rectal Balloon

With anorectal biofeedback, the physiological electromyography (EMG) activity of the anus and rectum and the maneuvers required to correct the patterns are shown to the patient on the computer screen. The aim of biofeedback in patients with defecation disorders is to practice defecation, to gain the ability to increase abdominal pressure when the anal sphincter is relaxed, and to gain the defecation function obtained by sensory training of the rectum [65] (Fig. 18.2). Before starting biofeedback, patients should be informed about the anatomy of the pelvic floor muscles, the diaphragmatic breathing technique, and defecation posture. The literature recommends that biofeedback treatment should be given once or twice a week for four to six ses-

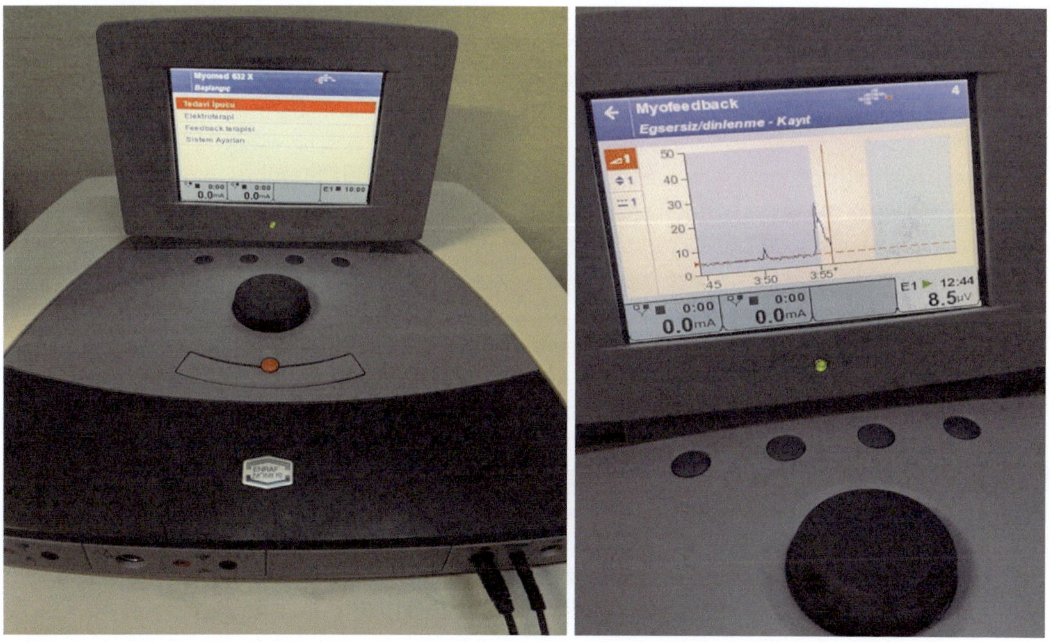

Fig. 18.2 EMG biofeedback device

sions, each lasting 30–60 min. In addition, patients should perform pelvic floor exercises with diaphragmatic breathing two to three times a day for 15–20 min as a home program [59, 62].

In older women with chronic constipation due to dyssynergic defecation, a total of six sessions of biofeedback every 15 days for 3 months was found to be more effective in improving bowel function and reducing the use of digital maneuvers compared with standard care and sham biofeedback [66]. A review of patients with functional constipation reported that biofeedback therapy was approximately six times more effective in improving constipation symptoms than laxative use, and EMG biofeedback was seven times more effective [67].

Rectal sensory training is used in patients with impaired rectal sensation. Healthy people are able to detect a balloon placed in the rectum and inflated with 15–20 ml of air. Patients with a hyposensitive rectum are trained to detect smaller volumes of rectal distension until a normal sensory threshold is reached or a plateau is reached. This allows patients to feel defecation sooner. Rectal balloon training can also be used in patients with urgency and rectal hypersensitivity. Patients with a hypersensitive rectum are trained to tolerate larger volumes until the sensation of urgency subsides. Patients with weak pelvic floor muscles learn to contract these muscles immediately and strongly in response to rectal filling [68].

Another biofeedback approach used for defecation disorders is the three-balloon system for training anal sphincter coordination. One large balloon is placed in the rectum, and the second and third balloons are placed above and below the anal canal. These balloons are connected to a manometric pressure recorder. When the larger balloon is inflated, the rectoanal inhibitory reflex is stimulated, and the patient can then be taught to perform a voluntary EAS contraction to counteract the involuntary relaxation of the IAS. This method teaches the patient how to perform an effective squeeze, during which the rectal pressure is shown to increase in the diagram. At the same time, the patient is encouraged to relax the EAS, as the diagram shows the pressure decreasing. The effectiveness of the treatment can be increased by adding abdominal breathing and core stabilization exercises to the biofeedback treatment program [21]. Three-balloon system applications are reported to have a therapeutic effect in terms of teaching voluntary anal compression and providing sufficient force and time for resting pressure to return to its initial level [69].

Pelvic Floor Muscle Training with Electrical Stimulation

Electrical stimulation is another modality recommended for the rehabilitation of AI. The aim of electrical stimulation is to passively increase pelvic floor muscle and anal sphincter strength and endurance and to improve awareness and isolated contraction of the anal sphincters. Electrical stimulation of the pelvic floor and anal sphincters can be applied in many different ways, including surface electrodes or intrarectal probes, and with many different stimulation parameters/treatment protocols [70]. Although amplitude-modulated mid-frequency stimulation has recently been recommended, low-frequency stimulation is usually used. When targeting EAS and the posterior pelvic floor compartment, it is recommended to use a 250 μs current duration and 35–40 Hz treatment frequency without causing fatigue [7]. Electrical stimulation is often used in combination with PTKE or biofeedback training. Electrical stimulation should not be used for anal and vaginal infections, rectal bleeding, sensory impairment, complete denervation of the pelvic floor muscles, hemorrhoids with edema and hematoma, dementia, pregnancy, painful palpation, or for the first 6 weeks after anal surgery [18].

18.4.4 Physical Activity and Exercise

Increased colonic mobility with regular physical activity, mechanical vibration of the body during aerobic exercise, and increased abdominal muscle pressure on the colon reduce anorectal symptoms [71]. A randomized controlled trial conducted to investigate the effect of regular physical activity in people with functional constipation reported that a 12-week physical activity program reduced total colonic transit time and improved constipation symptoms [72]. In addition, a regular aerobic exercise program (walking, cycling) has been reported to improve total and recto-sigmoid colonic transit time [72].

Patients with colorectoanal dysfunction may have high anal tone due to fear of pain and straining. Treatment of overactive pelvic floor muscles is aimed at restoring motor control and function, manually lengthening muscle fibers, and retraining muscle movement. Teaching the patient to lower or actively relax their muscles is called down training. Down training is usually done in combination with pelvic floor stretching and diaphragmatic breathing. Behavioral retraining using verbal and tactile cues improves colonic motility by improving kinesthetic and proprioceptive awareness of muscle contraction, active lengthening, and passive relaxation [73]. In addition, stretching exercises for the iliopsoas, piriformis, hamstrings, and hip adductors associated with the pelvic floor should be included in exercise programs [7] (Fig. 18.3).

It has a regulating effect on the nervous system, reducing the overactive sympathetic nervous system in patients with defecation disorders and anorectal pain and increasing the parasympathetic response through structured breathing control and the relaxing and calming effects of relaxation [47]. Breath control training teaches the patient to take slow, deep breaths and to pay attention to the relaxing sensations when exhaling. This relaxation technique is an effective treatment for correcting inappropriate breathing patterns (superficial chest breathing) in patients with stress-related physical disorders. The patient is taught to be aware of each breath, excluding all external stimuli. To increase its effectiveness, gender-neutral forms can be asked to do it slowly, thinking the word "calm" during the inhalation phase of deep breathing and the word "relax" during the exhalation phase. When teaching diaphragmatic breathing, the patient is asked to lie on gender-neutral forms back with gender-neutral forms knees bent, with one hand on gender-neutral forms chest and the other on his abdomen (on the rectus abdominis muscle), not moving the upper chest while breathing. The emphasis is on moving the abdomen outwards on inhalation and inwards on exhalation (Fig. 18.4). Gender-neutral forms can be asked to feel the pelvic floor displaced downwards while breathing [74]. Progressive relaxation techniques can be used for

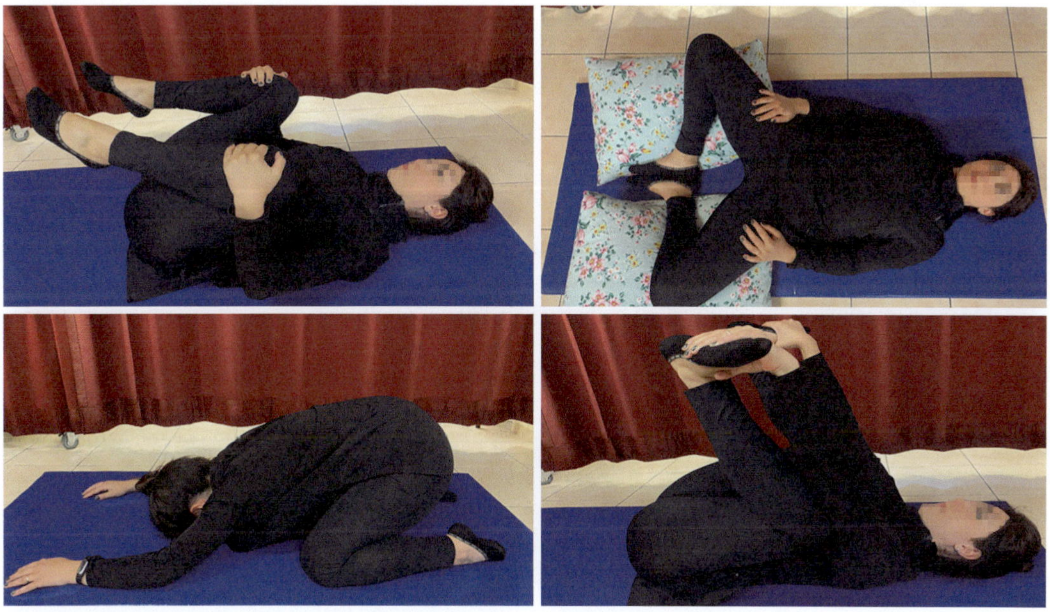

Fig. 18.3 Stretching exercises in colorectoanal dysfunction

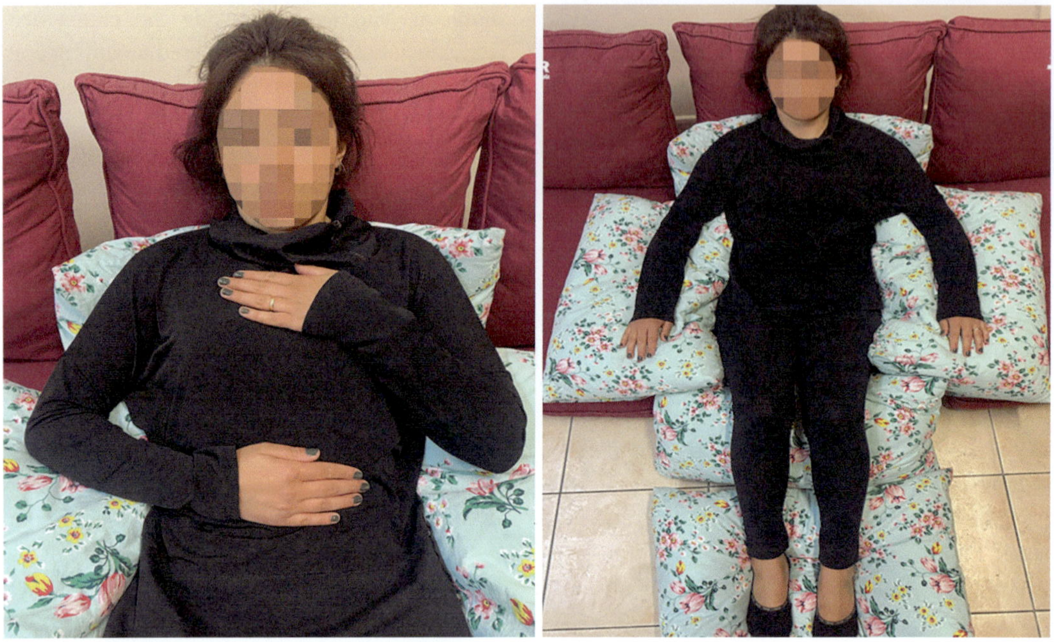

Fig. 18.4 Breathing awareness and relaxation training

the puborectalis and external anal sphincters, which are paradoxically contracted and unable to relax during dyssynergic defecation [73].

18.4.5 Manual Therapy

Classical Abdominal Massage
Classical abdominal massage is one of the most commonly used manual therapy methods for chronic constipation and defecation disorders. It is applied with clockwise massage techniques to the area where the ascending colon, transverse colon, descending colon, and sigmoid colon are located on the anterior abdominal wall. In abdominal massage, the digestive organs are compressed between the fingers and the posterior abdominal wall with manual pressure from the anterior abdominal wall, creating peristaltic stimulation. This causes feces to be redirected from the colon to the rectum (Fig. 18.5) [18]. Studies have reported that abdominal massage improves constipation symptoms by producing neurological and autonomic responses through mechanical stimulation. Abdominal massage reduces abdominal muscle tension by increasing local and visceral blood flow. It also stimulates colonic movements by accelerating peristaltic stimulation, thereby reducing the transit time of rectal contents through the colon [75]. Dogan et al. [76] reported significant improvements in constipation severity, bowel function scores, and quality of life in patients with functional constipation in the group receiving abdominal massage for 4 weeks compared with the placebo group receiving therapeutic ultrasound.

Connective Tissue Massage
Connective tissue massage (CTM) is a reflex therapy that stimulates autonomic nerve endings in the skin with specialized pulls applied to the connective tissue [75]. It is argued that CTM provides a balance between sympathetic and parasympathetic components of the autonomic nervous system [4]. In chronic constipation, CTM may increase intestinal motility by reflex stimulation of parasympathetic nerves. It has been reported in the literature that connective tissue massage applied to individuals with chronic constipation reduces the severity and clinical symptoms of constipation, improves health-related quality of life, and can be included in conservative treatment methods [75, 77]. Gürşen et al. [78] reported that

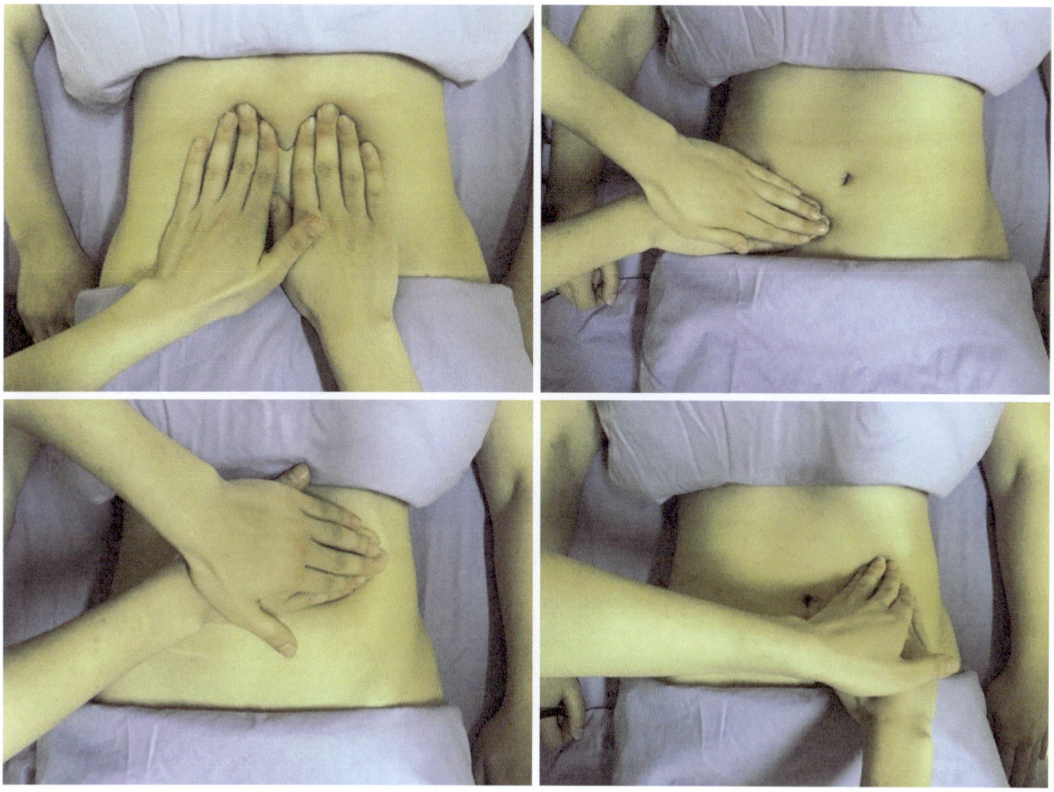

Fig. 18.5 Classical abdominal massage

in addition to lifestyle recommendations, CTM applied to the lumbosacral, lower thoracic, scapular, interscapular, and cervical regions 5 days a week for 4 weeks was more effective in improving chronic constipation symptoms and improving quality of life compared with lifestyle recommendations alone (Fig. 18.6).

Kinesio Taping

Finally, the kinesio taping method, which is frequently used in conservative physiotherapy, increases colonic motility and shortens colonic transit time when applied to the sacral and abdominal region, which is the reflex region of the intestine [18]. It can be applied on the sacrum and abdominal region in patients with chronic constipation. In a study, it was reported that the severity of constipation decreased and stool type and quality of life improved with taping application performed three times a week for 4 weeks in children with cerebral palsy with chronic constipation [77].

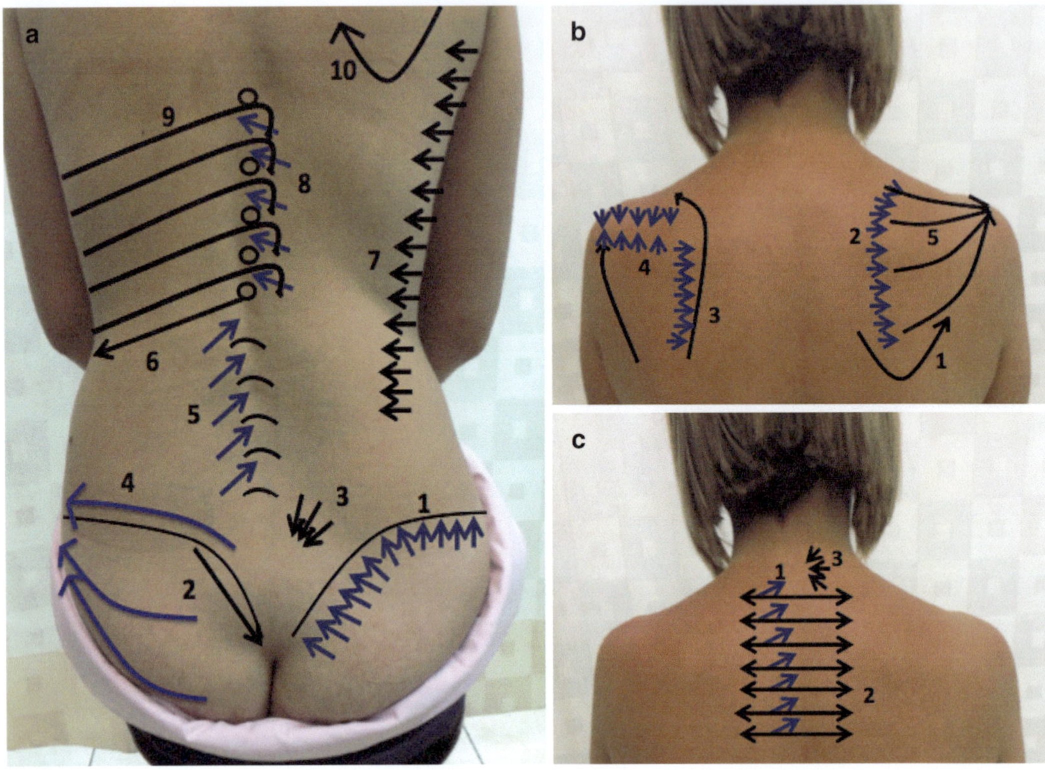

Fig. 18.6 Connective tissue massage. (**a**) Lumbosacral and lower thoracic regions, (**b**) scapular region, (**c**) interscapular region [75]

18.5 Conclusion

Problems affecting the colorectoanal region include anal incontinence, chronic constipation, defecation disorders, hemorrhoids, and anorectal pain. Patients with colorectal dysfunction should be assessed in detail based on history, disease-specific physiological tests, and physical and pelvic assessment, and treatment should include individualized approaches. The primary management of colorectoanal dysfunction is conservative. Conservative treatments include lifestyle changes, pharmacological treatment, and physiotherapy. Physiotherapy and rehabilitation methods, including patient education, bowel and defecation education, pelvic floor muscle training, pelvic floor training with biofeedback and rectal balloon, electrical pelvic floor stimulation applications, aerobic and stretching exercises, and specific manual therapy techniques, are used to achieve successful outcomes in functional status and quality of life in the treatment of colorectoanal dysfunction. To ensure optimal recovery in this group of patients, assessment and treatment should be carried out by a multidisciplinary team such as medical doctors, physiotherapists, and dieticians specialized in this area should be part of the multidisciplinary team.

References

1. Palit S, Lunniss PJ, Scott SM. The physiology of human defecation. Dig Dis Sci. 2012;57:1445–64.
2. Rao SS, Bharucha AE, Chiarioni G, Felt-Bersma R, Knowles C, Malcolm A, Wald A. Anorectal disorders. Gastroenterology. 2016;150(6):1430–1442. e1434.
3. Wieslander CK. Clinical approach and office evaluation of the patient with pelvic floor dysfunction. Obstet Gynecol Clin. 2009;36(3):445–62.
4. Baran E. Pelvis Anatomisi. In: Akbayrak T, editor. Kadın Sağlığında Fizyoterapi ve Rehabilitasyon. Pelikan Yayıncılık; 2016. p. 15–35.

5. Hohlschneider AM, Hustson JM. Anatomy and function of the Normal rectum and anus. In: Anorectal malformations in children: embryology, diagnosis, surgical treatment, follow-up; 2006. p. 143–60.
6. Shaw C, Wagg A. Urinary and faecal incontinence in older adults. Medicine. 2021;49(1):44–50.
7. Ceren Gürşen GG. Fekal İnkontinansta Fizyoterapi ve rehabilitasyon. In: Multidisipliner Bakış Temeli ile Pelvik Sağlıkta Fizyoterapi ve Rehabilitasyon. Ankara: Hedef Yayıncılık; 2023. p. 311–49.
8. Sultan AH, Monga A, Lee J, Emmanuel A, Norton C, Santoro G, Hull T, Berghmans B, Brody S, Haylen BT. An international Urogynecological association (IUGA)/international continence society (ICS) joint report on the terminology for female anorectal dysfunction. Int Urogynecol J. 2017;28:5–31.
9. Ruiz NS, Kaiser AM. Fecal incontinence-challenges and solutions. World J Gastroenterol. 2017;23(1):11.
10. Macmillan AK, Merrie AE, Marshall RJ, Parry BR. The prevalence of fecal incontinence in community-dwelling adults: a systematic review of the literature. Dis Colon Rectum. 2004;47(9):1341–9.
11. Pretlove S, Radley S, Toozs-Hobson P, Thompson P, Coomarasamy A, Khan K. Prevalence of anal incontinence according to age and gender: a systematic review and meta-regression analysis. Int Urogynecol J. 2006;17:407–17.
12. Lindberg G, Hamid SS, Malfertheiner P, Thomsen OO, Fernandez LB, Garisch J, Thomson A, Goh K-L, Tandon R, Fedail S. World gastroenterology organisation global guideline: constipation—a global perspective. J Clin Gastroenterol. 2011;45(6):483–7.
13. Sobrado CW, Corrêa Neto IJF, Pinto RA, Sobrado LF, Nahas SC, Cecconello I. Diagnosis and treatment of constipation: a clinical update based on the Rome IV criteria. J Coloproctol (Rio de Janeiro). 2018;38:137–44.
14. Schmidt FMQ, de Gouveia Santos VLC. Prevalence of constipation in the general adult population: an integrative review. J Wound Ostomy Cont Nurs. 2014;41(1):70–6.
15. Hayat U, Dugum M, Garg S. Chronic constipation: update on management. Cleve Clin J Med. 2017;84(5):397–408.
16. Drossman DA. Functional gastrointestinal disorders: history, pathophysiology, clinical features, and Rome IV. Gastroenterology. 2016;150(6):1262–1279. e1262.
17. Bharucha AE, Pemberton JH, Locke GR. American Gastroenterological Association technical review on constipation. Gastroenterology. 2013;144(1):218–38.
18. Ceren Orhan SK. Anorektal Disfonksiyonda Fizyoterapi ve Rehabilitasyon. In: Akbayrak T, editor. Kadın Sağlığında Fizyoterapi ve Rehabilitasyon, vol. 1. Pelikan Yayıncılık; Ankara, Türkiye, 2016. p. 141–67.
19. Lacy BE, Mearin F, Chang L, Chey WD, Lembo AJ, Simren M, Spiller R. Bowel disorders. Gastroenterology. 2016;150(6):1393–1407. e1395.
20. Schmulson MJ, Drossman DA. What is new in Rome IV. J Neurogastroenterol Motil. 2017;23(2):151.
21. Rao SS, Patcharatrakul T. Diagnosis and treatment of dyssynergic defecation. J Neurogastroenterol Motil. 2016;22(3):423.
22. Ortengren AR, Ramkissoon RA, Chey WD, Baker JR, Staller K, Iturrino J, Shah ED. Anorectal manometry to diagnose dyssynergic defecation: systematic review and meta-analysis of diagnostic test accuracy. Neurogastroenterol Motil. 2021;33(11):e14137.
23. Cerruto MA. Chronic pelvic pain and chronic pelvic pain syndrome: classification and epidemiology. In: Giammò A, Biroli A, editors. Chronic Pelvic Pain and Pelvic Dysfunctions: Assessment and Multidisciplinary Approach. Cham: Springer Nature Switzerland AG; 2021. p. 49–60.
24. Drossman DA, Li Z, Andruzzi E, Temple RD, Talley NJ, Grant Thompson W, Whitehead WE, Janssens J, Funch-Jensen P, Corazziari E. US householder survey of functional gastrointestinal disorders: prevalence, sociodemography, and health impact. Dig Dis Sci. 1993;38:1569–80.
25. Chiarioni G, Nardo A, Vantini I, Romito A, Whitehead WE. Biofeedback is superior to electrogalvanic stimulation and massage for treatment of levator ani syndrome. Gastroenterology. 2010;138(4):1321–9.
26. Gülören G, Çınar GN, Baran E, Gürşen C, Uzelpasacı E, Özgül S, Beksaç K, Fadıloglu E, Aydın E, Tanacan A. Hemorrhoids, anorectal symptoms, and related risk factors in pregnancy and the postpartum period: a follow-up study. J Women's Pelvic Health Phys Ther. 2024;48(3):184–93.
27. Çinar GN, Akbayrak T, Nakip G, Özgül S, Üzelpasacı E, Baran E, Gürşen C, Beksac K, Aydın E, Orgul G. Correlation between Various Anthropometric and Musculoskeletal Measurements and Hemorrhoids in Pregnancy. Türk Fizyoterapi ve Rehabilitasyon Dergisi. 2024;35(1):73–82.
28. Gardner IH, Siddharthan RV, Tsikitis VL. Benign anorectal disease: hemorrhoids, fissures, and fistulas. Ann Gastroenterol. 2020;33(1):9.
29. Wieslander CK. Clinical approach and office evaluation of the patient with pelvic floor dysfunction. Obstet Gynecol Clin N Am. 2009;36(3):445–62. https://doi.org/10.1016/j.ogc.2009.09.003.
30. Sbahi H, Cash BD. Chronic constipation: a review of current literature. Curr Gastroenterol Rep. 2015;17:1–13.
31. Menees S, Chey WD. Fecal incontinence: pathogenesis, diagnosis, and updated treatment strategies. Gastroenterol Clin. 2022;51(1):71–91.
32. Jorge MJ, Wexner SD. Etiology and management of fecal incontinence. Dis Colon Rectum. 1993;36(1):77–97.
33. Vaizey C, Carapeti E, Cahill J, Kamm M. Prospective comparison of faecal incontinence grading systems. Gut. 1999;44(1):77–80.
34. Rothbarth J, Bemelman WA, Meijerink WJ, Stiggelbout AM, Zwinderman AH, Buyze-Westerweel ME, Delemarre JB. What is the impact of fecal

incontinence on quality of life? Dis Colon Rectum. 2001;44:67–71.
35. Lewis SJ, Heaton KW. Stool form scale as a useful guide to intestinal transit time. Scand J Gastroenterol. 1997;32(9):920–4.
36. Mukhtar NB, Meeus M, Gursen C, Mohammed J, Dewitte V, Cagnie B. Development of culturally sensitive pain neuroscience education materials for Hausa-speaking patients with chronic spinal pain: a modified Delphi study. PLoS One. 2021;16(7):e0253757.
37. Droz J, Howard FM. Use of the short-form McGill pain questionnaire as a diagnostic tool in women with chronic pelvic pain. J Minim Invasive Gynecol. 2011;18(2):211–7.
38. Wijma AJ, van Wilgen CP, Meeus M, Nijs J. Clinical biopsychosocial physiotherapy assessment of patients with chronic pain: the first step in pain neuroscience education. Physiother Theory Pract. 2016;32(5):368–84.
39. Neblett R. The central sensitization inventory: a user's manual. J Appl Biobehav Res. 2018;23(2):e12123.
40. Darnall BD, Sturgeon JA, Cook KF, Taub CJ, Roy A, Burns JW, Sullivan M, Mackey SC. Development and validation of a daily pain catastrophizing scale. J Pain. 2017;18(9):1139–49.
41. Rockwood TH, Church JM, Fleshman JW, Kane RL, Mavrantonis C, Thorson AG, Wexner SD, Bliss D, Lowry AC. Fecal incontinence quality of life scale: quality of life instrument for patients with fecal incontinence. Dis Colon Rectum. 2000;43:9–16.
42. Yilmaz Sahin S, Oztas B, Kural E, Iyigun E. Transcultural adaptation and validation of the Turkish version of the gastrointestinal quality of life index. Indian J Surg. 2022;84(4):707–14.
43. Bengi G, Yalçın M, Akpınar H, Keskinoğlu P, Ellidokuz H. Validity and reliability of the patient assessment of constipation quality of life questionnaire for the Turkish population. Turk J Gastroenterol. 2015;26(4):309–14.
44. Bols E, Berghmans B, Hendriks E, Baeten C, Bie R. Physiotherapy ans surgery in faecal incontinence: an overview. Phys Ther Rev. 2008;13(2):1–20.
45. Igualada-Martinez P, Breslin E, Higgins D, Hainsworth A. Physiotherapy management of anorectal dysfunction. In: Seminars in colon and rectal surgery, vol. 1. Amsterdam: Elsevier; 2023. p. 100936.
46. Terra M, Deutekom M, Dobben A, Baeten C, Janssen L, Boeckxstaens G, Engel A, Felt-Bersma R, Slors J, Gerhards M. Can the outcome of pelvic-floor rehabilitation in patients with fecal incontinence be predicted? Int J Color Dis. 2008;23:503–11.
47. Bocchini R, Chiarioni G, Corazziari E, Pucciani F, Torresan F, Alduini P, Bassotti G, Battaglia E, Ferrarini F, Galeazzi F. Pelvic floor rehabilitation for defecation disorders. Tech Coloproctol. 2019;23:101–15.
48. Ortiz H, De Miguel M, Ciga MA. Clinical assessment of the incontinent patient. In: Fecal incontinence: diagnosis and treatment. New York: Springer; 2007. p. 89–93.
49. Deutekom M, Terra M, Dijkgraaf M, Dobben A, Stoker J, Boeckxstaens G, Bossuyt P. Patients' perception of tests in the assessment of faecal incontinence. Br J Radiol. 2006;79(938):94–100.
50. Azpiroz F, Puigdollers A, Amselem C. Evaluation of anorectal and pelvic floor muscle function. In: Urinary and fecal incontinence: an interdisciplinary approach. New York: Springer; 2005. p. 121–36.
51. Mateus-Vasconcelos ECL, Ribeiro AM, Antonio FI, Brito LGO, Ferreira CHJ. Physiotherapy methods to facilitate pelvic floor muscle contraction: a systematic review. Physiother Theory Pract. 2018;34(6):420–32.
52. Ferreira CHJ, Barbosa PB, de Oliveira Souza F, Antônio FI, Franco MM, Bø K. Inter-rater reliability study of the modified Oxford grading scale and the Peritron manometer. Physiotherapy. 2011;97(2):132–8.
53. Mazur-Bialy AI, Kołomańska-Bogucka D, Opławski M, Tim S. Physiotherapy for prevention and treatment of fecal incontinence in women—systematic review of methods. J Clin Med. 2020;9(10):3255.
54. Kim S-J. Diet, physical activity, and chronic constipation: unveiling the combined effects for better treatment strategies. J Neurogastroenterol Motil. 2024;30(3):255–6.
55. Badiali D, Corazziari E, Habib FI, Tomei E, Bausano G, Magrini P, Anzini F, Torsoli A. Effect of wheat bran in treatment of chronic nonorganic constipation: a double-blind controlled trial. Dig Dis Sci. 1995;40:349–56.
56. Benezech A, Bouvier M, Vitton V. Faecal incontinence: current knowledges and perspectives. World J Gastrointest Pathophysiol. 2016;7(1):59.
57. Dukas L, Willett WC, Giovannucci EL. Association between physical activity, fiber intake, and other lifestyle variables and constipation in a study of women. Off J Am Coll Gastroenterol|ACG. 2003;98(8):1790–6.
58. Sohrabi S, Malekzadeh R, Ansari R, Kamangar F. Squatting and risk of colorectal cancer: a case-control study. Middle East J Dig Dis. 2012;4(1):23.
59. Höder A, Stenbeck J, Fernando M, Lange E. Pelvic floor muscle training with biofeedback or feedback from a physiotherapist for urinary and anal incontinence after childbirth-a systematic review. BMC Womens Health. 2023;23(1):618.
60. Bols EM, Berghmans BC, Hendriks EJ, Baeten CG, de Bie RA. Physiotherapy and surgery in fecal incontinence: an overview. Phys Ther Rev. 2008;13(2):71–90.
61. Orhan C, Akbayrak T, Özgül S, Baran E, Üzelpasaci E, Nakip G, Özgül N, Beksaç MS. Effects of vaginal tampon training added to pelvic floor muscle training in women with stress urinary incontinence: randomized controlled trial. Int Urogynecol J. 2019;30:219–29.
62. Pun MY, Leung PH, Chan TC, Pang C, Chan KH, Kannan P. The effectiveness of physiotherapy interventions on fecal incontinence and quality of life following colorectal surgery: a systematic review

and meta-analysis of randomized controlled trials. Support Care Cancer. 2024;32(2):103.

63. Visser WS, Te Riele WW, Boerma D, Van Ramshorst B, Van Westreenen HL. Pelvic floor rehabilitation to improve functional outcome after a low anterior resection: a systematic review. Ann Coloproctol. 2014;30(3):109.
64. Lin YH, Yang HY, Hung SL, Chen HP, Liu KW, Chen TB, Chi SC. Effects of pelvic floor muscle exercise on faecal incontinence in rectal cancer patients after stoma closure. Eur J Cancer Care. 2016;25(3):449–57.
65. Sadeghi A, Akbarpour E, Majidirad F, Bor S, Forootan M, Hadian M-R, Adibi P. Dyssynergic defecation: a comprehensive review on diagnosis and management. Turk J Gastroenterol. 2023;34(3):182.
66. Rao SS, Seaton K, Miller M, Brown K, Nygaard I, Stumbo P, Zimmerman B, Schulze K. Randomized controlled trial of biofeedback, sham feedback, and standard therapy for dyssynergic defecation. Clin Gastroenterol Hepatol. 2007;5(3):331–8.
67. Koh C, Young C, Young J, Solomon M. Systematic review of randomized controlled trials of the effectiveness of biofeedback for pelvic floor dysfunction. J Br Surg. 2008;95(9):1079–87.
68. Scott KM. Pelvic floor rehabilitation in the treatment of fecal incontinence. Clin Colon Rectal Surg. 2014;27(03):99–105.
69. Whitehead WE. Medical and behavioral treatment of fecal incontinence. In: Urinary and fecal incontinence: an interdisciplinary approach. New York: Springer; 2005. p. 199–210.
70. Bates F, Bliss DZ, Bardsley A, Yeung WKW. Management of fecal incontinence in community-living adults. In: Bliss DZ, editor. Management of Fecal Incontinence for the Advanced Practice Nurse. Cham: Springer International Publishing AG; 2018. p. 93–126.
71. HP P, De Vries W, Vanberge-Henegouwen G, Akkermans L. Potential benefits and hazards of physical activity and exercise on the gastrointestinal tract. Gut. 2001;48(3):435–9.
72. De Schryver AM, Keulemans YC, Peters HP, Akkermans LM, Smout AJ, De Vries WR, Van Berge-Henegouwen GP. Effects of regular physical activity on defecation pattern in middle-aged patients complaining of chronic constipation. Scand J Gastroenterol. 2005;40(4):422–9.
73. Gao R, Tao Y, Zhou C, Li J, Wang X, Chen L, Li F, Guo L. Exercise therapy in patients with constipation: a systematic review and meta-analysis of randomized controlled trials. Scand J Gastroenterol. 2019;54(2):169–77.
74. Bartlett LM, Sloots KL, Nowak MJ, Ho Y-h. Impact of relaxation breathing on the internal anal sphincter in patients with faecal incontinence. Aust N Z Continence J. 2012;18(2):38–45.
75. Orhan C, Özgül S, Baran E, Üzelpasacı E, Akbayrak T. Comparison of connective tissue manipulation and abdominal massage combined with usual care vs usual care alone for chronic constipation: a randomized controlled trial. J Manip Physiol Ther. 2020;43(8):768–78.
76. Doğan İG, Gürşen C, Akbayrak T, Balaban YH, Vahabov C, Üzelpasacı E, Özgül S. Abdominal massage in functional chronic constipation: a randomized placebo-controlled trial. Phys Ther. 2022;102(7):pzac058.
77. Orhan C, Kaya Kara O, Kaya S, Akbayrak T, Kerem Gunel M, Baltaci G. The effects of connective tissue manipulation and Kinesio taping on chronic constipation in children with cerebral palsy: a randomized controlled trial. Disabil Rehabil. 2018;40(1):10–20.
78. Gürsen C, Günel MK, Kaya S, Kav T, Akbayrak T. Effect of connective tissue manipulation on symptoms and quality of life in patients with chronic constipation: a randomized controlled trial. J Manip Physiol Ther. 2015;38(5):335–43.

Physiotherapy and Rehabilitation for Common Problems During Pregnancy and Postnatal Period

19

Duygu Şahin Altaç and İlkim Çitak Karakaya

19.1 Introduction

Pregnancy is a process in which many anatomical, physiological, and hormonal changes occur. All these changes make the expectant mother sensitive to possible systemic problems. Physiotherapy applications during pregnancy aim to help the pregnant woman adapt to maternal changes, prevent or treat possible problems, and prepare the pregnant woman for birth. At the postnatal period, where pregnancy-related changes begin to return to the prepregnancy state, problems that occurred during pregnancy may continue, and some others due to childbirth may arise; therefore, the need for physiotherapy is retained. Given these objectives, it is crucial for physiotherapists to collaborate with expectant mothers and other healthcare professionals both during pregnancy and during the postnatal period. In this chapter, after informing the readers about types and possible etiologies of common pregnancy-related and postnatal problems, evidence-based approaches for their assessment and physiotherapy will be discussed in the light of the current literature.

19.2 Changes in the Body Systems During Pregnancy and at the Postnatal Period

The body of an expectant mother undergoes various anatomical and physiological changes during pregnancy to provide a convenient place for developing and supporting the fetus, to meet the increased metabolic requirements, and to prepare the body for birth. Postpartum is the period when these changes return to the nonpregnant state. Some authorities examine the postpartum period in three stages: the emergency (acute) period is the first 24–48 h after vaginal birth and the first 72 h after cesarean delivery; the early stage is the one-week period after birth; and the late period covers the period between 6 weeks and 6 months. Some other authorities consider the postpartum period as 6–8 weeks after birth since pregnancy-related anatomical and physiological changes mainly return to the prepregnancy state in this period [62]. The American College of Obstetricians and Gynecologists (ACOG) reports that this period extends up to 12 weeks and calls this period the "fourth trimester." Some investigators argue that the definition of the postnatal period should cover the year after birth, based on the necessity of continuing postpartum care and support [10].

D. Şahin Altaç (✉)
Department of Physiotherapy and Rehabilitation, Faculty of Health Sciences, Haliç University, Istanbul, Türkiye
e-mail: duygusahinaltac@halıc.edu.tr

İ. Çitak Karakaya
Department of Physiotherapy and Rehabilitation, Faculty of Health Sciences, Muğla Sıtkı Koçman University, Muğla, Türkiye
e-mail: ikarakaya@mu.edu.tr

T. Akbayrak, E. Üzelpasaci (eds.), *Physiotherapy and Rehabilitation in Pelvic and Women's Health-Related Problems*, https://doi.org/10.1007/978-3-032-28741-0_19

Table 19.1 provides information about maternal changes that occur during pregnancy and at the postnatal period [13, 21, 45, 48, 62, 63, 77]. This knowledge will provide physiotherapists a baseline for appropriate evaluation and specific management approaches to various problems that may occur in different systems both during pregnancy and in the postnatal period.

Table 19.1 Maternal changes during pregnancy and at the postnatal period

Test	Pregnancy	Postnatal period
Endocrine system	Menstruation disappears Secretion and amount of many hormones, such as beta-HCG, HPL, estrogen, progesterone, prolactin, oxytocin, adrenocorticotropic hormone, aldosterone, relaxin, thyroxins, and insulin, change through different stages of pregnancy Thyroid gland volume increases	Most of these hormones such as beta-HCG, estrogen, and progesterone return to prepregnancy state shortly after delivery, whereas relaxin takes approximately 12 months to return to baseline Menstruation usually reappears in 4–5 months Insulin sensitivity increases after delivery and is restored within 2–3 days Thyroid function returns to normal by 4 weeks postpartum
Musculoskeletal system	Increased body weight and body mass index Increased soft tissue laxity (especially the ligaments of the pelvis, low back, etc.) Postural changes (center of gravity shifts forward; kyphotic and lordotic curves increase, and pelvis tilts anteriorly, etc.) Shortening of the hip flexors and lumbar extensors and weakness of the abdominal musculature, hip extensors, etc.	A weight loss of 5–6 kg due to the expulsion of products of gestation and accompanying blood loss occurs shortly after giving birth. Further weight loss of 2–3 kg can be attributed to the brisk diuresis, which may continue up to 6 months after delivery Ligamentous laxity continues until the sixth week postpartum, and complete recovery takes 12 months postpartum Postural changes persist until the 12th week after birth
Hematologic and cardiovascular system	The heart is displaced upward and forward, the ventricular muscle mass increases, and the valve diameter expands Even though the heart expands physiologically, there is no significant change in the ejection fraction Cardiac output, stroke volume, and heart rate increase as pregnancy progresses Total peripheral vascular resistance decreases due to peripheral vasodilation Blood viscosity decreases, and plasma volume and red cell volume increase (plasma volume more than red cells) Vascularity increases in reproductive organs Systemic and pulmonary vascular resistances change throughout pregnancy Risk of thromboembolism increases	Cardiac output declines to prepregnancy values in 2 weeks postpartum Heart rate returns to pre-pregnant levels 6 weeks postpartum Systemic vascular resistance increases to pre-pregnant levels in 2 weeks postpartum The physiological hypertrophy of the ventricular system reverts to the pre-pregnant state in 4 weeks The hypercoagulable state resolves gradually after birth, as clotting factor levels normalize in 8–12 weeks postpartum Increased myometrial vascularity recovers spontaneously in most women at 6 weeks

(continued)

Table 19.1 (continued)

Test	Pregnancy	Postnatal period
Respiratory system	The mucosa of the nasopharynx becomes hyperemic and edematous Subcostal angle increases from 68 to 103 degrees The transverse diameter of the chest expands by 2 cm, and the chest circumference expands by 5–7 cm The level of the diaphragm rises 4 cm Respiratory muscle function is not affected and maximal expiratory and inspiratory pressures are unchanged Maternal oxygen consumption increases 20–40% The minute ventilation increases due to increased respiratory center sensitivity and drive; a low expiratory volume and compensated respiratory alkalosis occur Vital capacity remains unchanged Tidal volume and inspiratory capacity increase 30–40% and 5–10%, respectively Functional residual capacity (FRC) and residual volume decrease 20–25%	FRC changes return to normal 1–2 weeks postpartum, accompanying the reduction in uterine size All other respiratory parameters return to nonpregnant values within 6–12 weeks postpartum
Gastrointestinal system	Muscle tone throughout the digestive tract decreases Production of proinflammatory cytokines by Kupffer cells increases Gastric emptying is delayed Diaphragm rises due to enlarging uterus Bile composition changes Gastrointestinal transit time decreases Esophageal sphincter tone decreases Hypersecretion of acid due to high gastrin levels causes an increase in the incidence of acid reflux	Gastric activity returns to normal within 24–48 h following birth, while colonic activity returns to normal within 48–72 h Progesterone and gastrin levels decrease within 24 h, and gastroesophageal reflux and associated symptoms end over the next 3–4 days
Urogenital system	The volume of kidneys increases by 30% from the pre-pregnant state The ureters and renal pelvis dilate Renal plasma flow and glomerular filtration increase Intravesical pressure increases due to the increased weight of the uterus The risk of developing urinary tract infections increases In the second half of pregnancy, cervical dilation occurs, and increased relaxin hormone levels cause the collagen content of the cervix to soften The vagina appears purple and edematous during pregnancy due to the effect of ovarian hormones Vaginal pH decreases In addition to increased laxity, the need to support the fetal structures causes the pelvic floor to be under stress Glycogen in vaginal epithelium may increase	The dilated ureters and renal pelvis usually return to the pre-pregnant state within 4–8 weeks Size of the uterus gradually decreases in the postpartum period due to rapid changes in blood flow and the effect of lochia discharge, returning to its prepregnancy size within 4–8 weeks The cervix, which begins to shorten and thicken immediately after birth, never returns to its previous state The vagina regains its tone approximately 2 weeks after the postnatal period The greatest improvement in the pelvic floor occurs within 6 months postnatally

(continued)

Table 19.1 (continued)

Test	Pregnancy	Postnatal period
Integumentary system	Hyperpigmentation Striae or stretch marks over the abdomen The pigment changes accompanying pregnancy (melasma and linea nigra) Telangiectasia and spider angiomata Nonpitting edema and varicosities in the lower extremities	The pigment changes accompanying it usually disappear by 6–8 weeks The abdominal muscles regain their normal tone and elasticity, returning to prepregnancy levels by 6–8 weeks Divarication of recti and the striae or stretch marks over the abdomen and legs might not disappear

19.3 Musculoskeletal Problems

Factors such as increased body weight, displacement of the center of gravity due to the expansion of the uterus, and increased mechanical compression of joints and soft tissues due to fluid retention caused by hormonal changes make pregnant women susceptible to musculoskeletal problems [31]. Studies in the literature report that almost all women experience a musculoskeletal problem at least once during pregnancy [64]. Although musculoskeletal system problems in the postpartum period are mostly an extension of problems during pregnancy, they can also occur independently [62, 72]. The most common musculoskeletal problems of pregnancy are lumbopelvic pain (LPP), carpal tunnel syndrome (CTS), and diastasis recti abdominis (DRA). Thoracic outlet syndrome, De Quervain tenosynovitis, patellofemoral pain, osteonecrosis of the femoral head, and transient osteoporosis of the hip are other musculoskeletal problems that can occur during pregnancy. Among these, the LPP and DRA are the most common musculoskeletal problems that persist in the postnatal period [5].

19.3.1 Pregnancy-Related LPP

Pregnancy-related LPP is defined as pain localized to the lumbar spine and/or the pelvic girdle, which includes the symphysis pubis anteriorly and the sacroiliac joints (SIJ) posteriorly, for more than a week. LPP is a common problem that reaches its highest level of severity between 24 and 36 weeks of pregnancy and is experienced by approximately 86% of pregnant women [25, 62]. Although the main type of pregnancy-related LPP is the SIJ dysfunction, others include symphysis pubis dysfunction, lumbar disc herniation, and coccydynia [25, 40]. Pregnancy-related LPP continues to manifest itself in the postnatal period, especially in the first month after birth, at a rate of 35% [72]. LPP that occurs after birth, independent of pregnancy, usually includes causes such as delivering a large baby, having a small pelvic outlet, and the presence of diastasis of the symphysis pubis. Physiotherapy evaluation and management of LPP during pregnancy and at the postnatal period are generally parallel to each other [62].

Pain history, body diagram, adverse neural tension tests (passive straight leg raise/Lasegue), and provocation tests are of great importance in determining the type of pregnancy-related LPP (lumbar or pelvic girdle pain) (Fig. 19.1). Active straight leg raise (ASLR), posterior pelvic pain provocation (4P), Patrick-Faber (PF), pelvic compression and distraction, and Gaenslen and long dorsal sacroiliac ligament palpation (LDSL) tests are reliable and valid provocation tests used in the diagnosis of pelvic girdle pain. For the diagnosis of pregnancy-related pelvic girdle pain, pathologies originating from the lumbar vertebrae, nerve root symptoms, and urological and gynecological causes must be excluded [69, 78].

Physiotherapy programs for the LPP mainly include [14, 36, 60, 69, 75, 78, 78]:

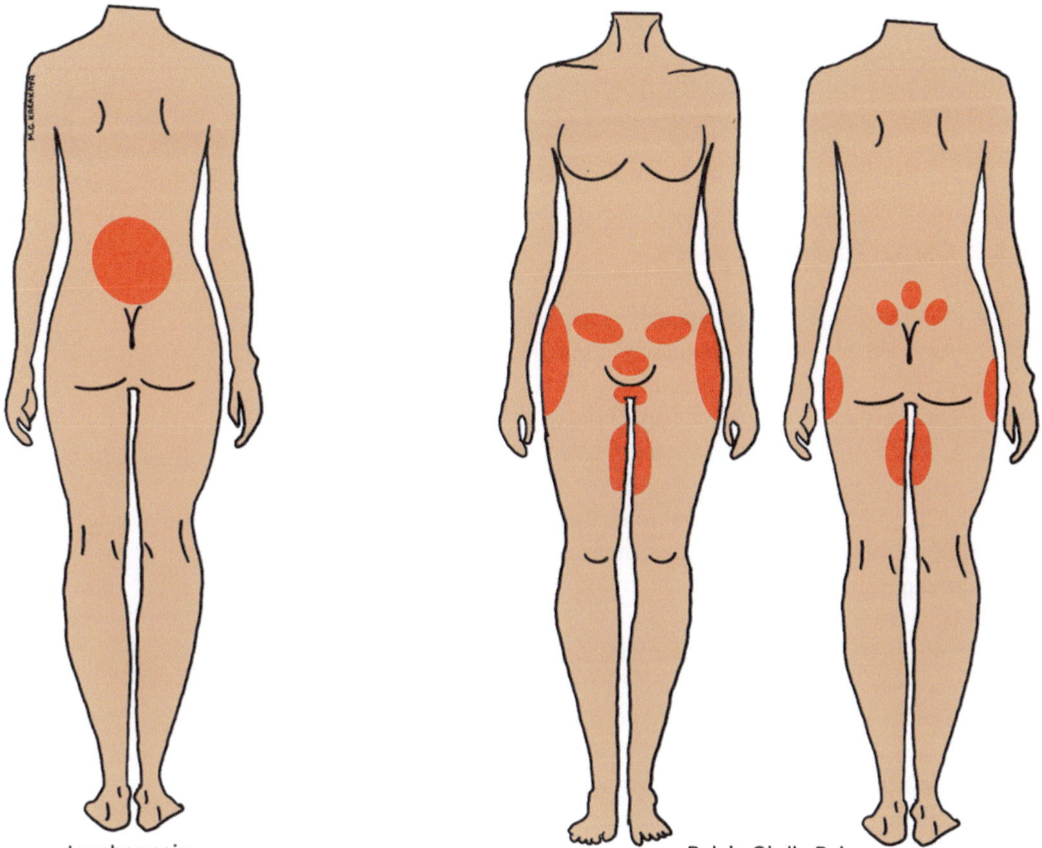

Fig. 19.1 Types of pregnancy-related LPP

- Patient education (covering topics on pain neuroscience, aligned posture, and modification of daily living activities)
- Exercise programs (aerobic exercises, aquatherapy, stabilization, strengthening and relaxation exercises, yoga, etc.)
- Manual therapy techniques (myofascial release, soft tissue massage, muscle-energy techniques, etc.)
- Use of pelvic belt and supports (Fig. 19.2)

In addition, the subject-related literature presents transcutaneous electrical nerve stimulation (TENS) and kinesiotaping as effective, safe (in the third trimester), low-cost, and suitable for home use methods that can be used to reduce pain in pregnancy-related LPP.

For postpartum women with LPP, physiotherapy programs have more alternatives since

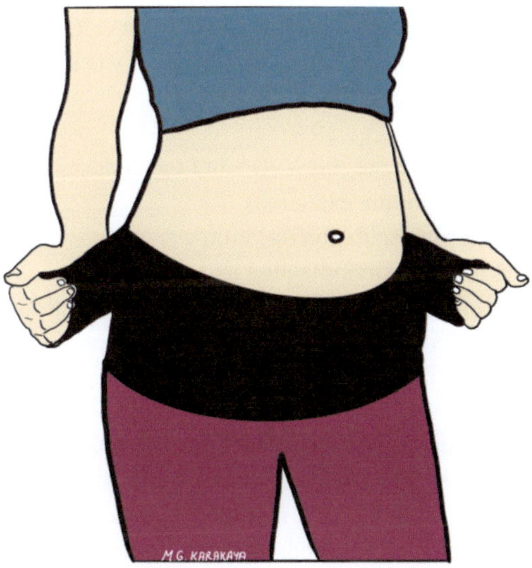

Fig. 19.2 Pelvic belt

electrophysical agents, which are contraindicated during pregnancy (diathermy, therapeutic ultrasound, neuromuscular electrical stimulation (NMES), etc.), are no longer contraindicated [74].

19.3.2 Carpal Tunnel Syndrome

As the most common entrapment neuropathy, CTS is reported to have a pregnancy-related prevalence of 1–62%. During pregnancy, CTS often occurs in the third trimester and bilaterally (Fig. 19.3). Although the etiology is not definite, it is thought that the symptoms are caused by local edema in the carpal tunnel as a result of hormonal changes during pregnancy. It usually disappears spontaneously after giving birth [52].

The evaluation of CTS in pregnancy includes sensory and motor testing, Tinel's and Phalen's tests, symptom severity, and functional status measures similar to the nonpregnant population [30]. Physiotherapy approaches mainly used for the treatment of pregnancy-associated CTS include [40, 82]:

- Patient education (appropriate sleeping position, avoiding excessive flexion movements during sleep, awareness of trigger activities, ergonomic modifications in the workplace, etc.)
- Splinting (Fig. 19.4)
- Exercise programs (including tendon and nerve gliding exercises)
- Neuromuscular reeducation
- Soft tissue mobilization and traction
- Kinesiotaping
- Cold application
- Compression and elevation

Besides these, subject-related literature presents laser and therapeutic ultrasound therapies, hot-sand bath therapy, iontophoresis, and phonophoresis as other modalities for CTS, although the available data on the safety and role of applying these physiotherapy procedures during pregnancy are limited (Cimpeanu et al. 2024).

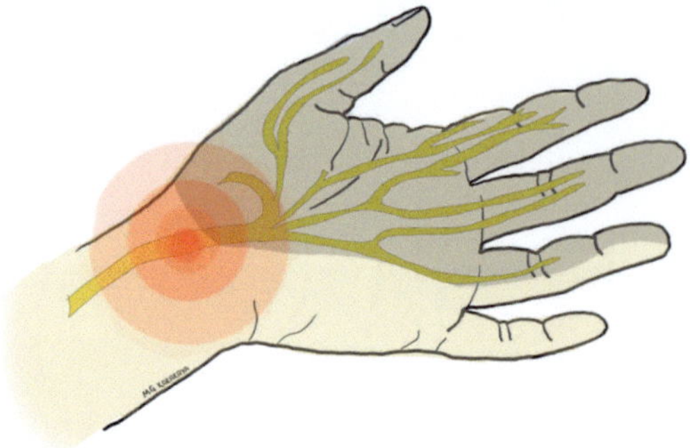

Fig. 19.3 Carpal tunnel syndrome

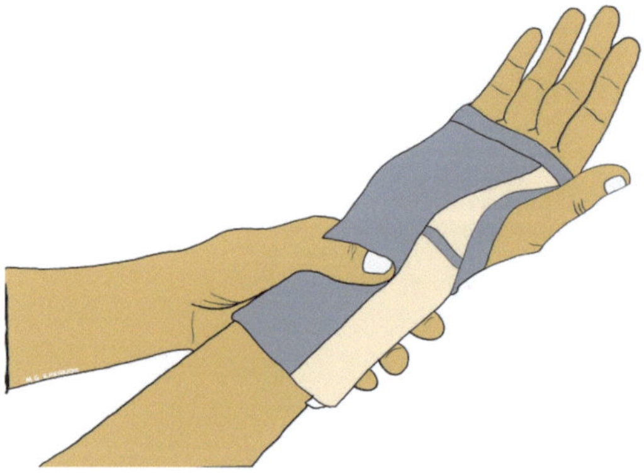

Fig. 19.4 Splinting for CTS

19.3.3 Diastasis Recti Abdominis

The musculoskeletal morphology of the anterolateral abdominal wall changes throughout pregnancy. The weight, dimensions, and capacity of the uterus increase, respectively, from 40 to 1000 g and from 4 to 4000 mL at term. To change the spatial connection between the upper and lower abdominal muscles, the length of the rectus abdominis muscle in particular increases by 115% compared to the beginning of pregnancy [54].

DRA is defined as the separation of the rectus abdominis muscles in the midline, creating a gap due to decreased tension resistance in the linea alba [2, 46]. Relaxation of the abdominal fascia due to hormonal fluctuations and the increased pressure of the enlarging uterus on the abdominal muscles lead to disruption of the integrity of the linea alba as pregnancy progresses, which causes DRA [2]. The prevalence of DRA increases from the 14th to the 21st weeks of pregnancy to an average of 33.1% and reaches 60% by the sixth week after delivery [68]. Generally, the inter-recti distance (IRD) naturally decreases after delivery and recovers completely within 6 months. However, some studies have shown that the inter-recti values in the postpartum period remain wider than in nulliparous women, and the prevalence of DRA is still very high at 6 months postpartum, suggesting that DRA may persist in the long term for some women [20, 54].

For DRA evaluation, the patient lying in the hook position is asked to lift her head and shoulders off the bed. During this movement, the number of fingers horizontally placed between the two rectus muscles at the level of the umbilicus and 3–5 cm below and above this level is recorded as the amount of DRA. The IRD ≥2 fingers indicates the presence of DRA [2, 46]. The IRD can also be measured by ultrasonographic imaging and calipers. In the ultrasonographic imaging, the inter-recti distance >2 mm at 3 cm below the umbilicus, >20 mm at the umbilicus, and >14 mm at 3 cm above indicates the presence of DRA [59]. Additionally, Beer et al. suggest that in nulliparous women, the linea alba should be considered "normal" when the IRD width is less than 15 mm at the xiphoid level, 22 mm at 3 cm above the umbilicus, and 16 mm at 2 cm below the umbilicus [9].

In the literature, it has been reported that physiotherapy is the only method that has the potential to both prevent and treat the DRA. The most commonly used physiotherapy methods include patient education (appropriate mobility and lifting techniques, correct posture, etc.), corset usage, taping (Fig. 19.5), and exercise programs (focused on strengthening the transversus abdominis and rectus abdominis muscles, as well as other core muscles including the pelvic floor, corrective exercises such as the Noble's technique, core stabilization exercises, hypopressive abdominal training, etc.) [53, 66]. For the prenatal period, a Delphi consensus study recommends [26]:

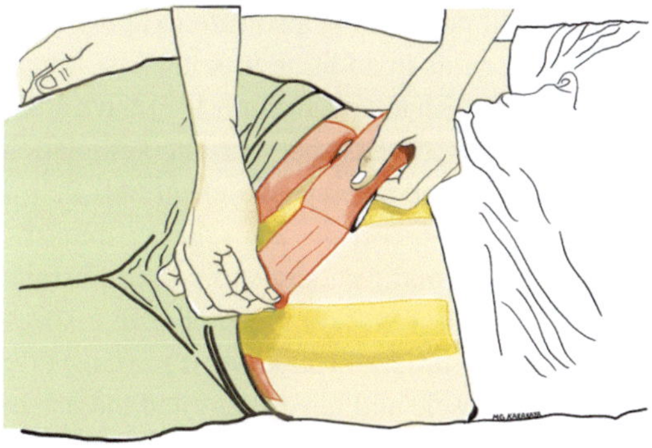

Fig. 19.5 Taping in DRA

- Emphasize static and dynamic postures that reduce excessive intra-abdominal pressures (i.e., maintaining a relaxed neutral spine).
- Encourage habitual activity patterns that reduce repeated increases in intra-abdominal pressure (i.e., rolling to the side to get up; avoid straining on the toilet).
- Commence inner unit exercises that facilitate optimal isolated and synergistic activation of the inner unit, and once control is achieved, progress with tailored outer unit and functionally oriented exercises.
- Avoid exercises that concentrically engage the superficial abdominal muscles (i.e., sit-ups).
- Encourage a breathing pattern that promotes a tension-free diaphragmatic pattern (e.g., downward motion of the diaphragm and lateral costal expansion on inhale).

In addition, if the IRD is more than three fingers, deep abdominal muscles should be trained first, and exercises that bend the trunk should be avoided to prevent herniation of internal structures [53]. Although many studies have reported that exercise training has a curative effect on DRA, a generally acceptable exercise protocol has not yet been established.

The physiotherapy methods that can be applied in the evaluation and treatment of DRA in the postnatal period are generally parallel to those in pregnancy. Fitriani et al. [32] have shown that postpartum mothers use abdominal fasteners, elastic corsets, massage, and herbal medicine to manage the symptoms of their condition. In the postnatal period, it is also safe to apply electrotherapy agents in addition to known treatment methods [40]. Khan and Bulbuli [43] have studied the effects of Russian current stimulation (two electrodes above and two electrodes below the umbilicus, on:off = 20 s:40 s, intensity adjusted based on the patient's tolerance, 30 min, 5 days/week for 4 weeks) together with a structured training program targeting the transverse abdominis muscle and have suggested the use of this approach when going through the postpartum recovery periods [43]. Tadmare et al. [71] have shown that NMES had a more significant effect on reducing DRA in postpartum women when compared with abdominal exercises.

In addition to all these treatments, it is reported that manual therapy techniques such as soft tissue mobilization and myofascial release, taping, and transcutaneous electrical acupoint stimulation (TEAS) can be used as components of physiotherapy programs in the treatment of DRA in the postnatal period [53].

19.4 Gastrointestinal Problems

The most common gastrointestinal system problems during pregnancy are nausea and vomiting, gastroesophageal reflux disease (GERD), and constipation [34].

19.4.1 Emesis Gravidarum

Emesis gravidarum (EG), which includes symptoms of pregnancy-related nausea, vomiting, and retching, is the most common pregnancy complication seen in 50–85% of pregnancies, usually starting in the fourth week of pregnancy and lasting until the 20th week. Although its etiology is not known exactly, it is thought that the inhibitory effect of progesterone on smooth muscles reduces gastrointestinal mobility and can lead to EG. Multiple and molar pregnancies and psychological factors such as anxiety, depression, and unwanted pregnancy are some of the related factors with this problem [34]. Although EG can be treated with antiemetic medications and herbal remedies containing ginger, the side effects of pharmacological interventions and concerns about fetal health lead pregnant women to choose non-pharmacological approaches [29]. Non-pharmacological approaches commonly used in the treatment of EG include various acustimulation methods (acupuncture, acupressure, acu-TENS, auriculotherapy, etc.), manual therapy, kinesiotaping, progressive relaxation and breathing exercises, hypnosis, cognitive therapy, music therapy, aromatherapy applications, diet and nutritional recommendations, and lifestyle interventions [19, 51, 61, 65, 70, 73]. In addition, ACOG reports that endurance training/aerobics, strength training, and stretching/relaxation exercise programs have positive effects on nausea and vomiting during pregnancy [37].

19.4.2 Gastroesophageal Reflux Disease

GERD is another condition that increases in prevalence as the third trimester progresses and affects approximately 80% of pregnant women. The most well-known symptoms of GERD are an acidic taste in the mouth and heartburn due to hormonal changes, increased intra-abdominal pressure, and decreased gastrointestinal transit time during pregnancy. Although GERD usually disappears after birth, approximately 20% of women continue to experience GERD symptoms even after birth [3]. The first step in treatment for a pregnant GERD patient includes lifestyle modifications, such as correct sleeping position (elevation of the head of the bed and the left lateral decubitus position) (Fig. 19.6), avoiding foods/drinks that may trigger the disease (fatty and spicy foods, citrus, carbonated beverages, and alcohol), and avoidance of lying down within 3 h of eating. However, if heartburn persists severely, medication can be started under the supervision of a physician. Inspiratory muscle training and increasing physical activity level to 150 min per week are among the physiotherapy methods that can be applied in the treatment of GERD [4, 23, 81].

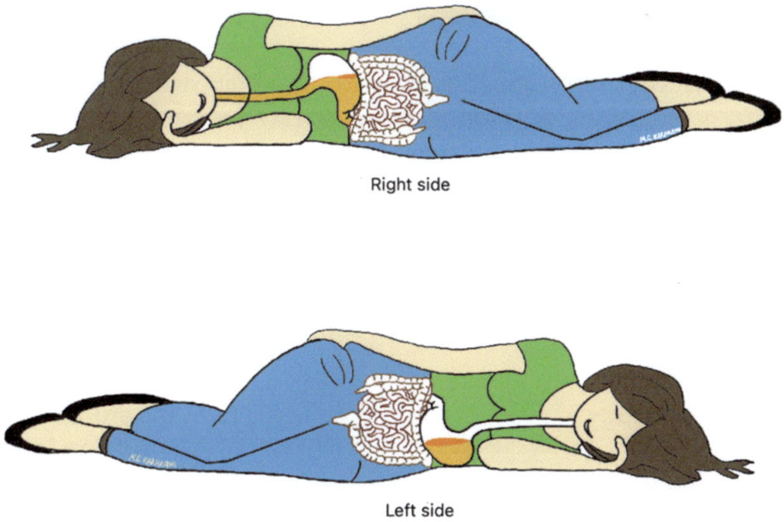

Fig. 19.6 Sleep position in GERD

19.4.3 Constipation

Constipation, i.e., functional bowel disorder, is a commonly observed problem during pregnancy (35%, 39%, and 20% in trimesters, respectively) and in the first 3–6 months postpartum (especially after cesarean section, 57%), which may persist in some cases up to a year. The high progesterone levels during pregnancy, which remain elevated for a few weeks after birth, result in hypomotility of the gastrointestinal tract and relaxation of the abdominal and pelvic muscles, therefore increasing constipation and gas production. The high intra-abdominal pressure, luminal obstruction due to an enlarged uterus, insufficient fiber intake, and hemorrhoids that hurt and restrict efficient bowel elimination are other factors exacerbating constipation [12]. Physiotherapy applications used in the treatment of constipation include patient education (increasing physical activity and fluid intake, eating less and frequently, consuming fibrous foods, avoiding foods and drinks containing caffeine, appropriate toileting position, etc.), abdominal and pelvic floor muscle training (PFMT) combined with anorectal biofeedback (BF), classical abdominal massage (may not be suitable for the early post-cesarean period), connective tissue massage, whole-body vibration therapy, and transcutaneous electrical tibial nerve stimulation. However, it should be noted that among these applications, connective tissue massage, whole-body vibration, and electrical tibial nerve stimulation should not be applied during pregnancy since their effects during this period are unknown [12, 28, 35, 62].

19.4.4 Gastrointestinal Function After Cesarean

Especially after cesarean section, accelerating the recovery of gastrointestinal function is important since from 5% to even 32% of women experience mild symptoms of delayed intestinal peristalsis recovery, referred to as postoperative ileus (POI), which prolongs hospitalization, causes bloating that exacerbates lower abdominal pain, and hinders breastfeeding and proper neonatal care [58]. Therefore, preventing POI and supporting the recovery of intestinal peristalsis are one of the priorities in the perioperative period. Studies on the effectiveness of physiotherapy programs after cesarean surgery have shown that TENS, connective tissue manipulation of the lumbosacral region, calm and deep breathing exercises, exercises resulting in gentle activation of the abdominal and pelvic muscles, assisting verticalization, and supporting early ambulation are effective in accelerating intestinal peristalsis recovery, in addition to their effects on post-cesarean pain [17, 58].

19.5 Urogenital Problems

Urogenital system problems during pregnancy and at the postpartum period generally include pelvic floor dysfunctions (PFDs). PFDs include urinary incontinence (UI), anal incontinence (AI), pelvic organ prolapse (POP), chronic pelvic pain, and sexual dysfunctions, which are characterized by tonus disturbances and/or impaired coordination of the pelvic floor muscles (PFM) that act as a sling.

19.5.1 Etiology

In addition to the effects of relaxin hormone on the ligamentous laxity of the pelvic region, the pelvic floor is constantly under stress during pregnancy due to increased intra-abdominal pressure (IAP) because of the growing uterus and the pelvic organs pushed inferiorly [8, 11, 47]. Pregnancy-related changes such as descent of the bladder neck, increase in bladder neck mobility, decrease in urethral resistance, and loss of pelvic floor contractility are compatible with changes in the mechanical properties of the fascial tissue and can be considered as physiological adaptations to the mechanical and hormonal changes of pregnancy [8, 11, 47].

19.5.2 Common Urogenital Problems During Pregnancy

Studies report that approximately one-third of women in the second and third trimesters of pregnancy have to deal with UI, which is the most common symptom associated with PFD [62]. While the incidence of AI is 7% in pregnant women, it is thought to be mostly related to accompanying comorbidities [39]. POP is defined as the prolapse of the pelvic organs into or out of the vagina due to a dysfunction in the tissues supporting the pelvic floor [16]. Studies report that POP occurring during pregnancy is usually asymptomatic and therefore does not present as a problem [62]. Female sexual dysfunction covers a group of psychosexual problems that include sexual desire, orgasm, and arousal disorders, as well as pain during intercourse [57]. Sexual dysfunctions during pregnancy manifest themselves for different reasons at different periods. While in the first trimester, the belief that sexual intercourse is associated with abortion is related to sexual dysfunction; frequent urination, increased pain parallel to the growth of the uterus, and strong uterine contractions may trigger this problem in the third trimester. Sexual dysfunction is less common in the second trimester compared to others [62].

19.5.3 Common Urogenital Problems During Postnatal Period

Factors such as episiotomy, operative delivery, perineal trauma, and prolonged second stage of labor cause UI in the postnatal period. The primary risk factor for AI in this period is anal sphincter injury during delivery. Risk factors for POP in the postnatal period include vaginal delivery using forceps and PFM damage during vaginal delivery, and studies report that the risk of POP doubles after the first delivery and increases by 10% for each subsequent delivery, depending on risk factors during pregnancy and delivery.

Micturition and defecation difficulties, such as urinary retention and constipation, frequently occur in the post-pregnancy period [62]. Urinary retention is defined as the inability to urinate after delivery, which is sudden in onset, painful or painless, and requires catheterization if it lasts more than 12 h.

The most common sexual dysfunctions in the postnatal period, dyspareunia, decreased libido, and orgasm problems, are frequently seen in the first 3 months after delivery, although studies show that problems persist for up to 12 months [62].

19.5.4 Recovery of the Pelvic Floor After Birth

Research shows that most of the recovery in the pelvic floor during the postpartum period occurs within 6 months. The degree and time of recovery are directly related to the amount of perineal trauma during birth. From this perspective, the best and fastest recovery occurs with cesarean birth or with the perineum remaining intact during vaginal delivery [33].

19.5.5 Assessment of Pelvic Floor Dysfunction During Pregnancy and After Birth

In similarity with all other PFD populations, evaluation of PFDs during pregnancy and the postnatal period generally includes a detailed anamnesis, inspection and palpation of the pelvic floor, sensory assessment, PFD strength and function tests, condition-specific symptom severity tests, voiding and defecation diaries, etc. However, evaluation of PFM strength and function during pregnancy is performed only with the index finger, and use of a perineometer is preferred because it carries a lower risk of infection compared to other methods [1, 24]. Although the evaluation of PFDs in the postnatal period is similar to the non-pregnant population, there is no consensus in the literature regarding the correct time to evaluate PFM intravaginally. A general recommendation is to wait approximately 6 weeks for the recovery of vaginal bleeding and discharge, episiotomy or rupture, perineal pain, etc., since they may lead to discomfort during the examination [62].

19.5.6 Physiotherapy of Pelvic Floor Dysfunctions During Pregnancy and After Birth

Physiotherapy methods used for PFDs in pregnancy generally start with patient education to increase knowledge and awareness of a healthy pelvic floor, teach the "knack maneuver," control weight gain, maintain aligned posture, provide correct use of ergonomics and body biomechanics, etc. PFMT can be applied alone or in combination with pressure/EMG-BF, as well as in combination with pelvic stabilization and core muscle exercises. Guidelines recommend that PFMT should be started from the antenatal period in order to prevent PFDs that may occur during pregnancy. It should be noted that electrical stimulation (ES) to the waist, abdomen, and acupuncture points; vaginal cones; pessaries; and clitoral vacuum devices should not be used during pregnancy since they may increase the risk of vaginal discharge and infection during this period [62]. In addition to PFMT, which aims to improve both contraction and relaxation functions of the perineal muscles, the use of perineal massage starting from the 35th gestational week decreases the risk of birth-related perineal trauma and facilitates recovery after birth [79] (Fig. 19.7).

Physiotherapy applications for UI, AI, POP, and sexual dysfunctions after birth are similar to those used during pregnancy. However, ES applications (NMES, interferential currents, high-voltage pulsed electrical stimulation, extracorporeal magnetic stimulation, etc.), which are contraindicated during pregnancy, can be safely used in the postnatal period, in combination with PFMT [27, 50]. Vaginal cones/balls and pessaries, which should be used only with caution during pregnancy because of the risk of infection and vaginal discharge, should also be used with caution in the early postpartum period, considering the numbness of the perineum that may occur in this period [62].

In addition to PFMT, pelvic floor-focused or whole-body-focused relaxation training can be used for sexual dysfunctions both during pregnancy and in the postpartum period. It is known that the most important reasons causing sexual dysfunction in the postnatal period are the decrease in PFM strength due to vaginal delivery, assisted delivery, perineal trauma, and episiotomy. Inspection of the perineal region during the postnatal period is important to find out any

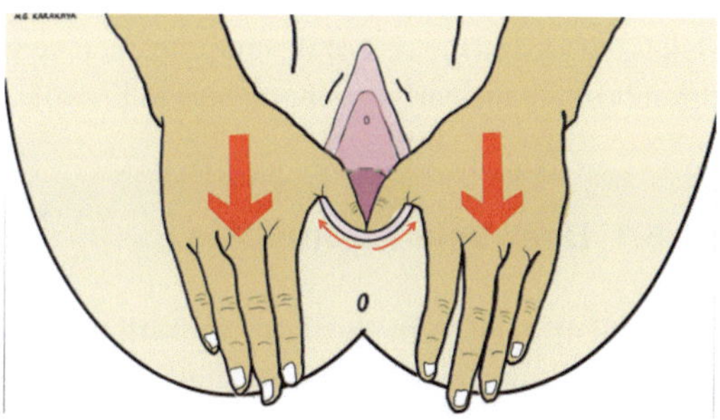

Fig. 19.7 Antenatal perineal massage

symptoms such as perineal tears, episiotomy, and edema, which may cause painful intercourse. In the presence of such symptoms, appropriate electrophysical agents (cold agents, therapeutic ultrasound, low-intensity laser therapy, etc.) and manual therapy techniques, in addition to PFMT, can be used to facilitate their recovery [15, 38]. In addition, pelvic floor-focused relaxation training with vaginal dilators and the Sniff, Flop, Drop technique are also used in the treatment of sexual dysfunctions in the postpartum period [62].

Physiotherapy practices used for the treatment of urinary retention primarily include ice application to the perineum to reduce periurethral edema, walking at a low pace, and hot baths. Spontaneous micturition occurs in approximately 50% of the cases in which these practices are applied [41]. Voiding training, controlled breathing, and PFMT combined with BF constitute other physiotherapy approaches that can be used in the treatment of urinary retention [62].

19.6 Vascular and Circulatory Problems

During pregnancy, increased blood volume, pressure of the growing uterus on the veins, and decreased vascular tonus due to the progesterone hormone make pregnant women more vulnerable to circulatory problems [42, 44]. The most common circulatory problems in pregnancy are varicose veins of the lower extremity and vulvovaginal region, hemorrhoids, and muscle cramps. Thrombosis and thromboembolism are also associated with vascular problems during pregnancy. In the postnatal period, the most common of these problems are varicose veins and hemorrhoids, as well as the risk of developing deep vein thrombosis in the early postnatal period [7, 40].

19.6.1 Deep Vein Thrombosis

To prevent deep vein thrombosis both during pregnancy and in the postnatal period, lower extremity muscle exercises and external compression methods can be used effectively [56]. Especially in the early postnatal period, pumping exercises of the foot and ankle in an elevated position, knee and hip flexion-extension, quadriceps and gluteal muscle contractions, compression stockings, elastic bandages, and external pneumatic compression devices are important in the prevention of this problem [6, 18].

19.6.2 Varicose Veins

Subject-related literature samples have emphasized that the incidence of varicose veins in the lower extremities during pregnancy varies between 20% and 50%, and especially advanced age and family history contribute significantly to their formation [22]. Varicose veins can be seen both during pregnancy and at any time in the postnatal period [7]. In the 2008 Guideline of the National Institute for Health and Care Excellence (NICE), the physiotherapy methods that can be applied in the treatment of lower extremity varicose veins are compression stockings, external pneumatic compression devices (Fig. 19.8), exercise programs performed with compression stockings, resting, especially in the left-lying position, and foot-ankle exercises [55].

Vulvovaginal varicose veins are less common (approximately 4%) than those in the lower extremities and usually occur in the second trimester of pregnancy [67]. Physiotherapy methods that can be applied in its treatment include resting positions with the elevated feet, compression garments, patient education/exercise approaches that prevent constipation, and PFMT [7, 40].

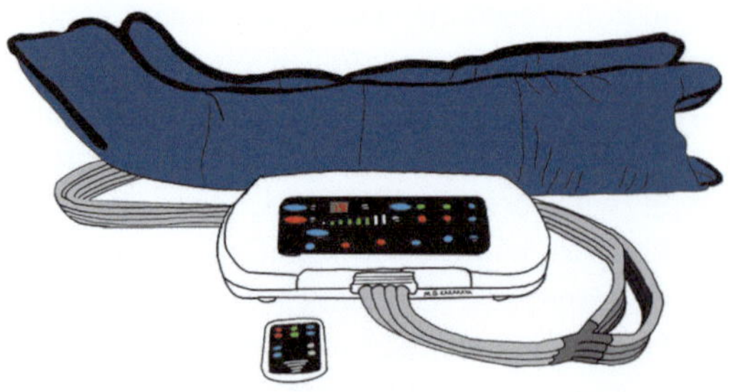

Fig. 19.8 External pneumatic compression device

19.6.3 Hemorrhoids

Hormonal changes and increased IAP during pregnancy pave the way for hemorrhoid formation. Studies report that women with hemorrhoids during pregnancy are usually asymptomatic and only 10% require treatment [62]. Physiotherapy methods that can be applied for the treatment of hemorrhoids occurring during pregnancy include sit baths to reduce pain, the use of sit-up pillows, and teaching correct defecation techniques to prevent constipation [7]. The strain and pressure exerted by the fetal head on the pelvic floor during birth also leads to an increase in existing complaints or the formation of new hemorrhoids in the postnatal period. Although hemorrhoids are more painful, especially in the early postnatal period, they shrink in the following days and their negative effects decrease. The treatment of hemorrhoids in the postnatal period is parallel to that in pregnancy and generally includes PFMT, sitz baths, local cold applications, and defecation training [7, 80].

19.6.4 Muscle Cramps

Muscle cramps, which occur primarily in the leg muscles and especially in the third trimester of pregnancy, are a common problem that impairs the quality of life of approximately 30–50% of pregnant women. Although the exact etiology and mechanism are not known, it is thought that conditions such as inactivity, electrolyte imbalance, and vitamin deficiency are associated with muscle cramps. In addition to medical treatments such as vitamin supplements and electrolyte support, physiotherapy methods that can be used in the treatment of muscle cramps during pregnancy include classical massage applications, stretching, relaxation, foot-ankle exercises (Fig. 19.9), and superficial heat agents [49].

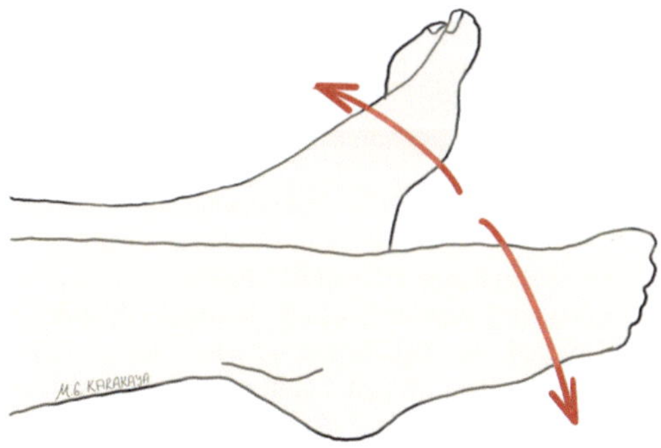

Fig. 19.9 Foot–ankle exercises

19.7 Conclusion

As the common ones explained above, women can experience many health problems during pregnancy and in the postnatal period, and physiotherapy remains a vital adjunct in their management. Therefore, collaborative care of patients by the physician and the physiotherapists can considerably enhance the health outcomes associated with these conditions. Recruitment of more physiotherapists in government hospitals and providing continuous in-service training opportunities will be valuable in improving healthcare services provided to the obstetric population.

Acknowledgments The authors would like to thank Prof. Dr. Mehmet Gürhan KARAKAYA for his valuable contributions to the drawings of the chapter.

References

1. Akbayrak T, Kaya S. Kadın Sağlığında Fizyoterapi ve Rehabilitasyon. Ankara: Hipokrat & Pelikan Kitabevi; 2016.
2. Akbayrak T, Akarcalı İ, Çıtak İ, et al. Relations of diastasis recti abdominis, rectus abdominus muscle strength and low back pain in pregnancy. JCOG. 2001;11:215–9.
3. Ali RAR, Hassan J, Egan LJ. Review of recent evidence on the management of heartburn in pregnant and breastfeeding women. BMC Gastroenterol. 2022;22:219.

4. Altuwaijri M. Evidence-based treatment recommendations for gastroesophageal reflux disease during pregnancy: a review. Medicine (Baltimore). 2024;101:e30487.
5. Ay S. Gebelikte görülen kas iskelet sistemi problemleri. Arch Rheumatol. 2008;23:056–9.
6. Bagaria SJ, Bagaria VB. Strategies for diagnosis and prevention of venous thromboembolism during pregnancy. J Pregnancy. 2011;2011:206858.
7. Baran E, Akbayrak T. Gebelikte Görülen Problemlerde Fizyoterapi ve Rehabilitasyon. In: Akbayrak T, Kaya S, editors. Kadın Sağlığında Fizyoterapi ve Rehabilitasyon. 1st ed. Ankara: Hipokrat Kitabevi & Pelikan Kitabevi; 2016. p. 189–213.
8. Barton S. The postnatal period. In: Polden M, Mantle J, editors. Physiotherapy in obstetrics and gynaecology. 2nd ed. Oxford: Butterwoth-Heinemann; 2004. p. 205–47.
9. Beer GM, Schuster A, Seifert B, et al. The normal width of the linea alba in nulliparous women. Clin Anat. 2009;22:706–11.
10. Berens P. Overview of the postpartum period: normal physiology and routine maternal care. UptoDate. 2020;15:1–34.
11. Bernard T, Cassidy J. The sacroiliac joint syndrome. In: Frymoyer JW, editor. The adult spine; principles and practise. 1st ed. Newyork: Raven; 1997. p. 2107–30.
12. Botla A, Saleh M, Ahmed W, et al. Bilateral transcutaneous tibial nerve stimulation: a promising treatment for women with postpartum constipation: a randomized controlled trial. Adv Rehab. 2024;38:16–24.
13. Chauhan G, Tadi P. Physiology, postpartum changes. Treasure Island (FL): StatPearls Publishing; 2020.
14. Chen L, Ferreira ML, Beckenkamp PR, et al. Management of "de novo" carpal tunnel syndrome in pregnancy: a narrative review. J Pers Med. 2024;14:240.
15. Chougala A, Mahishale A. A randomized clinical trial to evaluate the effect of therapeutic ultrasound and low-level laser therapy on perineal pain following vaginal delivery with episiotomy. JSAFOG. 2015;7:152–6.
16. Çıtak Karakaya İ. Pelvik Organ Prolapsusunda Fizyoterapi ve Rehabilitasyon. Turkiye Klinikleri J Physiother Rehabil-Special Topics. 2017;3:216–24.
17. Çıtak Karakaya İ, Yüksel İ, Akbayrak T, et al. Effects of physiotherapy on pain and functional activities after cesarean delivery. Arch Gynecol Obstet. 2012;285:621–7.
18. Clarke MJ, Broderick C, Hopewell S, et al. Compression stockings for preventing deep vein thrombosis in airline passengers. Cochrane Database Syst Rev. 2016;4:CD004002.
19. Committee on Practice Bulletins-Obstetrics. ACOG practice bulletin no. 189: nausea and vomiting of pregnancy. Obstet Gynecol. 2018;131:e15–30.
20. Critchley CJC. Physical therapy is an important component of postpartum care in the fourth trimester. Phys Ther. 2022;102:pzac021.
21. Datta S, Kodali BS, Segal S. Obstetric anesthesia handbook. New York: Springer; 2010.
22. de Barros Junior N, Perez MDCJ, Amorim JE, et al. Pregnancy and lower limb varicose veins: prevalence and risk factors. J Vasc Bras. 2010;9:29–35.
23. de Miranda Chaves RC, Navarro-Rodriguez T. Respiratory physiotherapy in gastroesophageal reflux disease: a review article. World J Respirol. 2015;5:28–33.
24. Dinç A, Kızılkaya Beji N. Pregnancy, intrapartum and postpartum period in the prevention and treatment of urinary incontinence. FNJN. 2008;16:143–9.
25. Döner Şİ, Gerçek H. Gebelikle İlişkili Lumbopelvik Ağrı ve Güncel Fizyoterapi Yöntemleri: Geleneksel Derleme. IGUSABDER. 2023;20:692–702.
26. Dufour SP, Bernard S, Murray-Davis B, et al. Establishing expert-based recommendations for the conservative management of pregnancy-related diastasis rectus abdominis: a Delphi consensus study. JWHPT. 2019;43:73–81.
27. Electrophysical agents – contraindications and precautions: an evidence based approach to clinical decision making in physical therapy. Physiother Can. 2010;62:1–80.
28. Elfatah Elhosary EA, ElAzab DR, Hanoura EM, et al. Effect of six weeks of whole-body vibration in treatment of postnatal constipation. J Pak Med Assoc. 2023;73:13–6.
29. Emami-Sahebi A, Elyasi F, Yazdani-Charati J. Psychological interventions for nausea and vomiting of pregnancy: a systematic review. TJOG. 2018;57:644–9.
30. Ertekin C. Pleksus Brakiyalisten Çıkan Sinirler: Santral ve Periferik EMG Anatomi-Fizyoloji-Klinik. İstanbul: Meta Basım Matbaacılık; 2006.
31. Fiat F, Merghes PE, Scurtu AD, et al. The main changes in pregnancy-therapeutic approach to musculoskeletal pain. Medicina (Kaunas). 2022;58:1115.
32. Fitriani H, Setyowati S, Afiyanti Y, et al. Traditional treatment for diastasis rectus abdominis in postpartum mothers: a phenomenological study. BJM. 2024;32:461–514.
33. Fonti Y, Giordano R, Cacciatore A, et al. Postpartum pelvic floor changes. J Prenat Med. 2009;3:57–9.
34. Gomes CF, Sousa M, Lourenço I, et al. Gastrointestinal diseases during pregnancy: what does the gastroenterologist need to know? Ann Gastroenterol. 2018;31:385–94.
35. Gürsen C, Kerem Günel M, Kaya S, et al. Effect of connective tissue manipulation on symptoms and quality of life in patients with chronic constipation: a randomized controlled trial. J Manip Physiol Ther. 2015;38:335–43.
36. Gutke A, Betten C, Degerskar K, et al. Treatments for pregnancy-related lumbopelvic pain: a systematic review of physiotherapy modalities. Acta Obstet Gynecol Scand. 2015;94:1156–67.
37. Haakstad LA, Torset B, Bø K. What is the effect of regular group exercise on maternal psychological out-

comes and common pregnancy complaints? An assessor blinded RCT. Midwifery. 2016;32:81–6.
38. Herrera I, Schneiderman R, Perez L. Therapy for management of childbirth perineal tears and postpartum pain. Pract Pain Manag. 2012;11:1–5.
39. Johannessen HH, Wibe A, Stordahl A, et al. Prevalence and predictors of anal incontinence during pregnancy and 1 year after delivery: a prospective cohort study. BJOG. 2014;121:269–79.
40. Kaya S. Prenatal, natal ve postnatal dönemde fizyoterapi ve rehabilitasyon. Turkiye Klinikleri J Physiother Rehabil-Special Topics. 2017;3:154–64.
41. Kaya YŞ, Kotun N. Postpartum urinary retention. Zeynep Kamil Med J. 2014;45:106–12.
42. Kepley JM, Bates K, Mohuiddin SS. Physiology, maternal changes. In: StatPearls [Internet]. Treasure Island (FL): StatPearls Publishing; 2023.
43. Khan N, Bulbuli A. Effect of Russian current and structured exercise program on postpartum diastasis recti abdominis: a case series. IJAHSP. 2024;22:1–9.
44. Klein HH, Pisch S. Cardiovascular changes during pregnancy. Herz. 2003;28:173–4.
45. Knight J. Pregnancy 3: effects of pregnancy on the musculoskeletal system and skin. Nurs Times [Online]. 2023;119:11.
46. Koçak YÇ, Bay H, Can HÖ. Doğum Sonu Muayenede Farkındalık: Diastazis Rekti ve Bakımı. J Nursology. 2020;23:304–10.
47. Kristiansson P, Svardsud K, Von Schoultz B. Serum relaxin, symphyseal pain and back pain during pregnancy. Am J Obstet Gynecol. 1996;175:1342–7.
48. Landon MB, Jauniaux ERM, Driscoll DA, et al. Gabbe's obstetrics normal and problem pregnancies. Philadelphia: Elsevier; 2024.
49. Luo L, Zhou K, Zhang J, et al. Interventions for leg cramps in pregnancy. Cochrane Database Syst Rev. 2020;12:Cd010655.
50. Ma X, Liu A. Effectiveness of electrical stimulation combined with pelvic floor muscle training on postpartum urinary incontinence. Medicine (Baltimore). 2019;98:e14762.
51. Matthews A, Haas DM, O'Mathuna DP, et al. Interventions for nausea and vomiting in early pregnancy. Cochrane Database Syst Rev. 2015;9:CD007575.
52. Meems M, Truijens S, Spek V, et al. Prevalence, course and determinants of carpal tunnel syndrome symptoms during pregnancy: a prospective study. BJOG. 2015;122:1112–8.
53. Michalska A, Rokita W, Wolder D, et al. Diastasis recti abdominis—a review of treatment methods. Ginekol Pol. 2018;89:97–101.
54. Mota P, Pascoal AG, Bo K. Diastasis recti abdominis in pregnancy and postpartum period. Risk factors, functional implications and resolution. Curr Womens Health Rev. 2015;11:59–67.
55. National Clinical Guideline Center (UK). Varicose veins in the legs: the diagnosis and management of varicose veins. London: National Institute for Health and Care Excellence (NICE); 2013.
56. Okumuş G, Özçelik B, Sasani H, et al. Do appropriate thromboprophylaxis and routine physiotherapy prevent venous thromboembolism in intensive care unit? TGKDC. 2015;23:92–7.
57. Özcan H, Kızılkaya Beji N. Female sexual function disorders: updating 2018. Androl Bul. 2018;20:133–7.
58. Pilch A, Jekielek M, Stach B, et al. Impact of obstetric physiotherapy and transcutaneous electrical nerve stimulation (TENS) on pain management and gastrointestinal function following cesarean birth: a randomized controlled trial. Eur J Midwifery. 2024;8:50.
59. Qu E, Wu J, Zhang M, et al. The ultrasound diagnostic criteria for diastasis recti and its correlation with pelvic floor dysfunction in early postpartum women. Quant Imaging Med Surg. 2021;11:706–13.
60. Quittan M, Bily M, Crevenna R, et al. Transcutaneous electrical nerve stimulation (TENS) in patients with pregnancy-induced low back pain and/or pelvic girdle pain. Phys Med Rehab Kuror. 2016;26:91–5.
61. Sahane P, Weljale B. Effectiveness of deep breathing exercise on nausea, vomiting among primigravida antenatal with hyperemesis gravidum admitted at antenatal ward of Pravara Rural Hospital, Loni (Bk). IJANM. 2020;8:300–4.
62. Şahin Altaç D, Çıtak Karakaya İ. Gebelikte ve Postnatal Dönemde Pelvik Fizyoterapi ve Rehabilitasyon. Turkiye Klinikleri J Physiother Rehabil-Special Topics. 2023a;9:46–54.
63. Şahin Altaç D, Çıtak Karakaya İ. Postpartum Pelvik Problemlerde Fizyoterapi ve Rehabilitasyon. In: Akbayrak T, Kaya S, Gürşen C, editors. "Multidisipliner Bakış Temeli" ile Pelvik Sağlıkta Fizyoterapi ve Rehabilitasyon. 1st ed. Ankara: Hedef CS Basın Yayın; 2023b. p. 49–81.
64. Sarıyıldız A, Benlidayı İC. Gebelik Dönemindeki Potansiyel Kas-İskelet Sistemi Sorunları. Arch Med Rev J. 2022;31:279–83.
65. Skarica B. Effectiveness of manual treatment on pregnancy symptoms: usefulness of manual treatment in treating pregnancy symptoms. Med Arch. 2018;72:131–5.
66. Skoura A, Billis E, Papanikolaou DT, et al. Diastasis recti abdominis rehabilitation in the postpartum period: a scoping review of current clinical practice. Int Urogynecol J. 2024;35:491–520.
67. Soule HM, Jayi S, Sano AA, et al. Vulvar varicose veins and pregnancy: childbirth management. PAMJ-Clin Med. 2020;3:1–4.
68. Sperstad JB, Tennfjord MK, Hilde G, et al. Diastasis recti abdominis during pregnancy and 12 months after childbirth: prevalence, risk factors and report of lumbopelvic pain. Br J Sports Med. 2016;50:1092–6.
69. Starzec M, Truszczynska-Baszak A. Pregnancy-related lumbopelvic pain: classification and diagnostics according to European guidelines and a review of literature. Med Rehabil. 2017;21:58–63.
70. Sushil Gawande SG, Madhuri Vaidya MV, Rahul Tadke RT, et al. Progressive muscle relax-

ation in hyperemesis gravidarum. J SAFOG. 2011;3:28–32.
71. Tadmare S, Bhatnagar G, Kamble R, et al. Comparison of abdominal exercises and neuromuscular electrical stimulation on diastasis recti abdominis muscle in postnatal females with caesarean section. Georgian Med News. 2024;346:63–7.
72. Terzi H, Terzi R, Altınbilek T. Pregnancy-related lumbopelvic pain in early postpartum period and risk factors. Int J Res Med Sci. 2015;3:1617–21.
73. Tsakiridis I, Mamopoulus A, Athanasiadis A, et al. The management of nausea and vomiting of pregnancy: synthesis of national guidelines. Obstet Gynecol Surv. 2019;74:161–9.
74. Tseng P, Puthussery S, Pappas Y, et al. A systematic review of randomised controlled trials on the effectiveness of exercise programs on lumbo pelvic pain among postnatal women. BMC Pregnancy Childbirth. 2015;15:316.
75. van Benten E, Pool J, Mens J, et al. Recommendations for physical therapists on the treatment of lumbopelvic pain during pregnancy: a systematic review. J Orthop Sports Phys Ther. 2014;44:464–73.
76. Van Geelen H, Ostergard D, Sand PA. A review of the impact of pregnancy and childbirth on pelvic floor function as assessed by objective measurement techniques. Int Urogynecol J. 2018;29:327–38.
77. Wise RA, Polito AJ, Krishnan V. Respiratory physiologic changes in pregnancy. Immunol Allergy Clin N Am. 2006;26:1–12.
78. Xue X, Chen Y, Mao X, et al. Effect of kinesio taping on low back pain during pregnancy: a systematic review and meta-analysis. BMC Pregnancy Childbirth. 2021;21:712.
79. Yetişmiş Y, Derya A. The effects of perineal massage performed during labor on childbirth comfort, perineal pain, and trauma in nulliparous women: a quasi-experimental study. JCOG. 2023;33:210–20.
80. Yikar S, Evsen N. Postpartum physical symptoms and nursing/midwifery care. J Midwifery Health Sci. 2022;5:79–84.
81. Yu C, Wang T, Gao Y, et al. Association between physical activity and risk of gastroesophageal reflux disease: a systematic review and meta-analysis. JSHS. 2024;13:687–98.
82. Cîmpeanu MC, Roman N, Grigorescu S, Grigorescu OD, Miclăuş RS. Management of "De Novo" Carpal Tunnel Syndrome in Pregnancy: A Narrative Review. J Pers Med. 2024;14(3):240. https://doi.org/10.3390/jpm14030240.

20 Physiotherapy and Rehabilitation in Infertility

Ege Nur Atabey Gerlegiz and Serap Özgül

20.1 Introduction

Infertility, a complex and widespread public health problem, has a direct impact on the quality of life of individuals and couples. According to the World Health Organization, infertility affects one in six people worldwide [1]. The main factors contributing to infertility include structural or functional disorders of the male and female reproductive systems, hormonal imbalances, and environmental factors [2, 3]. Traditional treatment approaches focus on pharmacological and assisted reproductive techniques [4]. The impact of physiotherapy and rehabilitation approaches in infertility management is being increasingly researched and emphasized. Exercise, manual therapy, electrical stimulation, and acupuncture as part of physiotherapy interventions have been shown to support reproductive health and improve outcomes when integrated with other infertility treatments [5, 6]. Physiotherapeutic approaches play a role in the management of infertility through their physical and psychosocial effects. This chapter discusses the definition and etiology of infertility and the physiotherapy and rehabilitation approaches that can be used in its management.

E. N. A. Gerlegiz (✉) · S. Özgül
Department of Fundamental Physiotherapy and Rehabilitation, Faculty of Physical Therapy and Rehabilitation, Hacettepe University, Ankara, Türkiye

20.2 Definition of Infertility

Infertility is defined as the inability to achieve pregnancy despite regular unprotected intercourse for at least 12 months. It is a condition associated with various biological, hormonal, and psychosomatic factors [1]. Primary infertility is defined as a woman who has never been pregnant, while secondary infertility is the inability to conceive after a previous pregnancy [7].

20.3 Epidemiology

Infertility is a significant public health problem affecting millions of individuals and couples worldwide [8]. The incidence of infertility has increased significantly, making it the third most serious health problem after cancer and cardiovascular disease [9]. It is estimated that approximately 186 million individuals and 48 million couples worldwide are affected by infertility [1, 8, 10].

The global prevalence of infertility ranges from 9% to 18%. The World Health Organization reports that one in six people (approximately 17%) will experience infertility at some point in their lives [1]. The prevalence of infertility is similar across countries, regardless of income level. In high-income countries, the infertility rate is reported to be 17.8%, compared with 16.5% in low- and middle-income countries [11].

T. Akbayrak, E. Üzelpasaci (eds.), *Physiotherapy and Rehabilitation in Pelvic and Women's Health-Related Problems*, https://doi.org/10.1007/978-3-032-28741-0_20

20.4 Etiology and Pathophysiology

Infertility can result from various problems within the male or female reproductive system. In men, the most common causes of infertility include insufficient or absent sperm, abnormal sperm shape, reduced motility, and ejaculation problems [2]. In women, abnormalities of the ovaries, uterus, fallopian tubes, and endocrine system can lead to infertility [2]. The main factors in the female reproductive system that can cause infertility include [3]:

Female reproductive system problems that can cause infertility	
Ovarian disorders	Polycystic ovary syndrome and other follicular disorders
Uterine disorders	Inflammatory conditions (e.g., endometriosis), congenital abnormalities (e.g., septate uterus), benign structural disorders (e.g., myomas)
Tubal disorders	Untreated sexually transmitted diseases, unsafe abortion procedures with low standards of hygiene, postpartum sepsis, presence of tubal occlusion due to complications of abdominal or pelvic surgery
Endocrine disorders	Hormonal imbalances, presence of pituitary tumors, or hypopituitarism

Infertility in men can develop due to various factors related to the male reproductive system, including [3, 12, 13]:

Conditions that can cause infertility in men	
Obstructions	Obstructions that cause problems with ejaculation. These blockages can occur in the tubes that carry sperm, such as the ejaculatory ducts and seminal vesicles. They are usually caused by injury or infection of the genital tract.
Hormonal disorders	Abnormalities in the hormones produced by the pituitary gland, hypothalamus, and testes.
Loss of testicular sperm production function (testicular failure)	Loss of testicular sperm production function due to various problems affecting the sperm-producing cells.
Abnormalities in sperm quality and function	Disorders in the shape and motility of sperm can adversely affect fertility.
Environmental and lifestyle factors	Factors such as smoking, excessive alcohol consumption, and obesity can affect fertility. In addition, exposure to environmental pollutants and toxins can have a direct toxic effect on gametes, reducing both their quantity and quality, thereby causing infertility.

For some infertile couples, no clear cause of infertility can be identified. In about 30% of infertile couples, a specific diagnosis can not be made, and this is known as "unexplained infertility." Unexplained infertility is defined as a condition where basic infertility investigations have been carried out and test results are normal [1]. It is important to assess each patient individually and accurately diagnose the factors causing infertility in order to provide appropriate treatment options.

20.5 Evaluation and Diagnosis

Early diagnosis of infertility, assessment of risk factors, elimination of these factors, and creation of supportive treatment plans are critical. The evaluation of infertility begins with a thorough medical history. As infertility can result from problems in the male, female, or both reproductive systems, a detailed assessment of both sexes is required [14].

20.5.1 Evaluation of Female Infertility

In female patients, a detailed history, physical examination, laboratory tests, and imaging techniques are used to identify factors that may contribute to infertility [14].

20.5.1.1 History Taking

When taking the history of infertility, the duration of infertility, previous investigations, and treatment outcomes should be elicited. The female's menstrual history should include age at menarche, cycle regularity, length, symptoms of molimina, and the onset and severity of dysmenorrhea, if present. Obstetric history should be reviewed, including previous pregnancies (gravidity), births (parity), time to conception, fertility treatments used, pregnancy outcomes, mode of delivery, and any complications during the process. In addition, previous contraceptive methods, frequency and timing of sexual intercourse, and sexual dysfunction should be discussed [15].

The patient's surgical history, particularly abdominal and pelvic surgery, should be obtained. Information on the type, indications, and outcomes of previous surgery is necessary. The gynecological history should include questions about pelvic inflammatory disease, sexually transmitted infections, endometriosis, and uterine fibroids [14, 15].

A review of systemic diseases is also an important part of the infertility evaluation. Thyroid disease, galactorrhea, and the presence of hirsutism should be assessed. Pelvic or abdominal pain and dyspareunia should also be investigated. Previous cervical cancer screening tests and results should be reviewed. A family history of birth defects, developmental delay, early menopause, or reproductive problems should be investigated. The patient's occupational history and exposure to known environmental hazards should be reviewed. Lifestyle habits such as nicotine, alcohol, and drug use should also be assessed. In addition, the use of potential teratogens, including allergies and current medications or supplements, should be addressed [14, 15].

20.5.1.2 Physical Examination

A detailed and focused physical examination is essential in the evaluation of female infertility. This should include an assessment of vital signs and body weight. The thyroid should be examined for enlargement, nodules, or tenderness. The breast examination should focus on breast secretions and their characteristics. To assess for androgen excess, symptoms such as acne and hirsutism should be evaluated. In addition, the condition of the breasts, groin, and axillary hair should be examined [16]. The pelvic examination should look for vaginal or cervical abnormalities and any discharge. The size, shape, position, and mobility of the uterus should be assessed. Adnexal masses, pelvic or abdominal tenderness, and organ enlargement or masses should be evaluated by palpation [14, 15].

20.5.1.3 Laboratory and Imaging Techniques

Laboratory tests and imaging techniques play an important role in the evaluation of infertility. Laboratory tests are used to assess ovarian reserve, ovulatory function, and hormonal imbalances. These tests include anti-Müllerian hormone (AMH) testing [17], measurement of follicle-stimulating hormone (FSH) [18], and estradiol (E2) levels on day 3, and measurement of thyroid-stimulating hormone (TSH) and prolactin [19]. Imaging techniques include transvaginal ultrasound, sonohysterography, hysterosalpingography, and hysteroscopy [14].

20.5.2 Evaluation of Male Infertility

As with women, the assessment of male infertility requires a comprehensive medical history. The history includes various parameters such as the individual's general health, previous medical and surgical interventions, medications, and substance use. In this context, systemic diseases, surgical history such as cryptorchidism, childhood diseases, history of infections, use of testosterone or gonadotoxic chemotherapeutic drugs, anabolic steroids, nicotine, alcohol, and marijuana should be questioned. Potential risk factors such as gonadal trauma or toxic exposure should also be considered. The frequency and timing of sexual intercourse, the presence of sexually transmitted infections, and erectile and ejaculatory dysfunction should be carefully assessed [14].

One of the most important diagnostic tools in male infertility is semen analysis. This procedure provides a quantitative microscopic assessment of sperm parameters. To increase the accuracy of the semen analysis, sexual abstinence for 2–5 days before semen collection is recommended, and the semen sample should ideally be collected by masturbation in a laboratory collection room. If abnormalities are found in the semen analysis, further tests and evaluations will be carried out. Patients with abnormalities in two separate analyses are referred to a urologist specializing in male infertility [14].

Prior to implementing physiotherapy and rehabilitation practices in infertility, additional physiotherapy and rehabilitation assessments should be performed beyond the basic assessments discussed above. The physical examination should include a detailed pelvic examination, particularly of the musculoskeletal system, in both male and female patients. Pelvic sensation, the presence of pain, myofascial trigger points, and the tone and symmetry of the pelvic floor muscles should be assessed [20]. In addition, muscle spasms and soft tissue mobility in the lower back, abdomen, and hips should be assessed, and a postural analysis performed [21].

20.6 Treatment Approaches

Infertility is emerging as a major public health problem worldwide, with serious implications for the physical, emotional, and social lives of individuals and couples. Common psychosocial problems associated with infertility include depression, anxiety, low self-esteem, marital conflict, and sexual dissatisfaction. In addition, infertility can lead to negative social outcomes such as social isolation, social discrimination, and exclusion [1]. Infertility treatment is a multidimensional process that should be planned according to the specific needs of the individual or couple. Various factors such as the woman's age, type of infertility, presence of male factor infertility, insurance coverage, history of genetic disorders, and desired family size are considered when planning treatment. Treatment options include lifestyle changes, pharmacotherapy and psychotherapy, assisted reproductive technologies, and, in advanced cases, surgery [4].

In the medical management of infertility, ovulation induction and ovarian stimulation are prominent approaches. Ovulation induction is one of the first-line methods for individuals with a history of anovulation. This method uses pharmacological agents to induce ovulation to regulate the timing of ovulation [22]. Ovarian stimulation is an approach used to promote the development of multiple mature ovarian follicles. These methods are usually supported by timed sexual intercourse or intrauterine insemination (IUI). However, assisted reproductive technologies offer effective solutions, particularly for unexplained infertility, endometriosis, tubal blockage, and male factor infertility. One of the most commonly used methods, in vitro fertilization (IVF), involves fertilizing eggs with sperm in a laboratory. The IVF process involves monitoring the development of the embryo in the laboratory and transferring it to the uterus at the appropriate time [23].

Approaches to male infertility, particularly in cases of azoospermia, include surgical methods to extract sperm from the testes. Techniques such as micro-TESE (testicular sperm extraction) increase the chances of finding sperm, and the samples obtained can be cryopreserved if necessary. Medical and surgical treatments to improve sperm functionality focus on improving sperm quality [24]. The process of managing infertility also increases psychological distress. Therefore, psychotherapy and psychosocial support should be an essential part of infertility management. Managing emotional states such as stress, anxiety, and depression can have a positive impact on treatment success. Methods such as cognitive behavioral therapy, support groups, and individual counseling can help couples maintain their psychological well-being [25].

20.7 Physiotherapy and Rehabilitation Approaches

Physiotherapy and rehabilitation approaches to infertility treatment have been increasingly studied in recent years. While there is no standard physiotherapy protocol, physiotherapists who specialize in pelvic and reproductive health provide important support to patients. The main roles of physiotherapists in this area include supporting patient education, raising awareness of physical activity and exercise, and implementing appropriate physiotherapy interventions. Other physiotherapy interventions include complementary and alternative methods such as manual therapy, electrical stimulation, and acupuncture. By applying their knowledge and skills in these methods, physiotherapists provide holistic support to individuals, which is crucial in improving the effectiveness of infertility treatment [5, 6].

20.7.1 Patient Education

In the process of infertility treatment, there is no standard approach to the scope, duration, or who is responsible for providing education to couples. However, the content of patient education should include the definition, anatomy, physiology, risk factors, treatment options, and possible outcomes of infertility, and the education should be tailored to the specific health conditions of the individuals/couples. The treatment process for infertility, which has a complex etiology, is lengthy. It is therefore important for individuals to be knowledgeable about the subject and the process, as this can help them to make informed decisions and develop positive attitudes. Inadequate information can have a negative impact on an individual's or couple's perception of self-efficacy and adherence to treatment. Patient education is essential to reduce anxiety and increase motivation during infertility treatment. Research has shown that lack of information about infertility and treatment processes leads to increased anxiety and lack of motivation for treatment. In this context, it is recommended that reproductive health education be considered a fundamental component of medical interventions [26].

The American College of Obstetricians and Gynaecologists (ACOG) [27] and the American Society for Reproductive Medicine (ASRM) [28] have published guidelines that guide preconception care and counseling. These guidelines suggest that every medical visit for individuals with reproductive potential should be viewed as an opportunity to improve reproductive health and obstetric outcomes. Preconception care aims to improve women's overall health by reducing modifiable risk factors and minimizing potential adverse effects on the fetus and neonate.

Key issues to be addressed during the preconception period include:

Key components of preconception education	
Pregnancy planning	Women should be advised to seek medical advice before trying to conceive, or as soon as they suspect they may be pregnant, and to adjust any current treatment as necessary
Chronic conditions	Conditions such as diabetes, hypertension, thyroid disease, and psychiatric disorders should be optimally managed before pregnancy
Medical history and medications	A detailed review of all medications and supplements used by the patient should be undertaken
Genetic screening	Appropriate genetic screening tests for hereditary conditions should be recommended before pregnancy
Vaccinations	Vaccination status for tetanus toxoid, reduced diphtheria toxoid, acellular pertussis (Tdap), measles-mumps-rubella, hepatitis B, and varicella should be reviewed annually. Routine influenza vaccination should be recommended to all patients, emphasizing the additional benefits for women during the influenza season in pregnancy
Infectious diseases	Patients at risk of sexually transmitted infections and Zika virus should be advised of precautions to take before planning a pregnancy
Substance use	Information should be provided on the harms and risks of alcohol, nicotine, and other harmful substances
Diet and vitamin supplementation	Guidance should be provided on the use of supplements such as folic acid, calcium, iron, and vitamins A, B12, and D
Body Mass Index (BMI)	Maintaining a normal BMI before pregnancy should be encouraged. Extreme BMI levels, whether high or low, are associated with infertility and pregnancy complications, so advice should be given in this area
Psychosocial factors	The need for psychosocial support and the risk of exposure to violence or coercion should be assessed

Patient education should be multifaceted, taking into account the different learning styles of individuals. Written materials, group sessions, one-to-one counseling, and resources provided through digital platforms are all important. Digital applications, in particular, are preferred because they provide constant access to information and allow individuals to learn at their own pace. Patient education plays a critical role in improving the clinical success of infertility treatment and ensuring active participation in the treatment process. Education provided to individuals planning a pregnancy facilitates a better understanding of the treatment process, adherence to lifestyle changes, and access to psychosocial support. In this context, patient education not only increases the individual's knowledge of the treatment but also facilitates the decision-making process [27, 28].

20.7.2 Physical Activity and Exercise Interventions

The World Health Organization defines physical activity as any physical movement that results in energy expenditure above the basal metabolic rate. A minimum of 150 min of moderate-to-vigorous physical activity per week is recommended to reduce reproductive health risks [29]. Appropriate physical activity is an inexpensive and accessible method of protecting and improving health with minimal side effects. Properly prescribed physical activity can improve antioxidant defenses, reduce inflammation, support immune function, and help prevent infertility [30]. Randomized controlled trials have shown that physical activity can have a beneficial effect on infertility by improving insulin resistance, free sex hormones, and immune function [31].

Meta-analyses have shown that physical activity can reduce the risk of endometriosis in women and improve reproductive performance in polycystic ovary syndrome [32]. High levels of physical activity have been shown to reduce the risk of infertility by 39%, and moderate levels by 30%. On the other hand, excessive physical activity at very high intensities has been observed to increase the risk of infertility compared with moderate levels [32].

Exercise is a planned and structured form of physical activity. In infertility treatment, exercise training is an important part of supporting physical and metabolic health. Physical inactivity or a sedentary lifestyle is a risk factor for infertility, while regular exercise can help reduce these risks [32].

A sedentary lifestyle increases the risk of infertility, whereas regular exercise may improve reproductive function through antioxidant and anti-inflammatory mechanisms. However, the role of variables such as type, duration, and intensity of exercise in these effects remains unclear. Observational studies suggest that cycling for more than 5 h per week may adversely affect sperm quality in men, while resistance exercise has been highlighted for its beneficial effects on male infertility [33]. A systematic review focusing on the fertile male population mentions that low- and moderate-intensity physical activity performed for recreational purposes may improve semen quality, while elite sports may negatively affect sperm motility [34, 35].

In infertile couples, male factors account for up to 50% of infertility, and infertility is often caused by disturbances in the spermatogenic process. Increased levels of cytokines in seminal plasma have been reported to negatively correlate with semen quality parameters and sperm DNA integrity [36, 37]. In addition, there is increasing evidence that inflammation in semen may be associated with oxidative stress [38, 39]. High levels of DNA fragmentation in sperm are a critical factor in pregnancy or embryo development [40]. Therefore, protective approaches against oxidative stress and inflammation are considered potentially beneficial in the treatment of male infertility.

A randomized controlled trial involving 433 sedentary infertile men evaluated the effects of 24 weeks of high-intensity exercise on pro-inflammatory cytokines, peroxidative and antioxidative biomarkers, semen quality, sperm DNA integrity, and pregnancy rates [34]. During the first 12 weeks of high-intensity exercise training, participants underwent a treadmill protocol three times a week for 40–50 min. This protocol consisted of a 10-min run at 70–75% of VO_2max, followed by a 3-min recovery period at 50–60% of VO_2max. For the final 12 weeks, participants followed a 50–60-min treadmill protocol three times a week. This protocol consisted of a 10-min run at 75–85% of VO_2max, followed by a 3-min recovery period at 50–60% of VO_2max. All exercise sessions included a 10–15-min warm-up and cool-down. The 24-week high-intensity exercise training improved reproductive function in previously sedentary infertile men, reduced markers of inflammation and oxidative stress, improved semen quality parameters, and increased pregnancy rates in infertile patients. Based on these findings, exercise training has been recommended as a potential intervention in the treatment of infertile men [34].

A randomized controlled trial involving 556 participants tested the hypothesis that a combination of aerobic and resistance exercise could reduce seminal inflammation and oxidative stress markers and improve semen quality, DNA integrity, and pregnancy rates in male factor infertility patients. The effects of combined aerobic and resistance exercise on seminal inflammation and oxidative stress markers were assessed over 24 weeks. The relationship between changes in these markers and semen quality, sperm DNA integrity, and pregnancy rates was also investigated [41].

The participants participated in the exercise training program for 24 weeks, with three sessions per week. Each session began with a 10-min warm-up that included walking, running, and flexibility exercises. After the warm-up, participants performed 30–35 min of alternating walking/running aerobic exercises, followed by 30–35 min of resistance exercises targeting large muscle groups. Upper-body exercises included bench presses, shoulder presses, biceps curls, and sit ups, while lower-body exercises included leg presses, calf raises, hip extensions, hamstring curls, and hip abduction/adduction. The exercises were initially performed at 50% of 1RM VO_2max, with the intensity gradually increased. Each session ended with a 10-min cool-down period consisting of slow walking and light muscle stretching. The control group received no exercise intervention. The exercise program significantly reduced seminal pro-inflammatory cytokines and markers of oxidative stress. In addition, improvements in the seminal antioxidant defense system were observed. The changes in inflammation and oxidative stress levels correlated with improvements in semen parameters, sperm DNA integrity, and pregnancy rates. Thus, the results of the study provide strong evidence for the beneficial effects of combined aerobic and resistance exercise on male factor infertility [41].

Exercise can affect the hypothalamic-pituitary-adrenal axis in women, potentially increasing hypothalamic-pituitary-gonadal activity and contributing to the resumption of ovulation. It may also have a beneficial effect on metabolic processes by regulating insulin and androgen levels [32]. Regular exercise in women can regulate the menstrual cycle and increase ovulation in women with polycystic ovary syndrome (PCOS), thereby increasing the chances of pregnancy. A study of obese and infertile women found that weight loss, improved physical fitness, and better mental health contributed to increased ovulation and pregnancy rates [42].

Research on female infertility has shown that regular, moderate exercise has a positive effect on fertility and assisted reproductive technology (ART) outcomes. A study of 26,955 women reported that vigorous exercise reduced the risk of ovulatory infertility [43, 44]. In a study of 216 obese women undergoing ART, those who exercised regularly had better outcomes than sedentary women, regardless of weight loss [45]. Exercise for 1 h at least three times a week improved implantation and pregnancy rates and reduced the risk of miscarriage in 436 women undergoing intracytoplasmic sperm injection (ICSI) [46]. In addition, low- to moderate-intensity aerobic exercise was associated with increased implantation and live birth rates in 131 ART patients [47].

A systematic review of the effects of exercise in overweight and obese women with polycystic ovary syndrome (PCOS) found that exercise improved menstrual regularity and ovulation frequency [48]. Compared with diet [49] or no treatment [50], exercise was shown to improve menstrual regulation and ovulation rates. Another trial showed that a combination of diet, aerobic exercise, or both aerobic and resistance exercise led to similar improvements [51]. In both PCOS and non-PCOS infertile women, 12–24-week lifestyle interventions involving diet, exercise, and/or behavioral changes improved ovulation and menstrual regularity and reduced the risk of miscarriage. Many of the interventions resulted in participants achieving pregnancy and giving birth by natural or assisted methods [52, 53]. As a result, exercise interventions have a direct impact on obesity and oocyte and sperm quality. Current data suggest that moderate-intensity exercise improves sperm quality in men and regulates ovulation in women, resulting in the release of higher-quality oocytes. In addition, regular moderate exercise may increase IVF success rates and provide general health benefits [54].

20.7.3 Yoga

Yoga is an ancient practice that focuses on the integration of body and mind to promote both physical and mental health. It has gained particular attention for its ability to reduce physiological stress and inflammation and is often considered an alternative to antidepressants. Yoga has positive effects on reproductive health in both women and men. The literature suggests that yoga contributes to hormonal balance, reduces abdominal tension, and increases blood flow to the uterus, ovaries, and fallopian tubes [55]. These effects improve the function of the reproductive organs and increase the chances of natural conception. Through the hypothalamic-pituitary-gonadal axis, yoga helps to balance hormonal profiles, reduce stress, and improve overall quality of life [56].

Regular yoga practice has been shown to regulate menstrual cycles and improve ovulation [57]. In men, yoga supports fertility potential by improving sperm quality [58]. Studies by Dhawan and Bisht have demonstrated the beneficial effects of yoga practices on sperm DNA, count, and quality [59, 60]. However, research in this area remains limited, and further studies are needed.

Systematic reviews investigating the effects of yoga on pregnancy outcomes suggest that yoga may improve IVF success rates as a complementary approach. Randomized controlled trials have shown that women who practice yoga have significantly higher pregnancy rates than control groups. For example, studies by Nayar and colleagues have shown that yoga practice not only improves pregnancy rates but also overall quality of life [61]. In a randomized controlled trial by Neelakshi, women undergoing ART who practiced yoga achieved higher rates of positive pregnancy outcomes [62]. In addition, research by Sharma and colleagues found that women undergoing yoga therapy had higher pregnancy rates than those treated with clomiphene [63]. Stress, anxiety, and depression are some of the most common psychological problems faced by infertile patients and have a direct impact on treatment success. Yoga and meditation improve the individual's ability to cope with stress and thus contribute positively to the treatment process. Studies by Galhardo and colleagues show that yoga practices reduce depression and anxiety, promote mental relaxation, and improve the quality of life associated with infertility [64]. Yoga is considered a complementary and effective approach to infertility treatment. In addition to reducing stress and promoting mental balance, yoga enhances fertility by improving hormonal regulation and physiological effects on the reproductive organs. As a natural, safe, and accessible method, yoga is a promising option for people undergoing infertility treatment.

20.7.4 Manipulative Treatment Interventions

Manual therapy is a method commonly used by physiotherapists in the treatment of various conditions. In infertility, manual therapy can be used for tubal obstruction, endometriosis, hormonal imbalances, and unexplained infertility. There are several studies in the literature that support the positive effects of manual therapy on infertility [65]. To understand the effects of manual therapy on infertility, it is important to understand the reproductive anatomy and the relationship of the peritoneum, pelvic fascia, and other connective tissues to the arterial, venous, and lymphatic circulations [66].

Fascia is a dynamic network that surrounds, protects, and supports all body structures [67]. The endopelvic fascia, which contains estrogen receptors, is subject to hormonal influences that affect its structure and function [67]. The peritoneum is a continuous serous membrane that covers the inner surface of the abdominal and pelvic walls and surrounds the abdominal visceral organs. It reduces friction between organs and provides the necessary conditions for the optimal functioning of the pelvic organs [68]. It is known that after surgery, the defense and repair mechanisms of the peritoneum can lead to adhesions, which can lead to infertility in women [69]. Studies have highlighted the potential of physiotherapy to reduce adhesions after surgery [70]. Four main manual therapy approaches that have been studied in the literature for their effects on infertility are the clear passage approach (CPA), the Mojzisova method, Mercier therapy, and osteopathic approaches [70].

20.7.4.1 Clear Passage Approach

The clear passage approach (CPA) was developed by Belinda and Larry Wurn. CPA is a patient-centered physiotherapy plan that focuses on reducing adhesions in the body and incorporates various manual therapy techniques. CPA uses myofascial release techniques, the Wurn technique, and visceral manipulation to release adhesions between visceral organs. The duration and intensity of the treatment depend on the patient's tolerance. The frequency and duration of treatment sessions can range from weekly one-hour sessions to intensive daily sessions lasting 2–4 h. The standard treatment protocol is approximately 20 hours. CPA has shown successful results in treating infertility, as well as reducing adhesions and pain in patients with small bowel obstruction and improving their quality of life [65, 71, 72]. However, most of the existing studies are retrospective and based on patient histories and incomplete data on male factors, indicating the need for further randomized controlled trials to investigate the effects of CPA.

20.7.4.2 Mojzisova Method

Developed by Ludmila Mojzisova, this method is based on reflexive interactions between the spinal cord and pelvic organs. This approach has shown positive effects on pelvic pain, dyspareunia, dysmenorrhea, spinal problems, and infertility. Although it has been hypothesized that it could be used for male infertility, there is no research to support this claim [73]. The therapy involves home exercise programs and manual therapy sessions with a physiotherapist. Women are instructed to do stretching and strengthening exercises at home twice a day. Manual therapy is given by a trained physiotherapist during the first half of the menstrual cycle, with one-hour sessions once a month. This therapy includes mobilization of the ribs, lumbar vertebrae, and sacroiliac joints; coccyx treatment; and internal rectal work. The treatment lasts for a total of six sessions over 6 months [74]. Although the number of trials on this method is limited, those that do exist show positive results. The age of the woman is an important factor in the success of the treatment. Success rates have been reported as 44.6% in women under 25 years of age, 22.6% in women aged 31–35 years, and 33.3% in women aged 36–40 years. Further studies are needed to investigate the effects and prognostic factors of this method in more detail [73, 74].

20.7.4.3 Mercier Therapy

Mercier therapy, developed by Dr. Jennifer Mercier, involves deep visceral manipulation of the pelvic organs. The aim of the therapy is to release restrictions between the reproductive organs and restore blood flow. Mercier therapy can be used alone or as a preparatory technique for assisted reproductive techniques. The treatment consists of 1-h sessions, with a protocol that includes a total of 6 h of therapy over a period of 1–6 weeks [75]. A study published in 2013 reported an 83% success rate in achieving pregnancy following treatment [75]. However, further research is needed to identify the factors that influence the outcomes and success of the therapy.

20.7.4.4 Osteopathic Approaches

Osteopathy, developed by Andrew Taylor Still in the mid-1800s, is recognized by the World Health Organization as a complementary and alternative medicine [76]. Osteopathy aims to restore normal mobility of the reproductive organs by releasing pelvic adhesions and improving circulation. Osteopathic approaches target the autonomic nervous system, which influences pelvic circulation. These approaches are thought to facilitate implantation and increase the chances of pregnancy by relieving adhesions, improving circulation and organ mobility, and reducing pain [77]. As fertility is a multifactorial process involving physiological, neuroendocrine, and mechanical aspects, the effects of osteopathic approaches on infertility are not yet fully understood. Although a limited number of heterogeneous studies highlight the potential effects of osteopathic approaches on infertility, further high-quality studies are needed [78].

20.7.5 Electrical Stimulation

In the field of physiotherapy and rehabilitation for women's health, electrotherapy modalities are widely used to reduce pain, strengthen muscles, and improve local awareness and circulation. However, the number of studies looking at neuromuscular electrical stimulation (NMES) about fertility is limited. NMES works by activating nerve fibers with electrical stimuli to induce muscle contractions [79]. Zhu et al. [80] evaluated the effects of combining NMES with Kuntai capsule therapy in infertile patients with thin endometrial lining who did not respond to long-term estrogen therapy. The results showed an increase in endometrial thickness, regulation of sex hormone levels, improvement in uterine hemodynamics, and improvement in clinical symptoms. Similarly, He et al. [81] investigated the combined effects of biomimetic electrical stimulation, low-intensity focused ultrasound, and acupuncture point stimulation. This combined approach was shown to increase endometrial blood flow, improve endometrial structure and receptivity, and increase clinical pregnancy rates. In infertile women with endometrial thickness of 7 mm or less, NMES application led to a significant increase in uterine blood flow and endometrial thickness. These results suggest that NMES is a promising method that can be used safely in the treatment of infertility [82].

In recent years, some studies have investigated the effects of TENS (transcutaneous electrical nerve stimulation) on fertilization. TENS has been shown to increase uterine blood flow and endometrial thickness, which helps the fertilized egg to implant. Current clinical trials support NMES as an effective physiotherapy method in the treatment of infertility. However, more research is needed to investigate the long-term effects of NMES [83].

Patients with spinal cord injury (SCI) are treated with electroejaculator stimulation (EES). In this method, a low-intensity electrical current is delivered through a rectal electrode, which stimulates the pelvic muscles to induce ejaculation. EES was first described in cats by Platz and Seager [84] and later applied to humans. Case reports and small studies have shown that pregnancy has been achieved using sperm from SCI patients [85]. The majority of men with SCI cannot achieve an antegrade ejaculation by masturbation or sexual stimulation. However, approximately 80% of SCI men with an intact ejaculatory reflex arc (T10 and above) can achieve antegrade ejaculation with penile vibratory stimulation (PVS). EES has been successfully used to obtain semen from SCI men, even those who lack key components of the ejaculatory reflex arc. It has also been successfully used to induce ejaculation in neurological conditions such as multiple sclerosis and diabetic neuropathy [86, 87].

Prior to intensive cancer treatment, PVS and EES have been successfully used in adolescent males for sperm retrieval and cryopreservation [86]. In addition, the use of PVS and EES in combination with assisted reproductive techniques such as intrauterine insemination or intracytoplasmic sperm injection (ICSI) is thought to play an important role in increasing male fertility potential [88].

20.7.6 Photobiomodulation (Laser Therapy)

In recent years, photobiomodulation therapy (laser therapy) has been widely used to support tissue healing, regeneration, and repair processes. This therapy activates the cell repair mechanisms, increasing ATP levels through energy absorbed by the cells. The increased ATP levels accelerate cell proliferation and differentiation, promoting healing processes [89]. Research shows that about two-thirds of infertility patients experiencing recurrent embryo implantation failure face issues related to the endometrium not being suitable for embryo implantation [90]. In a prospective randomized study by Tsai et al., 29 women received He-Ne laser irradiation before frozen-thawed embryo transfer, while 31 women received no pre-treatment. The study results showed that He-Ne laser irradiation supported the release of endometrial growth factors and cytokines during the implantation process, improved microcirculation, and thus increased endometrial receptivity and pregnancy rates [91].

Low-level laser therapy (LLLT) is another form of photobiomodulation treatment that can be absorbed by cells without creating thermal effects. In a study by El Faham et al., the potential of LLLT to enhance the proliferative capacity of the endometrium was investigated. In an in vitro setting, LLLT applied at a wavelength of 635 nm was observed to stimulate endometrial receptor gene expression and increase the differentiation and regeneration capabilities of endometrial cells [92]. Photobiomodulation therapy is still in the research phase and has not yet been fully integrated into mainstream medicine. However, the wavelength of the laser and the duration of application should be personalized for each patient. Further studies on laser therapy in infertility are needed [83].

20.7.7 Acupuncture

Acupuncture is a treatment method with over 2000 years of history, originating from Traditional Chinese Medicine and derived from the "Huangdi Neijing" (The Yellow Emperor's Inner Classic). Acupuncture involves inserting thin metal needles into specific acupuncture points on the body to prevent and treat disease. According to clinical studies, filiform acupuncture is the most preferred method in this area due to its simplicity and effectiveness [93, 94].

A 1999 study found that acupuncture could improve fertility, pregnancy rates, and the number of live births [95]. Other research has shown that acupuncture can support embryo implantation by increasing endometrial thickness and regulating uterine blood flow. It can also reduce stress and anxiety, improve quality of life, and improve pregnancy outcomes. In cases of infertility associated with thin endometrium, acupuncture's effectiveness in increasing endometrial receptivity has been confirmed in another study [83].

When acupuncture is combined with Chinese herbal treatments, more significant increases in endometrial thickness and pregnancy rates are observed. This combination works by increasing endometrial blood flow, which has a positive effect on embryo implantation and improves endometrial receptivity. Therefore, acupuncture combined with herbal treatments is a safe and effective complementary therapy for improving endometrial receptivity [96].

Acupuncture supports endometrial development through the hypothalamic-pituitary-ovarian axis, regulating uterine blood flow and increasing local circulation to create an optimal environment for embryo implantation [97]. It has also been shown to increase the levels of hormones such as estrogen and progesterone and to regulate the receptors for these hormones [98].

Li et al. [99] randomly divided 60 patients with infertility due to thin endometrium into two groups. The intervention group received acupuncture and Chinese herbal medicine, while the control group was treated with estradiol valerate tablets. The results showed a significant increase in endometrial thickness in the intervention group compared with the control group, and pregnancy rates were significantly higher in the treatment group. These findings support the use of acupuncture in combination with Chinese herbal treatments as an effective therapy for infertility caused by thin endometrium, promoting endometrial growth, improving receptivity, and increasing clinical pregnancy rates.

Xu et al. [100] conducted a study of 60 infertile patients with ovulatory dysfunction. The patients were randomly assigned to one of two groups. The control group received traditional ovulation induction, while the intervention group also received acupuncture at specific points (Baihui, Mingmen, Geshu, Guanyuan, and Qihai). The results showed that the intervention group had higher rates of embryo implantation and clinical pregnancy than the control group.

In conclusion, acupuncture is considered an effective complementary therapy, particularly for infertility associated with thin endometrium and problems with endometrial receptivity. However, the effects of these treatments need to be further supported by large sample studies, comprehensive and systematic research, and standardization of clinical protocols.

20.8 Conclusion

Infertility is a complex health issue that has a significant impact on the quality of life of individuals and couples. The management of infertility needs to be multidisciplinary, and a physiotherapist is an essential member of the multidisciplinary team. There is growing evidence to support the complementary role of physiotherapy and rehabilitation techniques alongside traditional medical treatments in the management of infertility. Pelvic health, and in particular, neuromusculoskeletal assessments, individualized exercise programs, manual therapeutic interventions, neuromuscular electrical stimulation management, and photobiomodulation techniques have the potential to support reproductive health and improve treatment outcomes. It should be noted that the physiotherapy and rehabilitation approaches discussed in this chapter not only support physical health but also contribute to the psychological and social well-being of individuals. Holistic and individualized physiotherapy approaches appear to have the potential to improve the effectiveness of infertility treatment and make a significant contribution to patients' quality of life. The evidence base for the effects of physiotherapy interventions, both alone and in combination, should be further strengthened by well-designed, randomized controlled trials with large sample sizes.

References

1. Organization Wh. WHO fact sheet on infertility. Lww; 2021. p. E52.
2. Harrison JE, Weber S, Jakob R, Chute CG. Icd-11: an international classification of diseases for the twenty-first century. BMC Med Inform Decis Mak. 2021;21:1–10.
3. Carson SA, Kallen AN. Diagnosis and management of infertility: a review. JAMA. 2021;326(1):65–76.
4. Devroey P, Fauser B, Diedrich K, Group Earw. Approaches to improve the diagnosis and management of infertility. Hum Reprod Update. 2009;15(4):391–408.
5. Salsabili N, Ansari NN, Berjis K, Sedighi A, Salsabili H. Effects of physiotherapeutic tens in a woman with unexplained infertility. Physiother Theory Pract. 2011;27(2):155–9.
6. Szafarowska M, Rosiński M, Segiet-Święcicka A, Jędrzejczyk S, Jerzak M, Jerzak M. Effect of physiotherapy on infertility treatment in polycystic ovary syndrome patients. Menopause Rev Przegląd Menopauzalny. 2024;23(1)
7. Jabeen F, Khadija S, Daud S. Prevalence of primary and secondary infertility. Saudi J Med. 2022;7(1):22–8.
8. Mascarenhas MN, Flaxman SR, Boerma T, Vanderpoel S, Stevens GA. National, regional, and global trends in infertility prevalence since 1990: a systematic analysis of 277 health surveys. PLoS Med. 2012;9(12):E1001356.
9. Cong J, Li P, Zheng L, Tan J. Prevalence and risk factors of infertility at a rural site of northern China. PLoS One. 2016;11(5):E0155563.
10. Inhorn MC, Patrizio P. Infertility around the globe: new thinking on gender, reproductive technologies and global movements in the 21st century. Hum Reprod Update. 2015;21(4):411–26.
11. Harris E. Infertility affects 1 in 6 people globally. JAMA. 2023;329(17):1443.
12. Gore AC, Chappell VA, Fenton SE, Flaws JA, Nadal A, Prins GS, et al. Edc-2: the Endocrine Society's

second scientific statement on endocrine-disrupting chemicals. Endocr Rev. 2015;36(6):E1–E150.
13. Segal TR, Giudice L. Before the beginning: environmental exposures and reproductive and obstetrical outcomes. Fertil Steril. 2019;112(4):613–21.
14. Walker Z, Gunn D. Review of infertility diagnosis and evaluation. Curr Obstet Gynecol Rep. 2021:1–6.
15. Penzias A, Azziz R, Bendikson K, Cedars M, Falcone T, Hansen K, et al. Fertility evaluation of infertile women: a committee opinion. Fertil Steril. 2021;116(5):1255–65.
16. Costello M, Misso M, Balen A, Boyle J, Devoto L, Garad R, et al. Evidence summaries and recommendations from the international evidence-based guideline for the assessment and management of polycystic ovary syndrome: assessment and treatment of infertility. Hum Reprod Open. 2019;2019(1):Hoy021.
17. Tsepelidis S, Devreker F, Demeestere I, Flahaut A, Gervy C, Englert Y. Stable serum levels of Anti-Müllerian hormone during the menstrual cycle: a prospective study in Normo-ovulatory women. Hum Reprod. 2007;22(7):1837–40.
18. Broekmans F, Kwee J, Hendriks D, Mol B, Lambalk C. A systematic review of tests predicting ovarian reserve and Ivf outcome. Hum Reprod Update. 2006;12(6):685–718.
19. Blickenstorfer K, Voelkle M, Xie M, Fröhlich A, Imthurn B, Leeners B. Are who recommendations to perform 2 consecutive semen analyses for reliable diagnosis of male infertility still valid? J Urol. 2019;201(4):783–91.
20. Wójcik M, Szczepaniak R, Placek K. Physiotherapy management in endometriosis. Int J Environ Res Public Health. 2022;19(23):16148.
21. Jędrzejczyk S, Szafarowska M, Rosiński M, Segiet-Święcicka A, Jerzak M, Jerzak M. Osteopathic approach as an additional therapy of infertility in women with Pcos. Eur J Obstet Gynecol Reprod Biol. 2024;293:94.
22. Messinis IE. Ovulation induction: a mini review. Hum Reprod. 2005;20(10):2688–97.
23. Choe J, Shanks Al. In vitro fertilization. 2020.
24. Achermann AP, Pereira TA, Esteves SC. Microdissection testicular sperm extraction (micro-tese) in men with infertility due to nonobstructive azoospermia: summary of current literature. Int Urol Nephrol. 2021;53(11):2193–210.
25. Abdolahi HM, Ghojazadeh M, Abdi S, Farhangi MA, Nikniaz Z, Nikniaz L. Effect of cognitive behavioral therapy on anxiety and depression of infertile women: a meta–analysis. Asian Pac J Reprod. 2019;8(6):251–9.
26. Bennett L, Wiweko B, Bell L, Shafira N, Pangestu M, Adayana IP, et al. Reproductive knowledge and patient education needs among Indonesian women infertility patients attending three fertility clinics. Patient Educ Couns. 2015;98(3):364–9.
27. Obstetricians Aco, Gynecologists. Acog committee opinion no. 762: prepregnancy counseling. Obstet Gynecol. 2019;133(1):E78–89.
28. Hill D. Prepregnancy counseling. Fertil Steril. 2019;111(1)
29. Gascoigne EL, Webster CM, Honart AW, Wang P, Smith-Ryan A, Manuck TA. Physical activity and pregnancy outcomes: an expert review. Am J Obstet Gynecol MFM. 2023;5(1):100758.
30. Maleki B, Tartibian B. Resistance exercise modulates male factor infertility through anti-inflammatory and antioxidative mechanisms in infertile men: a Rct. Life Sci. 2018;203:150–60.
31. Zhang H, Hua L, Liu D, Su X, Chen J, Chen J. Effects of physical activity on infertility in reproductive females. Reprod Biol Endocrinol. 2024;22(1):62.
32. Xie F, You Y, Guan C, Gu Y, Yao F, Xu J. Association between physical activity and infertility: a comprehensive systematic review and meta-analysis. J Transl Med. 2022;20(1):237.
33. Wise LA, Cramer DW, Hornstein MD, Ashby RK, Missmer SA. Physical activity and semen quality among men attending an infertility clinic. Fertil Steril. 2011;95(3):1025–30.
34. Maleki BH, Tartibian B. High-intensity exercise training for improving reproductive function in infertile patients: a randomized controlled trial. J Obstet Gynaecol Can. 2017;39(7):545–58.
35. Ibanez-Perez J, Santos-Zorrozua B, Lopez-Lopez E, Matorras R, Garcia-Orad A. An update on the implication of physical activity on semen quality: a systematic review and meta-analysis. Arch Gynecol Obstet. 2019;299:901–21.
36. Castiglione R, Salemi M, Vicari L, Vicari E. Relationship of semen hyperviscosity with Il-6, Tnf-A, Il-10 and Ros production in seminal plasma of infertile patients with prostatitis and Prostato-Vesiculitis. Andrologia. 2014;46(10):1148–55.
37. Furuya Y, Akashi T, Fuse H. Soluble Fas and Interleukin-6 and Interleukin-8 levels in seminal plasma of infertile men. Arch Androl. 2003;49(6):449–52.
38. Sanocka D, Jędrzejczak P, Szumała-Kaękol A, Frączek M, Kurpisz M. Male genital tract inflammation: the role of selected interleukins in regulation of pro-oxidant and antioxidant enzymatic substances in seminal plasma. J Androl. 2003;24(3):448–55.
39. Hajizadeh Maleki B, Tartibian B, Eghbali M, Asri-Rezaei S. Comparison of seminal oxidants and antioxidants in subjects with different levels of physical fitness. Andrology. 2013;1(4):607–14.
40. Zini A, Boman JM, Belzile E, Ciampi A. Sperm DNA damage is associated with an increased risk of pregnancy loss after IVF and ICSI: systematic review and meta-analysis. Hum Reprod. 2008;23(12):2663–8.
41. Hajizadeh Maleki B, Tartibian B. Combined aerobic and resistance exercise training for improving reproductive function in infertile men: a randomized controlled trial. Appl Physiol Nutr Metab. 2017;42(12):1293–306.
42. Hakimi O, Cameron L-C. Effect of exercise on ovulation: a systematic review. Sports Med. 2017;47:1555–67.

43. Hordern MD, Dunstan DW, Prins JB, Baker MK, Singh MAF, Coombes JS. Exercise prescription for patients with type 2 diabetes and pre-diabetes: a position statement from exercise and sport science Australia. J Sci Med Sport. 2012;15(1):25–31.
44. Rich-Edwards J, Spiegelman D, Garland M, Hertzmark E, Hunter DJ, Colditz GA, et al. Physical activity, body mass index, and ovulatory disorder infertility. Epidemiology. 2002;13(2):184–90.
45. Palomba S, Falbo A, Valli B, Morini D, Villani MT, Nicoli A, et al. Physical activity before IVF and ICSI cycles in infertile obese women: an observational cohort study. Reprod Biomed Online. 2014;29(1):72–9.
46. Ferreira RC, Halpern G, De Cássia Savio Figueira R, De Almeida Ferreira Braga DP, Iaconelli A Jr, Borges E Jr. Physical activity, obesity and eating habits can influence assisted reproduction outcomes. Womens Health. 2010;6(4):517–24.
47. Kucuk M, Doymaz F, Urman B. Effect of energy expenditure and physical activity on the outcomes of assisted reproduction treatment. Reprod Biomed Online. 2010;20(2):274–9.
48. Harrison C, Lombard C, Moran L, Teede H. Exercise therapy in polycystic ovary syndrome: a systematic review. Hum Reprod Update. 2011;17(2):171–83.
49. Palomba S, Giallauria F, Falbo A, Russo T, Oppedisano R, Tolino A, et al. Structured exercise training programme versus hypocaloric Hyperproteic diet in obese polycystic ovary syndrome patients with Anovulatory infertility: a 24-week pilot study. Hum Reprod. 2008;23(3):642–50.
50. Vigorito C, Giallauria F, Palomba S, Cascella T, Manguso F, Lucci R, et al. Beneficial effects of a three-month structured exercise training program on cardiopulmonary functional capacity in young women with polycystic ovary syndrome. J Clin Endocrinol Metabol. 2007;92(4):1379–84.
51. Thomson R, Buckley JD, Noakes M, Clifton PM, Norman RJ, Brinkworth GD. The effect of a hypocaloric diet with and without exercise training on body composition, cardiometabolic risk profile, and reproductive function in overweight and obese women with polycystic ovary syndrome. J Clin Endocrinol Metabol. 2008;93(9):3373–80.
52. Clark A, Thornley B, Tomlinson L, Galletley C, Norman R. Weight loss in obese infertile women results in improvement in reproductive outcome for all forms of fertility treatment. Hum Reprod. 1998;13(6):1502–5.
53. Miller PB, Forstein DA, Styles S. Effect of short-term diet and exercise on hormone levels and menses in obese, infertile women. J Reprod Med. 2008;53(5):315–9.
54. Topdağı YE, Öztürk Ş, Özdemir I, Çakına S. The role of regularly exercise in overcoming infertility barriers. J Sci Perspect. 2019;3(3):223–8.
55. Yıldırım A, Satılmış IG. The effects of yoga on pregnancy, stress, and anxiety in infertile individuals: a systematic review. Holist Nurs Pract. 2022;36(5):275–83.
56. Kochhar K, Oberoi A, Hazra S, Lal P. The role of traditional diet and yoga for infertility: a blend and balance of traditional knowledge and modern medicine. 2017.
57. Yadav VB, Chaudhari VS. Systemic review of yoga in infertile couple….. Current status and future direction Vd. 2017.
58. Dinçer Y, Şanlı Y, Kızılkaya Beji N. Infertilite Hemşireliğinde Kanıta Dayalı Yaklaşımlar. Androloji Bülteni. 2015;17(63):289–95.
59. Dhawan V, Kumar M, Deka D, Malhotra N, Dadhwal V, Singh N, et al. Meditation & Yoga: impact on oxidative DNA damage & dysregulated sperm transcripts in male partners of couples with recurrent pregnancy loss. Indian J Med Res. 2018;148(Suppl 1):S134–S9.
60. Bisht S, Banu S, Srivastava S, Pathak RU, Kumar R, Dada R, et al. Sperm Methylome alterations following yoga-based lifestyle intervention in patients of primary male infertility: a pilot study. Andrologia. 2020;52(4):E13551.
61. Nayar P, Nayar K, Singh M, Aggarwal N, Gupta M, Gupta R, et al., editors. Yoga as an adjuvant to enhance the outcome of IVF treatment, Human reproduction. Oxford: Oxford University Press; 2018.
62. Neelakshi G. Effectiveness of counseling and yoga on stress and coping among infertile women.
63. Sharma R, Shrivastava H, Kumar A. Comparative analysis of yoga and clomiphene in infertile women. Int J Pharmacol Ther. 2012;2(1)
64. Galhardo A, Cunha M, Pinto-Gouveia J. Mindfulness-based program for infertility: efficacy study. Fertil Steril. 2013;100(4):1059–67.
65. Breder Kp, Wurn BF, King Iii CR, Wurn LJ. Ten-year retrospective study on the efficacy of a manual physical therapy to treat female infertility. 2015.
66. Shermadou ES, Rahman S, Leslie SW. Anatomy, abdomen and pelvis, bladder. 2018.
67. Guimberteau JC, Armstrong C. Architecture of human living fascia: the extracellular matrix and cells revealed through endoscopy. Jessica Kingsley Publishers; 2024.
68. Van Der Wal J, Jeekel J. Biology of the peritoneum in normal homeostasis and after surgical trauma. Color Dis. 2007;9:9–13.
69. Capella-Monsonís H, Kearns S, Kelly J, Zeugolis DI. Battling adhesions: from understanding to prevention. BMC Biomed Eng. 2019;1:1–12.
70. Sayed AI, Yousef AM, Aly MG. Manual therapy and infertility: review of evidence. Turk J Physiother Rehabil. 32:3.
71. Rice AD, Patterson K, Reed ED, Wurn BF, Robles K, Klingenberg B, et al. Decreasing recurrent bowel obstructions, improving quality of life with physiotherapy: controlled study. World J Gastroenterol. 2018;24(19):2108.
72. Rice AD, Patterson K, Wurn BF, King CR, Wurn LJ. Update on "decreasing dyspareunia and dysmenorrhea in women with endometriosis via a manual physical therapy: results from 2 indepen-

dent studies". J Endometriosis Pelvic Pain Disord. 2014;6(3):161–2.
73. Konečná H. The physiotherapeutic method by Mojžíšová. Kontakt. 2007;9(2):422.
74. Volejnikovà H. Female infertility: a study of physical treatment by the method of L. Mojzisovà for functional disturbances of the pelvic region. J Orthop Med. 2001;23(2):47–9.
75. Mercier J, Miller K. Mercier therapy helps infertile women achieve pregnancy. Midwifery Today. 2013;105:40–68.
76. Organization Wh. Benchmarks for training in traditional. World Health Organization; 2010.
77. Stone C. Visceral and obstetric osteopathy. Elsevier Health Sciences; 2006.
78. Ruffini N, D'alessandro G, Cardinali L, Frondaroli F, Cerritelli F. Osteopathic manipulative treatment in gynecology and obstetrics: a systematic review. Complement Ther Med. 2016;26:72–8.
79. Enoka RM, Amiridis IG, Duchateau J. Electrical stimulation of muscle: electrophysiology and rehabilitation. Physiology. 2019;
80. Zhu Q. Analysis of the effect of bionic electrical stimulation combined with kuntai capsule on the thin endometrium with poor estrogen treatment. China Foreign Med Treat J. 2020;7:69–72.
81. He Zq Y, Liu P. Clinical effect of bionic electrostimulation combined with ultrasonic acupuncture on infertility patients with thin endometrium. Chin J Pract Gynecol Obstet. 2021;37:1254–8.
82. Bodombossou-Djobo MM, Zheng C, Chen S, Yang D. Neuromuscular electrical stimulation and biofeedback therapy may improve endometrial growth for patients with thin endometrium during frozen-thawed embryo transfer: a preliminary report. Reprod Biol Endocrinol. 2011;9:1–6.
83. Lin J, Ma H, Li H, Han J, Guo T, Qin Z, et al. The treatment of complementary and alternative medicine on female infertility caused by endometrial factors. Evid Based Complement Alternat Med. 2022;2022(1):4624311.
84. Platz C Jr, Seager S. Semen collection by electroejaculation in the domestic cat. J Am Vet Med Assoc. 1978;173(10):1353–5.
85. Brindley G. Electroejaculation: its technique, neurological implications and uses. J Neurol Neurosurg Psychiatry. 1981;44(1):9–18.
86. Müller J, Sønksen J, Sommer P, Schmiegelow M, Petersen PM, Heilman C, et al. Cryopreservation of semen from pubertal boys with cancer. Med Pediatr Oncol. 2000;34(3):191–4.
87. Gerig NE, Meacham RB, Ohl DA. Use of electroejaculation in the treatment of ejaculatory failure secondary to diabetes mellitus. Urology. 1997;49(2):239–42.
88. Sønksen J, Ohl DA. Penile vibratory stimulation and Electroejaculation in the treatment of ejaculatory dysfunction 1. Int J Androl. 2002;25(6):324–32.
89. Liebert A, Krause A, Goonetilleke N, Bicknell B, Kiat H. A role for Photobiomodulation in the prevention of myocardial ischemic reperfusion injury: a systematic review and potential molecular mechanisms. Sci Rep. 2017;7(1):42386.
90. Achache H, Revel A. Endometrial receptivity markers, the journey to successful embryo implantation. Hum Reprod Update. 2006;12(6):731–46.
91. Tsai H-W, Wang P-H, Hsu P-T, Chen S-N, Lin L-T, Li C-J, et al. Laser irradiation pretreatment improves endometrial preparation of frozen-thawed embryo transfer in recurrent implantation failure patients. Gynecol Endocrinol. 2020;36(8):734–8.
92. El Faham DA, Elnoury MAH, Morsy MI, El Shaer MA, Nour Eldin GM, Azmy OM. Has the time come to include low-level laser photobiomodulation as an adjuvant therapy in the treatment of impaired endometrial receptivity? Lasers Med Sci. 2018;33:1105–14.
93. Wang D, Jiang Y, Feng J, Gao J, Yu J, Zhao J, et al. Evidence for the use of complementary and alternative medicine for pelvic inflammatory disease: a literature review. Evid Based Complement Alternat Med. 2022;2022(1):1364297.
94. Zhenjiang Y, Zhiqin W, Jianbing Y, Xiaofei Z. Viewing the development of acupuncture and moxibustion from the successful "application for world heritage" of acupuncture and Moxibustion. J Hubei Univ Chin Med. 2011;13(4):42–4.
95. Stener-Victorin E, Waldenström U, Nilsson L, Wikland M, Janson PO. A prospective randomized study of electro-acupuncture versus Alfentanil as anaesthesia during oocyte aspiration in in-vitro fertilization. Hum Reprod. 1999;14(10):2480–4.
96. Fan S, Yang H-S, Fang Y-G, Hao M-Z, Liu S-Y, Feng Y-X, et al. Application status and thinking of acupuncture and Moxibustion therapy for assisted reproductive field in the United States. Zhongguo Zhen Jiu Chin Acupunct Moxibustion. 2022;42(2):237–40.
97. Luo M-H, Yan T, Zuo Y-C, Shi W-Y, Xin W, Zhang W. Effect of acupuncture and Moxibustion as the adjuvant therapy on frozen-thawed embryo transfer: a network meta-analysis. World J Acupunct Moxibustion. 2024;
98. Gu Y-E, Zhang X, Zhang Q, Dai M-C, Wu Y, Zhou Y, et al. The effects of acupuncture on pregnancy outcomes of in vitro fertilization with embryo transfer: an interdisciplinary systematic review. J Gynecol Obstet Hum Reprod. 2019;48(8):677–84.
99. Li Yc Y, Liao Y. Effect of acupuncture with nourishing kidney and filling essence formula on thin endometrial infertility. Shanghai J Acupunct Moxibustion. 2020;39:411–5.
100. Xu L-L, Zhou X, Zhang C-R, Zhang J-B. Effect of acupuncture on pregnancy outcomes of frozen embryo transfer in patients with anovulatory infertility. Zhongguo Zhen Jiu Chin Acupunct Moxibustion. 2022;42(2):150–4.

21 Physiotherapy and Rehabilitation in Menopause

Funda Demirtürk

21.1 Introduction

The word menopause originates from the Greek words "*men,*" meaning moon, and "*pausis,*" meaning pause [3]. Natural menopause is a normal condition that involves the permanent cessation of menstrual cycles due to the cessation of production of reproductive hormones from the ovaries for 12 months or more, without any other pathologic reasons [4]. But it may also occur due to surgical procedures such as bilateral oophorectomy or due to treatment of certain conditions such as endometriosis, after chemotherapy, radiation, or other therapies including antiestrogen agents [1, 5].

This transition period, which occurs between the ages of 45 and 55 years [6–10], varies from person to person, but the mean age of menopause is stated as 51 years in the literature [1, 7]. Genetic factors, smoking, and living at high altitude affect the age of menopause [11]. Menopause between the ages of 40 and 45 years is called premature menopause and it is a rare condition [1].

In women over the age of 45, the absence of menstrual bleeding for 1 year without any other reason is sufficient to diagnose menopause; in most cases, no other tests are required. Tests for menopause are usually necessary and performed on younger patients [1, 12].

Menopause is usually divided into phases such as *premenopause, perimenopause*, *menopause*, and *postmenopause* [1]. The *premenopause* is a stage where no noticeable changes in hormonal status suggestive of perimenopause or menopause occur, and menstrual cycles continue. *The perimenopause* stage is the last few years before menopause when women begin to experience irregular menstrual cycles and hot flashes as a result of changes in estrogen and follicle-stimulating hormone (FSH) levels. It usually occurs between the ages of 40 and 50, can last around 2–8 years, and ends with the last menstrual period. Menstrual irregularities are characterized by changes in either the amount of menstrual bleeding or the interval between menstrual periods [1].

Menopause encompasses a year without a monthly menstrual cycle, during which time many symptoms begin to appear. At the end of this process, menstruation and the woman's reproductive capacity end. It is accompanied by changes in the neuroendocrine and immunological systems [1, 13].

The postmenopause stage refers to the rest of a woman's life after menopause [1, 14]. It is divided into two stages: early and late. Early postmenopause is defined as the five-year period after the last menstrual period, during which ovarian hormone function declines further and

F. Demirtürk (✉)
Department of Physiotherapy and Rehabilitation, Faculty of Health Sciences, Tokat Gaziosmanpaşa University, Tokat, Türkiye
e-mail: funda.demirturk@gop.edu.tr

T. Akbayrak, E. Üzelpasaci (eds.), *Physiotherapy and Rehabilitation in Pelvic and Women's Health-Related Problems*, https://doi.org/10.1007/978-3-032-28741-0_21

reaches a permanent level, and rapid bone loss occurs. Late postmenopause begins 5 years after the last menstrual period and continues until the woman dies [13].

Climacterium, or life changes, is the physiological and psychological changes that occur during menopause. Climacteric is a popular term synonymous with perimenopause and is used as a more holistic concept that integrates the entire period of change, including psychological and other domains [13].

Apart from these definitions, a staging system, "Stages of Reproductive Aging Workshop (STRAW)," was developed considering data obtained from multiple longitudinal cohort studies, which stages the reproductive aging period of women as "*reproductive years, the menopausal transition, the final menstrual period, and postmenopause*" by taking into account the amount of bleeding, hormonal status, and symptoms. Although the STRAW system is used primarily for women's health research, of note, the STRAW staging criteria are not considered to represent diagnostic criteria for the menopausal transition or menopause [11, 12, 15].

Some hormonal changes are seen in the reproductive aging process, as also stated in the STRAW staging system. During the reproductive aging process, the number of follicles decreases. FSH rises as a result of declining levels of inhibin B, which is a dimeric protein that reflects the fall in ovarian follicle numbers. Loss of ovarian sensitivity to FSH and luteinizing hormone (LH) and loss of negative feedback of estradiol and inhibin B in the hypothalamic-pituitary unit cause increased production and release of gonadotropin-releasing hormone (GnRH), FSH, and LH. The changes in the hypothalamic-pituitary-ovarian axis can lead to hormone fluctuations, and anovulatory cycles become more common as the ovary becomes less responsive to gonadotropin stimulation. In the end, the endocrinological changes of the menopausal transition are an increase in serum FSH and a decrease in inhibin and estradiol [1, 16, 17].

Due to these reproductive aging and hormonal changes, most women in menopause may experience various symptoms that may affect their quality of life. The most common symptoms are *vasomotor symptoms* (*such as hot flashes and night sweats*), *osteoporosis*, *genitourinary symptoms*, *cognitive changes*, *sleep disorders*, *emotional changes* (anxiety and depression), and *cardiovascular system problems*. The number and severity of these symptoms vary according to many factors, such as the woman's age at menopause, the way she entered menopause, her knowledge and attitudes, the culture she lives in, and the woman's social gender roles [18–20].

Questionnaires and scales can be used to identify and quantify menopausal symptoms to facilitate diagnosis and indicate and monitor treatment. Kupperman Index, Menopause Rating Scale, Menopause-Specific Quality of Life Questionnaire, and Greene Climacteric Scale are some of them [21]. The most commonly used one is the Menopause Rating Scale, which was first developed by Schneider and colleagues in Germany in 1992. The scale is used to determine the severity of menopausal symptoms and their effects on quality of life and includes 11 items across three domains: *somatic-vegetative* (hot flashes or sweating, heart discomfort, sleeping problems, and muscle and joint problems), *psychological* (depressive mood, irritability, anxiety, and fatigue), and *urogenital* (sexual problems, bladder problems, and vaginal dryness) [22–24].

Considering the life expectancy of women, this means that a woman spends approximately one-third of her life in menopause [25]. Therefore, factors that develop due to menopause and affect the woman's quality of life should be taken seriously, and necessary interventions should be made [1, 26]. The World Health Organization (WHO) recommends social, psychological, and physical health support during the menopausal transition and after menopause and emphasizes that it should be an integral part of health services [26]. After women are informed and lifestyle changes are made, treatment options such as hormonal or nonhormonal medical treatments, physiotherapy applications, and complementary approaches can be used to relieve menopause symptoms and improve quality of life [20].

In this section, some of the symptoms and conditions frequently encountered in relation to menopause for which physiotherapy approaches can be effective will be discussed in the light of evidence-based literature.

21.2 Physiotherapy and Rehabilitation in Menopausal Symptoms and Problems

21.2.1 Vasomotor Symptoms (VMS)

During and after the menopause transition, the most common complaints that most women suffer from are hot flashes (*or hot flushes*) (HF) and night sweats. Hot flashes are defined as a sudden feeling of heat in the chest, neck, and face and are reported to be seen in approximately 80% of women during the late transition. They may be accompanied by reddening of the skin and sweating and may be followed by chills and shivering in some women. When they occur at night, they are called "night sweats" and disrupt sleep patterns. This symptom usually lasts 1–5 min but can last up to 15 min in some cases. The severity of HF varies from person to person and can be seen in the same person at different times and with different severities [27]. The prevalence and severity of vasomotor symptoms vary according to obesity [28], race, smoking, living in higher temperatures, and lower altitudes [29] and physical activity level [30–33].

Peak prevalence of hot flashes occurs during the late menopausal transition and during early postmenopause [31, 34, 35]. VMS subside and stop in most women within a few years of onset [36]. However, recent findings suggest that symptoms often last much longer. "Study of Women across the Nation" (SWAN) indicates that the median total VMS duration was 7.4 years [37]. There are study results showing that frequent and severe hot flashes are associated with an increased risk of hypertension and cardiovascular disease in women [38].

The mechanism underlying hot flashes is the disruption of the thermoregulatory function of the hypothalamus due to estrogen withdrawal. Hormonal changes in menopausal women disrupt the balance of norepinephrine and dopamine neurotransmitters, leading to vasomotor instability [39]. As estrogen levels decrease in postmenopausal women, hypothalamic opioids such as beta-endorphins also decrease [40]. Both human and animal studies have shown that estrogen concentrations are related to beta-endorphin concentrations in the hypothalamus. Furthermore, beta-endorphin concentrations in the cerebrospinal fluid are lower in postmenopausal women than in women of childbearing age and are related to serum estrogen concentrations. The decrease in beta-endorphins is thought to cause dysfunction of the body's thermoregulatory center and is suggested to be the cause of hot flashes [41].

Elevated sympathetic activation, acting through central alpha-2 adrenergic receptors, contributes to the initiation of hot flashes. Small elevations in core body temperature can trigger hot flashes [42, 43], and clonidine was found to consistently and significantly reduce hot flash frequency [43].

Estrogen supplementation as hormone therapy (HT) has positive effects on quality of life, especially in postmenopausal women with vasomotor symptoms [44]. Baerug et al. [45] showed that estrogen therapy relieved VMS and reduced the number of hot flashes by as much as 95% in menopausal women [45]. HT is usually recommended for menopausal women aged younger than 60 years, within 10 years of their final menstrual periods, and without contraindications [46]. Despite its benefits for menopausal symptoms, the rate of women using HT decreased after the publication of the Women's Health Initiative (WHI) study, which pointed out its side effects and increased risk of certain diseases (e.g., venous thromboembolism, ischemic stroke, breast cancer) [47]. For this reason, it should be well decided to whom it should be given and for what periods.

The choice of treatment should be determined according to the patient's expectations and the severity of symptoms. While women with mild symptoms may not require pharmacologic treatment, women with moderate to severe symptoms may. Low-dose estrogen plus progestin therapy (or estrogen alone if no uterus) is recommended for postmenopausal women with moderate to severe VMS. But women with a history of an estrogen-sensitive cancer (including breast cancer), coronary heart disease, myocardial infarction, stroke, venous thromboembolism, or an inherited high risk of thromboembolic disease are not good candidates for HT [48].

Nonhormonal therapies may be appropriate in situations where estrogen is contraindicated, not well tolerated, or not preferred by the woman. However, it should not be forgotten that nonhormonal pharmacological agents, herbal, or dietary remedies that will be applied as an alternative to hormone therapy may also have various side effects [48].

Non-pharmacological methods include behavioral strategies such as adjusting room temperature, dressing in layers to allow removal when necessary, applying cooling, and using a fan [49]. In addition to these, physiotherapy approaches such as exercise, connective tissue massage, and relaxation training can be applied.

21.2.1.1 Physiotherapy in Vasomotor Symptoms

21.2.1.1.1 Physical Activity, Exercise, and Yoga

As well as its benefits on overall health, physical activity or exercise is considered a potentially effective treatment for hot flashes and night sweats and is recommended for women in the reproductive aging process. According to the "Women in Sport" report, despite their low physical activity levels, menopausal women have been shown to be more willing to be active and increase their activity levels if recommended by their health professionals [49, 50]. There are studies in the literature that demonstrate the relationship between the activity level of menopausal women and hot flash complaints [51–56] and indicate the acute and long-term effects of exercise on hot flashes.

Ivarsson et al. [30], in their study, grouped 793 women who had reached a natural menopause into sedentary, moderately, or highly active women, based on a physical activity score. They found that only 5% of women with high levels of physical activity had severe hot flashes. Among those who did little or no exercise, the rate of those who complained of severe hot flashes was determined to be 14–16% [30].

The Royal College of Obstetricians and Gynecologists (RCOG 2006) in the United Kingdom (UK) has advised (Scientific Advisory Committee Opinion Paper 6) that women who are more active tend to suffer less from the symptoms of menopause and that the best type of activity is aerobic, sustained, regular exercise such as swimming and running [57].

In a randomized controlled study, it was determined that the frequency of HF and depression decreased and quality of life and lean muscle mass increased in symptomatic sedentary women who did 50 min of aerobic exercise four times a week, for 6 months, compared to the control group [58].

In the study conducted by Elavsky et al. [56], it was determined that VMSs decreased objectively and subjectively 24 h after moderate-intensity physical activity [56].

Berin et al. [59], in their randomized controlled study, investigated the effect of 15 weeks of resistance training on the frequency of moderate to severe hot flashes in postmenopausal women. Postmenopausal women with at least four moderate or severe hot flashes or night sweats per day were randomized to a 15-week resistance training intervention (n = 29) or unchanged physical activity (n = 29). The resistance training was performed three times per week, and the program contained eight exercises performed with 8 to 12 repetitions in two sets. The women did not use any therapy for hot flashes 2 months prior to study entry. A diary was used to observe hot flashes. The longitudinal analysis showed that HF decreased significantly after 3 weeks of resistance training, whereas the control group did not change. It was found that the frequency of moderate and severe HF decreased by 44% in women randomized to 15 weeks of resistance training in the postmenopausal period, while no significant change was observed in the control group. In theory, resistance training may decrease HF by induction of central β-endorphin production through activation of large muscle groups, which would be a much-needed addition to the few existing treatment options [59].

A Cochrane systematic review of five randomized controlled trials reported insufficient evidence to determine whether exercise significantly reduces vasomotor symptoms [60].

Some studies have focused on the conclusion that aerobic or low-intensity exercise has no or modest effects on hot flashes [61]. In a study of 280 women, increasing physical activity has not been found to be effective on vasomotor and sexual symptoms of menopause [62]. The Australian Women's Health Longitudinal Study, involving 3330 women, suggested that there was no improvement in vasomotor or psychological symptoms and only marginal improvements in somatic symptoms when physical activity was introduced as a factor affecting these symptoms [63]. It is thought that poor compliance with exercise, high dropout rates, and lack of outcome data may explain the weak effects of exercise on hot flashes [59].

But recent evidence suggests that structured exercise, including aerobic and resistance interventions and yoga, has a positive but limited effect for reducing menopausal symptoms [10].

The effect of exercise in reducing hot flashes in postmenopausal women may be explained by several mechanisms. It is well established with research that physical exercise involving major muscle groups increases energy expenditure and leads to the release of beta-endorphin, both in the central nervous system and peripherally [64]. However, there are many different opinions in the literature regarding the intensity, type, and duration of exercise. Since postmenopausal women have lower beta-endorphin concentrations than fertile women and exercise increases beta-endorphin release in the central nervous system and the periphery, exercise may help stabilize thermoregulation [65]. This may explain the decreased frequency and intensity of hot flashes with increased physical activity. However, the fact that women who exercise regularly are accustomed to and comfortable with the sensation of being hot and sweaty must be taken into consideration. Therefore, they may report less intense hot flashes [30].

Exercise helps a woman maintain her optimal body composition, body fat distribution, and slow weight gain. Therefore, the effects of physical activity in relieving hot flashes may be due to its effects on body composition [66].

In 3201 women aged 42–52 years, followed annually for 8 years, hot flashes were associated with higher cholesterol, triglyceride, and apolipoprotein A levels [67]. Another study indicated a strong correlation between hot flashes and insulin resistance in 3075 women [68]. Since studies have shown that hot flashes are associated with high cholesterol, triglyceride, apolipoprotein A, and glucose levels, it can be said that regular exercise is effective in reducing hot flashes by reducing the levels of these parameters.

Yoga is an ancient Eastern technique that aims to integrate the mind, body, and spirit and is thought to benefit women in menopause by regulating the autonomic nervous system and the hypothalamic-pituitary axis [69]. Yoga reduces stress and balances hormones by activating the parasympathetic nervous system [70]. In addition, yoga promotes relaxation, improves sleep quality, improves muscle and joint health, and supports cardiovascular health. These effects can contribute to the relief of menopausal symptoms and enable women to get through this transition period more easily and comfortably [71].

In the umbrella review of Shepherd-Banigan et al. [72], yoga was found to have small to moderate benefits on reduced hot flash severity and psychological symptoms [72].

A review of 13 randomized controlled studies involving 1306 participants found yoga to be effective in reducing total menopausal symptoms, psychological, somatic, vasomotor, and urogenital symptoms compared with no treatment. In this regard, Cramer's results support the umbrella review results [73].

In a study conducted by Susanti et al. [74], 208 menopausal women were equally divided into intervention and control groups, and the women in the intervention group underwent a total of 60 sessions of yoga, each lasting 75 minutes, for 20 weeks. The Depression, Anxiety, and Stress Scale; the Multidimensional Scale of Perceived Social Support; the Menopause Rating

Scale; and the Pittsburgh Sleep Quality Index were used to assess menopausal symptoms. They found that yoga significantly improved VMS and sleep quality [74].

Money et al. [75], in their "overview of reviews," assessed the effectiveness of physical activity and exercise interventions for menopausal women. They examined 17 reviews that included 80 unique relevant primary studies with 8983 participants. Their results indicated that there is evidence showing improvement of physical, urogenital, and total symptoms following yoga interventions, but the evidence for vasomotor and psychological symptoms was inconclusive. Although aerobic exercises had beneficial effects on total and vasomotor symptoms, the effects were not conclusive. Evidence was very limited for other types of physical activity and its impact on physical, sexual, and urogenital symptoms. In conclusion, they suggest that there is some evidence that yoga and aerobic exercise may be beneficial for some menopause symptoms, but there is insufficient evidence to recommend a particular form of exercise [75].

Another systematic review and meta-analysis study published by Wang et al. [76] showed similar results to those of Money et al. [75]. The authors included 24 studies (2028 subjects) and examined the effects of yoga on menopausal symptoms and stated that yoga may have beneficial effects on improving total menopausal symptoms in postmenopausal women, including subscales of psychological, somatic, and urogenital symptoms; sleep quality; anxiety; depressive symptoms; body mass index; systolic blood pressure; and diastolic blood pressure. However, no significant effects were found for hot flashes and quality of life [76]. This result was interpreted as being consistent with the results previously done by Freedman [77] and Irvin [78], who showed that behavioral control interventions (such as muscle relaxation, biofeedback, or reading) do not produce significant improvement in hot flashes.

The effects obtained with exercise may vary depending on the type, frequency, and intensity of exercise. It is stated that aerobic exercises mainly increase maximal oxygen consumption (VO_2 max) and work capacity, while resistance training leads to increased strength and muscle volume. Although both exercise modalities activate muscle groups, different muscle fibers are recruited in response to the different demands during exercise, with more muscle fibers being activated during resistance training than aerobic exercise. However, it is not known whether resistance training affects the endogenous opioid system differently from aerobic exercise. It has been suggested that exercise needs to be performed at a certain intensity to be effective and that the lack of effect of many interventions such as walking or yoga may be due to their low intensity [59].

It seems that more studies are needed to reveal the effects of exercise on vasomotor symptoms more clearly.

21.2.1.1.2 Connective Tissue Massage

Connective tissue massage (CTM), or in other words, connective tissue manipulation, is a special technique developed by a German physiotherapist, Elisabeth Dicke, in the 1930s [79].

CTM is a reflex therapy in which traction force is applied to the connective tissue interfaces in the skin in a way that stimulates autonomic nerve endings in order to regulate the balance between the sympathetic and parasympathetic parts of the autonomic nervous system (ANS), usually moving in a parasympathetic direction. The principles of CTM are based on the fact that a disorder in an internal organ is reflected externally by increased tone in the superficial muscles (Mackenzie areas), especially in the back region, and by a change in the character of the interstitial fluid in the subcutaneous tissues (head areas), accompanied by hypersensitivity to touch. Such signs are generally distributed within the dermatomes that are suitable for the segmental innervation of the affected organ. The therapeutic effect in CTM is also directed to the diseased organ by mechanically stimulating the appropriate dermatomes. The dermatome is primarily stimulated from the dorsal surface of the body. The therapeutic effects obtained occur as a result of changes in blood flow in the deep tissues or the suppression of pain. This connection between deep and superficial tissues is provided by neural mechanisms known as "cutaneovisceral reflexes," which include autonomic pathways and rich somatosensory plexuses in the skin and subcutaneous tissues [80, 81].

Ebner and Schliack attempted to explain the mechanism of action of the technique as follows: CTM produces local mechanical effects in the connective tissue and its associated cells (mast cells and fibroblasts) and reduces sympathetic activity, thereby eliciting reflex mechanisms that cause vasodilation. As a result, circulation in the associated tissues, including the parasympathetic ganglion, increases, which in turn increases circulation throughout the body. Such an increase in circulation accelerates wound healing, increases collateral circulation, normalizes or increases the elasticity of the connective tissue, improves the response to exercise, reduces muscle spasms, and provides balance within the autonomic nervous system [82].

Research, including CTM therapy, has investigated the effects of the technique on various circulatory problems (e.g., peripheral arterial disease, cellulitis, and diabetic foot), autonomic, visceral, and multisystem dysfunctions (e.g., systemic sclerosis and chronic constipation), painful conditions (e.g., chronic spinal pain, fibromyalgia, migraine, and tension-type headache), gynecological and hormonal disorders (e.g., primary dysmenorrhea), and anxiety [83–94].

Despite the widespread use of CTM in many situations, the number of studies investigating its effectiveness in climacteric symptoms in menopausal women is very limited.

Akarcali applied CTM to 19 postmenopausal cases for 15 sessions and evaluated hormone values and climacteric complaints. As a result of the study, she observed that there was a significant decrease in the total scores of the Blatt Menopausal Index after CTM. When the Blatt Menopausal Index was examined in more detail, it was determined that there was a significant decrease in 11 climacteric complaints, including hot flashes, sweating, paresthesia, insomnia, fatigue, headache, irritability, depression, shortness of breath, palpitations, and psycholability, and that there was no significant change in musculoskeletal pain and vertigo symptoms. In addition, in the hormone tests performed before and after CTM, a significant increase was found in LH and estradiol, while no significant change was observed in FSH and prolactin values. With these data obtained, it was concluded that CTM is an effective method in the treatment of climacteric symptoms and ensures the regular functioning of the neuroendocrine system through the autonomic nervous system [95].

In another study by Albayrak et al. [96], the effects of CTM on postmenopausal symptoms, menopause-specific quality of life, and insomnia were evaluated [96]. A total of 57 postmenopausal women were randomly allocated to either the CTM group or the control group (sham therapeutic ultrasound), and participants received massage or the sham intervention in three sessions per week for 4 weeks, each session lasting 15 min. Hot flash frequency, hot flash score (frequency × severity), menopause-specific quality of life, emotional state, insomnia, and satisfaction with the intervention, as well as menopause symptom severity with the Menopause Assessment Scale, were assessed. The CTM group showed greater improvements in all primary and secondary outcome measures, except for insomnia severity, compared to the control group. The researchers noted that CTM could be used as a first-line approach to improve physical and emotional health in the short term in postmenopausal women [96].

VMS is generally associated with an increase in sympathetic nervous system activity, but it has also been associated with a decrease in parasympathetic nervous system activity or changes in both systems in opposite directions at the same time [97]. So, it has been reported in the literature that approaches that reduce sympathetic discharge, such as breathing and relaxation exercises, may be effective in alleviating VMS [98]. Based on the mechanism suggested by Ebner and Schliack, it can be said that CTM may be effective in menopause-related vasomotor symptoms. However, more studies are needed to demonstrate its effectiveness.

21.2.1.1.3 Relaxation Techniques

Relaxation techniques, a behavioral intervention, appear to reduce sympathetic activity and venous norepinephrine concentrations [99, 100] while lowering blood pressure. This effect may be explained by reduced plasma norepinephrine levels [99].

There are different relaxation techniques used widely that target the muscles, mind, nervous system, part of the body, or the whole body, such as (a) Jacobson progressive relaxation, (b) modified version of Jacobson progressive relaxation, known as Bernstein and Borkovec's version, (c) Everly and Rosenfeld's passive relaxation, (d) Madder release, (e) Ost's applied relaxation, (f) Poppen's behavioral relaxation training, (g) the Mitchell method, (h) the Alexander technique, and (i) Benson's relaxation response [101].

Paced respiration (slow, controlled diaphragmatic breathing) and muscle relaxation are two well-known somatic relaxation techniques for vasomotor symptoms. The most common forms of muscle relaxation are progressive muscle relaxation and passive muscle relaxation [102].

Some clinical trials have shown that paced respiration and progressive relaxation are beneficial in treating menopausal symptoms [78, 103–106].

But a Cochrane study by Saensak et al. [107] reviewed the evidence on the effects of these techniques on hot flashes, night sweats, and sleep disturbances in menopausal women [107]. In four randomized controlled studies, with 281 participants, relaxation was compared with electroacupuncture, superficial needling, paced respiration, placebo, and no treatment. After the analyses, it was concluded that the evidence is insufficient to show the effectiveness of relaxation techniques as a treatment for menopausal vasomotor symptoms or to determine whether this treatment is more effective than no treatment, placebo, acupuncture, superficial needle insertion, or paced respiration. But no data on night sweats and sleep disturbances were reported [107].

21.2.2 Osteoporosis

Osteoporosis is one of the most common problems among women during menopause. It is defined as a decrease in bone density, deterioration in the microarchitectural structure of bone, and an increase in fragility. History of fragility fracture, bone mineral density (BMD), or calculated 10-year fracture risk are used for diagnosis [108].

Fragility Fracture In the presence of a fragility fracture, particularly at the spine, hip, wrist, humerus, and pelvis, fragility fracture history can be used for the diagnosis without measurement of BMD. Fractures of the skull, cervical spine, hands, and feet are not considered fragility fractures. Stress fractures are also not considered fragility fractures because they usually result from repetitive injuries in individuals with healthy bones.

Bone Mineral Density (BMD) Dual-energy x-ray absorptiometry (DXA) is the gold standard for diagnosis in the absence of fragility fracture [109]. The World Health Organization indicates that a BMD that is 2.5 standard deviations (SD) or more below the mean BMD of the young adult reference population (i.e., T-score ≤ -2.5) is appropriate for the diagnosis of osteoporosis, provided that other causes of low BMD are excluded [110].

Fracture risk assessment tools are also used in the United States to clinically diagnose and determine the threshold for intervention [111, 112].

Postmenopausal estrogen decline is said to cause accelerated bone apoptosis due to decreased osteoprotegerin production by osteoblasts and increased bone marrow receptor activator of nuclear factor kappa-B ligand (RANKL) [113].

21.2.2.1 Treatment

All postmenopausal women should be counseled on general lifestyle measures and changes to reduce bone loss. Recommendations include adequate calcium and vitamin D intake, regular exercise, smoking cessation, and avoidance of heavy alcohol use. Women should also be counseled on fall prevention and advised to avoid medications that increase bone loss (e.g., glucocorticoids) [114–124].

Falling is a major health problem that can have devastating or even fatal consequences in the elderly [125]. The consequences of fractures (particularly hip fractures) include loss of independence, chronic pain, hospitalization, reduced quality of life, and increased mortality [126]. Although not every fall results in injury, falling anxiety or fear resulting from a previous fall experience can negatively impact a person's mobility and participation in social environments and can lead to social isolation and depression [127]. For this reason, it is important and vital to take precautions against these conditions that may develop in further years and to implement strategies that will strengthen bones.

Menopausal women have greater limitations in walking, leg and grip strength, joint range of motion, flexibility, and balance compared to premenopausal women. In addition, visceral and abdominal fat accumulation caused by estrogen deficit and relative hyperandrogenism, a body mass index over 25 kg/m^2, and muscle dysfunction are among the factors that increase the risk of falling [128–130].

Antiresorptive and anabolic bone medications are said to increase bone mineral density and reduce the risk of fractures but do not prevent falls [131–134].

21.2.2.2 Exercise

Exercise is the most effective non-pharmacological strategy for fall prevention [135] and has been shown to significantly reduce fracture risk [136]. Exercise not only increases bone mineral density, but it also improves muscle strength, power, and balance, which are factors associated with fall risk.

The beneficial effects of exercise on bones are well known. The literature contains results on the effects of various types, durations, intensities, and frequencies of exercise on BMD values in different bones (spine, hips, wrist, etc.). Exercises generally applied in osteoporosis are walking, aerobic, weight-bearing, aquatic exercises, resistance exercises, tai chi, impact activities, and/or different combinations of these exercises [124, 137–150]. However, it is necessary to clearly define which approach should be applied to prevent osteoporosis or slow its progression in menopausal women [151, 152].

Exercise might be more effective during early than in late postmenopause, at least with respect to trabecular bone loss [153].

Kemmler et al. (2020) found that all types of exercise (weight-bearing exercises, dynamic resistance exercises, or a combination of them) significantly affected BMD at the lumbar spine, femoral neck, and total hip [154].

Body et al. [155], in their consensus article (consensus of the Belgian Bone Club), reviewed the literature on non-pharmacological prevention and treatment of osteoporosis in men and women, and as a general recommendation, they reported that exercises should be performed two to three times per week and must include 15–60 min of aerobic exercises and a set of strength training. The exercise intensity should be at 70–80% of functional capacity or maximum strength. In preventing osteoporosis, high-impact exercises (e.g., jumping rope and running) have the greatest potential to improve BMD, while low- to moderate-impact exercises (e.g., step aerobics and interval running) are more suitable for those who are not accustomed to exercise and for people over the age of 50. In patients with osteoporosis, strength training should be site specific. Weight-bearing exercises should be performed to load the bone areas predominantly affected by the osteoporotic fracture. Exercise programs should start at an easy level and be gradual in intensity and impact, and emphasis should be placed on regularity [155].

Fischbacher et al. [156], in their two-part review series, examined the issue from many perspectives. They aimed first to summarize and critically evaluate existing evidence of exercise's effect on bone mass, bone structure, and bone turnover markers (BTMs) in healthy postmenopausal women and, second, to examine the influence of intensity on bone response to exercise. The first part of their study (systematic review) involved one hundred trials, investigating a total of 120 exercise interventions. Each exercise intervention was classified as low, moderate, or high intensity based on predefined classification criteria. Of those, 57 interventions were low intensity, 57 were moderate, and six were high intensity. The classification criteria for resistance training (RT) interventions were based on a published load-repetition relationship and intensity classification scheme. RT programs with sets of fewer than six repetitions at >80% of 1-repetition maximum (1 RM) load were classified as high intensity, 8 to 15 repetitions at 65–80% of 1 RM were classified as moderate, and >15 repetitions at <65% of 1 RM were classified as low intensity. Classification of impact and other physical activities was based on ground reaction forces (GRFs). For interventions that combined multiple activities, classification was based on the activity with the highest intensity. All studies they reviewed included postmenopausal women with a mean age of 45–81 years. They found that low-intensity exercise was not effective in increasing bone mass. Higher-quality evidence suggests that moderate-to-high-intensity interventions, particularly those combining high-intensity resistance and impact training, are most beneficial for bone mass. Only high-intensity exercise appears to improve structural parameters of bone strength, but data are limited. Only low- and moderate-intensity interventions reported significant improvements in BTMs, but no significant benefit was observed. In conclusion, it is stated that exercise intensity is positively associated with adaptive bone response [156].

In the second part of their study (meta-analysis), they aimed to determine the effects of low, moderate, and high-intensity exercise on BMD at the spine and hip in postmenopausal women. Fifty-three trials testing 63 interventions (19 low, 40 moderate, 4 high intensity) were included, and all trials were conducted in healthy postmenopausal women with a mean age between 51.4 and 79.3 years. Data from a total of 3941 participants were included in the analyses, of which 1948 were in the exercise group and 1582 were in the control group. A further 209 participants on antiresorptive medication received an exercise intervention compared to 202 control participants on medications. In conclusion, it was observed that high-intensity exercise was a more effective stimulus for lumbar spine BMD than low or moderate-intensity exercise, but these effects did not occur in the femoral neck. It was stated that moderate-intensity exercise was superior to ineffective low-intensity exercise for total hip BMD, but there was insufficient data for meta-analysis of high-intensity exercises [157].

Animal studies have shown that the critical attributes of mechanical stimuli to trigger an osteogenic response are dynamic [158], high magnitude [159], rapidly applied [160], and short term [161]. Despite these characteristics being recognized for over 30 years [158, 162], most human studies of exercise interventions for osteoporosis have focused on low- to moderate-intensity loading only. A meta-analysis (June 2020) examining the effects of exercise on BMD in postmenopausal women found that effect sizes across included trials varied widely and could not be explained by subgroup analyses based on exercise type, force type (e.g., ground and joint reaction forces), duration of intervention, or menopausal status [149]. It was concluded that important variables, including training frequency and intensity across exercise protocols, played a role in this outcome. This finding seems to be consistent with the study results of Zitzmann et al. [163], who showed higher effects of higher training frequency ($2 \geq$ sessions/week) vs. low training frequency (1- < 2 times a week) [163].

The paucity of trials testing high-intensity exercise has been attributed to the traditionally conservative approach to exercise intervention in this age group. The perception of an increased risk of injury associated with high-magnitude loading in postmenopausal women may have led to a cautious approach to such interventions, although data from high-intensity exercise do not suggest a greater risk of adverse events compared with lower-intensity exercise [156].

The optimal exercise prescription for postmenopausal bone health in healthy individuals is thought to include moderate- to high-intensity progressive resistance training alone or in combination with weight-bearing impact training. But if the risk of fracture is very high or if there are accompanying diseases or extreme weaknesses, it may be difficult to recommend this exercise prescription. In this case, it may be a safer approach to apply an exercise program specially prepared for the individual under the supervision of a physiotherapist [164].

Traditional Chinese exercises like tai chi (TC), Baduanjin, Wuqinxi, and Yijinjing are applied to prevent osteoporosis as they enhance muscle strength, improve balance ability, reduce the risk of falls, and reduce the incidence of fractures caused by osteoporosis. The mechanism of action of TC on bone mineral density in postmenopausal women is to continuously adjust the position of the body's center of gravity to maintain balance and emphasize breathing during exercise. Long-term exercise increases the stress on the subject's waist and lower extremity muscles, thereby promoting the increase of bone mass and affecting bone mineral density. Because these exercises are mostly carried out outdoors, it is thought that they can increase the conversion of vitamin D and promote the absorption of calcium through sunlight. In addition, their other advantages are that they are easy to apply, economical, and safe, and therefore they can quickly alleviate bone loss and improve the quality of life of patients with bone loss [165].

The effects on BMD in postmenopausal women were presented in a systematic review and meta-analysis study, and as a result, in the analysis of 20 RCTs including 1933 cases, it was seen that all of the techniques were effective in partially improving BMD indicators in postmenopausal women, while TC was effective for all BMD indicators and was recommended as the most appropriate exercise method for postmenopausal women [166].

The Pilates method is a combination of exercises that focus on lumbopelvic stabilization and activation of the deep muscles of the trunk, creating a complete connection between mind and body. It includes six fundamental principles: centering, concentration, control, precision, breath, and flow. Pilates exercise is said to be a useful tool in the prevention and management of falls in women during the second half of their lives. It is recommended as an effective and safe method for the improvement of both static and dynamic balance. Physical capacities, quality of life, and some psychological factors related to fear of falling may be improved by the practice of Pilates. But a systematic review and a meta-analysis study by de Oliveira et al. (2022) reported that Pilates exercises had no significant effects on BMD in postmenopausal women [167]. Although its effects on BMD have not been demonstrated, the use of Pilates for fall prevention in menopausal women may be encouraged due to its effects on muscle strength and balance.

21.2.3 Genitourinary Syndrome of Menopause

The new term "genitourinary syndrome of menopause" (GSM) was introduced by the International Society for the Study of Women's Sexual Health and the Menopause Society in 2014 [168, 169]. This term covers all of the atrophic symptoms patients may have in the vulvovaginal and bladder–urethral areas due to estrogen deficiency during menopause.

Estrogen is a vasoactive hormone that increases blood flow. Vaginal lubrication is caused by fluid transudation from blood vessels and endocervical and Bartholin glands. The loss of estrogen leads to a *Lactobacillus* reduction, causing vaginal fluid to become alkaline and making it vulnerable to urinary tract infections [170].

Estrogen receptors in the bladder trigone and urethra are thought to help increase the sensory threshold when the bladder is distended. Estrogen deficiency lowers the threshold and impairs urethral closure pressure and the Valsalva leak point pressure, contributing to urinary urgency [171]. Estrogen deficiency also impairs connective tissue and leads to urethral sphincter dysfunction and stress incontinence [172], as well as pelvic organ prolapse [173].

Vulvovaginal symptoms include vaginal dryness, burning, itching, dyspareunia, vaginal discharge, bleeding, or spotting. Urinary tract symptoms include dysuria, frequent urination, urethral discomfort, or, rarely, hematuria [174].

Some women do not seek treatment for these problems due to shame, cultural, religious, or societal beliefs, or a lack of awareness about safe and effective treatments [175].

21.2.3.1 Treatment

Vaginal moisturizers and lubricants can be used for vaginal dryness. Moisturizers can be used 2–3 days a week, not just during sexual activity, but lubricants should be used before coitus. They may increase coital comfort but cannot reverse atrophic changes [176]. Women can also perform pelvic floor exercises for this problem [174, 177]. If nonhormonal vaginal moisturizers and lubricants do not provide adequate symptom relief, vaginal estrogen therapy or other hormonal medications may be prescribed for patients without contraindications to their use [178]. Estrogen therapy may also help provide some relief in urinary tract symptoms, such as stress or urgency incontinence in the absence of infection [179].

Vaginal hormone therapy may work for most patients with GSM, but other modes of treatment, such as physical therapy or vaginal dilators, may be used for refractory symptoms or if hormone therapy is contraindicated. Vaginal dilators may be particularly effective for patients who avoid intercourse due to pain (since vaginal dilators are available in sets of graduated sizes and a narrow dilator can be used initially) or for patients with levator spasm, as they can help relax the spasm [174].

In a case report, a 77-year-old woman with stress urinary incontinence and severe vulvovaginal atrophy underwent pelvic floor muscle training for 12 weeks. After 12 weeks of the training program, the patient reported a reduction in vaginal dryness and dyspareunia symptoms, as well as a better quality of sexual life. On posttreatment physical evaluation, the pelvic floor muscles' tone and elasticity were improved, although some other vulvovaginal atrophy signs remained unchanged. The improvement in GSM symptoms resulting from pelvic floor training is thought to be due to improved blood flow in the vulvovaginal tissues, improved pelvic floor function, and increased vulvovaginal tissue elasticity [180].

There are a lot of risk factors that play a role in the etiology of pelvic floor dysfunction (urinary incontinence and pelvic organ prolapse), such as aging, parity, a history of pelvic and/or perineal surgery, obesity, as well as chronic conditions such as diabetes [181, 182]. Pelvic floor muscle exercises, electrotherapy, biofeedback, and vaginal cones are physiotherapy methods applied in pelvic dysfunction and aim to strengthen the pelvic floor muscles [183, 184]. Pelvic floor dysfunction and physiotherapy are discussed in detail in other chapters (Chaps. 14, 15, and 17) of this section, so further information will not be provided in this section.

21.2.4 Cognitive Symptoms, Sleep Disorders, Anxiety, and Depression in Menopause

Complaints of cognitive and psychological problems such as brain fog and depressive symptoms are common during the menopausal transition. However, there is less evidence of an objective long-term accelerated decline in mental health and cognitive function after menopause. These transient effects appear to be most obvious in verbal memory and learning. However, long-term beneficial effects on cognition have not been demonstrated in randomized controlled trials of HT. The role of vasomotor symptoms (VMS) and sleep deprivation in both memory and mood needs to be investigated more closely. The fact that VMS are worse at night, with hot flashes and sweating, and lead to sleep disruption, suggests that these effects may mediate complaints of cognitive function and mood [185].

Cognitive aging affects cognitive functions such as memory, processing speed, and understanding. Lower cognitive function and cognitive decline have been associated with decreased functional capacity regarding daily life activities, disability, poor quality of life, and increased risk of mortality [186, 187].

Depression and insomnia are seen as common during the menopausal transition. These symptoms can negatively affect health, well-being, and daily activities, leading to a decline in overall quality of life [11]. Insomnia may be present as difficulty falling asleep or staying asleep. Even if a woman does not have depression before menopause, the rate of being newly diagnosed with depression in the postmenopausal process has been reported to be 16%. Fluctuations and decreases in estrogen are said to play a role in these conditions [188].

21.2.4.1 Physiotherapy

Many examples of studies can be found in the literature in which different physiotherapy methods are applied for the management of these problems. In a systematic review study conducted by Lialy and colleagues, the effects of practices such as exercise, reflexology, aromatherapy, massage, craniofacial massage, and foot baths on insomnia and depression in menopausal women were examined. In conclusion, it is stated that using non-pharmaceutical interventions such as therapeutic and manual physiotherapy has an overall positive impact on reducing insomnia and depression in menopausal women [14].

There are some mechanisms that explain the effects of physiotherapy on mental health and sleep. Physiotherapy practices are said to reduce depression and improve sleep without any changes in oxidative stress by increasing the levels of hormones such as serotonin and the serum concentration of brain-derived neurotrophic factor [189, 190]. Takashi et al. [190] suggested that increasing daily physical activity significantly increased brain-derived neurotrophic factor (BDNF) concentrations in postmenopausal women. BDNF plays an important role in reducing symptoms of depression in older adults and is also associated with memory impairment. Therefore, increasing physical activity is important for increasing BDNF levels and positively affecting mental well-being [190]. Aging has been associated with impaired brain serotonin transmission, which may contribute to the development of depressive symptoms. Therefore, long-term participation in physical activity may increase serotonin levels in the brain, thereby improving mental health and reducing the risk of depressive disorders. In addition, studies have shown that regular exercise training positively affects oxidative stress status. Physical activity increases antioxidant capacity, which in turn reduces oxidative stress and, therefore, depression [191], as high oxidative stress has been associated with the development of depression [192].

It can be said that moderate-to-vigorous intensity or light intensity physical activity relieves depressive symptoms. Therefore, women can choose the intensity level that suits their preferences and circumstances; however, it has been suggested that participating in moderate-to-vigorous physical activity or a combination of intensities may provide greater benefits than light intensity alone [14].

Because of the relationship between insomnia and depression, it is suggested that stretching exercises done before going to sleep will have positive effects on insomnia and, therefore, depression. Stretching exercises performed before bedtime have been shown to reduce sleep latency and contribute to better sleep quality, thus positively affecting menopausal and depressive symptoms. Acute stretching also suppresses sympathetic nerve activity and increases parasympathetic activity, promoting better sleep. Daily stretching routines over a 28-day period are said to have chronic effects on the autonomic nervous system [14].

For menopausal women who have time during the day, engaging in physical activities such as walking (e.g., aiming for at least 10,000 steps per day) and aerobic exercises is suggested; however, for women with limited time or work commitments, focusing on stretching before bedtime alone can still be beneficial [14].

Some studies show that low- and moderate-intensity aerobic exercise interventions, three times a week, 70–90 min/time, and 8–10 weeks have the best effects on improving sleep disorders. Although an individual exercise method is more effective, group exercises can also be preferred because social support increases the continuity of exercise [193].

Yoga may also be considered as part of symptom management in menopausal women due to its positive effects on menopausal symptoms, sleep quality, anxiety, and depressive symptoms [72, 76].

Garcia-Garro et al. [194], in their randomized controlled study, investigated the effects of a

Pilates exercise program on cognitive and physical functioning of postmenopausal women over 60 years of age. The exercise group did Pilates exercises for 12 weeks (twice weekly). Functional flexibility, lower body strength, and cognitive functions were assessed. They stated that women in the Pilates group experienced improvements across all variables examined except for global cognitive function. The Pilates training program was beneficial for cognitive abilities such as verbal fluency and executive function. In addition, improvements in functional flexibility and lower body strength were found. When compared with the control group, the analysis revealed significant benefits in the Pilates group for all measures except for global cognitive function and functional flexibility (Back Scratch Test). In conclusion, they suggested that Pilates has the potential to improve both cognitive and functional abilities among postmenopausal women [194].

21.2.5 Cardiovascular Symptoms

During the reproductive age, estrogen provides protection against cardiovascular disease (CVD) in women, as it is essential for vasodilation, maintaining healthy lipid levels, suppressing inflammation, and exerting vital protective and regulatory effects on the cardiovascular system. Estrogen withdrawal in postmenopausal women may lead to lipid metabolism disorders, decreased vascular elasticity, and endothelial dysfunction, increasing the risk of atherosclerosis, hypertension, and arteriosclerosis. In estrogen deficiency, low-density lipoprotein (LDL), total cholesterol, and triglyceride levels increase, while high-density lipoprotein (HDL) levels decrease. The increase in risk is also due to the increase in fat, change in body composition, and insulin resistance that occurs in menopausal women [195]. Epicardial fat is positively associated with obesity and body mass index (BMI). Myocardial steatosis and accumulation of fat in epicardial adipose tissue enhance the development of insulin resistance and type II diabetes mellitus, hypertension, and dyslipidemia, all of which also lead to more cardiovascular risk in women after menopause [195–197].

While the prevalence of cardiovascular disease in premenopausal women is lower than in men, it increases significantly after menopause, even exceeding the risk in men of the same age [198, 199]. It is stated that the risk is even higher in surgical menopause [200]. Females who experience VMS are more likely to have adverse cardiovascular disease risk profiles compared with individuals without VMS [201, 202]. Therefore, it is very important to address cardiovascular health problems in women during menopause.

21.2.5.1 Physiotherapy

Physical exercise is a common lifestyle modification and is recommended as a first-line or adjunctive therapy [203]. Studies show that exercise reduces cardiovascular disease risk in menopausal women through the mechanisms below:

- Exercise improves lipid metabolism (an increase in HDL and a decrease in LDL, triglycerides, and cholesterol) [204], endothelial function (increasing nitric oxide (NO) levels), and vascular elasticity [205] and positively impacts vascular health [206].
- It promotes an increase in antioxidant biomarkers such as superoxide dismutase and catalase, which play a crucial role in oxidative stress modulation [207].
- The most apparent cardiovascular effect of exercise is lowering blood pressure. Cardiovascular autonomic regulation and an increase in baroreflex sensitivity with exercise may play a role in this situation [208, 209].
- Exercise influences BMI, fat mass, lean mass, visceral adipose tissue area, adiponectin level, serum lipids, and metabolic status, which may be important for cardiovascular disease [210, 211].
- A progressive decrease in muscular mass and strength, known as sarcopenia, is associated with increased risk for cardiovascular diseases and all-cause mortality. So, apart from the effects of exercise on the cardiovascular parameters mentioned above, its inde-

pendent effect on muscle strength is also important in the prevention and treatment of CVDs [212].

Different types of training programs, including aerobic, resistance, endurance, high- intensity interval training, or the combined forms, are applied [213]. The type, duration, intensity, and frequency of exercise play an important role in the mechanism of action mentioned above.

Loaiza-Betancur et al. (2021), in their systematic review, aimed to examine the effect of exercise training on systolic blood pressure (SBP), diastolic blood pressure (DBP), and mean arterial pressure (MAP) in menopausal and postmenopausal women. Compared with the control group, exercise training resulted in clinically significant reductions in SBP, DBP, and MAP. Aerobic training did not result in significant reductions in SBP, DBP, and MAP, whereas combined training produced larger reductions. They stated that exercise training produced small but clinically significant reductions in SBP, DBP, and MAP in menopausal and postmenopausal women younger than or older than 65 years of age with prehypertension or hypertension. Aerobic exercise did not result in clinically significant improvements in blood pressure (BP) in this population, whereas combined exercise produced the largest reductions in SBP, DBP, and MAP [214].

In a systematic review and meta-analysis study, He et al. [215] examined resistance training effects on lipid profiles in postmenopausal women. They determined that resistance training can decrease total cholesterol, low-density lipoprotein cholesterol, and triglyceride levels in postmenopausal females. The impact of resistance training on high-density lipoprotein cholesterol levels was small and was only observed in individuals with obesity. In terms of intervention duration, randomized controlled trials lasting <16 weeks and enrolling patients younger than 60 years were more successful in reducing TC levels. These results were explained by the fact that compliance with physical exercise-based interventions may be higher if the duration of the program is shorter [215].

There are examples of studies that say a combination of aerobic and resistance exercise produces the best results in cardiorespiratory fitness and arterial stiffness [216] or blood pressure values in menopausal women [217].

It is said that combined resistance and aerobic exercises performed at moderate intensity (40–60% of heart rate reserve or 40–60% of heart rate max) three times a week, each training session approximately 60 min, for 12 weeks can produce a clinically significant difference in the cardiovascular system [218].

In a network meta-analysis and systematic review of 32 randomized controlled trials, including 1427 women, the effect of five different types of exercise on vascular function was analyzed in postmenopausal women. The authors concluded that interval training and aerobic combined with resistance training are the most effective exercise interventions for improving vascular function in postmenopausal women, while continuous endurance training and resistance training are less effective. Therefore, interval training and aerobic exercise combined with resistance training are the recommended exercise modalities for improving vascular function in postmenopausal women [213].

21.3 Conclusion

Although it is a natural part of aging, the transition to menopause and the many changes experienced during this process can affect a woman's quality of life. It is essential for women to be informed about the process, the problems that may be experienced during this period, and how to solve these problems. As a support or alternative to medical treatments, physiotherapy approaches should be considered to diminish menopausal problems and improve women's quality of life because they are low-cost, have fewer side effects, and are easy to apply.

References

1. Gatenby C, Simpson P. Menopause: physiology, definitions, and symptoms. Best Pract Res Clin Endocrinol Metab. 2024;38(1):101855.
2. Nelson HD. Menopause. Lancet. 2008;371(9614):760–70.
3. Stojanovska L, Apostolopoulos V, Polman R, Borkoles E. To exercise, or, not to exercise, during menopause and beyond. Maturitas. 2014;77(4):318–23.
4. Harlow SD, Gass M, Hall JE, Lobo R, Maki P, Rebar RW, Sherman S, Slus PM, de Villiers TJ. Executive summary of the stages of reproductive aging workshop + 10: addressing the unfinished agenda of staging reproductive aging. J Clin Endocrinol Metab. 2012;97:1159–68.
5. Peacock K, Carlson K, Ketvertis KM. Menopause. [Updated 2023 Dec 21]. In: StatPearls [Internet]. Treasure Island (FL): StatPearls Publishing; 2024 Jan-. Available from: https://www.ncbi.nlm.nih.gov/books/NBK507826/
6. Choudhry DN, Saleem S, Hatim S, Irfan R. The effect of resistance training in reducing hot flushes in post-menopausal women: a meta-analysis. J Bodyw Mov Ther. 2024;39:335–42.
7. Strand NH, D'Souza RS, Gomez DA, Whitney MA, Attanti S, Anderson MA, Moeschler SM, Chadwick AL, Maloney JA. Pain during menopause. Maturitas. 2025;191:108135. https://doi.org/10.1016/j.maturitas.2024.108135. Epub 2024 Oct 31
8. Brockie J, Lambrinoudaki I, Ceausu I, et al. EMAS position statement: menopause for medical students. Maturitas. 2014;78(1):67–9.
9. Brinton RD, Yao J, Yin F, Mack WJ, Cadenas E. Perimenopause as a neurological transition state. Nat Rev Endocrinol. 2015;11:393–405. https://doi.org/10.1038/nrendo.2015.82.
10. Liu T, Chen S, Mielke GI, McCarthy AL, Bailey TG. Effects of exercise on vasomotor symptoms in menopausal women: a systematic review and meta-analysis. Climacteric. 2022;25(6):552–61. https://doi.org/10.1080/13697137.2022.2097865. Epub 2022 Jul 29
11. Santoro N, Roeca C, Peters BA, Neal-Perry G. The menopause transition: signs, symptoms, and management options. J Clin Endocrinol Metab. 2021;106(1):1–15. https://doi.org/10.1210/clinem/dgaa764.
12. UpToDate; Clinical manifestations and diagnosis of menopause. Author: Robert F Casper, MD. Section Editors: Robert L Barbieri, MD, William F Crowley, Jr, MD. Deputy Editor: Kathryn A Martin, MD, Literature review current through: Nov 2024. This topic last updated: Jun 29, 2023. https://www.uptodate.com/contents/clinical-manifestations-and-diagnosis-of-menopause?search=menopause&source=search_result&selectedTitle=1%7E150&usage_type=default&display_rank=1
13. Roush K. What nurses know-menopause. New York: Demos Medical Publishing; 2011. p. 1–24.
14. Lialy HE, Mohamed MA, AbdAllatif LA, Khalid M, Elhelbawy A. Effects of different physiotherapy modalities on insomnia and depression in perimenopausal, menopausal, and post-menopausal women: a systematic review. BMC Womens Health. 2023;23(1):363. https://doi.org/10.1186/s12905-023-02515-9. Erratum in: BMC Womens Health. 2023 23(1):419. doi:10.1186/s12905-023-02573-z
15. Harlow SD, Gass M, Hall JE, Lobo R, Maki P, Rebar RW, et al. Executive summary of the stages of reproductive aging workshop + 10: addressing the unfinished agenda of staging reproductive aging. Menopause. 2012;19(4):387–95. https://doi.org/10.1097/gme.0b013e31824d8f40.
16. Davis SR, Lambrinoudaki I, Lumsden M, Mishra GD, Pal L, Rees M, et al. Menopause. Nat Rev Dis Primers. 2015;1:15004. https://doi.org/10.1038/nrdp.2015.4.
17. Burger HG, Dudley EC, Robertson DM, Dennerstein L. Hormonal changes in the menopause transition. Recent Prog Horm Res. 2002;57:257–75. https://doi.org/10.1210/rp.57.1.257.
18. Takahashi TA, Johnson KM. Menopause. Med Clin North Am. 2015;99(3):521–34. https://doi.org/10.1016/j.mcna.2015.01.006.
19. Talaulikar V. Menopause transition: physiology and symptoms. Best Pract Res Clin Obstet Gynaecol. 2022;81:3–7. https://doi.org/10.1016/j.bpobgyn.2022.03.003. Epub 2022 Mar 16
20. Voedisch AJ, Dunsmoor-Su R, Kasirsky J. Menopause: a global perspective and clinical guide for practice. Clin Obstet Gynecol. 2021;64(3):528–54. https://doi.org/10.1097/GRF.0000000000000639.
21. Sourouni M, Zangger M, Honermann L, Foth D, Stute P. Assessment of the climacteric syndrome: a narrative review. Arch Gynecol Obstet. 2021;304(4):855–62. https://doi.org/10.1007/s00404-021-06139-y. Epub 2021 Jul 6
22. Hauser GA, Huber IC, Keller PJ, Lauritzen C, Schneider HPG. Evaluation der klinischen Beschwerden (Menopause Rating Scale). Zentralbl Gynakol. 1994;116:16–23.
23. Potthoff P, Heinemann LAJ, Schneider HPG, Rosemeier HP, Hauser GA. Menopause-Rating Skala (MRS): Methodische Standardisierung in der deutschen Bevölkerung. Zentralbl Gynakol. 2000;122:280–6.
24. Schneider HP, Heinemann LA, Rosemeier HP, Potthoff P, Behre HM. The menopause rating scale (MRS): comparison with Kupperman index and quality-of-life scale SF-36. Climact J Int Menopause Soc. 2000;3(1):50–8.
25. Hand A, Gray T, Simpson P. Diagnosis and management of the menopause. InnovAiT. 2021;14(10):590–8.
26. World Health Organization. WHO consolidated guideline on self-care interventions for health:

sexual and reproductive health and rights. Geneva: World Health Organization; 2019.
27. Kronenberg F. Hot flashes. In: Lobo RA, editor. Treatment of the postmenopausal woman: basic and clinical aspects. 2nd ed. Philadelphia: Lippincott Williams & Wilkins; 1999. p. 157–77.
28. North American Menopause Society. Consumer Education Committee. Treating hot flushes. 2012. http://www.menopause.org/docs/for-women/mnflushes.pdf.
29. Hunter MS, Gupta P, Chedraui P, Blümel JE, Tserotas K, Aguirre W, et al. The international menopause study of climate, altitude, temperature (IMS-CAT) and vasomotor symptoms. Climacteric. 2013;16(1):8–16. https://doi.org/10.3109/13697137.2012.699563. Epub 2012 Sep 4
30. Ivarsson T, Spetz AC, Hammar M. Physical exercise and vasomotor symptoms in postmenopausal women. Maturitas. 1998;29(2):139–46. https://doi.org/10.1016/s0378-5122(98)00004-8.
31. Thurston RC, Joffe H. Vasomotor symptoms and menopause: findings from the study of women's health across the nation. Obstet Gynecol Clin. 2011;38(3):489–501.
32. McKinlay SM, Brambilla DJ, Posner J. The normal menopause transition. Maturitas. 1992;14:103–15.
33. Freeman EW, Sammel MD, Lin H, Gracia CR, Pien GW, Nelson DB, et al. Symptoms associated with menopausal transition and reproductive hormones in midlife women. Obstet Gynecol. 2007;110:230–40.
34. Gold EB, Block G, Crawford S, Lachance L, FitzGerald G, Miracle H, et al. Lifestyle and demographic factors in relation to vasomotor symptoms: baseline results from the study of women's health across the nation. Am J Epidemiol. 2004;159:1189–99.
35. Williams E, Kalilani L, DiBenedetti B, Zhou X, Granger AL, Fehnel SE, et al. Frequency and severity of vasomotor symptoms among perimenopausal and postmenopausal women in the United States. Climacteric. 2008;11(1):32–43.
36. Kronenberg F. Hot flashes: epidemiology and physiology. Ann N Y Acad Sci. 1990;592:52.
37. Avis NE, Crawford SL, Greendale G, Bromberger JT, Everson-Rose SA, Gold EB, et al. Duration of menopausal vasomotor symptoms over the menopause transition. JAMA Intern Med. 2015;175(4):531–9.
38. Thurston RC, Aslanidou Vlachos HE, Derby CA, Jackson EA, Brooks MM, Matthews KA, et al. Menopausal vasomotor symptoms and risk of incident cardiovascular disease events in SWAN. J Am Heart Assoc. 2021;10(3):e017416. https://doi.org/10.1161/JAHA.120.017416. Epub 2021 Jan 20
39. Randolph JF Jr, Sowers M, Bondarenko I, Gold EB, Greendale GA, Bromberger JT, et al. The relationship of longitudinal change in reproductive hormones and vasomotor symptoms during the menopausal transition. J Clin Endocrinol Metab. 2005;90(11):6106–12.
40. Hammar ML, Hammar-Henriksson MB, Frisk J, Rickenlund A, Wyon YA. Few oligo-amenorrheic athletes have vasomotor symptoms. Maturitas. 2000;34(3):219–25.
41. Nappi C, Petralgia F, Gambardella A, De Masellis G, Di Carlo C, Genazanni AR, et al. Relationship between cerebrospinal fluid b-endorphin and plasma pituitary-gonadal hormone levels in women. J Endocrinol Investig. 1990;13:149–53.
42. Bruck K, Hinckel P. Thermoregulatory noradrenergic and serotonergic pathways to hypothalamic units. J Physiol. 1980;304:193–202.
43. Freedman EW, Sammel MD, Lin H, Gracia CR, Kapoor S, Ferdousi T. The role of anxiety and hormonal changes in menopausal hot flashes. Menopause. 2005;12:258–66.
44. MacLennan A, Lester S, Moore V. Oral estrogen replacement therapy versus placebo for hot flushes: a systematic review. Climacteric. 2001;4(1):58–74.
45. Baerug U, Winge T, Nordland G, Faber-Swensson E, Heldaas K, Norling B, et al. Do combinations of 1mg estradiol and low doses of NETA effectively control menopausal symptoms? Climacteric. 1998;1:219–28.
46. Manson JE, Crandall CJ, Rossouw JE, Chlebowski RT, Anderson GL, Stefanick ML, et al. The women's health initiative randomized trials and clinical practice: a review. JAMA. 2024;331(20):1748–60. https://doi.org/10.1001/jama.2024.6542.
47. Crawford SL, Crandall CJ, Derby CA, El Khoudary SR, Waetjen LE, Fischer M, Joffe H. Menopausal hormone therapy trends before versus after 2002: impact of the Women's Health Initiative study results. Menopause. 2018;26(6):588–97. https://doi.org/10.1097/GME.0000000000001282.
48. The 2023 Nonhormone Therapy Position Statement of the North American Menopause Society Advisory Panel. The 2023 nonhormone therapy position statement of the North American Menopause Society. Menopause. 2023;30(6):573–90.
49. Sport, England. Women in Sport. Silver Linings – Understanding women's relationship with sport and physical activity in later life [Internet]. 2017. https://womeninsport.org/wp-content/uploads/2017/10/-Silver-Linings-report.pdf.
50. Women in Sport. 2018. Menopause, me and physical activity: Exploring the impact of menopause on physical activity behaviour. Accessed September 24, 2023. https://womeninsport.org/wp-content/uploads/2018/05/Menopause-report-PDF-final-1-2.pdf
51. Hammar M, Berg G, Lindgren R. Does physical exercise influence the frequency of postmenopausal hot flushes? Acta Obstet Gynecol Scand. 1990;69(5):409–12. https://doi.org/10.3109/00016349009013303.
52. Col NF, Guthrie JR, Politi M, Dennerstein L. Duration of vasomotor symptoms in middle-aged women: a longitudinal study. Menopause. 2009;16(3):453–7. https://doi.org/10.1097/gme.0b013e31818d414e.

53. Di Donato P, Giulini NA, Bacchi Modena A, Cicchetti G, Comitini G, Gentile G. Factors associated with climacteric symptoms in women around menopause attending menopause clinics in Italy. Maturitas. 2005;52(3–4):181–9. https://doi.org/10.1016/j.maturitas.2005.01.008.
54. Moilanen J, Aalto AM, Hemminki E, Aro AR, Raitanen J, Luoto R. Prevalence of menopause symptoms and their association with lifestyle among Finnish middle-aged women. Maturitas. 2010;67(4):368–74. https://doi.org/10.1016/j.maturitas.2010.08.007. Epub 2010 Sep 24
55. Gold EB, Sternfeld B, Kelsey JL, Brown C, Mouton C, Reame N, Salamone L, Stellato R. Relation of demographic and lifestyle factors to symptoms in a multi-racial/ethnic population of women 40-55 years of age. Am J Epidemiol. 2000;152(5):463–73. https://doi.org/10.1093/aje/152.5.463.
56. Elavsky S, Gonzales JU, Proctor DN, Williams N, Henderson VW. Effects of physical activity on vasomotor symptoms: examination using objective and subjective measures. Menopause. 2012;19(10):1095–103.
57. Royal College of Obstetricians and Gynaecologists. Scientific Advisory Committee. Alternatives to HRT for the management of symptoms of the menopause. Royal College of Obstetricians and Gynaecologists, www.rcog.org.uk/index.asp?pageid=1561. Accessed 23 Feb 2006.
58. Luoto R, Moilanen J, Heinonen R, Mikkola T, Raitanen J, Tomas E, et al. Effect of aerobic training on hot flushes and quality of life – a randomized controlled trial. Ann Med. 2012;44(6):616–26.
59. Berin E, Hammar M, Lindblom H, Lindh-Åstrand L, Rubér M, Spetz Holm AC. Resistance training for hot flushes in postmenopausal women: a randomised controlled trial. Maturitas. 2019;126:55–60. https://doi.org/10.1016/j.maturitas.2019.05.005.
60. Daley A, Stokes-Lampard H, Thomas A, MacArthur C. Exercise for vasomotor menopausal symptoms. Cochrane Database Syst Rev. 2014;2014(11):CD006108. https://doi.org/10.1002/14651858.CD006108.pub4.
61. Daley AJ, Thomas A, Roalfe AK, Stokes-Lampard H, Coleman S, Rees M, Hunter MS, MacArthur C. The effectiveness of exercise as treatment for vasomotor menopausal symptoms: randomised controlled trial. BJOG. 2015;122(4):565–75. https://doi.org/10.1111/1471-0528.13193. Epub 2014 Dec 17
62. McAndrew LM, Napolitano MA, Albrecht A, Farrell NC, Marcus BH, Whiteley JA. When, why and for whom there is a relationship between physical activity and menopause symptoms. Maturitas. 2009;64(2):119–25.
63. Van Poppel MNM, Brown WJ. "It's my hormones, doctor"–does physical activity help with menopausal symptoms? Menopause. 2008;15(1):78–85.
64. Schwarz L, Kindermann W. Changes in b-endorphin levels in response to aerobic and anaerobic exercise. Rev Sports Med. 1992;13:25–36.
65. Shanafelt TD, Barton DL, Adjei AA, Loprinzi CL. Pathophysiology and treatment of hot flashes. İçinde: Mayo Clinic Proceedings. Elsevier; 2002. pp. 1207–18.
66. Sternfeld B, Bhat AK, Wang H, Sharp T, Charles P, Quesenberry J. Menopause, physical activity, and body composition/fat distribution in midlife women. Med Sci Sports Exerc. 2005;37(7):1195–202.
67. Thurston RC, El Khoudary SR, Sutton-Tyrrell K, Crandall CJ, Gold EB, Sternfeld B, et al. Vasomotor symptoms and lipid profiles in women transitioning through menopause. Obstet Gynecol. 2012;119(4):753–61. https://doi.org/10.1097/AOG.0b013e31824a09ec.
68. Thurston RC, El Khoudary SR, Sutton-Tyrrell K, Crandall CJ, Sternfeld B, Joffe H, et al. Vasomotor symptoms and insulin resistance in the study of women's health across the nation. J Clin Endocrinol Metab. 2012;97(10):3487–94. https://doi.org/10.1210/jc.2012-1410. Epub 2012 Jul 31
69. Tellhed U, Daukantaite D, Maddux RE, Svensson T, Melander O. Yogic breathing and mindfulness as stress coping mediate positive health outcomes of yoga. Mindfulness. 2019;10(12):2703–15. https://doi.org/10.1007/s12671-019-01225-4.
70. Pascoe MC, Bauer IE. A systematic review of randomised control trials on the effects of yoga on stress measures and mood. J Psychiatr Res. 2015;68:270–82.
71. Kanchibhotla D, Harsora P, Subramanian S. Influence of yogic breathing in increasing social connectedness among Indian adults. Acta Psychol. 2024;243:104164. https://doi.org/10.1016/j.actpsy.2024.104164. Epub 2024 Feb 2
72. Shepherd-Banigan M, Goldstein KM, Coeytaux RR, McDuffie JR, Goode AP, Kosinski AS, et al. Improving vasomotor symptoms; psychological symptoms; and health-related quality of life in peri- or post-menopausal women through yoga: an umbrella systematic review and meta-analysis. Complement Ther Med. 2017;34:156–64. https://doi.org/10.1016/j.ctim.2017.08.011. Epub 2017 Aug 24.
73. Cramer H, Peng W, Lauche R. Yoga for menopausal symptoms-a systematic review and meta-analysis. Maturitas. 2018;109:13–25. https://doi.org/10.1016/j.maturitas.2017.12.005. Epub 2017 Dec 6
74. Susanti HD, Sonko I, Chang PC, Chuang YH, Chung MH. Effects of yoga on menopausal symptoms and sleep quality across menopause statuses: a randomized controlled trial. Nurs Health Sci. 2022;24(2):368–79. https://doi.org/10.1111/nhs.12931. Epub 2022 Mar 21
75. Money A, MacKenzie A, Norman G, Eost-Telling C, Harris D, McDermott J, et al. The impact of physical activity and exercise interventions on symptoms for women experiencing menopause: overview of reviews. BMC Womens Health. 2024;24(1):399. https://doi.org/10.1186/s12905-024-03243-4.

76. Wang H, Liu Y, Kwok JYY, Xu F, Li R, Tang J, et al. The effectiveness of yoga on menopausal symptoms: a systematic review and meta-analysis of randomized controlled trials. Int J Nurs Stud. 2025;161:104928. https://doi.org/10.1016/j.ijnurstu.2024.104928. Epub 2024 Oct 11
77. Freedman RR, Woodward S. Behavioral treatment of menopausal hot flushes: evaluation by ambulatory monitoring. Am J Obstet Gynecol. 1992;167(2):436–9. https://doi.org/10.1016/s0002-9378(11)91425-2.
78. Irvin JH, Domar AD, Clark C, Zuttermeister PC, Friedman R. The effects of relaxation response training on menopausal symptoms. J Psychosom Obstet Gynaecol. 1996;17(4):202–7. https://doi.org/10.3109/01674829609025684.
79. Goats GC, Keir KAI. Connective tissue massage. Br J Sp Med. 1991;25(3):131–3.
80. Holey AE. Connective tissue massage: a bridge between complementary and orthodox approaches. J Bodyw Mov Ther. 2000;4(1):72–80.
81. Holey LA, Dixon J. Connective tissue manipulation: a review of theory and clinical evidence. J Bodyw Mov Ther. 2014;18(1):112–8. https://doi.org/10.1016/j.jbmt.2013.08.003. Epub 2013 Sep 8
82. Reed BV, Held JM. Effects of sequential connective tissue massage on autonomic nervous system of middle-aged and elderly adults. Phys Ther. 1988;68(8):1231–4.
83. Celenay ST, Kaya DO, Ucurum SG. Adding connective tissue manipulation to physiotherapy for chronic low back pain improves pain, mobility, and well-being: a randomized controlled trial. J Exerc Rehabil. 2019;15(2):308–15. https://doi.org/10.12965/jer.1836634.317.
84. Ekici G, Bakar Y, Akbayrak T, Yuksel I. Comparison of manual lymph drainage therapy and connective tissue massage in women with fibromyalgia: a randomized controlled trial. J Manip Physiol Ther. 2009;32(2):127–33. https://doi.org/10.1016/j.jmpt.2008.12.001.
85. Toprak Celenay S, Coban O, Mete O, Karahan N. An investigation of the effects of connective tissue massage in women with migraine: a controlled clinical trial. J Bodyw Mov Ther. 2023;33:112–9. https://doi.org/10.1016/j.jbmt.2022.09.008. Epub 2022 Sep 23
86. Akbayrak T, Akarcali I, Karabudak R, Demirtürk F. The results of connective tissue manipulation in the treatment of tension type headache. Pain Clin. 2002;13:343–7.
87. Castro Sánchez AM, Moreno Lorenzo C, Matarán-Peñarrocha GA, Feriche-Fernández-Castanys B, Granados-Gámez G, Quesada-Rubio JM. Connective tissue reflex massage for type 2 diabetic patients with peripheral arterial disease: randomized controlled trial. Evid Based Complement Alternat Med. 2011;2011:804321. https://doi.org/10.1093/ecam/nep171. Epub 2011 Mar 13
88. Özgül S, Nalan Çinar G, Gürşen C, Baran E, Üzelpasaci E, Nakip G, et al. The effects of connective tissue manipulation in primary dysmenorrhea: a randomized placebo-controlled study. Reprod Sci. 2023;30(1):181–91. https://doi.org/10.1007/s43032-022-00964-5. Epub 2022 May 13
89. Bongi SM, Del Rosso A, Galluccio F, Sigismondi F, Miniati I, Conforti ML, et al. Efficacy of connective tissue massage and mc Mennell joint manipulation in the rehabilitative treatment of the hands in systemic sclerosis. Clin Rheumatol. 2009;28(10):1167–73. https://doi.org/10.1007/s10067-009-1216-x. Epub 2009 Jun 25.
90. Orhan C, Özgül S, Baran E, Üzelpasacı E, Akbayrak T. Comparison of connective tissue manipulation and abdominal massage combined with usual care vs usual care alone for chronic constipation: a randomized controlled trial. J Manip Physiol Ther. 2020;43(8):768–78. https://doi.org/10.1016/j.jmpt.2019.05.013. Epub 2020 Sep 3
91. Bayrakci Tunay V, Akbayrak T, Bakar Y, Kayihan H, Ergun N. Effects of mechanical massage, manual lymphatic drainage and connective tissue manipulation techniques on fat mass in women with cellulite. J Eur Acad Dermatol Venereol. 2010;24(2):138–42. https://doi.org/10.1111/j.1468-3083.2009.03355.x. Epub 2009 Jul 13
92. Joseph LH, Paungmali A, Dixon J, Holey L, Naicker AS, Htwe O. Therapeutic effects of connective tissue manipulation on wound healing and bacterial colonization count among patients with diabetic foot ulcer. J Bodyw Mov Ther. 2016;20(3):650–6. https://doi.org/10.1016/j.jbmt.2016.01.010. Epub 2016 Feb 2. Erratum in: J Bodyw Mov Ther. 2019 23(3):440. doi:10.1016/j.jbmt.2019.03.007
93. McKechnie AA, Wilson F, Watson N, Scott D. Anxiety states: a preliminary report on the value of connective tissue massage. J Psychosom Res. 1983;27(2):125–9. https://doi.org/10.1016/0022-3999(83)90088-0.
94. Horstkotte W, Klempien EJ, Scheppokat KD. Skin temperature and blood flow changes in occlusive arterial disease under physiological and pharmacological therapy. Angiology. 1967;18:1–5.
95. Akarcalı İ. Klimakterik sendromda konnektif doku masajının etkinliği. Türk J Med Res. 1992;10(3):167–74.
96. Albayrak G, Çağlıyan Türk A, Özgül S. Effects of connective tissue massage on physical and emotional symptoms, insomnia, and quality of life in postmenopausal women: a randomized, sham-controlled trial. Maturitas. 2025;191:108149. https://doi.org/10.1016/j.maturitas.2024.108149. Epub 2024 Nov 7
97. Thurston RC, Christie IC, Matthews KA. Hot flashes and cardiac vagal control: a link to cardiovascular risk? Menopause. 2010;17(3):456–61. https://doi.org/10.1097/gme.0b013e3181c7dea7.
98. Lindh-Åstrand L, Nedstrand E. Effects of applied relaxation on vasomotor symptoms in postmenopausal women: a randomized con-

trolled trial. Menopause. 2013;20(4):401–8. https://doi.org/10.1097/gme.0b013e318272ce80.
99. Hjemdahl P, Fagius J, Freyschusss U. Muscle sympathetic activity and norepinephrine release during mental challenge in humans. Am J Physiol. 1989;257:341–7.
100. Lee DD, Kimura S, DeQuattro V, Davison G. Relaxation therapy lowers blood pressure more effectively in hypertensives with raised plasma norepinephrine and blunts pressor response to anger. Clin Exp Hypertens A. 1989;11(Suppl 1):191–8. https://doi.org/10.3109/10641968909045423.
101. Payne RA. Relaxation techniques: a practical handbook for the health care professional. 3rd ed. China: Elsevier Limited; 2005.
102. Benson H, Klipper MZ. The relaxation response. New York: Harper Collins Publishers; 2000.
103. Germaine LM, Freedman RR. Behavioral treatment of menopausal hot flashes: evaluation by objective methods. J Consult Clin Psychol. 1984;52:1072–9.
104. Freedman R, Woodward S. Behavioral treatment of menopausal hot flushes: evaluation by ambulatory monitoring. Am J Obstet Gynecol. 1992;167:436–9.
105. Hunter M, Liao KL. Evaluation of a four-session cognitive behavioural intervention for menopausal hot flushes. Br J Health Psychol. 1996;1:113–25.
106. Wijma K, Melin A, Nedstrand E, Hammar M. Treatment of menopausal symptoms with applied relaxation: a pilot study. J Behav Ther Exp Psychiatry. 1997;28:251–64.
107. Saensak S, Vutyavanich T, Somboonporn W, Srisurapanont M. Relaxation for perimenopausal and postmenopausal symptoms. Cochrane Database Syst Rev. 2014;(7):CD008582. https://doi.org/10.1002/14651858.CD008582.pub2.
108. UpToDate: Overview of the management of low bone mass and osteoporosis in postmenopausal women. Authors: Harold N Rosen, MD E Michael Lewiecki, MD Section Editors: Clifford J Rosen, MD Kenneth E Schmader, MD Deputy Editor: Katya Rubinow, MD, Literature review current through: Nov 2024. This topic last updated: Sep 11, 2024. https://www.uptodate.com/contents/overview-of-the-management-of-low-bone-mass-and-osteoporosis-in-postmenopausal-women?search=osteoporosis&source=search_result&selectedTitle=2%7E150&usage_type=default&display_rank=2.
109. Meeta LD, Agarwal N, Vaze N, Shah R, Malik S. Clinical practice guidelines on menopause: an executive summary and recommendations. J Health. 2013;4(2):77–106.
110. WHO Study Group. Assessment of fracture risk and its application to screening for postmenopausal osteoporosis (technical report series). Geneva: World Health Organization; 1994.
111. Siris ES, Adler R, Bilezikian J, Bolognese M, Dawson-Hughes B, Favus MJ, et al. The clinical diagnosis of osteoporosis: a position statement from the National Bone Health Alliance Working Group. Osteoporos Int. 2014;25(5):1439–43. https://doi.org/10.1007/s00198-014-2655-z.
112. LeBoff MS, et al. The clinician's guide to prevention and treatment of osteoporosis. Osteoporos Int. 2022;33(10):2049–102. https://doi.org/10.1007/s00198-021-05900-y. Epub 2022 Apr 28. Erratum in: Osteoporos Int. 2022 33(10):2243. doi:10.1007/s00198-022-06479-8
113. Mederle OA, Balas M, Ioanoviciu SD, Gurban C-V, Tudor A, Borza C. Correlations between bone turnover markers, serum magnesium and bone mass density in postmenopausal osteoporosis. Clin Interv Aging. 2018;13:1383–9.
114. Kanis JA, Johansson H, Johnell O, Oden A, De Laet C, Eisman JA, et al. Alcohol intake as a risk factor for fracture. Osteoporos Int. 2005;16(7):737–42.
115. Eastell R. Treatment of postmenopausal osteoporosis. N Engl J Med. 1998;338(11):736–46.
116. Ward KD, Klesges RC. A meta-analysis of the effects of cigarette smoking on bone mineral density. Calcif Tissue Int. 2001;68(5):259–70.
117. Brooke-Wavell K, Skelton DA, Barker KL, Clark EM, De Biase S, Arnold S, et al. Strong, steady and straight: UK consensus statement on physical activity and exercise for osteoporosis. Br J Sports Med. 2022;56:837–46.
118. Gregg EW, Cauley JA, Seeley DG, Ensrud KE, Bauer DC. Physical activity and osteoporotic fracture risk in older women. Study of osteoporotic fractures research group. Ann Intern Med. 1998;129(2):81–8. https://doi.org/10.7326/0003-4819-129-2-199807150-00002.
119. Turner CH. Exercise as a therapy for osteoporosis: the drunk and the street lamp, revisited. Bone. 1998;23:83.
120. Giangregorio LM, Papaioannou A, Macintyre NJ, et al. Too fit to fracture: exercise recommendations for individuals with osteoporosis or osteoporotic vertebral fracture. Osteoporos Int. 2014;25:821.
121. Feskanich D, Willett W, Colditz G. Walking and leisure-time activity and risk of hip fracture in postmenopausal women. JAMA. 2002;288:2300.
122. Kemmler W, Häberle L, von Stengel S. Effects of exercise on fracture reduction in older adults: a systematic review and meta-analysis. Osteoporos Int. 2013;24(7):1937–50. https://doi.org/10.1007/s00198-012-2248-7.
123. Hoffmann I, Shojaa M, Kohl M, von Stengel S, Becker C, Gosch M, et al. Exercise reduces the number of overall and major osteoporotic fractures in adults. Does supervision make a difference? Systematic review and meta-analysis. J Bone Miner Res. 2022;37(11):2132–48. https://doi.org/10.1002/jbmr.4683.
124. Howe TE, Shea B, Dawson LJ, et al. Exercise for preventing and treating osteoporosis in post-

menopausal women. Cochrane Database Syst Rev. 2011;2011:CD000333.
125. Finlayson ML, Peterson EW. Falls, aging, and disability. Phys Med Rehabil Clin N Am. 2010;21:357–73.
126. Cummings SR, Melton LJ. Epidemiology and outcomes of osteoporotic fractures. Lancet. 2002;359(9319):1761–7. https://doi.org/10.1016/S0140-6736(02)08657-9.
127. Zijlstra GA, van Haastregt JC, van Rossum E, van Eijk JT, Yardley L, Kempen GI. Interventions to reduce fear of falling in community-living older people: a systematic review. J Am Geriatr Soc. 2007;55:603–15.
128. Lee CG, Carr MC, Murdoch SJ, Mitchell E, Woods NF, Wener MH, et al. Adipokines, inflammation, and visceral adiposity across the menopausal transition: a prospective study. J Clin Endocrinol Metab. 2009;94(4):1104–10. https://doi.org/10.1210/jc.2008-0701.
129. Perez-Lopez FR. Androgens in menopausal women. Med Clin (Barc). 2003;120:31–6.
130. Hita-Contreras F, Martínez-Amat A, Lomas-Vega R, Álvarez P, Mendoza N, Romero-Franco N, et al. Relationship of body mass index and body fat distribution with postural balance and risk of falls in Spanish postmenopausal women. Menopause. 2013;20(2):202–8. https://doi.org/10.1097/gme.0b013e318261f242.
131. Byun JH, Jang S, Lee S, Park S, Yoon HK, Yoon BH, Ha YC. The efficacy of bisphosphonates for prevention of osteoporotic fracture: an update meta-analysis. J Bone Metab. 2017;24(1):37–49. https://doi.org/10.11005/jbm.2017.24.1.37.
132. Cummings SR, San Martin J, McClung MR, Siris ES, Eastell R, Reid IR, et al. FREEDOM trial. Denosumab for prevention of fractures in postmenopausal women with osteoporosis. N Engl J Med. 2009;361(8):756–65. https://doi.org/10.1056/NEJMoa0809493.
133. Zhu L, Jiang X, Sun Y, Shu W. Effect of hormone therapy on the risk of bone fractures: a systematic review and meta-analysis of randomized controlled trials. Menopause. 2016;23(4):461–70. https://doi.org/10.1097/GME.0000000000000519.
134. Riggs BL, Hartmann LC. Selective estrogen-receptor modulators-mechanisms of action and application to clinical practice. N Engl J Med. 2003;348(7):618–29. https://doi.org/10.1056/NEJMra022219. Erratum in: N Engl J Med. 2003 348(12):1192
135. Sherrington C, Fairhall NJ, Wallbank GK, Tiedemann A, Michaleff ZA, Howard K, et al. Exercise for preventing falls in older people living in the community. Cochrane Database Syst Rev. 2019;1(1):CD012424. https://doi.org/10.1002/14651858.CD012424.pub2.
136. Kemmler W, Bebenek M, Kohl M, von Stengel S. Exercise and fractures in postmenopausal women. Final results of the controlled Erlangen fitness and osteoporosis prevention study (EFOPS). Osteoporos Int. 2015;26(10):2491–9. https://doi.org/10.1007/s00198-015-3165-3.
137. Martyn-St James M, Carroll S. Meta-analysis of walking for preservation of bone mineral density in postmenopausal women. Bone. 2008;43:521–31.
138. Ma D, Wu L, He Z. Effects of walking on the preservation of bone mineral density in perimenopausal and postmenopausal women: a systematic review and meta-analysis. Menopause. 2013;20:1216–26.
139. Liu F, Wang S. Effect of tai chi on bone mineral density in postmenopausal women: a systematic review and meta-analysis of randomized control trials. J Chin Med Assoc. 2017;80(12):790–5. https://doi.org/10.1016/j.jcma.2016.06.010.
140. Sun Z, Chen H, Berger MR, Zhang L, Guo H, Huang Y. Effects of tai chi exercise on bone health in perimenopausal and postmenopausal women: a systematic review and meta-analysis. Osteoporos Int. 2016;27(10):2901–11. https://doi.org/10.1007/s00198-016-3626-3.
141. Simas V, Hing W, Pope R, Climstein M. Effects of water-based exercise on bone health of middle-aged and older adults: a systematic review and meta-analysis. Open Access J Sports Med. 2017;8:39–60. https://doi.org/10.2147/OAJSM.S129182.
142. Zhao R, Zhao M, Xu Z. The effects of differing resistance training modes on the preservation of bone mineral density in postmenopausal women: a meta-analysis. Osteoporos Int. 2015;26(5):1605–18. https://doi.org/10.1007/s00198-015-3034-0.
143. Martyn-St James M, Carroll S. High-intensity resistance training and postmenopausal bone loss: a meta-analysis. Osteoporos Int. 2006;17(8):1225–40. https://doi.org/10.1007/s00198-006-0083-4.
144. Shojaa M, von Stengel S, Kohl M, Schoene D, Kemmler W. Effects of dynamic resistance exercise on bone mineral density in postmenopausal women: a systematic review and meta-analysis with special emphasis on exercise parameters. Osteoporos Int. 2020;31(8):1427–44. https://doi.org/10.1007/s00198-020-05441-w.
145. Marín-Cascales E, Alcaraz PE, Ramos-Campo DJ, Rubio-Arias JA. Effects of multicomponent training on lean and bone mass in postmenopausal and older women: a systematic review. Menopause. 2018;25(3):346–56. https://doi.org/10.1097/GME.0000000000000975.
146. Kelley GA, Kelley KS, Kohrt WM. Effects of ground and joint reaction force exercise on lumbar spine and femoral neck bone mineral density in postmenopausal women: a meta-analysis of randomized controlled

trials. BMC Musculoskelet Disord. 2012;13:177. https://doi.org/10.1186/1471-2474-13-177.
147. Zhao R, Zhang M, Zhang Q. The effectiveness of combined exercise interventions for preventing postmenopausal bone loss: a systematic review and meta-analysis. J Orthop Sports Phys Ther. 2017;47(4):241–51. https://doi.org/10.2519/jospt.2017.6969.
148. Mohammad Rahimi GR, Smart NA, Liang MTC, Bijeh N, Albanaqi AL, Fathi M, et al. The impact of different modes of exercise training on bone mineral density in older postmenopausal women: a systematic review and meta-analysis research. Calcif Tissue Int. 2020;106(6):577–90. https://doi.org/10.1007/s00223-020-00671-w.
149. Shojaa M, Von Stengel S, Schoene D, Kohl M, Barone G, Bragonzoni L, et al. Effect of exercise training on bone mineral density in post-menopausal women: a systematic review and meta-analysis of intervention studies. Front Physiol. 2020;11:652. https://doi.org/10.3389/fphys.2020.00652.
150. Marques EA, Mota J, Carvalho J. Exercise effects on bone mineral density in older adults: a meta-analysis of randomized controlled trials. Age (Dordr). 2012;34:1493–515.
151. Blake J, Cosman FA, Lewiecki EM, McClung MR, Pinkerton JV, Shapiro M, et al. Management of osteoporosis in postmenopausal women: the 2021 position statement of the North American Menopause Society. Menopause J N Am Menopause Soc. 2021;28:973–97. https://doi.org/10.1097/gme.0000000000001831.
152. Kanis JA, Cooper C, Rizzoli R, Reginster JY. European guidance for the diagnosis and management of osteoporosis in postmenopausal women. Osteoporos Int. 2019;30(1):3–44. https://doi.org/10.1007/s00198-018-4704-5. Epub 2018 Oct 15. Erratum in: Osteoporos Int. 2020 31(1):209. doi:10.1007/s00198-019-05184-3. Erratum in: Osteoporos Int. 2020 31(4):801. doi:10.1007/s00198-020-05303-5
153. Beck BR, Snow CM. Bone health across the lifespan–exercising our options. Exerc Sport Sci Rev. 2003;31:117–22.
154. Kemmler W, Shojaa M, Kohl M, von Stengel S. Effects of different types of exercise on bone mineral density in postmenopausal women: a systematic review and meta-analysis. Calcif Tissue Int. 2020;107(5):409–39. https://doi.org/10.1007/s00223-020-00744-w. Epub 2020 Aug 12. PMID: 32785775; PMCID: PMC7546993
155. Body JJ, Bergmann P, Boonen S, Boutsen Y, Bruyere O, Devogelaer JP, et al. Non-pharmacological management of osteoporosis: a consensus of the Belgian bone Club. Osteoporos Int. 2011;22(11):2769–88. https://doi.org/10.1007/s00198-011-1545-x. Epub 2011 Mar 1. PMID: 21360219; PMCID: PMC3186889
156. Kistler-Fischbacher M, Weeks BK, Beck BR. The effect of exercise intensity on bone in postmenopausal women (part 1): a systematic review. Bone. 2021;143:115696. https://doi.org/10.1016/j.bone.2020.115696. Epub 2020 Dec 24
157. Kistler-Fischbacher M, Weeks BK, Beck BR. The effect of exercise intensity on bone in postmenopausal women (part 2): a meta-analysis. Bone. 2021;143:115697. https://doi.org/10.1016/j.bone.2020.115697. Epub 2020 Dec 24
158. Lanyon LE, Rubin CT. Static vs dynamic loads as an influence on bone remodelling. J Biomech. 1984;17:897–905.
159. Mosley JR, March BM, Lynch J, Lanyon LE. Strain magnitude related changes in whole bone architecture in growing rats. Bone. 1997;20(3):191–8. https://doi.org/10.1016/s8756-3282(96)00385-7.
160. Rubin CT, Lanyon LE. Regulation of bone mass by mechanical strain magnitude. Calcif Tissue Int. 1985;37:411–7.
161. Robling AG, Burr DB, Turner CH. Recovery periods restore mechanosensitivity to dynamically loaded bone. J Exp Biol. 2001;204:3389–99.
162. O'Connor JA, Lanyon LE, MacFie H. The influence of strain rate on adaptive bone remodelling. J Biomech. 1982;15:767–81.
163. Zitzmann AL, Shojaa M, Kast S, Kohl M, von Stengel S, Borucki D, et al. The effect of different training frequency on bone mineral density in older adults. A comparative systematic review and meta-analysis. Bone. 2022;154:116230. https://doi.org/10.1016/j.bone.2021.116230. Epub 2021 Oct 5
164. Manaye S, Cheran K, Murthy C, Bornemann EA, Kamma HK, Alabbas M, et al. The role of high-intensity and high-impact exercises in improving bone health in postmenopausal women: a systematic review. Cureus. 2023;15(2):e34644.
165. Zhao J. Effects of tai chi Chuan on the changes of bone mineral density of perimenopausal women. Chin J Tissue Eng Res. 2020;24:176–80. https://doi.org/10.3969/j.issn.2095-4344.1908.
166. Hou J, Mao H, Xie P, Cui Y, Rong M. The effect of different traditional Chinese exercises on bone mineral density in menopausal women: a systematic review and network meta-analysis. Front Public Health. 2024;12:1430608. https://doi.org/10.3389/fpubh.2024.1430608.
167. de Oliveira RG, Anami GEU, Coelho EA, de Oliveira LC. Effects of Pilates exercise on bone mineral density in postmenopausal women: a systematic review and meta-analysis. J Geriatr Phys Ther. 2022;45(2):107–14. https://doi.org/10.1519/JPT.0000000000000309.

168. Portman DJ, Gass ML. Vulvovaginal atrophy terminology consensus conference panel. Genitourinary syndrome of menopause: new terminology for vulvovaginal atrophy from the International Society for the Study of women's sexual health and the North American Menopause Society. J Sex Med. 2014;11:2865–72.
169. The North American Menopause Society Is Now The Menopause Society. The Menopause Society, 2023. https://www.menopause.org/docs/default-source/press-release/name-change-announcement.pdf. Accessed on 16 Oct 2023.
170. Willhite LA, O'Connell MB. Urogenital atrophy: prevention and treatment. Pharmacotherapy. 2001;21:464–80.
171. Robinson D, Cardozo LD. The role of estrogens in female lower urinary tract dysfunction. Urology. 2003;62(Suppl):45–51.
172. Hyun HS, Park BR, Kim YS, Mun ST, Bae DH. Urodynamic characterization of postmenopausal women with stress urinary incontinence: retrospective study in incontinent pre- and postmenopausal women. J Korean Soc Menopause. 2010;16:148–52.
173. Jackson SR, Avery NC, Tarlton JF, Eckford SD, Abrams P, Bailey AJ. Changes in metabolism of collagen in genitourinary prolapse. Lancet. 1996;347(9016):1658–61. https://doi.org/10.1016/s0140-6736(96)91489-0.
174. UpToDate: Genitourinary syndrome of menopause (vulvovaginal atrophy): Treatment. Authors: Gloria Bachmann, MD, MMS, JoAnn V Pinkerton, MD, FACOG, MSCP, Section Editors: Robert L Barbieri, MD, Harold J Burstein, MD, PhD Deputy Editor: Alana Chakrabarti, MD. Literature review current through: Nov 2024. This topic last updated: Nov 13, 2024. https://e1c9b1a9cc9b2679354d789c7627a4c889c411cc.vetisonline.com/contents/genitourinary-syndrome-of-menopause-vulvovaginal-atrophy-treatment?search=menopause%2C%20genitourinary&source=search_result&selectedTitle=1%7E150&usage_type=default&display_rank=1.
175. Kingsberg SA, et al. Female sexual health: barriers to optimal outcomes and a roadmap for improved patient-clinician communications. J Womens Health. 2019;28(4):432–43. https://doi.org/10.1089/jwh.2018.7352.
176. Edwards D, Panay N. Treating vulvovaginal atrophy/genitourinary syndrome of menopause: how important is vaginal lubricant and moisturizer composition? Climacteric. 2016;19:151.
177. Sarmento ACA, Costa APF, Lírio J, Eleutério J Jr, Baptista PV, Gonçalves AK. Efficacy of hormonal and nonhormonal approaches to vaginal atrophy and sexual dysfunctions in postmenopausal women: a systematic review. Rev Bras Ginecol Obstet. 2022;44(10):986–94. https://doi.org/10.1055/s-0042-1756148. Epub 2022 Nov 29
178. Mitchell CM, Reed SD, Diem S, Larson JC, Newton KM, Ensrud KE, et al. Efficacy of vaginal estradiol or vaginal moisturizer vs placebo for treating postmenopausal vulvovaginal symptoms: a randomized clinical trial. JAMA Intern Med. 2018;178(5):681–90. https://doi.org/10.1001/jamainternmed.2018.0116.
179. Rahn DD, Carberry C, Sanses TV, Mamik MM, Ward RM, Meriwether KV, et al. Vaginal estrogen for genitourinary syndrome of menopause: a systematic review. Obstet Gynecol. 2014;124(6):1147–56. https://doi.org/10.1097/AOG.0000000000000526.
180. Mercier J, Morin M, Lemieux MC, Reichetzer B, Khalifé S, Dumoulin C. Pelvic floor muscles training to reduce symptoms and signs of vulvovaginal atrophy: a case study. Menopause. 2016;23(7):816–20. https://doi.org/10.1097/GME.0000000000000620.
181. Reigota RB, Pedro AO, et al. Prevalence of urinary incontinence and its association with multimorbidity in women aged 50 years or older: a population-based study. Neurourol Urodyn. 2016;35(1):62–8.
182. Jacob L, Lopez-Sanchez GF, Oh H, Shin JI, Grabovac I, Soysal P, et al. Association of multimorbidity with higher levels of urinary incontinence: a crosssectional study of 23 089 individuals aged ≥ 15 years residing in Spain. Br J Gen Pract. 2020;71(702):e71–7.
183. Malinauskas AP, Bressan EFM, de Melo AMZRP, Brasil CA, Lordêlo P, Torelli L. Efficacy of pelvic floor physiotherapy intervention for stress urinary incontinence in postmenopausal women: systematic review. Arch Gynecol Obstet. 2023;308(1):13–24.
184. Marcellou EG, Stasi S, Giannopapas V, Bø K, Bakalidou D, Konstadoulakis M, et al. Effect of pelvic floor muscle training on urinary incontinence symptoms in postmenopausal women: a systematic review and meta-analysis. Eur J Obstet Gynecol Reprod Biol. 2025;304:134–40. https://doi.org/10.1016/j.ejogrb.2024.11.040. Epub 2024 Nov 26
185. Hogervorst E, Craig J, O'Donnell E. Cognition and mental health in menopause: a review. Best Pract Res Clin Obstet Gynaecol. 2022;81:69–84. https://doi.org/10.1016/j.bpobgyn.2021.10.009. Epub 2021 Nov 30
186. Batty GD, Deary IJ, Zaninotto P. Association of Cognitive Function with cause-specific mortality in middle and older age: follow-up of participants in the English longitudinal study of ageing. Am J Epidemiol. 2016;183:183–9.
187. Plassman BL, Williams JW, Burke JR, Holsinger T, Benjamin S. Systematic review: factors associated with risk for and possible prevention of cognitive decline in later life. Ann Intern Med. 2010;153:182–93.

188. Soares CN. Depression in peri- and postmenopausal women: prevalence, pathophysiology and pharmacological management. Drugs Aging. 2013;30(9):677–85.
189. Stuenkel CA, Davis SR, Gompel A, Lumsden MA, Murad MH, Pinkerton JV, et al. Treatment of symptoms of the menopause: an endocrine society clinical practice guideline. J Clin Endocrinol Metab. 2015;100(11):3975–4011. https://doi.org/10.1210/jc.2015-2236.
190. Takahashi M, Lim PJ, Tsubosaka M, Kim HK, Miyashita M, Suzuki K, et al. Effects of increased daily physical activity on mental health and depression biomarkers in postmenopausal women. J Phys Ther Sci. 2019;31(4):408–13.
191. Fatouros IG, Jamurtas AZ, Villiotou V, Pouliopoulou S, Fotinakis P, Taxildaris K, et al. Oxidative stress responses in older men during endurance training and detraining. Med Sci Sports Exerc. 2004;36(12):2065–72.
192. Liu T, Zhong S, Liao X, Chen J, He T, Lai S, et al. A meta-analysis of oxidative stress markers in depression. PLoS One. 2015;10(10):e0138904. https://doi.org/10.1371/journal.pone.0138904.
193. Jing Y, Liu M, Tang H, Kong N, Cai J, Yin Z. The effect of aerobic exercise on sleep disorder in menopausal women: a systematic review and meta-analyses. BMC Womens Health. 2024;24(1):635. https://doi.org/10.1186/s12905-024-03477-2.
194. García-Garro PA, Hita-Contreras F, Martínez-Amat A, Achalandabaso-Ochoa A, Jiménez-García JD, Cruz-Díaz D, et al. Effectiveness of a Pilates training program on cognitive and functional abilities in postmenopausal women. Int J Environ Res Public Health. 2020;17(10):3580. https://doi.org/10.3390/ijerph17103580.
195. Carr MC. The emergence of the metabolic syndrome with menopause. J Clin Endocrinol Metab. 2003;88:2404–11. https://doi.org/10.1210/jc.2003-030242.
196. Wu Y, Zhang A, Hamilton DJ, Deng T. Epicardial fat in the maintenance of cardiovascular health. Debakey Cardiovasc J. 2017;13:20–4.
197. Gonzalez N, Moreno-Villegas Z, Gonzalez-Bris A, Egido J, Lorenzo O. Regulation of visceral and epicardial adipose tissue for preventing cardiovascular injuries associated to obesity and diabetes. Cardiovasc Diabetol. 2017;16(1):44. https://doi.org/10.1186/s12933-017-0528-4.
198. Gersh F, O'Keefe JH, Elagizi A, Lavie CJ, Laukkanen JA. Estrogen and cardiovascular disease. Prog Cardiovasc Dis. 2024;84:60–7. https://doi.org/10.1016/j.pcad.2024.01.015.
199. Teoh J, Li X, Simoncini T, Zhu D, Fu X. Estrogen-mediated gaseous signaling molecules in cardiovascular disease. Trends Endocrinol Metab. 2020;31(10):773–84. https://doi.org/10.1016/j.tem.2020.06.001.
200. Zhu D, Chung HF, Dobson AJ, Pandeya N, Giles GG, Bruinsma F, et al. Age at natural menopause and risk of incident cardiovascular disease: a pooled analysis of individual patient data. Lancet Public Health. 2019;4(11):e553–64. https://doi.org/10.1016/S2468-2667(19)30155-0. Epub 2019 Oct 3
201. Gast G-CM, Grobbee DE, Pop VJM, Keyzer JJ, Samsioe GN, et al. Menopausal complaints are associated with cardiovascular risk factors. Hypertension. 2008;51:1492–8. https://doi.org/10.1161/HYPERTENSIONAHA.107.106526.
202. Lee E, Anselmo M, Tahsin CT, Vanden Noven M, Stokes W, Carter JR, et al. Vasomotor symptoms of menopause, autonomic dysfunction, and cardiovascular disease. Am J Physiol Heart Circ Physiol. 2022;323(6):H1270–80. https://doi.org/10.1152/ajpheart.00477.2022. Epub 2022 Nov 11
203. Lin YY, Lee SD. Cardiovascular benefits of exercise training in postmenopausal hypertension. Int J Mol Sci. 2018;19(9):2523. https://doi.org/10.3390/ijms19092523.
204. Yin Y, Yu Z, Wang J, Sun J. Effects of the different tai chi exercise cycles on patients with essential hypertension: a systematic review and meta-analysis. Front Cardiovasc Med. 2023;10:1016629. https://doi.org/10.3389/fcvm.2023.1016629.
205. Dai DF, Rabinovitch PS, Ungvari Z. Mitochondria and cardiovascular aging. Circ Res. 2012;110(8):1109–24. https://doi.org/10.1161/CIRCRESAHA.111.246140.
206. Seals DR, Nagy EE, Moreau KL. Aerobic exercise training and vascular function with ageing in healthy men and women. J Physiol. 2019;597(19):4901–14. https://doi.org/10.1113/JP277764.
207. Jarrete AP, Novais IP, Nunes HA, Puga GM, Delbin MA, Zanesco A. Influence of aerobic exercise training on cardiovascular and endocrine-inflammatory biomarkers in hypertensive postmenopausal women. J Clin Transl Endocrinol. 2014;1:108–14.
208. Novais IP, Jarrete AP, Puga GM, Araujo HN, Delbin MA, Zanesco A. Effect of aerobic exercise training on cGMP levels and blood pressure in treated hypertensive postmenopausal women. Mot Rev Educação Física. 2017;23:1–6.
209. Shimojo GL, Palma RK, Brito JO, Sanches IC, Irigoyen MC, De Angelis K. Dynamic resistance training decreases sympathetic tone in hypertensive ovariectomized rats. Braz J Med Biol Res. 2015;48:523–7.
210. Wu S, Park KS, McCormick JB. Effects of exercise training on fat loss and lean mass gain in mexican-american and korean premenopausal women. Int J Endocrinol. 2017;2017:5465869. https://doi.org/10.1155/2017/5465869.
211. Lee JA, Kim JW, Kim DY. Effects of yoga exercise on serum adiponectin and metabolic syndrome factors in obese postmenopausal women. Menopause. 2012;19:296–301.
212. Khalafi M, Sakhaei MH, Habibi Maleki A, Rosenkranz SK, Pourvaghar MJ, Fang Y, et al. Influence of exercise type and duration on cardiorespiratory fitness and muscular strength in

post-menopausal women: a systematic review and meta-analysis. Front Cardiovasc Med. 2023;10:1190187. https://doi.org/10.3389/fcvm.2023.1190187.

213. Sun W, Han Y, Gu S. Effects of five types of exercise on vascular function in postmenopausal women: a network meta-analysis and systematic review of 32 randomized controlled trials. PeerJ. 2024;12:e17621. https://doi.org/10.7717/peerj.17621.

214. Loaiza-Betancur AF, Chulvi-Medrano I, Díaz-López VA, Gómez-Tomás C. The effect of exercise training on blood pressure in menopause and postmenopausal women: a systematic review of randomized controlled trials. Maturitas. 2021;149:40–55. https://doi.org/10.1016/j.maturitas.2021.05.005. Epub 2021 May 24

215. He M, Hu S, Wang J, Wang J, Găman MA, Hariri Z, et al. Effect of resistance training on lipid profile in postmenopausal women: a systematic review and meta-analysis of randomized controlled trials. Eur J Obstet Gynecol Reprod Biol. 2023;288:18–28. https://doi.org/10.1016/j.ejogrb.2023.06.023. Epub 2023 Jun 24

216. Ferreira L, Abrantes C, Alves ME, Moreira C, Moreira H. Effects of exercise programs on cardiorespiratory fitness and arterial stiffness on postmenopausal women: a systematic review study. Maturitas. 2024;181:107917. https://doi.org/10.1016/j.maturitas.2024.107917. Epub 2024 Jan 19

217. Xi H, He Y, Niu Y, Sui X, Zhang J, Zhu R, et al. Effect of combined aerobic and resistance exercise on blood pressure in postmenopausal women: a systematic review and meta-analysis of randomized controlled trials. Exp Gerontol. 2021;155:111560. https://doi.org/10.1016/j.exger.2021.111560. Epub 2021 Sep 22

218. Manojlović M, Protić-Gava B, Maksimović N, Šćepanović T, Poček S, Roklicer R, et al. Effects of combined resistance and aerobic training on arterial stiffness in postmenopausal women: a systematic review. Int J Environ Res Public Health. 2021;18(18):9450. https://doi.org/10.3390/ijerph18189450.

22 Physiotherapy and Rehabilitation in Andropause

Betül Erbay, Gözde Tekin, and Esra Üzelpasacı

22.1 Introduction

While fertility rates are decreasing all over the world, the life expectancy of individuals is increasing, and the world is getting older. In recent years, healthy and active aging has gained importance in parallel with the increase in the life expectancy of individuals. The aging male population is threatened by chronic diseases associated with loss of function and reduced quality of life. Age-related diseases gain importance in this process. The transition from adulthood to old age in men marks a turning point, leading to numerous physiological, psychological, and social changes. Andropause, one of the most significant yet often unnoticed changes, refers to an age-related decline in testosterone levels in men, which becomes more common as the global population ages. Physiotherapy and rehabilitation practices have an important place as inexpensive, easily applicable, noninvasive, and effective methods in the prevention and treatment of sexual, physical, cardiometabolic, and psychological symptoms associated with andropause.

B. Erbay (✉)
Department of Therapy and Rehabilitation, Health Services Vocational School, Bartın University, Bartin, Türkiye
e-mail: berbay@bartin.edu.tr

G. Tekin
Healthcare Services Department, Vocational School of Health Services, Muş Alparslan University, Muş, Türkiye
e-mail: g.tekin@alparslan.edu.tr

E. Üzelpasacı
Gülhane Faculty of Physiotherapy and Rehabilitation, University of Health Sciences, Ankara, Türkiye
e-mail: esra.uzelpasaci@sbu.edu.tr

22.2 Definition of Andropause

The term andropause is a combination of the Greek words "andras" (male) and "pause" (stop). This term is used to describe the clinical picture in which there are physical and psychological changes due to decreased concentrations of androgen hormones in aging men, similar to menopause in women. The worsening of the general and sexual condition associated with decreased testosterone levels in men was first described by Hellers and Meyers in 1944 with the term "male climacteric." In the literature, the terms male menopause, androgen deficiency in the aging man, partial androgen deficiency in the aging man, aging man syndrome, hypogonadism, functional hypogonadism, and late-onset hypogonadism, which have been more accepted and used more frequently in the last two decades, are used instead of andropause. Despite all these different nomenclatures, the term andropause is basically a serious and complex syndrome for the aging male population, which negatively affects many organ functions and the quality of life of

T. Akbayrak, E. Üzelpasaci (eds.), *Physiotherapy and Rehabilitation in Pelvic and Women's Health-Related Problems*, https://doi.org/10.1007/978-3-032-28741-0_22

the individual, characterized by androgen deficiency [1].

Unlike the sharp and dramatic change in menopause in women, men do not experience a sudden stop in gonadal function. Andropause is characterized by an insidious onset and slow progression. Hypothalamus-pituitary-gonadal axis function gradually decreases with aging in men. As a result, testosterone levels decrease through both central (pituitary) and peripheral (testicular) mechanisms, resulting in a loss of the circadian rhythm of testosterone secretion [2, 3]. Conditions affecting the testes lead to primary hypogonadism, whereas issues with the hypothalamus or pituitary gland result in secondary hypogonadism. Additionally, hypogonadism may arise from problems that impact both the testes and the hypothalamus-pituitary axis. Both primary and secondary forms of hypogonadism result in diminished testosterone levels and complications related to sperm production. In addition, primary hypogonadism causes high gonadotropin levels, while secondary hypogonadism causes low or inappropriate gonadotropin levels. Causes of primary hypogonadism include Klinefelter syndrome, cryptorchidism, some types of cancer chemotherapy, trauma or radiation therapy to the testicles, HIV infection, anorchidism, and myotonic dystrophy. Causes of secondary hypogonadism include severe obesity, iron overload syndromes, nutritional deficiency/excessive exercise, some sleep problems, systemic disease, excessive alcohol consumption, organ failure (liver, heart, and lung), opioid/anabolic steroid/glucocorticoid use, and hypothalamic/pituitary tumors [4].

Circulating serum testosterone levels are progressively decreasing, and symptoms are thought to depend on the aging process. In a significant proportion of men over 50, testosterone levels fall below the threshold values typically used to diagnose testosterone deficiency in younger men. Studies show that approximately 25% of men over 70 years of age meet the laboratory criteria for hypogonadism [2, 3]. Furthermore, the aging process in men is associated with a decline in testosterone as well as other hormones such as melatonin, growth hormone, dehydroepiandrosterone (DHEA), and insulin-like growth factor-1 (IGF-1) [5].

Andropause can often be a silent threat to men's health after the age of 40. According to the European Male Ageing Study, which evaluated more than 3000 men, the incidence of andropause in men aged 40 to 79 is 2.1%. The European Study of Male Aging found the prevalence of andropause to be 0.1%, 0.6%, 3.2%, and 5.1% in men aged 40–49, 50–59, 60–69, and 70–79 years, respectively. Despite the high prevalence of low testosterone concentrations in older men (up to 68% in their 70s and up to 91% in their 80s and beyond), the clinical signs and symptoms of andropause may remain unnoticed in the early stages. Symptoms of andropause are usually mild and difficult to distinguish from those associated with normal aging [6, 7]. In aging men, hypogonadal conditions cause harmful effects on the metabolic functioning of many organs in the body and lead to serious health problems. The effects of decreased testosterone due to aging include sexual dysfunction, metabolic diseases, diabetes mellitus, cardiovascular diseases, osteoporosis, hypertension, hyperlipidemia, decreased physical performance, and an increased risk of kidney disease. In addition, all-cause mortality was found to be elevated in men with low testosterone levels [8].

The threshold of testosterone at which symptoms become evident varies from person to person, and many men are not symptomatic despite having low testosterone levels. A decrease in testosterone and other anabolic hormones in men from their mid-30 s may contribute to aging-related impairments in body functions (e.g., weakness, obesity, osteopenia, cognitive decline, and erectile failure), and testosterone deficiency in older men has been shown to be associated with an increased risk of death over the next 20 years, regardless of multiple risk factors and several preexisting health issues [9].

22.3 Andropause Diagnosis

The diagnosis of andropause requires the presence of both clinical symptoms and low serum testosterone levels. The European Study of Male Aging stated that the minimum criteria for the diagnosis of late-onset hypogonadism are a total testosterone level <11 nmol/L, a free testosterone level <220 pmol/L, and the presence of three sexual symptoms: decreased libido, impaired morning erections, and erectile dysfunction [10, 11]. Symptoms of late-onset hypogonadism include not only sexual symptoms but also a number of symptoms such as sarcopenia, muscle atrophy, increased body fat, type 2 diabetes, anemia, osteoporosis, depressive mood, impaired concentration, insomnia, daytime sleepiness, decreased vitality, sweating, and hot flashes. Although most of these symptoms are nonspecific, their severity may vary from person to person, and since these symptoms may have origins outside of andropause, the exclusion of other potential disease entities exclusion of other disease entities and subnormal serum testosterone levels is necessary for accurate diagnosis [12]. Diagnosis of andropause is difficult and complex because testosterone gradually decreases over several years and lacks easily identifiable signs and symptoms. Furthermore, the signs and symptoms of andropause are similar to or occur concurrently with other diseases of aging and may be misdiagnosed by clinicians or go unnoticed by patients [2].

22.4 Testosterone Physiology and Its Functions in the Body

Androgens are hormones synthesized from cholesterol in the testes (Leydig cells) and adrenal glands, which regulate primary and secondary sexual characteristics in men. Testosterone is the most potent and abundant androgen and is the primary male sex hormone. Testosterone is converted to two active metabolites in target cells: dihydrotestosterone (DHT) and estradiol. Dihydrotestosterone, which is more metabolically active than testosterone, is formed in the presence of the enzyme 5α-reductase in the liver, kidneys, skin, and prostate. Estradiol is formed in the liver, kidneys, brain, and adipose tissue. In adult men, the testicles produce about 95% of circulating testosterone, and the adrenal glands produce the remaining 5%. Approximately 98% of testosterone in a healthy man is bound to sex hormone-binding globulin (SHBG). The remaining 2% of circulating testosterone is bioavailable or free. Sex hormone-binding globulin increases with age, resulting in increased testosterone binding and less bioavailability of testosterone. Testosterone in the blood is regulated through negative feedback by a complex system between the hypothalamus, anterior pituitary, and testes. It releases gonadotropin-releasing hormone (GnRH), luteinizing hormone (LH), and follicle-stimulating hormone (FSH) secreted from the hypothalamus by the anterior pituitary. LH stimulates Leydig's interstitial cells in the testes to synthesize and secrete testosterone. Testosterone secretion occurs in pulsating bursts that reach their highest level in the morning and their lowest level in the evening, about six times a day [2, 13–15].

Testosterone plays an important role in the descent of the testicles during embryonic development, as well as in the development of male excretory ducts and external genital organs. The development of male genitals and masculine secondary sexual characteristics, such as broad shoulders, narrow hips, increased body hair, hardening of the skin, increased sebaceous gland secretion, and thickening of the voice in adolescence, is driven by testosterone and DHT. In addition, testosterone has a positive effect on sexual function, such as libido, arousal, and spermatogenesis, and plays a role in the formation of sexual behavior in men [16]. However, testosterone is not only a male sex hormone but also plays a key role in many important physiological effects across various organs in the body, beyond sexual function. The other physiological effects of testosterone in the body are summarized as follows [14]:

22.4.1 Bones

Testosterone has two key effects on bones. The first effect inhibits osteoclastic activity and bone resorption by converting to estradiol via the testosterone aromatase enzyme. Second, it stimulates osteoblastic activity and increases bone formation by converting to DHT through 5-α-reductase. Hypogonadal men face the risk of osteopenia or osteoporosis, which may result in fractures [16].

22.4.2 Muscles

Testosterone plays a role in maintaining normal muscle metabolism and muscle mass by promoting nitrogen retention in the body. Decreased muscle mass and strength in hypogonadal men may result in muscle weakness, fatigue, and risk of falling [16].

22.4.3 Cognition and Mood

Testosterone supports psychological traits linked to a positive mood and quality of life. Studies report that elderly men with low testosterone levels have a higher rate of irritability, decreased self-confidence, dysphoria, and depression than the healthy population. It is suggested that this is due to the involvement of testosterone, which affects mood, appetite, and serotonin release in its neuroactive activity and in the neuroplasticity processes of hippocampal formation. Testosterone's role in psychological factors is not limited to negative or positive mood. In addition, testosterone also plays a role in the emergence of diverse and complex behaviors such as unconscious fear, anxiety, social dominance, intergroup cooperation, and out-group hostility in the individual [17].

22.4.4 Erythropoiesis and Anemia

Testosterone is a hematopoiesis stimulator in the bone marrow and thus increases hematocrit. Testosterone levels of men with unexplained anemia should be measured [16].

22.4.5 Cardiovascular System

Testosterone plays an important role in cardiovascular homeostasis by exerting a cardioprotective effect with its activity on lean body mass, body composition, lipid profile, and insulin resistance. Several studies have shown a direct relationship between testosterone deficiency and increased risk of cardiovascular disease in men. In a large-scale meta-analysis, it was shown that individuals with cardiovascular disease had significantly lower testosterone and higher levels of 17β-estradiol [17]. In addition, the presence of other risk factors for early atherosclerosis, increased visceral adipose tissue, hyperinsulinemia, and myocardial infarction has been reported in hypogonadal men [16].

22.4.6 Autoimmune Disease

Testosterone is one of the body's natural anti-inflammatory agents through its inhibition of both the hormonal and cellular immune response. It is also responsible for the inhibition of inflammatory reactions in autoimmune rheumatic diseases [16].

22.5 Pathophysiology of Andropause

Andropause is a gradual process in men's lives, and its symptoms often manifest more prominently in middle age and beyond. Testosterone levels decrease by 1% per year with aging, and this decrease is more pronounced in the bioavailable testosterone due to changes in sex hormone-binding globulin (SHBG). In a 75-year-old male, the bioavailable testosterone level was found to be less than half that of a healthy male in the 20–30 age group. The rate of decline in testosterone levels is not the same for everyone, and there are many factors that influence this decline.

Age-related comorbidities such as diabetes, heart disease, kidney disease, obesity, metabolic syndrome, and glucocorticoid use, severe emotional stress, smoking, alcohol use, and some medications also play a role in lowering testosterone levels. Despite all these adverse factors, this decline in testosterone can be slowed down by the management of health and lifestyle factors [1, 9, 18].

The reasons for the decrease in testosterone production in men are multifactorial. The most common cause is the structural change or decrease in the number of testosterone-producing Leydig cells and decreased sensitivity to regulation by pituitary hormones such as luteinizing hormone (LH) [2]. Other causes that play a role in the pathophysiology of andropause include lifestyle factors such as age, body mass index (BMI), physical activity, smoking, and alcohol use. In contrast to female menopause, it is noteworthy that age-related decline in testosterone in older men is not inevitable and can be prevented by lifestyle modifications [19].

22.5.1 Age

In men, circulating testosterone reaches its highest concentration in the third decade of life and then gradually decreases with age. The annual decrease in testosterone ranges from 0.3% to 1.8%. Circulating testosterone concentrations remain within the reference range of young men in the majority of aging men and fall clearly into the hypogonadal range only in a small fraction of the elderly population [19]. While aging-related SHBG, follicle-stimulating hormone (FSH), and luteinizing hormone (LH) levels increase, free testosterone, bioavailable testosterone, and total testosterone decrease. Low TT and high LH levels indicate a decrease in Leydig cell mass or a decrease in the capacity to produce testosterone and a decrease in sensitivity to LH. Age-related FSH increase was independently associated with more androgen decrease, and high FSH levels were associated with low testicular volume [20]. The total number of Leydig cells decreases by about 50% between the ages of 20 and 80. Structural changes are observed in certain Leydig cells with aging in the testicles. It has been determined that there is a significant relationship between the number of Leydig cells whose function is impaired as a result of degenerative changes and the decrease in testosterone production. Despite the decrease in the number of functional Leydig cells due to aging, circulating testosterone concentrations remain within the physiological range in most aging men thanks to increased LH. Generally, in 1.8% of men over 70 years of age, Leydig cell capacity is eventually depleted, and primary hypogonadism occurs. Additionally, the function of the hypothalamus-pituitary-testicular (HPT) axis is affected by aging [19]. Additional factors that accompany aging, such as obesity, unhealthy lifestyle, and poor health, can disrupt the HPT axis, further exacerbating this age-related decline in testosterone concentrations [7].

22.5.2 Body Mass Index (BMI)

BMI is negatively associated with total testosterone, free testosterone, biologically active testosterone, and SHBG. This inverse relationship between SHBG and BMI is believed to be caused by the inhibition of SHBG hepatic synthesis due to hyperinsulinemia [20]. Furthermore, as an anabolic hormone, testosterone plays a role in reducing visceral adiposity and increasing lean body mass [17]. In men with a body mass index (BMI) >30 kg/m^2, serum testosterone is, on average, 30% lower than in men with a BMI <25 kg/m^2 at any age [21].

22.5.3 Physical Activity

Studies have found a nonlinear relationship between physical activity and testosterone. While high physical activity was associated with higher testosterone and extreme activity with lower testosterone, no relationship was found between moderate physical activity and testosterone. Excessive physical activity is associated with lower testosterone, considering that it causes degenerative changes in the hypothalamus-pituitary-gonadal axis [20].

22.5.4 Smoking and Alcohol Use

In smokers, higher total testosterone, free testosterone, biologically active testosterone, and SHBG were detected. Acute increases in LH caused by tobacco are blamed for this condition. In addition, the presence of lower body fat in smokers also supports the positive relationship between smoking and SHBG. A nonlinear relationship is reported between alcohol consumption and T. Moderate alcohol consumption (up to six drinks per week) is associated with an increase in total and free testosterone. In those who consume high levels of alcohol, a decrease in androgen levels is observed as a result of possible Leydig cell damage or hypothalamus-pituitary-gonadal axis damage [20].

22.6 Physiological Effects and Symptoms of Andropause

Testosterone plays a crucial role in the functioning of various systems and organs in aging men. In the aging man, circulating testosterone concentrations decrease by 0.3–1.8% per year. Testosterone deficiency is common in older men and is characterized by various signs and symptoms that can significantly impact the aging process and quality of life. There are many specific and non-specific symptoms and signs associated with the diagnosis of andropause in men and suggestive of androgen deficiency [19, 22] (Table 22.1). Although signs and symptoms are primarily related to sexual function, they may also include fatigue, muscle and joint pain, muscle atrophy, memory impairment, decreased mental focus, difficulty coping with stress, negative mood, sleep disorders, hot flashes, prostatitis, gynecomastia, anemia, short stature, anxiety, accelerated osteoporosis, and urinary frequency and incontinence. While most of these symptoms are nonspecific, they negatively affect both the mental and physical health and quality of life of men [9, 17].

Many signs and symptoms of andropause are multifactorial and can be associated with lifestyle factors, psychological factors, and normal aging. Therefore, these symptoms may also be observed in men with normal testosterone levels. Although it is commonly stated that testosterone decreases with age, more than 80% of men maintain normal testosterone levels in old age. The age-related increase in SHBG causes a decrease in free testosterone and bioavailable testosterone, but the increase in andropause rates in older men is primarily associated with an increase in the prevalence of obesity, type 2 diabetes mellitus, and chronic disease. Signs and symptoms of andropause vary greatly from person to person, depending on the age of on set, duration, severity, and underlying pathophysiology. Although the preva-

Table 22.1 Symptoms and findings associated with the diagnosis of andropause and suggestive of androgen deficiency

More specific symptoms	Less specific symptoms	Less specific signs
Decreased libido	Easy fatigue, decreased energy	Reduction in body and facial hair
Decreased spontaneous erections	Decreased physical activity, strength, and function	Increase in body fat, waist circumference, and BMI (obesity)
Erectile dysfunction	Decreased self-confidence and motivation	Decreased muscle mass
	Mood swings and irritability	Gynecomastia
	Decreased concentration and memory problems	Osteoporosis (loss of height, mildly traumatic fracture) /low bone density
	Insomnia and daytime sleepiness	Unexplained anemia
	Hot flashes	

lence of andropause increases with advancing age, it can occur in adult males of all ages. The more signs and symptoms a man has, the more likely he is to have true andropause [23]. There are many studies examining the symptoms and signs of andropause in different categories. In the literature, andropause signs and symptoms are generally examined under four main headings [23, 24].

- Sexual symptoms
- Physical symptoms
- Cardiometabolic symptoms
- Psychological symptoms

22.6.1 Sexual Symptoms

Sexual dysfunctions, especially low sexual desire, decreased morning and night erections, and erectile dysfunction, are at the forefront, showing symptoms suggestive of andropause, especially when they are related to each other. Delayed puberty, small testicles, infertility, decreased sexual activity, decreased frequency of sexual thought, delayed ejaculation, and decreased amount of ejaculate are also among the sexual symptoms [23].

22.6.2 Physical Symptoms

Decrease in body hair, gynecomastia, decrease in muscle mass and strength (sarcopenia), flushing or sweating, sleep disturbances, fatigue, osteoporosis, loss of height, and fractures with low trauma are examples of physical symptoms of andropause. Fine skin wrinkles can also be seen, especially around the mouth [23]. Sarcopenia adversely affects the ability to exercise, causing limitations in mobility. Furthermore, low testosterone concentrations are associated with low bone mineral density and high risk for osteoporotic fractures. After all, negative body composition exacerbates weakness and further increases morbidity and mortality [25]. Studies show that normal serum testosterone is essential for maintaining bone mineral density at various stages of life [26]. As men age, they are increasingly likely to experience sleep disorders, particularly sleep apnea. The literature indicates that sleep duration has an effect on testosterone levels in men. Reducing sleep duration to 5 h per day resulted in a 10–15% decrease in testosterone levels. However, the evidence confirming the effect of sleep deprivation or circadian rhythm disturbances on testosterone is inconclusive. Sleep deprivation may be a symptom of hypogonadism. In individuals with sleep deprivation and hypogonadism who were receiving hormone replacement therapy, sleep quality improved after a period of 12 months [27].

22.6.3 Cardiometabolic Symptoms

Cardiometabolic symptoms include increased body mass index or obesity, visceral obesity, metabolic syndrome, insulin resistance, and type 2 diabetes. Testosterone deficiency in men is often associated with increased waist circumference, obesity, metabolic syndrome, and impaired health. Especially visceral obesity, decreases in muscle mass, and bone mineral density are frequently observed. Obesity contributes to the development of metabolic syndrome and increases the risk of cardiovascular complications. Metabolic syndrome associated with andropause is an umbrella term encompassing associated comorbidities such as obesity, dyslipidemia, low high-density lipoprotein, hypertension, and type II diabetes mellitus and/or insulin resistance [7, 23, 28]. There exists an inverse correlation between testosterone levels and glucose metabolism. Conditions like metabolic syndrome and insulin resistance can lead to decreased serum testosterone, which, in turn, contributes to visceral fat buildup, further insulin resistance, and abnormal lipid levels. Research indicates that serum testosterone levels can be a strong predictor of metabolic syndrome and type 2 diabetes mellitus. Therefore, measuring serum testosterone should be part of the diagnostic process for assessing metabolic syndrome and type 2 diabetes [8].

A bidirectional relationship between hypogonadism and metabolic disorders has been reported in the literature. Decreased testosterone causes high expression of lipoprotein lipase and an increase in visceral adipose tissue. The accumulation of visceral adipose tissue causes the release of proinflammatory cytokines (TNF-α, IL-1β, leptin), which exert a direct inhibitory effect on both the hypothalamic-pituitary-gonadal (HPG) axis and the testicular Leydig cells responsible for testosterone production. In addition, visceral adipose tissue causes elevated levels of aromatase and leads to insulin resistance and reduces myogenesis through an androgen receptor-mediated pathway [28].

Overweight and obesity affect more than a third of men worldwide. Studies show that individuals who consume sugar-sweetened beverages with a high glycemic load experience a significant decrease in total testosterone and free testosterone. In addition, carbohydrate-rich diets instead of protein have been shown to increase testosterone and/or SHBG [28]. Obesity-associated hypogonadism is typically secondary hypogonadism, often referred to as male obesity-associated secondary hypogonadism. Various mechanisms have been proposed as the pathogenesis of secondary hypogonadism associated with male obesity, such as increased aromatase activity, adipokine production, and leptin resistance in the hypothalamus, which facilitates estradiol peripheral aromatization of T in adipose tissue. It is thought that the decrease in sex hormone-binding globulin (SHBG) levels previously shown in obese men also contributes to this situation by reducing total testosterone levels [29]. A study of 100 men with moderate to severe obesity found that about 45% of them were diagnosed with secondary hypogonadism associated with obesity [30]. Overall, weight loss has been linked to increased testosterone levels in men with hypogonadism [31]. In addition, excessive body mass causes higher cortisol levels and negatively affects testosterone levels. According to the hair analysis of people with different body mass, higher cortisol levels and lower testosterone levels were detected in obese people [27].

22.6.4 Psychological Symptoms

Mood changes such as anger, irritability, sadness, and depression, along with decreased quality of life, poor self-assessment of health, and impaired cognitive functions (including concentration, verbal memory, and spatial performance), are common [23]. Psychological stressors induce cortisol secretion, leading to a decrease in testosterone levels in the body. Although the physiological fluctuation of cortisol in the body does not disrupt the body's homeostasis, if cortisol levels exceed physiological values over a long period of time in the case of chronic stress, this causes negative consequences related to testosterone secretion. When cortisol levels are excessively high, membrane transport is impaired, oxidation potential increases, and catabolic reactions accelerate [27].

22.7 Differences and Similarities Between Andropause and Menopause

Menopause is defined as the cessation of spontaneous menstruation for 12 months in women. Worldwide, most women go through menopause between the ages of 49 and 52 [32]. It is accepted that women in the menopause process exhibit changes in behavior, thinking, and actions compared to other stages of their lives. However, this is not the case for men, who experience symptoms similar to those of female menopause. Although andropause symptoms are known to be caused by testosterone deficiency, there remain differing beliefs and uncertainties surrounding the condition [33].

Hormonal changes occur in both aging men and women. However, addressing andropausal changes similarly to those accompanying menopause remains a subject of debate today. In women, the hormonal function of the ovaries begins to disappear, which is associated with a loss of reproductive capacity, while in men, the hormonal function of the testicles is preserved into old age. Changes in gonadal hormone concentration in men are related to a decrease in testosterone concentration, are continuous, and show individual differences. Furthermore, the slow development of andropause, especially between the ages of 40 and 55, and the lack of clear evaluation criteria further complicate the situation. This suggests that these symptoms may result not only from hormonal changes but also from other factors associated with aging. There is debate about the safety of diagnosing andropause based solely on low testosterone levels. The literature indicates that certain chronic diseases and medications contribute to the decrease in testosterone concentration. Studies show that only a small group of men experience the severe symptoms of andropause. It is accepted that andropause occurs after the age of 50. The decrease in testosterone in men accelerates between the ages of 45 and 50, while menopause occurs in a more specific age range (usually after the age of 48), and the changes are more pronounced than in men. Hormonal changes in women begin as early as the age of 40, ultimately leading to the cessation of ovulation, which significantly impacts quality of life [34].

The biological mechanism of serum testosterone decline in aging men is distinct from that of menopause. Lower serum testosterone levels in older men can be explained, in part, by the aging of the neuroendocrine system and less efficient production of LH and testosterone by the testicle. A significant portion of the decline can be attributed to the effects of metabolic syndrome, particularly obesity, on testosterone production. The effects are not only limited to men of "menopausal" age but are also seen in younger men [8].

Although there are differences in the physiological mechanisms of andropause and menopause, some similar symptoms can be seen in both women and men. These symptoms can be summarized as follows:

- Decreased sexual desire and sexual activity
- Decreased bone mineral density and increased risk of osteoporosis
- Fat accumulation in the abdominal region
- Hot flashes and sweating
- Difficulty sleeping
- Increased psychological symptoms such as anxiety, depressive symptoms, nervousness, concentration problems, fatigue, inability to enjoy life, resentment, and mood swings
- Increased risk of cardiovascular diseases, such as diabetes and hypertension
- Elevation of cholesterol, triglyceride, and insulin levels [35]

22.8 Clinical Evaluation in Andropause

Hypogonadism is a clinical syndrome caused by a decrease in the production of androgens, especially in middle-aged and elderly men, and is linked to the appearance of sarcopenia. This syndrome is also observed in young men, leading to sexual dysfunctions [1]. Hypogonadism is associated with visceral obesity, metabolic syndrome, early atherosclerosis, type 2 diabetes, osteoporosis, decreased muscle mass, reduced energy levels, diminished mental focus, decreased ability to cope with stress, anxiety, and an increased frequency of incontinence. Although most of these symptoms are not specific, they negatively affect men's physical health and quality of life [36, 37].

According to the European Study of Male Aging, the minimum diagnostic criteria for andropause include: total testosterone levels below 11 nmol/L, free testosterone levels below 220 pmol/L, decreased libido, loss of morning erections, and at least three sexual symptoms such as erectile dysfunction. These findings are considered indicators of hormonal changes caused by aging [11].

The Androgen Decline in Aging Male Questionnaire (ADAM-Q), the Aging Male Symptom-Questionnaire (AMS-Q), and the Male Andropause Symptoms Self-Assessment Questionnaire (MASS-Q) are scales developed to assist in the evaluation and diagnosis of andropause in men. Despite their high sensitivity, these scales alone are not sufficient in the diagnosis of andropause due to their low specificity, and they should be supported by laboratory tests to confirm the diagnosis [38].

The Androgen Decline in Aging Male Questionnaire (ADAM-Q) has 88% sensitivity and 44% specificity. It consists of ten questions that assess the symptoms associated with low testosterone levels. Positive answers to the first and seventh questions, or any other three questions suggest the presence of andropause [39].

The Aging Male Symptom-Questionnaire (AMS-Q) has a 96% sensitivity and 30% specificity. It consists of 17 questions and three main headings: psychological, somatic, and sexual. Each question is scored between 1 and 5. A total score between 17 and 26 indicates that the individual is asymptomatic, meaning no obvious symptoms are experienced. A score between 27 and 36 indicates mild symptoms, a score between 37 and 49 indicates moderate symptoms, and a score above 50 indicates severe symptoms [40].

It evaluates the individual in terms of sexual, somatic, psychological, and behavioral aspects. The Cronbach α value of the scale was found to be 0.89, and the criterion validity was found to be 0.67, as reported by Asadollahi et al. MASS-Q consists of 25 questions. Each question is scored between 1 and 5. As the score increases, the severity of the symptoms experienced by the person increases. A score below 40 means "You probably don't need testosterone therapy," while a score between 40 and 84 is interpreted as "You may benefit from testosterone therapy." A score above 85 means "You are most likely to benefit from testosterone replacement therapy" [41, 42].

22.9 Physiotherapy and Rehabilitation in Individuals with Andropause

In line with the symptoms of andropause, it is necessary to take steps to alleviate and prevent the symptoms of this period and its negative effects on health. The role of physiotherapy and rehabilitation is crucial during andropause. Low-cost, side-effect-free physiotherapy methods that do not require advanced technology should be considered in the treatment of problems that occur during this period. In addition, it is an important advantage that physiotherapy methods can be applied together with other treatment options. Studies on the effectiveness of physiotherapy and rehabilitation for treating andropause-related symptoms are limited in the literature. Physiotherapy approaches recommended during this period include exercise training, breathing and relaxation exercises, and massage [43].

Before physiotherapy approaches are applied, clinical and physiotherapy evaluations of individuals should be made in detail.

22.9.1 Physiotherapy and Rehabilitation Evaluation in Andropause

The evaluation of a man in the period of andropause in terms of physiotherapy and rehabilitation covers various parameters, including the examination of both the problems that may arise due to andropause and the problems associated with aging.

22.9.1.1 History

In the physiotherapy evaluation process, the process typically begins with a comprehensive patient history. Starting the history-taking process with questions assessing the patient's mental status helps evaluate the reliability of their responses. The patient's complaints, medical history, social history, system inquiry for multifaceted and geriatric syndromes, nutritional status, family history, sexual history, and functional status should be reviewed. The drugs used and body mass index should be noted [44].

22.9.1.2 Evaluation of Cognitive Disorders

The prevalence of dementia increases in individuals over the age of 60. In the evaluation of a patient with possible dementia, the history-taking process is the most important stage. In this process, there is an opportunity to evaluate both close and distant memories while telling the patient's story. The progressive course of forgetfulness, language problems, personality changes, and psychiatric symptoms should definitely be evaluated [45].

It is recommended to apply standardized and validated screening tests in the evaluation of memory problems and dementia. The mini-mental state assessment test is the most commonly used test in the assessment. This test, which consists of 11 questions, is evaluated over 30 points. While 24 to 30 points are considered normal, 18 to 23 points are associated with mild dementia, and 17 points and below are associated with severe dementia [46].

22.9.1.3 Mood Assessment

Andropause is a stage in which a man experiences changes in his emotional health. A decrease in testosterone levels has been associated with a decrease in the capacity to cope with stress, negative mood, and sleep disorders [1]. A comparable number of studies have shown that depressed men have lower testosterone levels compared to controls. However, some studies have revealed that there is no difference in testosterone levels between depressed individuals and controls. No studies have reported higher testosterone levels in the depressed state [47, 48].

In men with andropause, standardized questionnaires, including the Beck Depression Inventory, Hamilton Depression Scale, and Hamilton Anxiety Scale, can be used to evaluate mood [49, 50].

22.9.1.4 Evaluation of Sexual Life

Andropause can present sexual challenges in some individuals. Male sexual dysfunction can include a wide range of issues, from low libido to erectile dysfunction, premature ejaculation, and others [10].

The International Erectile Function Index and the Sexual Health Inventory for Men (SHIM) scales can be used to evaluate erectile function in men [51, 52].

22.9.1.5 Evaluation of Muscle Strength

Muscle mass loss occurs in men as a result of andropause, and muscle strength should be evaluated [53]. Manual muscle testing, dynamometric methods, or isokinetic devices can be used to evaluate muscle strength [54].

22.9.1.6 Evaluation of the Cardiopulmonary System

Low androgen levels have been associated with increased rates of cardiovascular diseases in men [55]. Therefore, heart rate, respiratory rate, systolic and diastolic blood pressure, and O_2 saturation should be evaluated before and after exercise.

Exercise tests are essential for evaluating the cardiopulmonary system. The 12-m walking test, bicycle ergometer, and 6-m walking test are frequently used in clinics. The 6-m walking test is considered a valid and reliable test to assess the exercise capacity of patients with chronic heart failure and chronic obstructive pulmonary disease. It is preferred due to its ease of use and reliability [56].

The cardiopulmonary exercise test (CPET) is a maximal exercise test with simultaneous gas exchange analysis, providing a comprehensive assessment of physiological responses to exercise and cardiovascular fitness. Noninvasive determination of direct oxygen uptake and carbon dioxide output during rest and exercise provides accurate and reproducible data on ventilation, gas exchange, and interaction of cardiovascular and musculoskeletal system functions and enables the determination of deviations from normal [57].

22.9.1.7 Evaluation of Physical Activity

Studies show that there is a relationship between a decrease in serum testosterone levels and a decrease in physical activity levels in men [58]. Physical activity logs, accelerometers, pedometers, or questionnaires can be used to evaluate the level of physical activity. The most frequently used questionnaire in the evaluation is the International Physical Activity Questionnaire (IPAQ) [59].

22.9.1.8 Evaluation of Urinary Incontinence

Individuals should be evaluated for urinary incontinence. Three-day bladder diaries, pad tests, or questionnaires can be used for evaluation. The Incontinence Severity Index (ISI) can be used to assess the extent of urinary incontinence [60].

22.9.1.9 Assessment of Quality of Life

In men with andropause, decreased energy levels, deterioration in sexual performance, and mood changes contribute to a reduced quality of life [61]. The Nottingham Health Profile (NSP), Short Form-36 (SF-36), or King's Health Questionnaire can be used to assess quality of life [62, 63].

22.9.2 Physiotherapy and Rehabilitation

22.9.2.1 Patient Training

Patient education should constitute the first step of treatment in order for individuals to effectively manage the treatment adherence process and symptoms. Effective patient education should be tailored to the needs, age, condition, expectations, and sociocultural characteristics of the individual. The goals of patient education are to inform the individual about the disease, its symptoms, and risk factors; to explain the treatment process; and to promote healthy living habits. In particular, individuals with insulin resistance, obesity, decreased bone mineral density, arterial hypertension, and metabolic syndrome, as risk factors for andropause, should be encouraged to improve their nutrition and physical activity levels [53].

Studies show that men over 40 have low awareness of andropause. Training on andropause should be provided in community health centers, universities, and other public platforms to raise awareness about this important issue [64].

22.9.2.2 Massage Therapy

Massage therapy provides relaxation, improving body functions and overall health through targeted manipulation of muscles and connective tissue. This technique focuses on applying pressure to muscles, tendons, ligaments, skin, joints, lymph vessels, and other connective tissues. The benefits of massage include activating the parasympathetic nervous system, reducing anxiety, improving blood circulation, regulating blood pressure, relieving fatigue, and strengthening immune function. Research suggests that massage therapy reduces cortisol levels, relieves pain, improves immune response, and reduces symptoms of depression [65].

Studies conducted on women with menopause suggest that massage therapy reduces hot flashes and has positive effects on mental health, body image, and quality of life [66, 67]. There are no studies proving the effectiveness of massage therapy in men with andropause. However, massage therapy may be beneficial in mood and sleep disorders that are frequently seen during andropause. Further studies are needed to confirm the effectiveness of massage therapy during andropause.

22.9.2.3 Relaxation Training

Relaxation training involves a variety of practices, such as progressive muscle relaxation and diaphragm breathing, to reduce somatic tension or uncomfortable thoughts. It is easy to implement [68]. Relaxation techniques are effectively applied in the treatment of many health problems, such as sleep disorders, headaches, cancer treatment, asthma, and clinical depression [69, 70]. In recent years, relaxation training has been included in treatment programs aimed at relieving menopausal symptoms in women. Clinical studies have shown that progressive relaxation techniques are useful in relieving menopausal symptoms [71, 72]. It is believed that these methods could also be effective in treating symptoms of andropause, which share similarities with those of menopause. Further studies are needed to confirm the effectiveness of relaxation training during andropause.

22.9.2.4 Low-Energy Shockwave Therapy (LESWT)

Recently, the use of LESWT in the treatment of erectile dysfunction has become increasingly widespread thanks to the increase in data on its effectiveness. It is assumed that the shock wave can increase penile blood flow and improve endothelial function by stimulating angiogenesis in the corpus cavernosum [73]. However, in studies evaluating the efficacy of LESWT in erectile dysfunction, individuals with hypogonadism were excluded. In only one study, individuals with hypogonadism were not excluded, and it was observed that erectile function increased [74]. Therefore, considering the effect of testosterone on erectile function, there is a need for studies evaluating the effects of LESWT on erectile dysfunction in individuals with hypogonadism [75].

22.9.2.5 Exercise Training

Symptoms associated with andropause should be reviewed before planning exercise training. Exercise training may be useful in improving sarcopenia, cardiovascular diseases, decreased bone mineral density, insulin resistance, obesity, mood disorders, and cognitive decline associated with andropause. After a detailed evaluation of the individual's symptoms and condition, personalized exercise programs should be developed. In addition, group exercises may be recommended, when appropriate, to increase social interaction among individuals [76].

22.9.2.5.1 Aerobic Training

Aerobic exercise training refers to exercises in which the body's large muscles move rhythmically over long periods of time. It includes activities such as walking, swimming, dancing, tennis, and cycling. Aerobic exercises are endurance activities that do not require excessive speed or force. However, aerobic exercise requires changes in parameters such as heart rate, blood pressure, and respiratory frequency to meet the demands of the cardiovascular system during increased workloads [77].

Aerobic exercises reduce total cholesterol, triglycerides, and low-density lipoproteins; reduce adipose tissue; increase muscle tissue; and improve sexual functions [78, 79]. At the same time, aerobic exercises help reduce depression through hormonal changes. It reduces the risk of developing diseases such as coronary artery disease, hypertension, type 2 diabetes, and osteoporosis [80].

In men, exercise stimulates testosterone production from the testicles [81]. However, high-intensity exercise or lack of exercise may cause a decrease in testosterone levels. Therefore, it is recommended to start with moderate-intensity exercise for 30 m three times a week for men in the andropause period [76].

One of the most important risk factors associated with andropause is secondary osteoporosis. Aerobic exercises and muscle contraction during physical activity, as well as increased muscle mass, exert an anabolic effect on bone through mechanical load. Exercise may increase serum testosterone levels after a short time, thus serum testosterone may prevent bone loss [82]. For all these reasons, prescribing physical activity and exercise to guarantee bone health and prevent fractures may be part of the therapeutic approach for older men with andropause.

There are a few studies examining the effectiveness of aerobic exercise in men in the andropause period. In the study conducted by Stout MSc et al., it was shown that combining testosterone therapy and exercise rehabilitation in male patients with chronic heart failure and low testosterone levels had positive effects, such as increased exercise capacity, decreased body mass index, and increased hand grip strength [83]. In their study, Chasland et al. revealed that a regular exercise program is more effective than testosterone therapy to improve body composition and strength in middle-aged men with slightly low testosterone levels [84]. In the study conducted by Lovell et al., it was observed that cortisol levels decreased while testosterone levels increased during exercise in elderly men who exercised regularly. They reported that the positive effects of exercise on hormonal levels were partially lost in men who stopped exercising [85].

22.9.2.5.2 Resistance Training

In men with andropause, loss of muscle strength, sarcopenia, and a decrease in bone mineral density occur. Strength is required to perform daily activities, maintain/improve functional capacity, and reduce disability. To achieve these goals,

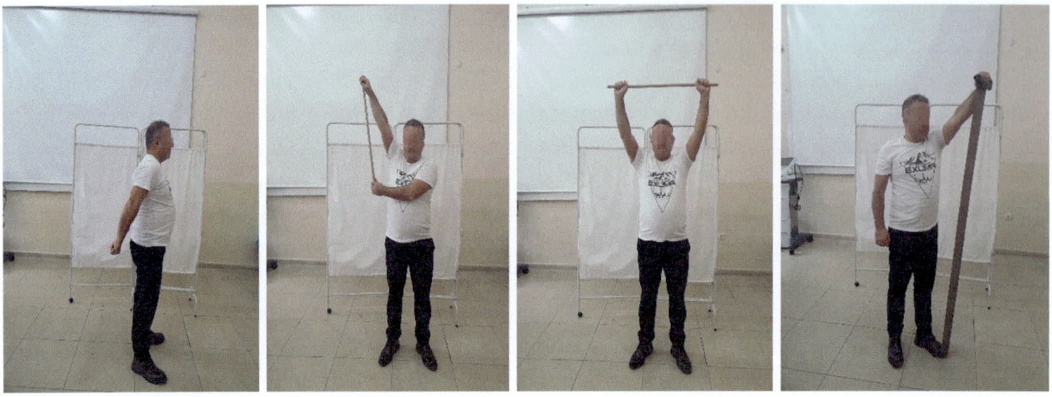

Fig. 22.1 Example strengthening exercise applications

resistance exercises should be included in the exercise program of individuals. Resistance exercises involve working muscles against a certain load using equipment such as body weight, exercise balls, free weights, and elastic bands (Fig. 22.1). Resistance exercises are considered one of the most effective strategies for promoting muscle hypertrophy and improving muscle function and strength in older adults [86, 87].

Resistance exercises aimed at maintaining and increasing muscle mass in aging men are more effective than testosterone replacement therapy alone. In a study conducted by Kerry L. Hildreth et al., it was reported that resistance exercises were effective in improving body composition and strength in elderly men with low testosterone levels, and testosterone supplementation could provide additional benefits in body composition, but its effect on functional performance and strength was limited [88].

Resistance training plays a crucial role in regulating testosterone levels in the blood [89]. Exercise-induced changes in testosterone levels are generally more closely associated with moderate- and high-intensity exercises. When the number of repetitions remains constant, higher intensity resistance exercises lead to a more pronounced increase in testosterone levels. In order to support testosterone increase with exercise, it is important to diversify the muscle groups exercised [90].

22.9.2.5.3 Balance and Proprioception Exercises

Recurrent falls are common among aging individuals and pose a significant healthcare burden. A decrease in serum testosterone levels leads to muscle strength loss, sarcopenia, and a decline in physical performance, resulting in an increased risk of falling. In a study, a gradual increase was observed in the risk of falling with lower testosterone levels. The severity of injuries from falls varies significantly, from minor skin injuries to major fractures and, in some cases, fatal traumas [91].

In order to maintain independence in men in the andropause period, it is very important to increase physical function, improve balance, and reduce the risk of falls and fractures. Simple balance exercises on the floor, exercises using an exercise ball, and balance board exercises can be incorporated into the exercise program to support the development of balance and proprioception (Fig. 22.2). Advanced studies examining the effectiveness of balance and proprioception exercises in men in the andropause period are needed in the literature [76].

22.9.2.5.4 Pelvic Floor Muscle Training

Testosterone deficiency is associated with erectile dysfunction, spontaneous loss of erection, hypoactive sexual desire, urinary incontinence, and a positive relationship with overactive blad-

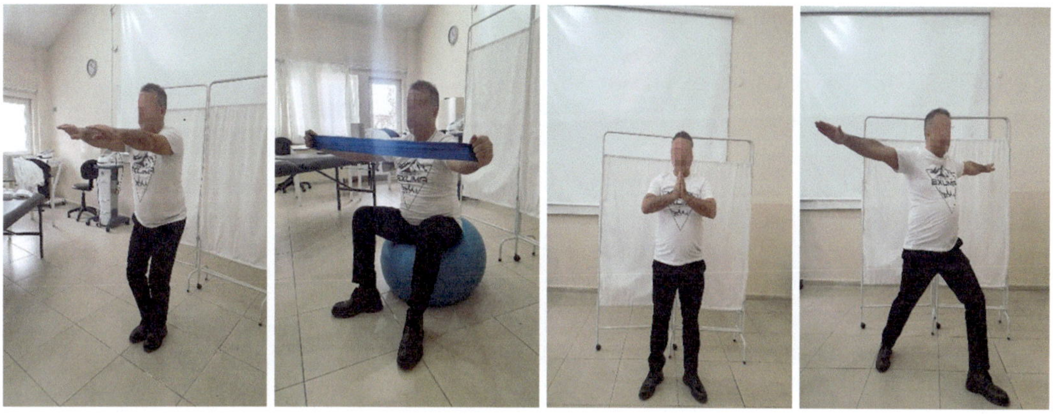

Fig. 22.2 Example balance and proprioception exercise applications

der [1]. A study has reported that hypogonadism causes a decrease in the width of the bulbocavernosus, ischiocavernosus, and levator ani muscles [92].

Pelvic floor muscle training increases urethral closure pressure, allowing stress urinary incontinence to heal and inhibiting involuntary detrusor contractions. The function of the pelvic floor muscles is associated with erectile function. Especially the bulbocavernous and ischiavernous muscles play an important role in the erectile process. These muscles become active during penile erection, contracting and increasing penile stiffness, thus allowing intracorporeal pressure to exceed systemic systolic pressure. It can also improve sexual function by increasing blood flow to the penis, enhancing sensory perception, and delaying ejaculation. Therefore, pelvic floor muscle exercises offer a non-pharmacological approach to addressing sexual dysfunction in men [93].

22.9.2.5.5 In-Water Exercises

In-water exercises help apply postural corrections more comfortably by reducing the load on the spine and other joints. The tension on the surface of the water and the internal friction (viscosity) between the water molecules create the water resistance. Water resistance makes the aquatic environment ideal for exercise. It stimulates turbulence, proprioception, and balance reactions caused by movement in water and reduces the load-bearing effect on bones. Research shows that high-intensity in-water exercise programs improve physical conditioning and body balance and reduce fall rates [94].

Resistance training in water has been shown to increase salivary testosterone levels in both young and older adults. Water-based exercise, which focuses on strength development, has been found to lead to a more pronounced and acute increase in salivary testosterone levels than water-based aerobic exercises due to the higher intensity used [95]. Therefore, it is important to schedule intensive training sessions to stimulate anabolic hormones to increase strength and possibly muscle mass, especially in elderly individuals [96].

22.9.2.5.6 Dual Task Exercises

Cognitive problems such as forgetfulness, difficulty focusing, and decision-making difficulties may also occur in men in the andropause period. In a study by Yaffe et al., it was suggested that there is a relationship between testosterone level and cognitive capacity. However, it has not yet been fully clarified whether this relationship is due to the aging process or low testosterone levels [97]. Cognitive-motor dual task is defined as the simultaneous completion of cognitive and motor tasks. Cognitive-motor intervention refers to the overload of attention abilities, resulting in a decrease in the performance of one or both tasks. Aging is associated with a decrease in motor and cognitive functions or an increased risk of falling with increased cognitive-motor intervention [98]. For this reason, in recent years, interventions that require the performance of a simultaneous motor and cognitive task have been used in studies. These studies have shown that dual task exercises can increase balance, walking speed, and cognitive performance, and consequently reduce the risk of falling [99].

22.9.3 Points to Consider in Exercise Training in Men in the Andropause Period

There are some important points to be considered in the exercise programs prepared for men in the andropause period. First, it is important to determine whether the individual has previously received testosterone replacement therapy or is currently undergoing it. While such hormone therapies can improve the quality of life in men with low testosterone levels in many ways, they may also pose certain risks during exercise. The most common risks include increased hematocrit levels and edema. Elevated hematocrit levels may cause an increase in heart rate and blood pressure, affecting cardiovascular responses to exercise. This has the potential to increase the risk of stroke and myocardial infarction. Therefore, a history of testosterone replacement therapy should be carefully assessed before establishing an exercise program to assess cardiovascular risks in men in the andropause period, and the program should be planned individually, in a controlled manner. In addition, dietary habits should be assessed when designing an exercise program. Adequate protein intake and balanced carbohydrate consumption should be ensured for the effectiveness of the exercise program, as malnutrition can be a limiting factor in participation in exercise in older men in the andropause period. In terms of overcoming this barrier and the sustainability of the program, it will be beneficial to direct individuals to the dietitian [76].

22.10 Conclusion

Andropause is defined as an age-related decline in testosterone levels in men, becoming more common as the global population ages. With andropause, symptoms such as low sexual desire, reduced morning and night erections, erectile dysfunction, premature ejaculation, loss of muscle mass and strength (sarcopenia), fever, sweating, sleep disturbances, fatigue, osteoporosis, increased body mass index or obesity, visceral obesity, metabolic syndrome, insulin resistance, anger, irritability, sadness, and depression can occur in men. Physiotherapy and rehabilitation practices play an important role in the prevention and management of these symptoms. Physiotherapy and rehabilitation approaches, which have no side effects and do not require advanced equipment when delivered by skilled, cost-effective physiotherapists, should be considered for managing the issues associated with this period and, if possible, should be preferred as the first option after a comprehensive evaluation. In addition, the fact that physiotherapy approaches can be used in combination with other treatment methods offers an important advantage. However, there is a limited number of studies in the literature investigating the effectiveness of physiotherapy and rehabilitation practices during andropause, and more randomized controlled trials are needed in this area.

References

1. Singh P. Andropause: current concepts. Ind J Endocrinol Metab. 2013;17(Suppl 3):S621–9.
2. Harvey J, Berry JA. Andropause in the aging male. J Nurse Pract. 2009;5(3):207–12.
3. Seidman SN. Androgens and the aging male. Psychopharmacol Bull. 2007;40(4):205–18.
4. Bhasin S, Brito JP, Cunningham GR, Hayes FJ, Hodis HN, Matsumoto AM, et al. Testosterone therapy in men with hypogonadism: an endocrine society clinical practice guideline. J Clin Endocrinol Metabol. 2018;103(5):1715–44.
5. Schreiber G, Ziemer M. The aging male–diagnosis and therapy of late-onset hypogonadism. JDDG: J Dtsch Dermatol Ges. 2008;6(4):273–9.
6. Nikjou R, Ajri-Khameslou M, Jegargoosheh S, Momeni P, Nemati-Vakilabad R. The severity of andropause symptoms and its relationship with social

well-being among retired male nurses: a preliminary cross-sectional study. BMC Geriatr. 2024;24(1):184.
7. Kanakis GA, Goulis DG. Addressing andropause: challenges and strategies for healthy aging in men. Maturitas. 2024;192:108041.
8. Saad F, Gooren LJ. Late onset hypogonadism of men is not equivalent to the menopause. Maturitas. 2014;79(1):52–7.
9. Rezaei N, Azadi A, Pakzad R. Prevalence of andropause among Iranian men and its relationship with quality of life. Aging Male. 2020;23:369.
10. Wu FC, Tajar A, Beynon JM, Pye SR, Silman AJ, Finn JD, et al. Identification of late-onset hypogonadism in middle-aged and elderly men. N Engl J Med. 2010;363(2):123–35.
11. Tajar A, Huhtaniemi IT, O'Neill TW, Finn JD, Pye SR, Lee DM, et al. Characteristics of androgen deficiency in late-onset hypogonadism: results from the European male aging study (EMAS). J Clin Endocrinol. 2012;97(5):1508–16.
12. Nieschlag E. Late-onset hypogonadism: a concept comes of age. Andrology. 2020;8(6):1506–11.
13. Baulieu EE. Androgens and aging men. Mol Cell Endocrinol. 2002;198(1–2):41–9.
14. Bansal V. Andropause a clinical entity. J Univ Coll Med Sci. 2013;1(2):54–68.
15. Seidman S. Normative hypogonadism and depression: does 'andropause' exist? Int J Impot Res. 2006;18(5):415–22.
16. Bain J. The many faces of testosterone. Clin Interv Aging. 2007;2(4):567–76.
17. Barone B, Napolitano L, Abate M, Cirillo L, Reccia P, Passaro F, et al. The role of testosterone in the elderly: what do we know? Int J Mol Sci. 2022;23(7):3535.
18. Mohammadi M, Allahverdipour H, Ghanbari Moghaddam A, Matlabi H. The prevalence of andropause and its relationship with sexual quality of life among older Iranian men. Am J Mens Health. 2023;17(2):15579883231161050.
19. Huhtaniemi IT, Wu FC. Ageing male (part I): pathophysiology and diagnosis of functional hypogonadism. Best Pract Res Clin Endocrinol Metab. 2022;36(4):101622.
20. Samaras N, Frangos E, Forster A, Lang PO, Samaras D. Andropause: a review of the definition and treatment. Eur Geriatr Med. 2012;3(6):368–73.
21. Jakiel G, Makara-Studzińska M, Ciebiera M, Słabuszewska-Jóźwiak A. Andropause–state of the art 2015 and review of selected aspects. Menopause Rev/Przegląd Menopauzalny. 2015;14(1):1–6.
22. Corona G, Goulis DG, Huhtaniemi I, Zitzmann M, Toppari J, Forti G, et al. European academy of andrology (EAA) guidelines on investigation, treatment and monitoring of functional hypogonadism in males: endorsing organization: European society of endocrinology. Andrology. 2020;8(5):970–87.
23. Hackett G, Kirby M, Edwards D, Jones TH, Wylie K, Ossei-Gerning N, et al. British Society for Sexual Medicine guidelines on adult testosterone deficiency, with statements for UK practice. J Sex Med. 2017;14(12):1504–23.
24. Giagulli VA, Castellana M, Lisco G, Triggiani V. Critical evaluation of different available guidelines for late-onset hypogonadism. Andrology. 2020;8(6):1628–41.
25. Lane D, L. Stovall J. Effects of testosterone replacement therapy on cognitive function in older men. J Clin Endocrinol Metab. 2019;104(4):1185–95.
26. Popovic V, M.D. Vukic A. Andropause: clinical and biological aspects. Maturitas. 2018;112:74–9.
27. Kim S, Seale RJ, S. FA. Testosterone and its implications for cardiovascular health. Endocr Rev. 2017;38(5):434–54.
28. Rosner W, H. P. Castracane A. The role of testosterone in the aging male. Mol Cell Endocrinol. 2015;405:121–35.
29. Zegers S, Goulis DG. Andropause and the metabolic syndrome. Diabetes Metab. 2020;46(3):185–93.
30. Marsh JW, Caruso MD, B. Testosterone supplementation and age-related decline in men's health. J Aging Health. 2022;34(3):316–30.
31. Dobs AS, Storer FS. The androgen effects on male health. J Androl. 2014;25(2):206–15.
32. Holman MS, D. J. Holt P. Hypogonadism and its impact on mental health. Psychiatry Res. 2021;301:113–20.
33. Hamilton JR, P. S. Marks G. Testosterone replacement in men with low levels: a systematic review of the evidence. J Clin Endocrinol Metab. 2022;107(4):1082–90.
34. Allen S, Wolk RR. The effects of testosterone in elderly men: a review of the literature. Endocrinol Metab Clin. 2019;48(2):249–58.
35. Chen S, L. R. M. Green L. Andropause and quality of life in older men. Geriatr Psychiatry. 2017;15(2):111–20.
36. Stevens P, K. Harris E. Clinical and therapeutic approaches to andropause: a comprehensive overview. Ageing Res Rev. 2018;46:35–41.
37. Morales AD, Gonzalez-Carreno P. The relationship between testosterone therapy and cardiovascular events in older men: a meta-analysis. Cardiovascular Reviews. 2021;32(4):467–76.
38. Taylor D, F. M. Yung M. Mechanisms of androgen action in aging and age-related diseases. Current Opinion in Geriatric Medicine. 2020;28(6):441–9.
39. Bertoldo ML, M. Trivedi L. Understanding testosterone regulation and the role in late-life depression. Am J Psychiatry. 2023;180(8):638–44.
40. Cummings S, Hughes PG, D. Aging and androgen decline: a comprehensive review. Endocr Pract. 2024;30(2):214–26.
41. Asadollahi A, Saberi LF, Faraji N. Validity and reliability of male andropause symptoms self-assessment questionnaire among elderly males in Khuzestan province of Iran. J Midlife Health. 2013;4:233–7.
42. Çetin AM, Baylan B, Imamoglu MA, Akbayrak T. Validity and reliability of the Turkish male andropause symptoms self-assessment questionnaire. J Mid-life Health. 2023;14(1):21–7.
43. Bacevičienė R, Valonytė L, Čeponis J. The effect of physiotherapy in addition to testosterone replacement

therapy on the efficiency of the motor system in men with hypogonadism. Medicina. 2013;49(2):13.
44. Savaş S, Akçiçek F. Kapsamlı geriatrik değerlendirme. Ege Tıp Dergisi. 2010;49(3):19–30.
45. Sink KM, Yaffe K. Cognitive impairment and dementia. In: Landefeld CS, Palmer RM, Johnson MA, et al., editors. Current geriatric diagnosis and treatment. Columbus: McGraw-Hill; 2004. p. 60–73.
46. Folstein MF, Folstein SE, McHugh PR. "Mini-mental state". A practical method for grading the cognitive state of patients for the clinician. J Psychiatr Res. 1975;12(3):189–98.
47. Fischer S, Ehlert U, Amiel Castro R. Hormones of the hypothalamic-pituitary-gonadal (HPG) axis in male depressive disorders - a systematic review and meta-analysis. Front Neuroendocrinol. 2019;55:100792.
48. Khera M, Bhattacharya RK, Blick G, et al. The effect of testosterone supplementation on depression symptoms in hypogonadal men from the Testim registry in the US (TRiUS). Aging Male. 2012;15:14–21.
49. Aydogan U, Aydogdu A, Akbulut H, Sonmez A, Yuksel S, Basaran Y, et al. Increased frequency of anxiety, depression, quality of life and sexual life in young hypogonadotropic hypogonadal males and impacts of testosterone replacement therapy on these conditions. Endocr J. 2012;59(12):1099–105.
50. Wilkinson P, Ruane C, Tempest K. Depression in older adults. Br Med J Publ Group; 2018.
51. Rosen RC, Cappelleri JC, Smith MD, et al. Constructing and evaluating the 'sexual health inventory for men: IIEF-5' as a diagnostic tool for erectile dysfunction (ED). Int J Impot Res. 1998;10(Suppl 3):Abstract 256, 35.
52. Alwaal A, Awad M, Boggs N, et al. Sexual health inventory for men questionnaire as a screening method for erectile dysfunction in a general urology clinic. Sex Med. 2020;8:660–3.
53. Lunenfeld B, Mskhalaya G, Zitzmann M, Arver S, Kalinchenko S, Tishova Y, Morgentaler A. Recommendations on the diagnosis, treatment and monitoring of hypogonadism in men. Aging Male. 2015;18(1):5–15.
54. Toraman NF. Yaşlılarda kas ve iskelet sistemi sorunları. GeroFam. 2011;2(2):1–17.
55. Armeni E, Lambrinoudaki I. Androgens and cardiovascular disease in women and men. Maturitas. 2017;104:54–72.
56. Bautmans I, Lambert M, Mets T. The six-minute walk test in community dwelling elderly: influence of health status. BMC Geriatr. 2004;4(6) 1–9.
57. Glaab T, Taube C. Practical guide to cardiopulmonary exercise testing in adults. Respir Res. 2022;12(23):9.
58. Wu FCW, Tajar A, Pye SR, Silman AJ, Finn JD, O'Neill TW, et al. Hypothalamic-pituitary-testicular axis disruptions in older men are differentially linked to age and modifiable risk factors: the European male aging study. J Clin Endocrinol Metabol. 2008;93(7):2737–45.
59. Van Poppel MNM, Chinapaw MJM, Mokkink LB, van Mechelen W, Terwee CB. Physical activity questionnaires for adults. Sports Med. 2010;40(7):565–600.
60. Martin JL, Williams KS, Abrams KR, Turner DA, Sutton AJ, Chapple C, Assassa RP, Shaw C. Systematic review and evaluation of methods of assessing urinary incontinence. Health Technol Assess. 2006;10(6):1.
61. Haren MT, Kim MJ, Tariq SH, Wittert GA, Morley JE. Andropause: a quality-of-life issue in older males. Med Clin North Am. 2006;90(5):1005–23.
62. Shiraishi K, Oka S, Matsuyama H. Assessment of quality of life during gonadotrophin treatment for male hypogonadotrophic hypogonadism. Clin Endocrinol. 2014;81(2):259–65.
63. Haywood K, Garratt A, Fitzpatrick R. Quality of life in older people: a structured review of generic self-assessed health instruments. Qual Life Res. 2005;14(7):1651–68.
64. Samipoor F, Pakseresht S, Rezasoltani P, Kazemnajad Leili E. Awareness and experience of andropause symptoms in men referring to health centers: a cross-sectional study in Iran. Aging Male. 2017:1–8.
65. Murphy JT. A review of complementary and alternative care for infertility issues. J Clin Chiropractic Pediatr. 2010;11(2):804–10.
66. Mehrnoush V, Darsareh F, Roozbeh N, Ziraeie A. Efficacy of the complementary and alternative therapies for the management of psychological symptoms of menopause: a systematic review of randomized controlled trials. J Menopausal Med. 2021;14(3):115–31.
67. Espí-López GV, Monzani L, Gabaldón-García E, Zurriaga R. The beneficial effects of therapeutic craniofacial massage on quality of life, mental health and menopausal symptoms and body image: a randomized controlled clinical trial. Complement Ther Med. 2020;51:102415.
68. Bernstein DA, Borkovec TD. Progressive relaxation training: a manual for the helping professions. Champaign, Illinois: Research Press; 1973.
69. Wang Y, Yang L, Lin G, Huang B, Sheng X, Wang L, Chen L, Qiu X, Wu X, Lin R. The efficacy of progressive muscle relaxation training on cancer-related fatigue and quality of life in patients with cancer: a systematic review and meta-analysis of randomized controlled studies. Int J Nurs Stud. 2024;152:104694.
70. Cooley C, Park Y, Ajilore O, Leow A, Nyenhuis SM. Impact of interventions targeting anxiety and depression in adults with asthma. J Asthma. 2020:1–24.
71. Aksu SP, Erenel AŞ. Effects of health education and progressive muscle relaxation on vasomotor symptoms and insomnia in perimenopausal women: a randomized controlled trial. Patient Educ Couns. 2022;105(11):3279–86.
72. Karaman A, Karakaş D, Aslan R. Impact of progressive muscle relaxation on anxiety and depression levels among the elderly: a systematic review and meta-analysis. Aging Ment Health. 2023;27(1):30–40.

73. Chisholm D, Stone T. Anxiety and depression in the elderly: a review. J Geriatr Psychiatry Neurol. 2019;32(3):157–65.
74. Sramkova T, Motil I, Jarkovsky J, Sramkova K. Erectile dysfunction treatment using focused linear low-intensity extracorporeal shockwaves: single-blind, sham-controlled, randomized clinical trial. Urol Int. 2019;104(5–6):417–24.
75. Kałka D, Biernikiewicz M, Gebala J, Sobieszczańska M, Jakima S, Pilecki W, Rusiecki L. Diagnosis of hypogonadism in patients treated with low energy shock wave therapy for erectile dysfunction: a narrative review. Transl Androl Urol. 2020;9(6):2786–96.
76. Janot JM. Andropause: man's problem for the ages. Male menopause currently affects up to 10 million American men, who can benefit from a customized exercise program. IDEA Fit J. 2005;2(5):52–60.
77. Voet NB, van der Kooi EL, Riphagen II, Lindeman E, van Engelen BG, Geurts AC. Strength training and aerobic exercise training for muscle disease. Cochrane Database Syst Rev. 2013;2013(7):CD003907.
78. Unnikrishnan R. Aquatic exercise as an adjunct therapy for erectile dysfunction: a narrative review. Asian J Pharm Res Health Care. 2022;14(3):142–8.
79. Misic MM, Rosengren KS, Woods JA, Evans EM. Muscle quality, aerobic fitness and fat mass predict lower-extremity physical function in community-dwelling older adults. Gerontology. 2007;53(5):260–6.
80. Jerome L, Fleg E. Aerobic exercise in the elderly: a key to successful aging. Discov Med. 2012;13(70):223–8.
81. Khoo J, Tian HH, Tan B, et al. Comparing effects of low- and high-volume moderate-intensity exercise on sexual function and testosterone in obese men. J Sex Med. 2013;10:1823–32.
82. Zouhal H, Jayavel A, Parasuraman K, Hayes LD, Tourny C, Rhibi F, Laher I, Abderrahman AB, Hackney AC. Effects of exercise training on anabolic and catabolic hormones with advanced age: a systematic review. Sports Med. 2021;52(6):1353–68.
83. Stout M, Tew GA, Doll H, Zwierska I, Woodroofe N, Channer KS, Saxton JM. Testosterone therapy during exercise rehabilitation in male patients with chronic heart failure who have low testosterone status: a double-blind randomized controlled feasibility study. Am Heart J. 2012;164(6):893–901.
84. Chasland C, Yeap B, Maiorana AJ, Chan YX. Testosterone and exercise: effects on fitness, body composition, and strength in middle-to-older aged men with low-normal serum testosterone levels. Am J Phys Heart Circ Phys. 2021;320:1985–98.
85. Lovell DI, Cuneo R, Wallace J, McLellan C. The hormonal response of older men to sub maximum aerobic exercise: the effect of training and detraining. Steroids. 2012;77(5):413–8.
86. Liu CJ, Chang WP, Araujo de Carvalho I, Savage KEL, Radford LW, Thiyagarajan JA. Effects of physical exercise in older adults with reduced physical capacity: meta-analysis of resistance exercise and multimodal exercise. Int J Rehabil Res. 2017;40(4):303–14.
87. Peterson MD, Rhea MR, Sen A, Gordon PM. Resistance exercise for muscular strength in older adults: a meta-analysis. Ageing Res Rev. 2010;9(3):226–37.
88. Hildreth KL, Barry DW, Moreau KL, Vande Griend J, Meacham RB, Nakamura T, Schwartz RS. Effects of testosterone and progressive resistance exercise in healthy, highly functioning older men with low-normal testosterone levels. J Clin Endocrinol Metabol. 2013;98(5):1891–900.
89. Corona G, Rastrelli G, Sparano C, Vignozzi L, Sforza A, Maggi M. Advances in the treatment of functional male hypogonadism. Expert Rev Endocrinol Metab. 2024;19(2):163–77.
90. Vingren JL, Kraemer WJ, Ratamess NA, Anderson JM, Volek JS, Maresh CM. Testosterone physiology in resistance exercise and training. Sports Med. 2010;40(12):1037–53.
91. Orwoll E, Lambert LC, Marshall LM. Endogenous testosterone levels, physical performance, and fall risk in older men. Arch Intern Med. 2006;166(19):2124–31.
92. Rathi N, Blake Z, Hyman J, Nemirovsky DR, Gelikman DG, Hesswani C et al. Castration levels of testosterone results in atrophy of androgen-sensitive perineal muscles: a potential biomarker for male hypogonadism. Urology. 2024;196:313–20.
93. Roostayi M, Rahdar N. The role of physiotherapy in the treatment of men's sexual dysfunction (erectile dysfunction and premature ejaculation): a review. Physiother Q. 2022;30(2):30–7.
94. Demirdal ÜS. Benefits of aquatic exercises in patients with osteoporosis. Turk J Osteoporosis. 2012;18:37–9.
95. Cadore EL, Lhullier FLR, Alberton CL, Almeida AP, Sapata KB, Korzenowski AL, Kruel LF. Salivary hormonal responses to different water-based exercise protocols in young and elderly men. J Strength Cond Res. 2009;23:2695–701.
96. Borreani S, Colado JC, Calatayud J, Pablos C, Moya-Nájera D, Triplett N. Aquatic resistance training. Strength Cond. J. 2014;36(3):48–61.
97. Yaffe K, Lui LY, Zmuda J, Cauley J. Sex hormones and cognitive function in older men. J Am Geriatr Soc. 2002;50(4):707–12.
98. Yogev-Seligmann G, Rotem-Galili Y, Mirelman A, Dickstein R, Giladi N, Hausdorff JM. How does explicit prioritization alter walking during dual-task performance? Effects of age and sex on gait speed and variability. Phys Ther. 2010;90(2):177–86.
99. Gallou-Guyot M, Mandigout S, Bherer L, Perrochon A. Effects of exergames and cognitive-motor dual-task training on cognitive, physical and dual-task functions in cognitively healthy older adults: an overview. Ageing Res Rev. 2020;63:101135.

23 Physiotherapy and Rehabilitation in Cancer Specific to Pelvic and Women's Health

Alper Tuğral and Yeşim Bakar

23.1 Introduction

According to the World Cancer Research report, nearly 17% of all types of cancer are diagnosed in women. Gynecological cancers in women refer to a broad spectrum of malignancies associated with different tumors and locations, such as the vulva, cervix, uterus, and ovary. It is known that gynecologic cancers affect women between 50 and 60 years of age, and these types of cancers represent nearly 15% of all new cancers in females worldwide [1]. The most common type of gynecologic cancer in women is endometrial cancer [2]. On the other hand, the US data report that 21% of all new cancers are in women, and female breast cancer takes the first place according to its incidence [3]. GLOBOCAN data reported that breast cancer is also reported to be the most frequent type of cancer, with 11.6% of all cancers globally [1].

A. Tuğral (✉)
Department of Physiotherapy and Rehabilitation, Faculty of Health Sciences, Izmir Bakircay University, Izmir, Türkiye
e-mail: alper.tugral@bakircay.edu.tr

Y. Bakar
Department of Physiotherapy and Rehabilitation, Institute of Postgraduate Education, Izmir Bakircay University, Izmir, Türkiye
e-mail: yesim.bakar@bakircay.edu.tr

Although the rates of disease and progression-free survival of urogynecological cancer have increased thanks to early screening, referrals, improved awareness, and advances in the treatment, there is still a growing need for the management of short and long-term consequences of the treatment of urogynecological cancers [4]. Survivors of gynecological cancers are reported to have suffered from a wide range of problems due to the multifactorial nature of gynecological cancer treatment, such as surgery, chemotherapy, and radiotherapy; thus, the problems experienced can remarkably differ in the context of physical, psychological, emotional, and functional aspects [5]. Since these problems can affect women detrimentally not only during and/or after treatment but also during survivorship, it is of utmost importance to manage these problems as early as possible to preserve functional capacity, physical and emotional stability, and so on. Research suggests that survivors have also outlined the need for further information and awareness about coping strategies for these potential prolonged side effects of gynecologic cancer treatment [6, 7].

This chapter tries to emphasize the management options for the side effects associated with the treatment of urogynecological cancers in the context of physiotherapy and rehabilitation.

T. Akbayrak, E. Üzelpasaci (eds.), *Physiotherapy and Rehabilitation in Pelvic and Women's Health-Related Problems*, https://doi.org/10.1007/978-3-032-28741-0_23

23.2 Common Problems Associated with Gynecological Cancers: Survivorship Issues

The pelvic girdle and pelvic floor, which are the main regions covering a complex set of functions such as continence, micturition, defecation, sexual function, delivery, and being a support base for internal organs (bladder) by being exposed to perpendicular forces against gravity, play a key role in the symptoms of urogynecological cancer treatment. Due to the complexity and diversity of duties and functions of the pelvic girdle and pelvic floor, problems can be diverse, such as urinary incontinence, fecal incontinence, sexual dysfunction, pelvic organ prolapse, and dyspareunia [8]. As outlined previously, the combination of different treatment modalities can cause diverse problems and may impact their severity. For instance, hysterectomy, brachytherapy, and teletherapy and/or chemotherapy can frequently be applied in patients with endometrial cancer, and even radiation itself can cause sexual dysfunction and dyspareunia via the creation of mucosal toxicity, vaginal stenosis, adhesions, loss of elasticity, vaginal atrophy, dryness, and narrowing and shortening the vaginal length, and therefore, all of those all contribute to the perceiving pain during intercourse as described "dyspareunia" [9, 10]. It was stated that vaginal length is 2 cm shorter after hysterectomy in patients with cervical cancer compared to those with a positive hysterectomy history without cancer [11, 12]. The reported rates of dyspareunia can be as high up to nearly 40–60%, after cervical and endometrial cancer treatment [8]. Notably, not only for treatment but also the late effects of radiation treatment alter the morphometry of the pelvic musculature via increased muscle tone and deterioration of muscle contractile properties, which can also account for the perceived symptom burden [13]. On the other hand, one of the most prominent dysfunctions of the bladder after gynecologic cancer surgery is urinary incontinence, which can be seen in up to 76% of endometrial and cervical cancer survivors [8]. Studies also reported that nearly half of them (47%) suffer from moderate to severe stress urinary incontinence [14]. It is known that the possible neural damage during surgery might affect the optimal sensation and functioning of the bladder [15]. In terms of the musculoskeletal point of view, pain is one of the most frequent symptoms among gynecologic cancer survivors. It was stated that nearly 50% of patients requested information and/or strategies for the management of pain. Physical therapy is reported to be one of the safest and most effective modalities for pain management in that patient cohort. Determining trigger points and pressure-sensitive regions may elucidate the actions that need to be taken. For instance, the levator ani, suprapubic muscles, obturator internus, and iliopsoas muscles are common regions for trigger points in non-cancer populations [16, 17].

Gynecologic cancers and their related treatment might impact the function of the pelvic girdle and/or pelvic floor variably. Pelvic floor dysfunction (PFD) refers to the umbrella term of problems/symptoms associated with gynecologic cancer treatment, in which bladder, bowel, sexual, and musculoskeletal functions of the pelvis are affected.

23.3 The Key Role of Pelvic Floor Architecture on the Background Pathophysiology of Pelvic Floor Dysfunction

The pelvic floor and pelvic girdle consist of complex contractile (muscles) and noncontractile (ligaments, soft tissue, etc.) features along with neurovascular supply. Impairments associated with the pelvic floor (PF), such as prolapse, myofascial, and neuropathic pain, can originate from potential damage associated with gynecologic cancer treatment, specifically with surgical treatment. Post-surgical scarring, surgical resection of specific tissues and organs, and neurovascular damage may play a role in deteriorated PF function. Therefore, ongoing chronic complications related to the treatment of gynecologic cancers are directly linked to PF musculature [18].

The contraction and relaxation mechanisms of PF muscles are generally characterized by ventral-cephalic and dorso-caudad directions, respectively. According to the definition of the International Continence Society, normal PF function not only refers to the optimal voluntary contraction and relaxation but also to involuntary contraction and relaxation [18]. PF muscles represent themselves as supporting bases for visceral organs such as the bladder, as well as acting roles on continence, elimination, and trunk stability, and play a key role in different functional activities and load transfer; the distribution of muscle fibers, whether type I or type II in PF muscles, carries great importance, just like other muscle groups [13]. Therefore, not only voluntary contraction but also preserved contraction of associated muscles of the pelvic floor play a role in diverse functional capabilities of the pelvic floor, such as maintaining continence and micturition [13]. In addition, involuntary relaxation of pelvic floor muscles is important for allowing vaginal penetration in the context of sexual dysfunction.

A great proportion of gynecologic cancer survivors suffer from a wide variety of symptoms associated with disrupted pelvic floor function, such as urinary incontinence, dyspareunia, pelvic organ prolapses, and so forth. De Noronha et al. [11] reported that only 20–25% of cervical cancer survivors had good and/or normal pelvic floor muscle contraction. Moreover, it was stated that endometrial cancer survivors had reduced pelvic floor muscle contraction force more than 1 year after completion of primary treatment compared to those with a positive nonmalignant hysterectomy history [19]. As detailed above, remarkable proportions of gynecologic cancer survivors suffer from different chronic complications related to pelvic floor musculature [12], and pelvic floor muscle therapy (PFMT) has been reported to be the most commonly applied and evidence-based approach to these problems in this patient group [13].

23.4 Multimodal Pelvic Physical Therapy

Multimodal pelvic physical therapy refers to a broad range of applications and modalities, including manual therapy, stretching, neuromuscular re-education, exercise, pain management modalities, lifestyle and behavioral modifications, and PFMT. PFMT has been reported to be the most common approach in patients with gynecologic cancer, as well as in the non-cancer population due to its proven efficacy on different symptoms related to pelvic floor dysfunctions. PFMT tries to improve muscular coordination, contraction, endurance, and relaxation [20, 21]. For instance, a study reported that PFMT improved pelvic floor muscle strength at the three-month follow-up [22]. Cyr et al. [10] reported improved muscle contractility and decreased muscle tone after multimodal PFMT in gynecologic cancer survivors who suffer from dyspareunia. Brennen et al. [23] reported a moderate level of evidence for PFMT regarding its efficacy in improving sexual function and quality of life after gynecological cancer treatment. Moreover, Araya-Castro et al. [9] reported that PFMT, along with education, could prevent vaginal stenosis in patients with cervical cancer undergoing radiotherapy. On the other hand, there are also studies in which no significant change was reported in pelvic floor muscle strength after PFMT [24], yet it is believed that increased awareness of PFMT among cervical patients can act as a protective factor for potential urinary incontinence. Nevertheless, it should be noted that even a standardized PFMT can impact differently in patients with the same diagnosis; therefore, patient characteristics should be taken into account when implementing a multimodal PFMT program.

Briefly, PFMT should be started in a lying position and should incrementally be modified to a sitting and standing position. The vast majority of literature suggests that two to six sets of PFMT should be performed a day [9, 10, 15, 20, 22, 24]. Maximal pelvic floor muscle contraction, rapid maximal contraction, relaxation, and voluntary precontraction of pelvic muscles prior to physical activities are generally reported as steps that should be performed during PFMT. However, it is important to note that contractions of gluteal, adductor, and abdominal muscles should be strictly avoided during PFMT [22]. To this end, teaching the correct contraction of pelvic floor muscles is of utmost importance prior to PFMT. Biofeedback devices can be used to teach proper contraction and relaxation in order to optimize the most effective and correct contraction of pelvic floor muscles [25]. Literature suggests that PFMT with biofeedback can yield better results [26].

There is no strictly standardized treatment for pelvic floor dysfunctions in gynecological cancer populations, yet physiotherapy modalities, including different interventions such as extracorporeal magnetic innervation (ExMI), biofeedback, exercise, and electrophysical agents, or in combination, have been shown to be effective in improving pelvic floor dysfunctions [21]. Sun et al. [27] reported improvements in urinary incontinence according to the nearly 50% decrease in pad test via ExMI that was applied for a total of 12 weeks with 50 and 10 Hz each for 10 min in patients with uterine cervical cancer who had a radical hysterectomy.

Electrical stimulation is been known to be used for bladder-related disorders such as urinary retention and urinary incontinence due to its recognized efficacy [28]. Transcutaneous electric nerve stimulation (TENS), which is known as the most frequent type of electrical stimulation used in bladder dysfunction, has been reported to be efficacious via proven nerve fiber regeneration, angiogenesis, and expression of collagen in detrusor and urethral sphincter muscles in rats [29]. In prostate cancer, TENS was also reported to have improved bladder function [30, 31]. Nevertheless, electrical stimulation is not recommended due to reported potential risks such as the growth of cancer and metastasis via stimulating cell replication and DNA synthesis in gynecological cancer survivors even after 5 years of completion of primary treatment [32]. Since Wang et al. [33] reported no significant effect of electrostimulation on the proliferation of cancer cells in a mouse model, studies indicated that electrostimulation could be used in women after surgery due to the elimination of tumors via hysterectomy [15]. Li et al. [28] reported that TENS was able to improve maximum flow rate, yet it did not improve urination function and residual urine volume in patients with gynecologic malignancies after radical hysterectomy.

Exercise has been recognized broadly as a noninvasive, non-pharmacological approach for managing diverse side effects of cancer treatment. A growing body of research has proven that exercise is a safe and effective option for different types of cancer. Exercise is suggested with a strong level of evidence in clinical oncology guidelines, including strength training [34]. Though there is a relative scarcity of the role of exercise in gynecologic cancer survivors, it was also reported that exercise was capable of improving physical activity levels and improving body composition [35]. Rose et al. [36] also reported that exercise significantly improved physical capacity and muscular strength in gynecological cancer survivors. Not only physical function but also depression, fatigue, and quality of life were shown to be improved via exercise in gynecologic cancer survivors [37]. Since the effect of exercise is dose-dependent and its clinical outcomes are mostly based on adherence [38], it should be noted that the best outcomes can be reached via tailored and individualized exercise programs. Because dramatically lower levels of adherence to exercise and/or physical activity among cancer survivors are a well-known point globally [39], we can kindly suggest that supervised exercise yields better adherence to exercise according to our clinical experience.

23.5 Lower Extremity Lymphedema due to Gynecologic Cancers

Lymphedema can be described as the accumulation of protein-rich fluid in interstitial spaces due to disrupted lymphatic function. Though there are two main types of lymphedema that exist, primary and secondary, secondary lymphedema is a more common condition that is characterized by external damage to lymphatic function, such as cancer surgery, trauma, infection, radiation, and so forth [40] (Fig. 23.1).

Over 90% of secondary lymphedema occurs due to cancers. Incidence and prevalence of secondary lower extremity lymphedema can vary based on the extent of surgical procedures (i.e.,

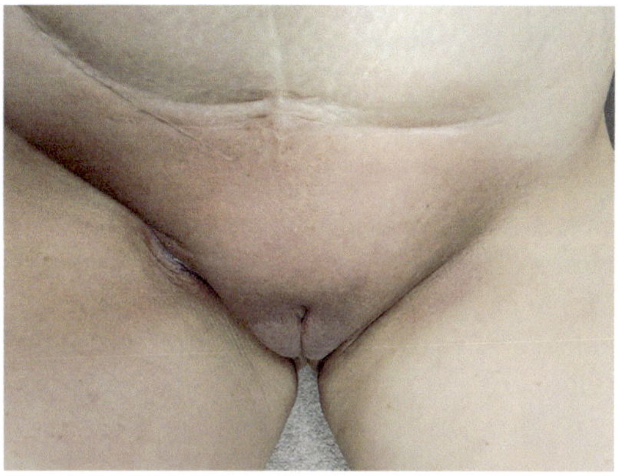

Fig. 23.1 Genital area after radiotherapy

lymphadenectomy) as well as the additional adjuvant modalities (i.e., chemotherapy and/or radiotherapy). Lymphatic circulation of gynecologic organs and tissues is primarily in close association with the following three regional lymph nodes, which are generally sampled and/or completely excised according to the standard surgical procedure: inguinofemoral, para-aortic, and pelvic lymph nodes [41]. In this regard, the literature suggests that there are two main issues that can be considered the major contributors to lower extremity lymphedema, as follows: lymphadenectomy and radiation therapy [40, 41]. As it is well recognized, the total number of excised lymph nodes is positively correlated with the risk of lower extremity lymphedema. For instance, Lim et al. [42] reported that 55% of their sample had lower extremity lymphedema after lymphadenectomy for early-stage ovarian cancer, in which over half of them had more than 35 lymph nodes excised. On the other hand, some of the additional surgical procedures, such as sentinel lymph node sampling or saphenous vein sparing, can mitigate the risk of lower extremity lymphedema [40]. Dardarian et al. [43] reported that the saphenous vein-sparing technique decreased the risk of lower extremity lymphedema from 38% to 11%. In another study, the risk of lower extremity lymphedema in sentinel lymph node sampling was 1.9%, while it was 25.3% in lymphadenectomy [44]. Besides, radiation alone can also account for nearly a 7% incidence of lower

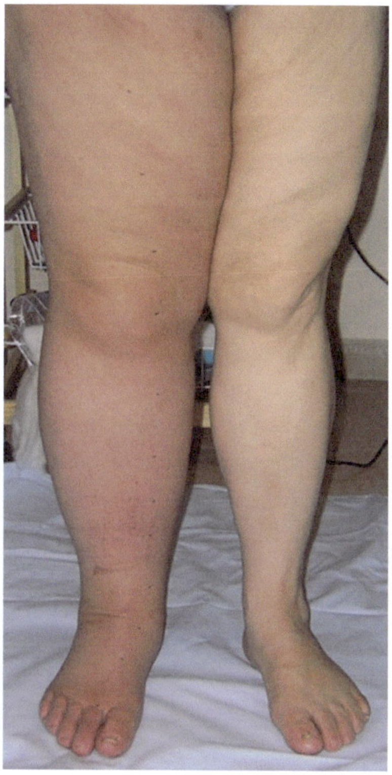

Fig. 23.2 Lower extremity lymphedema after endometrial cancer

extremity lymphedema in vulvar cancer [45]. Overall, the rate of lower extremity lymphedema is reported to be about nearly 25%, while this rate can be as high as 70% [46] (Fig. 23.2).

Lower extremity lymphedema can cause secondary and even tertiary complications such as skin reactions and ulcerations, repetitive infections, increased financial burden, decreased functionality in daily life activities, and so forth [40, 47, 48]. Therefore, prevention and early diagnosis of lower extremity lymphedema are of utmost importance since the aggravation of the severity of the condition linearly deteriorate the aforementioned problems and symptoms that may be suffered by gynecologic cancer survivors with lymphedema. Though there are some surgical and microsurgical procedures for preventing and/or treating lower extremity lymphedema, such as lympho-lymphatic and lymphoveno anastomoses as well as lymph node transplantations, the long-term results of these procedures still need to be explored further [49, 50]. However, this chapter will focus on the conservative management of lower extremity lymphedema.

23.6 Conservative Management of Lower Extremity Lymphedema

In the literature, CDP is reported as the gold standard for the conservative management of lymphedema. CDP consists of two main phases: the "intensive phase" and the "maintenance phase." The two phases are characterized by manual lymph drainage, skin care, compression, and exercise. Compression is applied to the affected extremity(ies) by short-stretch multilayer compression bandages in the first phase, while compression stockings are used to provide continued compression in the second phase. The aim of this concept is to provide maximal reduction of lymphedema in phase I while preserving the clinically reduced lymphedema via compression stockings and exercise, along with self-manual lymph drainage (MLD), self-bandage, and skin care in the second phase [51]. Below, these subdomains of CDP are tried to be explained briefly (Figs. 23.3 and 23.4).

23.6.1 Manual Lymph Drainage

Manual lymph drainage (MLD) was introduced in 1936 by Emil Vodder, who characterized it by gentle pressures without any friction on the skin in order to facilitate lymph flow via increasing

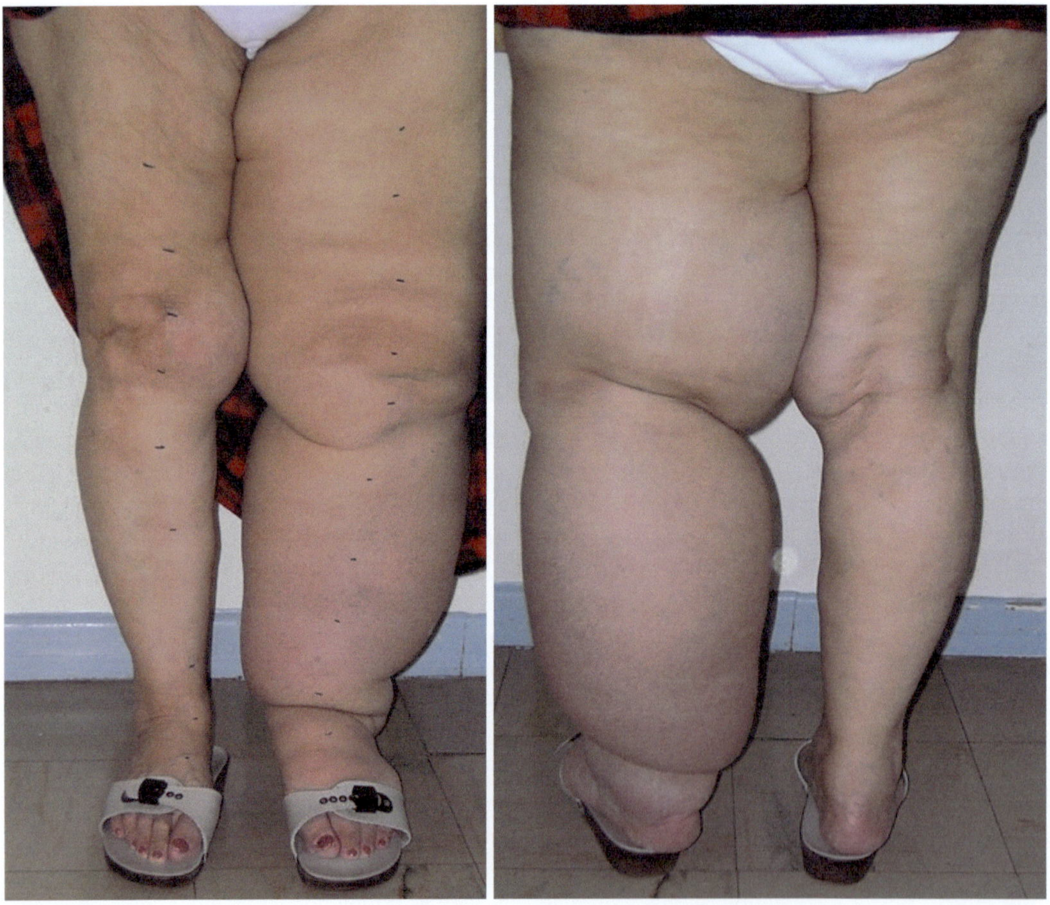

Fig. 23.3 Unilateral lower extremity lymphedema

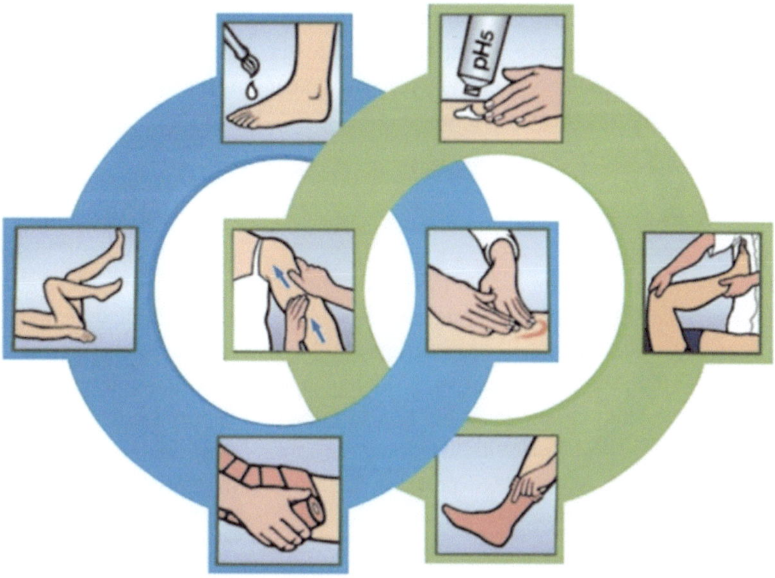

Fig. 23.4 Schematic illustration of CDP

lymphatic contraction in the affected extremities. In this regard, the schematic representation of MLD should be individualized, whether ventral or dorsal pathways, as well as following the inter-anastomotic ways such as axillo-inguinal or interinguinal. In addition, studies indicated that MLD can increase lympho-lymphatic and lympho-venous anastomoses. MLD is one of the vital parts of the CDP concept, and its acute effect on increased lymph flow is generally supported by compression; therefore, it can be concluded that MLD acts as a synergistic component of CDP prior to compression. Besides, MLD was reported to be useful in different regions, specifically where compression cannot be properly available, such as the breast and trunk region [51, 52].

23.6.2 Skin Care

Since the basic definition of lymphedema starts with the "*accumulation of protein-rich fluid..,*" this protein-rich fluid hinders oxygen and nutritional transport to the tissues. In addition, changing this hydrostatic pressure gradient can cause cell death, inflammation, and infiltration of CD4+ and T cells; thereafter, fibroblast and smooth muscle proliferation can finally result in deteriorated adipose deposition [40, 41]. Especially in lower extremity lymphedema, chronic tissue swelling can cause advanced skin changes and even open wounds such as lymphatic ulcerations. These secondary problems not only prevent the gain of the best clinical outcomes but also can cause additional financial and clinical burdens. To this end, skin care with proper moisturizers should be provided both in the intensive phase and the maintenance phase in lower extremity lymphedema.

23.6.3 Compression

Compression is the mainstay of lymphedema reduction due to the mechanism characterized by increased interstitial pressure that can be achieved via compression. Increased interstitial pressure improves resorption; therefore, reduction of extracellular fluid presents itself as decreased swelling. Multilayer inelastic compression bandages and flat-knitted compression garments/stockings should be used to provide compression in the intensive phase and maintenance phase, respectively. Since lymphedema is a chronic condition, sustainable compression is of utmost importance to preserve a stabilized lower extremity lymphedema. Compression class II (23–32 mmHg) or higher is generally acceptable and tolerable in patients with lower extremity lymphedema after gynecologic cancer treatment [48, 53] (Figs. 23.5 and 23.6).

23.6.4 Exercise

Exercise is an important part of the CDP concept. It is suggested that doing exercise while wearing compression stockings or compression bandages during CDP due to short-stretch inelastic bandages has lower resting pressure, whereas they exert higher pressure during activity. By doing so, a tolerably increased sub-bandage pressure improves the reduction of edema. On the other hand, clinical guidelines for exercise in cancer generally recommend the same level of physical activity as those with no sign of malignancy. Rose et al. [36] reported that exercise improved exercise capacity and muscular strength in post-gynecological cancer survivors. Moreover, a growing body of research outlined that all types of exercise can be safely applied to patients with cancer, including gynecological cancers. Aerobic exercise is reported to be feasible without any adverse effects as well as effective in improving perceived fatigue, depression, and quality of life, which are quite evident due to the multifactorial nature of treatment in gynecological cancer patients [37].

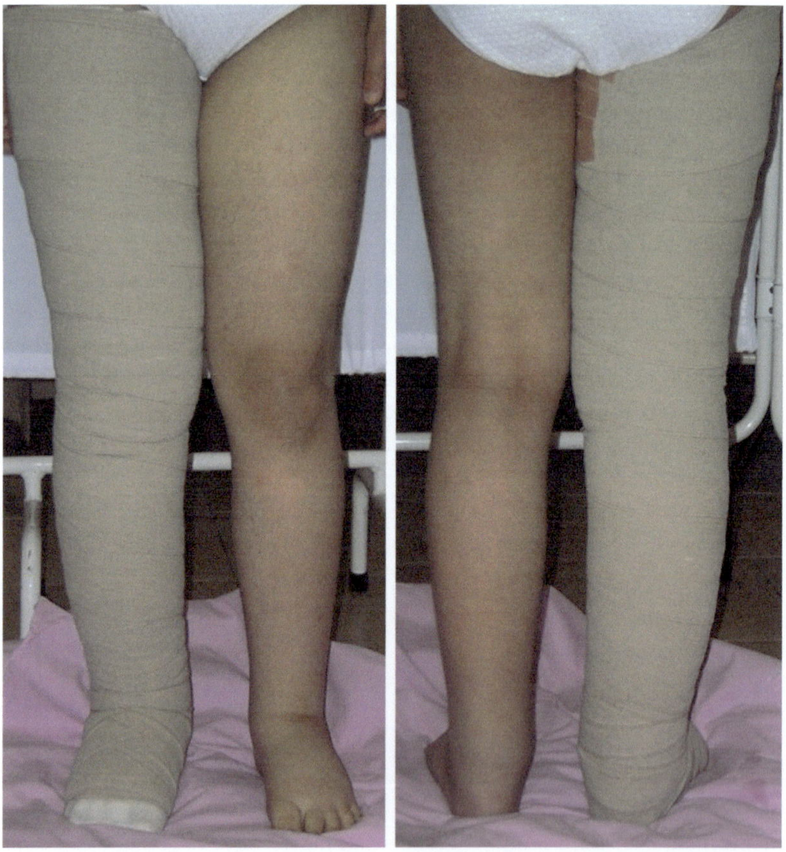

Fig. 23.5 Multilayer compression bandages in a patient with lower extremity lymphedema

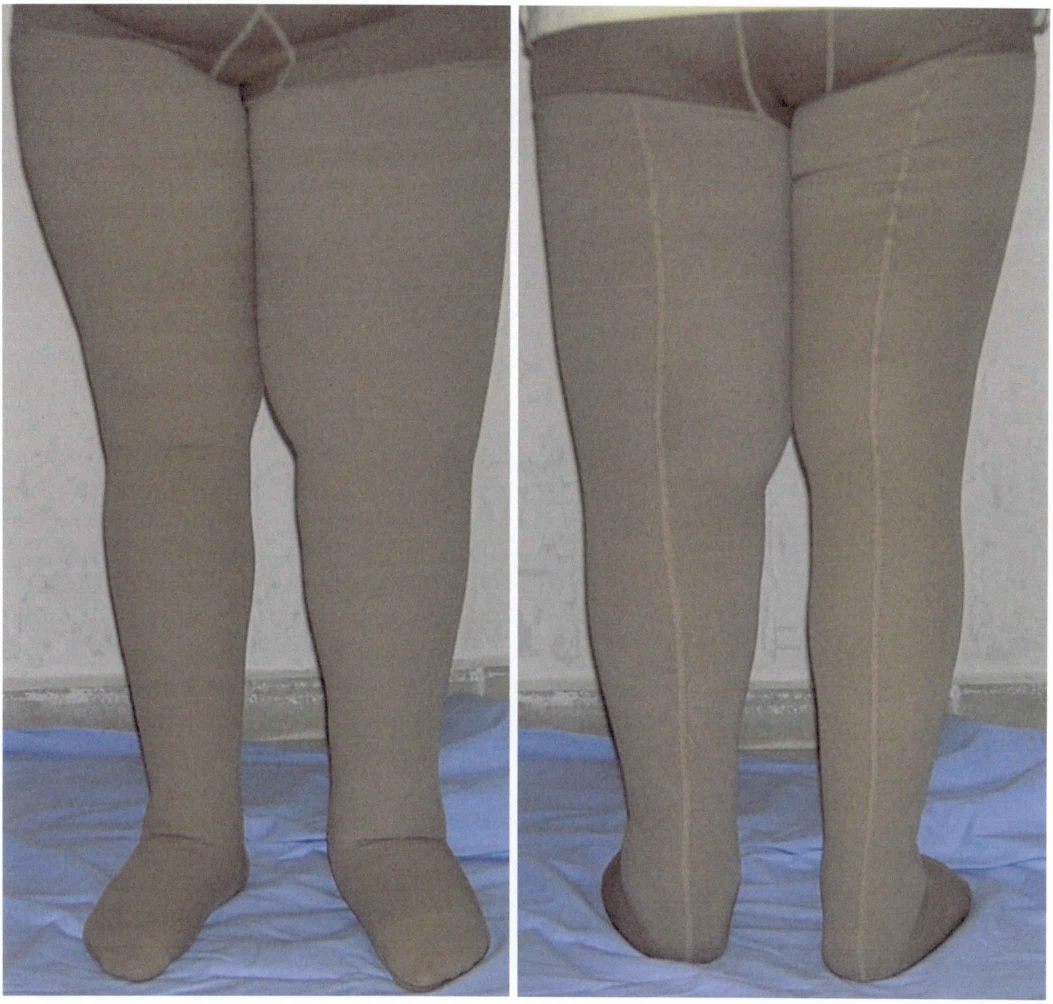

Fig. 23.6 Compression stocking

23.7 Genital Lymphedema

Genital lymphedema, which is in close association with lower extremity lymphedema, is an overwhelming situation after gynecologic cancer treatment. In females, the labia majora and minora, as well as the mons pubis, can be affected, and genital lymphedema can present either symmetrically or asymmetrically. Discomfort, pruritus, lymphorrhea, papillomatosis, deteriorated hygiene, and sexual dysfunction/discomfort can be major issues that should be considered in the context of genital lymphedema [54]. Since there is no option to assess its presence due to a lack of any validated measurement options or specific questions, being aware of potential latent symptoms, specifically in the genital area, for those with lower extremity lymphedema, is of utmost importance. Nearly one and a half years were reported to be the median time from the onset of genital lymphedema to consulting with a specialist [55]. Neverthcless, the Genital Lymphedema Score (GLS) [56] has been reported to be useful for assessing genital lymphedema, comprising six items, each of which should be scaled from 0 to 9 as follows: the sensation of heaviness, tension, swelling, urinary disorders, lymphatic cysts, and lymphorrhea (Fig. 23.7).

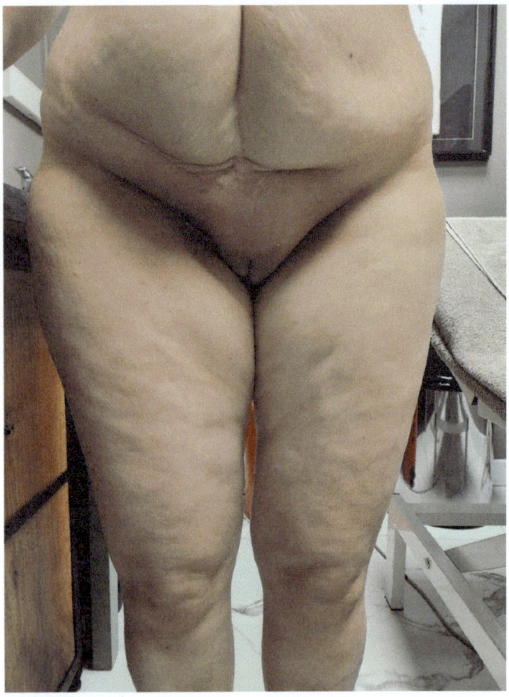

Fig. 23.7 Genital lymphedema associated with right lower extremity lymphedema

The conservative management options for genital lymphedema are quite limited due to the inability to apply compression compared to the extremities. Besides, adjusting the compression level as well as tolerance to compression of the vulva is generally reported to be poor. However, hypoallergenic pads within the underwear can be used to apply compression for the intensive maintenance of CDP. Along with compression, MLD by using ventrodorsal axillo-inguinal anastomosis should be used prior to compression. It should be noted that patient education, maintaining daily hygiene, skin care, self-MLD, and self-compression carry great importance in managing genital lymphedema in the long term [54].

23.8 Physiotherapy and Rehabilitation in Breast Cancer: Special Focus on the Most Frequent Type of Cancer Associated with Women's Health

Breast cancer (BC) is the most frequent type of cancer seen in women globally. According to the GLOBOCAN data, over two million new cases of BC were reported in 2022, which comprised nearly 12% of all types of cancer cases [1]. BC was also stated to be responsible for the leading cause of death among women in 157 countries, according to this report [1]. However, nearly 90% of five-year disease-free survival rates have been reached in BC thanks to early screening, advancements in treatment, and awareness [57]. Not only increased survival rates but also a wide variety of perceived symptoms in BC survivorship bring a growing need for prospective management strategies in order to improve one's physical, psychological, and functional well-being and quality of life [58]. In the following sections, the functional aspect of BC survivorship issues that should be approached within physical therapy and rehabilitation will be discussed further.

23.8.1 Common Problems in Breast Cancer Survivorship

Treatment of BC entails a multimodal approach, including surgery, chemotherapy, radiotherapy, and hormone replacement therapy. Since these treatment strategies can act quite differently on perceived symptoms by patients, there is a wide variety of symptoms and problems that can be experienced by BC survivors that may impede their functional life [13, 46, 58]. Cancer-related fatigue, breast cancer-related lymphedema

(BCRL), alterations in the musculoskeletal system (i.e., decreased muscle strength and endurance, decreased functional and cardiorespiratory capacity, deteriorated function of the shoulder complex), prolonged pain in the affected site and thorax, axillary web syndrome, and aromatase inhibitor-related musculoskeletal syndrome (AIMSS) are those that should be considered further to better understand functional decline and draw a rehabilitation program for the ones who suffer from those problems [59, 60].

23.8.2 Shoulder Complex and Upper Quadrant Dysfunction

Though BC surgery has evolved to a lesser extent from modified radical mastectomy toward breast-conserving surgery, the sampling methodology of nodal status, whether axillary lymph node dissection (ALND) or sentinel lymph node biopsy (SLNB), is a standard treatment protocol to uncover the grade of BC. Specifically, patients who underwent ALND have been reported to suffer from more shoulder dysfunction than those with SLNB. Studies also suggest that up to 60% of BC survivors experience upper quadrant (including the neck) dysfunction, and ALND was reported to be one of the risk factors for this dysfunction [57, 61–63]. Cumulative and adaptive alterations in muscle groups associated with the upper quadrant can cause deteriorated scapular kinematics, which can further affect activities of daily living and function [63]. Besides, studies also highlighted the reduced activity of the pectoralis major muscle along with the increased activity of the serratus anterior muscle during arm elevation [64, 65]. These altered activities were also confirmed via EMG studies; thus, potential predisposing factors of future problems related to the upper quadrant should also be considered. On the other hand, not only surgery but also adjuvant radiotherapy is stated to be responsible for the potential decline in shoulder function. For instance, more than 7 Gy dose of radiotherapy has been found to be associated with a nearly 30° reduction of shoulder abduction range of motion, which was also in parallel with the impaired Disabilities of Arm, Shoulder and Hand (DASH) questionnaire score [62, 66, 67]. Interventions to improve upper quadrant biomechanics include postural training, shoulder mobility exercises, and breathing exercises (i.e., diaphragmatic), and it has been shown that the short-term effects of these modalities have been favorable results [61].

23.8.3 Pain

Though the surgical procedure for BC has been performed to a lesser extent recently, persistent pain can be perceived in the axilla, extremity, and surgical site, and it is one of the most cumbersome complications in BC survivors [13]. Studies indicated that pain can last for up to 5 years, and it affects 60% of BC survivors [68]. Surgical procedures modified radical mastectomy (MRM or breast-conserving surgery) as well as axillary procedures (ALND or SLNB) can affect the severity of pain along with radiotherapy and psychosocial factors. Because perceived pain impacts the functional use of upper extremities, preventing and/or managing pain as early as possible is important to minimize future functional declines in BC survivors. On the other hand, we were also able to show the effect of handedness on pain in BC survivors, in which pain tolerance of the trapezius muscle was significantly lower in BC survivors whose surgical site and dominant site are the same [69]. This finding is important to consider further regarding handedness when planning a rehabilitation program. Since there is a lack of evidence about the use of laser therapy, thermal therapy, and electrotherapy to manage pain in BC survivors, relaxation methods and exercise are the ones that should be taken into account in these patients [70]. De Groef et al. [66] reported that the interventions, including postural and resistance training, and PNF techniques, along with passive mobilizations, yielded promising results in improving upper extremity morbidity. Yet, the same authors also highlighted that there is still a lack of specific recommendations and prescriptions on exercise features. Therefore, it might be plausible to conclude that individualized planning of rehabilitation as early as possible can yield the best clinical outcomes.

23.8.4 Bone Health, Osteoporosis, and Aromatase Inhibitor-Related Musculoskeletal Syndrome (AIMSS)

Systemic chemotherapy is a standard treatment for invasive BC, and it has been proven to be effective in improving survival. Nevertheless, chemotherapy-related bone loss due to ovarian failure and adjuvant aromatase inhibitor therapy was shown to be responsible for up to eightfold higher bone loss compared to natural menopause [71]. Since these types of drugs should be used to prevent the aggravation of estrogen-dependent tumors, monitoring potential detrimental effects on bone health is important in BC survivors. The National Comprehensive Cancer Network recommends screening for osteoporosis via dual energy X-ray absorptiometry (DEXA) scans in BC survivors [72]. Rehabilitation strategies generally focus on resistance training along with fall risk reduction modalities. To this end, high-risk BC survivors should not only be monitored regularly but also individualized resistance exercise training should be adjusted according to regular monitoring [13]. On the other hand, aromatase inhibitor-related musculoskeletal syndrome (AIMSS) has been well recognized among BC survivors, which is characterized by increased arthralgia and myalgia along with secondary consequences such as soft tissue problems and tenosynovitis [73]. A vicious cycle of pain perception can be evident since estrogen depletion is known to be associated with increased pro-inflammatory cytokines. Besides, estrogen depletion is also related to decreased vitamin D, and it cannot be treated with supplementation; therefore, strict monitoring of bone health among BC survivors is a prerequisite prior to rehabilitation [73, 74].

23.8.5 Breast Cancer-Related Lymphedema

Breast cancer-related lymphedema (BCRL) is one of the most fearsome and chronic complications of BC treatment. The incidence of BCRL was reported to be 40%, yet varied rates have also been attributed to the different assessment modalities [75]. ALND and increased body mass index take the lion's share in increasing the risk of BCRL. Decreased functionality, heaviness feeling, advanced secondary complications (i.e., skin reactions, infections, etc.) [58], deteriorated posture and scapular kinematics [63], impaired cutaneous sensation [76], depression, and kinesiophobia [77] are well-known symptoms associated with BCRL.

The conservative management of BCRL is CDP, as outlined and detailed previously. Yet, specific points should be taken into account in detail when compared to those with lower extremity lymphedema. For instance, patients with left-sided BCRL generally cannot tolerate the higher-pressure compression bandage as expected according to the Laplace law [78]. Breast lymphedema [79], deteriorated pulmonary function [80], and trunk lymphedema [81] should additionally be considered further in patients with BCRL (Fig. 23.8).

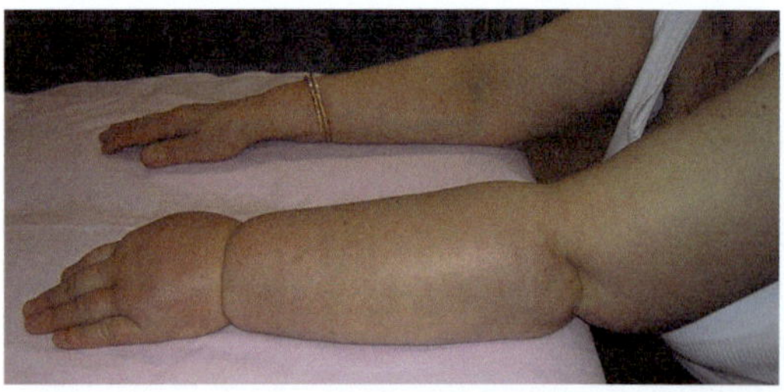

Fig. 23.8 Breast cancer-related lymphedema

23.8.6 Fatigue and Cardiorespiratory Decline

Fatigue is one of the most frequent symptoms of all cancer survivors [82]. Though different origins can be mentioned in terms of fatigue, such as systemic chemotherapy, decreased physical activity, and physical and psychological consequences of multimodal cancer treatment, patients can perceive fatigue even after years of completion of primary treatment [83]. Not only does fatigue impede participation in functional activities and daily life but also contributes to increased physical inactivity. Since fatigue can be multifactorial, approaching how to manage fatigue should also be detailed and multifaceted. Exercise has been recommended as the best non-pharmacological option to manage fatigue in all types of cancer [84]. Healthcare professionals, especially physical therapists, should be strictly aware of potential fatigue-related consequences such as falls, inability to adhere to an exercise program, and physical activity recommendations prior to, during, and after the rehabilitation program. On the other hand, cardiorespiratory decline due to cardiotoxic effects of systemic chemotherapy should also be noted among BC survivors. It was reported that cardiotoxicity and related disorders and deaths are the leading reasons for long-term mortality and morbidity among BC survivors [85].

23.8.7 Exercise: The Milestone of Managing Functional Decline in BC Survivors

Exercise has been well-acquainted with being the best option for cancer survivors, not only during active treatment but also for the survivorship continuum [84, 86]. Since multimodal cancer treatment impairs the function of BC survivors in the context of physical, psychological, and emotional aspects, BC survivors tend to decrease their physical activity level, perceive increased fatigue, and experience decreased muscle strength, and all of these create a vicious cycle of symptom aggravation, which could further impede one's functional ability [87]. According to the American College of Sports Medicine (ACSM) guideline, two to three times weekly, at least 30–60 min of exercise has shown strong evidence of improvement in fatigue, quality of life, physical function, anxiety, and so forth [86].

In the context of BCRL or the ones with the risk of BCRL, it has been well established that the beneficial effects of aerobic and resistance exercise are without adverse or harmful effects [88]. In addition, exercise is also shown to be beneficial for gynecologic cancer survivors [37]. It should be noted that exercise prescription should be carefully planned to manage potential adverse effects as well as provide stable adherence. For instance, patients who suffer from urinary incontinence should avoid plyometric and/or explosive types of exercise that can instantly increase intra-abdominal pressure. Patients with BCRL should exercise while wearing or providing compression on their affected extremity [89].

23.9 Conclusion

The incidence of women's cancers, including gynecological and breast cancer, seems to be increasing, and managing their long-term side effects is of utmost importance not only to improve one's ability to function and participate in social and work life but also to create a sustainable and optimal survivorship outcome. In this regard, objective conservative modalities such as PFMT, as well as exercise prescription, are important since they act as noninvasive, non-pharmacological options to improve cancer survivorship. As outlined before, there is a growing need to increase awareness of PFMT and exercise, not only for healthcare professionals but also for patients. Therefore, it is plausible to conclude that multidisciplinary teamwork should be embraced to enhance the best clinical outcomes. Complex decongestive physiotherapy (CDP), multimodal PFMT, and exercise have been well-acquainted with objective modalities to manage the side effects of cancer treatment. Even though they might share the same diagnosis, individualized management approaches should be adopted for each patient in the rehabilitation process.

References

1. Bray F, Laversanne M, Sung H, Ferlay J, Siegel RL, Soerjomataram I, et al. Global cancer statistics 2022: GLOBOCAN estimates of incidence and mortality worldwide for 36 cancers in 185 countries. CA Cancer J Clin. 2024;74(3):229–63.
2. Braun MM, Overbeek-Wager EA, Grumbo RJ. Diagnosis and management of endometrial cancer. Am Fam Physician. 2016;93(6):468–74.
3. Fund WCR. Worldwide cancer data, Global Cancer Statistics for the Most Common Cancers. World Cancer Research Fund International; 2018.
4. Sankaranarayanan R, Ferlay J. Worldwide burden of gynaecological cancer: the size of the problem. Best Pract Res Clin Obstet Gynaecol. 2006;20(2):207–25.
5. Brennen R, Lin K-Y, Denehy L, Soh S-E, Frawley H. Patient and clinician perspectives of pelvic floor dysfunction after gynaecological cancer. Gynecol Oncol Rep. 2022;41:101007.
6. Sekse RJT, Dunberger G, Olesen ML, Østerbye M, Seibæk L. Lived experiences and quality of life after gynaecological cancer—an integrative review. J Clin Nurs. 2019;28(9–10):1393–421.
7. ALJ L, Butow PN, Philp S, Hobbs K, Phillips E, Robertson R, et al. Age-related supportive care needs of women with gynaecological cancer: a qualitative exploration. Eur J Cancer Care. 2019;28(4):e13070.
8. Ramaseshan AS, Felton J, Roque D, Rao G, Shipper AG, Sanses TV. Pelvic floor disorders in women with gynecologic malignancies: a systematic review. Int Urogynecol J. 2018;29:459–76.
9. Araya-Castro P, Sacomori C, Diaz-Guerrero P, Gayan P, Roman D, Sperandio FF. Vaginal dilator and pelvic floor exercises for vaginal stenosis, sexual health and quality of life among cervical cancer patients treated with radiation: clinical report. J Sex Marital Ther. 2020;46(6):513–27.
10. Cyr M-P, Dumoulin C, Bessette P, Pina A, Gotlieb WH, Lapointe-Milot K, et al. Changes in pelvic floor morphometry and muscle function after multimodal physiotherapy for gynaecological cancer survivors suffering from dyspareunia: a prospective interventional study. Physiotherapy. 2022;114:54–62.
11. Noronha AF, Figueiredo EM, Franco TMRF, Cândido EB, Silva-Filho AL. Treatments for invasive carcinoma of the cervix: what are their impacts on the pelvic floor functions? Int Braz J Urol. 2013;39:46–54.
12. Bernard S, Ouellet M-P, Moffet H, Roy J-S, Dumoulin C. Effects of radiation therapy on the structure and function of the pelvic floor muscles of patients with cancer in the pelvic area: a systematic review. J Cancer Surviv. 2016;10:351–62.
13. Oza S, Badillo SA, Breevoort S, Florendo J. Women's cancer rehabilitation: a review of functional impairments and interventions among breast and gynecologic cancer survivors. Curr Phys Med Rehabil Rep. 2020;8:217–28.
14. Segal S, John G, Sammel M, Andy UU, Chu C, Arya LA, et al. Urinary incontinence and other pelvic floor disorders after radiation therapy in endometrial cancer survivors. Maturitas. 2017;105:83–8.
15. Li H, Zhou C-K, Song J, Zhang W-Y, Wang S-M, Gu Y-L, et al. Curative efficacy of low frequency electrical stimulation in preventing urinary retention after cervical cancer operation. World J Surg Oncol. 2019;17:1–7.
16. FitzGerald M, Kotarinos R. Rehabilitation of the short pelvic floor. I: background and patient evaluation. Int Urogynecol J. 2003;14:261–8.
17. Akkuzu G, Kurt G, Guvenc G, Kok G, Simsek S, Dogrusoy S, et al. Learning needs of gynecologic cancer survivors. J Cancer Educ. 2018;33:544–50.
18. Messelink B, Benson T, Berghmans B, Bo K, Corcos J, Fowler C, et al. Standardization of terminology of pelvic floor muscle function and dysfunction: report from the pelvic floor clinical assessment group of the international continence society. Neurourol Urodyn. 2005;24(4):374.
19. Bernard S, Moffet H, Plante M, Ouellet M-P, Leblond J, Dumoulin C. Pelvic-floor properties in women reporting urinary incontinence after surgery and radiotherapy for endometrial cancer. Phys Ther. 2017;97(4):438–48.
20. Yang EJ, Lim J-Y, Rah UW, Kim YB. Effect of a pelvic floor muscle training program on gynecologic cancer survivors with pelvic floor dysfunction: a randomized controlled trial. Gynecol Oncol. 2012;125(3):705–11.
21. Tim S, Mazur-Bialy AI. Physiotherapy interventions in the treatment of pelvic floor dysfunctions after gynaecological oncology procedures: a systematic review. J Gynecol Obstet Hum Reprod. 2024;53(1):102688.
22. Rutledge TL, Rogers R, Lee S-J, Muller CY. A pilot randomized control trial to evaluate pelvic floor muscle training for urinary incontinence among gynecologic cancer survivors. Gynecol Oncol. 2014;132(1):154–8.
23. Brennen R, Lin K-Y, Denehy L, Frawley HC. The effect of pelvic floor muscle interventions on pelvic floor dysfunction after gynecological cancer treatment: a systematic review. Phys Ther. 2020;100(8):1357–71.
24. Sacomori C, Araya-Castro P, Diaz-Guerrero P, Ferrada IA, Martínez-Varas AC, Zomkowski K. Prerehabilitation of the pelvic floor before radiation therapy for cervical cancer: a pilot study. Int Urogynecol J. 2020;31:2411–8.
25. Bernard S, McLean L, Boucher S, Hébert LJ, Plante M, Grégoire J, et al. An in-home rehabilitation program for the treatment of urinary incontinence symptoms in endometrial cancer survivors: a single-case experimental design study. Int Urogynecol J. 2021;32:2947–57.
26. Cyr M-P, Dumoulin C, Bessette P, Pina A, Gotlieb WH, Lapointe-Milot K, et al. Feasibility, acceptability and effects of multimodal pelvic floor physical therapy for gynecological cancer survivors suffering from painful sexual intercourse: a multicenter

prospective interventional study. Gynecol Oncol. 2020;159(3):778–84.
27. Sun MJ, Sun R, Chen LJ. The therapeutic efficiency of extracorporeal magnetic innervation treatment in women with urinary tract dysfun ction following radical hysterectomy. J Obstet Gynaecol. 2015;35(1):74-8. https://doi.org/10.3109/01443615.2014.935721.
28. Li X-W, Gao L, Wang Q, Lv Q-B, Xia Z-j, Wen H-W, et al. Long-term effect of early post-operative transcutaneous electrical stimulation on voiding function after radical hysterectomy: a multicenter, randomized, controlled trial. Front Med. 2021;8:677029.
29. Cao T, Xie B, Yang S, Wang J, Yang X, Shen B, et al. Low-frequency intravesical electrical stimulation for the treatment of acute urinary retention: a promising therapeutic approach. Front Med. 2021;8:572846.
30. Mariotti G, Sciarra A, Gentilucci A, Salciccia S, Alfarone A, Pierro GD, et al. Early recovery of urinary continence after radical prostatectomy using early pelvic floor electrical stimulation and biofeedback associated treatment. J Urol. 2009;181(4):1788–93.
31. Yamanishi T, Mizuno T, Watanabe M, Honda M, Yoshida K-I. Randomized, placebo controlled study of electrical stimulation with pelvic floor muscle training for severe urinary incontinence after radical prostatectomy. J Urol. 2010;184(5):2007–12.
32. Sandy Rennie. ELECTROPHYSICAL AGENTS - Contraindications And Precautions: An Evidence-Based Approach To Clinical Decision Making In Physical Therapy Physiother Can. 2011;62(5):1–80. https://doi.org/10.3138/ptc.62.5 PMID:21886384.
33. Wang S, Sun X, Cheng W, Zhang J, Wang J. Pilot in vitro and in vivo study on a mouse model to evaluate the safety of transcutaneous low-frequency electrical nerve stimulation on cervical cancer patients. Int Urogynecol J. 2019;30:71–80.
34. Campbell KL, Winters-Stone K, Wiskemann J, May AM, Schwartz AL, Courneya KS, et al. Exercise guidelines for cancer survivors: consensus statement from international multidisciplinary roundtable. Med Sci Sports Exerc. 2019;51(11):2375.
35. Lin K, Frawley H, Denehy L, Feil D, Granger CL. Exercise interventions for patients with gynaecological cancer: a systematic review and meta-analysis. Physiotherapy. 2016;102(4):309–19.
36. Rose GL, Stewart EM, Clifford BK, Bailey TG, Rush AJ, Abbott CR, et al. Efficacy of exercise interventions for women during and after gynaecological cancer treatment–a systematic scoping review. Support Care Cancer. 2023;31(6):342.
37. Ma RC, Li XJ, Liu R, Xu XX. Effects of physical exercise interventions for individuals with gynecologic cancer: a systematic review and meta-analysis. Oncol Nurs Forum. 2023;50(4):531–43
38. Schoenfeld BJ, Ogborn D, Krieger JW. Dose-response relationship between weekly resistance training volume and increases in muscle mass: a systematic review and meta-analysis. J Sports Sci. 2017;35(11):1073–82.
39. Ackah M, Barakou I, Abonie US, Hettinga FJ. Adherence to exercise in breast cancer survivors during and after active treatment: a systematic review and meta-analysis. JSAMS Plus. 2024;4:100071.
40. Dessources K, Aviki E, Leitao MM Jr. Lower extremity lymphedema in patients with gynecologic malignancies. Int J Gynecol Cancer. 2020;30(2):252.
41. Grada AA, Phillips TJ. Lymphedema: pathophysiology and clinical manifestations. J Am Acad Dermatol. 2017;77(6):1009–20.
42. Lim MC, Lee JS, Nam BH, Seo S-S, Kang S, Park S-Y. Lower extremity edema in patients with early ovarian cancer. J Ovarian Res. 2014;7:1–8.
43. Dardarian TS, Gray HJ, Morgan MA, Rubin SC, Randall TC. Saphenous vein sparing during inguinal lymphadenectomy to reduce morbidity in patients with vulvar carcinoma. Gynecol Oncol. 2006;101(1):140–2.
44. Van der Zee AG, Oonk MH, De Hullu JA, Ansink AC, Vergote I, Verheijen RH, et al. Sentinel node dissection is safe in the treatment of early-stage vulvar cancer. J Clin Oncol. 2008;26(6):884–9.
45. Berger J, Scott E, Sukumvanich P, Smith A, Olawaiye A, Comerci J, et al. The effect of groin treatment modality and sequence on clinically significant chronic lymphedema in patients with vulvar carcinoma. Int J Gynecol Cancer. 2015;25(1):119.
46. Cormier JN, Askew RL, Mungovan KS, Xing Y, Ross MI, Armer JM. Lymphedema beyond breast cancer: a systematic review and meta-analysis of cancer-related secondary lymphedema. Cancer. 2010;116(22):5138–49.
47. Ryan M, Stainton MC, Slaytor EK, Jaconelli C, Watts S, MacKenzie P. Aetiology and prevalence of lower limb lymphoedema following treatment for gynaecological cancer. Aust N Z J Obstet Gynaecol. 2003;43(2):148–51.
48. Bakar Y, Tuğral A. Lower extremity lymphedema management after gynecologic cancer surgery: a review of current management strategies. Ann Vasc Surg. 2017;44:442–50.
49. Jørgensen MG, Toyserkani NM, Sørensen JA. The effect of prophylactic lymphovenous anastomosis and shunts for preventing cancer-related lymphedema: a systematic review and meta-analysis. Microsurgery. 2018;38(5):576–85.
50. Campisi C, Bellini C, Campisi C, Accogli S, Bonioli E, Boccardo F. Microsurgery for lymphedema: clinical research and long-term results. Microsurgery. 2010;30(4):256–60.
51. Földi M, Földi E, Strößenreuther C, Kubik S. Földi's textbook of lymphology: for physicians and lymphedema therapists. Elsevier Health Sciences; 2012.
52. Kim S, Yi CH, Kwon O. Effect of complex decongestive therapy on edema and the quality of life in breast cancer patients with unilateral lymphedema. Lymphology. 2007;40(3):143–51.
53. Partsch H. Compression therapy: clinical and experimental evidence. Ann Vasc Dis. 2012;5(4):416–22.

54. Vignes S. Genital lymphedema after cancer treatment: a narrative review. Cancer. 2022;14(23):5809.
55. Simon L, Trévidic P, Denis P, Vignes S. Vulvar lymphangioma circumscriptum: comparison of primary and acquired forms in a cohort of 57 patients. J Eur Acad Dermatol Venereol. 2018;32(2):e56–e8.
56. Yamamoto T, Yamamoto N, Furuya M, Hayashi A, Koshima I. Genital lymphedema score: genital lymphedema severity scoring system based on subjective symptoms. Ann Plast Surg. 2016;77(1):119–21.
57. Tao X, Li T, Gandomkar Z, Brennan PC, Reed WM. Incidence, mortality, survival, and disease burden of breast cancer in China compared to other developed countries. Asia Pac J Clin Oncol. 2023;19(6):645–54.
58. Cho J, Jung S-Y, Lee JE, Shim E-J, Kim NH, Kim Z, et al. A review of breast cancer survivorship issues from survivors' perspectives. J Breast Cancer. 2014;17(3):189.
59. Fisher MI, Capilouto G, Malone T, Bush H, Uhl TL. Comparison of upper extremity function in women with and women without a history of breast cancer. Phys Ther. 2020;100(3):500–8.
60. Lovelace DL, McDaniel LR, Golden D. Long-term effects of breast cancer surgery, treatment, and survivor care. J Midwifery Womens Health. 2019;64(6):713–24.
61. Singh C, De Vera M, Campbell KL. The effect of prospective monitoring and early physiotherapy intervention on arm morbidity following surgery for breast cancer: a pilot study. Physiother Can. 2013;65(2):183–91.
62. Ribeiro IL, Camargo PR, Alburquerque-Sendin F, Ferrari AV, Arrais CL, Salvini TF. Three-dimensional scapular kinematics, shoulder outcome measures and quality of life following treatment for breast cancer–a case control study. Musculoskelet Sci Pract. 2019;40:72–9.
63. Rezende MS, Rossi DM, de Lima AMR, Clemente GS, de Oliveira AS, de Oliveira Guirro EC. Shoulder and scapulothoracic impairments in women with breast cancer-related lymphedema in the upper limb: a cross-sectional study shoulder and breast cancer-related lymphedema. J Bodyw Mov Ther. 2024;37:177–82.
64. Marazzi F, Masiello V, Marchesano D, Boldrini L, Luzi S, Ferrara PE, et al. Shoulder girdle impairment in breast cancer survivors: the role of range of motion as predictive factor for dose distribution and clinical outcome. Tumori J. 2019;105(4):319–30.
65. Johansen S, Fosså K, Nesvold IL, Malinen E, Fosså SD. Arm and shoulder morbidity following surgery and radiotherapy for breast cancer. Acta Oncol. 2014;53(4):521–9.
66. De Groef A, Van Kampen M, Dieltjens E, Christiaens M-R, Neven P, Geraerts I, et al. Effectiveness of postoperative physical therapy for upper-limb impairments after breast cancer treatment: a systematic review. Arch Phys Med Rehabil. 2015;96(6):1140–53.
67. Shamley D, Srinaganathan R, Oskrochi R, Lascurain-Aguirrebeña I, Sugden E. Three-dimensional scapulothoracic motion following treatment for breast cancer. Breast Cancer Res Treat. 2009;118:315–22.
68. Mejdahl MK, Andersen KG, Gärtner R, Kroman N, Kehlet H. Persistent pain and sensory disturbances after treatment for breast cancer: six year nationwide follow-up study. BMJ. 2013;346:f1865.
69. Tuğral A, Bakar Y, Akyol M. The characteristics of pain tolerance in patients who underwent unilateral breast cancer surgery: the effect of handedness and surgical site to assess the potential musculoskeletal symptoms and function. Clin Breast Cancer. 2022;22(7):e729–e35.
70. Harris SR, Schmitz KH, Campbell KL, McNeely ML. Clinical practice guidelines for breast cancer rehabilitation: syntheses of guideline recommendations and qualitative appraisals. Cancer. 2012;118(S8):2312–24.
71. Shapiro CL, Manola J, Leboff M. Ovarian failure after adjuvant chemotherapy is associated with rapid bone loss in women with early-stage breast cancer. J Clin Oncol. 2001;19(14):3306–11.
72. Gralow JR, Biermann JS, Farooki A, Fornier MN, Gagel RF, Kumar R, et al. NCCN task force report: bone health in cancer care. J Natl Compr Cancer Netw. 2013;11(suppl_3):S-1–S-50.
73. Anand K, Niravath P. Acupuncture and vitamin D for the management of aromatase inhibitor-induced arthralgia. Curr Oncol Rep. 2019;21:1–8.
74. Schaible HG, Von Banchet GS, Boettger M, Bräuer R, Gajda M, Richter F, et al. The role of proinflammatory cytokines in the generation and maintenance of joint pain. Ann N Y Acad Sci. 2010;1193(1):60–9.
75. DiSipio T, Rye S, Newman B, Hayes S. Incidence of unilateral arm lymphoedema after breast cancer: a systematic review and meta-analysis. Lancet Oncol. 2013;14(6):500–15.
76. Baran E, Özçakar L, Özgül S, Aksoy S, Akbayrak T. Upper limb sensory evaluations and ultrasonographic skin measurements in breast cancer–related lymphedema receiving complex decongestive physiotherapy. Support Care Cancer. 2021;29:6545–53.
77. Malchrowicz-Mośko E, Nowaczyk P, Wasiewicz J, Urbaniak T, Siejak W, Rozmiarek M, et al. The level of kinesiophobia in breast cancer women undergoing surgical treatment. Front Oncol. 2023;13:1010315.
78. Karakashian K, Pike C, van Loon R. Computational investigation of the Laplace law in compression therapy. J Biomech. 2019;85:6–17.
79. Tuğral A, Akyol M, Bakar Y. The effect of adjuvant radiotherapy on skin biophysical properties in patients with breast cancer at risk for breast lymphedema: a prospective study. Clin Physiol Funct Imaging. 2023;43(4):263–70.
80. Tuğral A, Arıbaş Z, Akyol M, Bakar Y. Understanding changes in pulmonary function and functional status in breast cancer patients after systemic chemotherapy

and radiotherapy: a prospective study. BMC Pulm Med. 2024;24(1):83.

81. Koehler LA, Mayrovitz HN. Tissue dielectric constant measures in women with and without clinical trunk lymphedema following breast cancer surgery: a 78-week longitudinal study. Phys Ther. 2020;100(8):1384–92.
82. Gerber LH. Cancer-related fatigue: persistent, pervasive, and problematic. Phys Med Rehabil Clin. 2017;28(1):65–88.
83. Fernandez C, Firdous S, Jehangir W, Behm B, Mehta Z, Berger A, et al. Cancer-related fatigue: perception of effort or task failure? Am J Hosp Palliat Med. 2020;37(1):34–40.
84. Belloni S, Arrigoni C, Caruso R. Effects from physical exercise on reduced cancer-related fatigue: a systematic review of systematic reviews and meta-analysis. Acta Oncol. 2021;60(12):1678–87.
85. Patnaik JL, Byers T, DiGuiseppi C, Dabelea D, Denberg TD. Cardiovascular disease competes with breast cancer as the leading cause of death for older females diagnosed with breast cancer: a retrospective cohort study. Breast Cancer Res. 2011;13:1–9.
86. Chyu C, Halnon N. Exercise training in cancer survivors. Curr Oncol Rep. 2016;18:1–9.
87. Clifford BK, Mizrahi D, Sandler CX, Barry BK, Simar D, Wakefield CE, et al. Barriers and facilitators of exercise experienced by cancer survivors: a mixed methods systematic review. Support Care Cancer. 2018;26:685–700.
88. Luan B, Li Z, Yang Q, Xu Z, Chen Y, Wang M, et al. The effects of ACSM-based exercise on breast cancer-related lymphoedema: a systematic review and meta-analysis. Front Physiol. 2024;15:1413764.
89. Gülören G, Doğan Y, Özgül S, Gürşen C, Çinar GN, İpekten F, et al. Acute effects of remedial exercises with and without compression on breast-cancer-related lymphedema. Healthcare. 2023;11(22):2949. MDPI

Part IV

Special Topics in Pelvic and Women's Health

Sports in Pelvic and Women's Health

24

Caglar Soylu and Emre Serdar Atalay

24.1 Introduction

Pelvic health is a critical but often overlooked aspect of sports medicine, particularly in the context of women's health. The pelvic region—encompassing the pelvis, pelvic floor muscles, and associated organs—plays a fundamental role in stability, movement, and overall athletic performance. Women, in particular, face unique challenges and risks related to pelvic health due to anatomical, hormonal, and biomechanical differences [12]. This introduction aims to provide an evidence-based overview of the importance of pelvic health in sports, focusing on its implications for performance, injury prevention, and overall well-being.

24.1.1 Pelvic Anatomy and Function in Athletes

During physical activity, the pelvis is the central structure for load transfer between the upper and lower body. The pelvic floor muscles, a group of striated muscles spanning the bottom of the pelvis, contribute to core stability, continence, and support for pelvic organs. Studies have highlighted the dynamic interaction between the pelvic floor, diaphragm, and abdominal muscles during running, jumping, and weightlifting [12, 30]. Dysfunction in this region can lead to issues like urinary incontinence, pelvic organ prolapse, and low back pain, all of which may compromise athletic performance and quality of life [70].

24.1.2 Prevalence of Pelvic Health Issues in Female Athletes

Research has shown that female athletes are disproportionately affected by pelvic health issues compared to their male counterparts. Conditions such as stress urinary incontinence and pelvic girdle pain are prevalent among high-impact sports participants. For instance, Nygaard et al. [70] reported that up to 70% of female athletes experience urinary incontinence during sports, yet only a fraction seek medical intervention [70].

Despite the multifactorial pathophysiology, physical effort from high-impact sports is an important risk factor that could explain a higher prevalence in athletes compared to the sedentary population. Athletes involved in these sports frequently experience continuous ground impacts and/or abdominal contractions that cause sudden increases in intra-abdominal pressure (IAP), placing stress on the pelvic floor (PF) muscles.

C. Soylu (✉) · E. S. Atalay
Gulhane Faculty of Physiotherapy and Rehabilitation, University of Health Sciences, Ankara, Türkiye
e-mail: caglar.soylu@sbu.edu.tr; emreserdar.atalay@sbu.edu.tr

T. Akbayrak, E. Üzelpasaci (eds.), *Physiotherapy and Rehabilitation in Pelvic and Women's Health-Related Problems*, https://doi.org/10.1007/978-3-032-28741-0_24

These physical demands are common among high-impact athletes who specialize in various track and field events [54, 68]. The exertion required during their training routines can potentially alter the physiological urethrovesical angle, leading to urine leakage that may impact their social and personal lives [46].

Previous research has indicated that self-reported urinary incontinence (UI) is prevalent among both elite and amateur athletes, with objective measures such as urine leakage being more common in elite athletes compared to their non-elite counterparts ([23]) and significantly higher than in the non-athletic population [17, 18]. Factors such as greater physical exhaustion, higher training volumes, and the intensity of elite-level training may contribute to the increased prevalence of UI symptoms in this group. [3, 23, 51].

In a study examining urinary incontinence in female CrossFit athletes, urinary incontinence was reported by 1,637 of 4,823 women, corresponding to a prevalence rate of 33.9%. The most common type is stress incontinence at 81.2%. The likelihood of urinary incontinence (UI) was found to be higher for factors such as age, body mass index, and parity. Jump-based exercises were frequently linked to urine leakage. Additionally, CrossFit practitioners exhibited a greater prevalence of UI compared to control groups [27].

A systematic review and meta-analysis conducted in 2020 reported a prevalence of urinary incontinence (UI) among female athletes at approximately 25.9% across various sports, with stress urinary incontinence (SUI) being the most common type. Notably, volleyball players had the highest prevalence rate of 75.6% [77, 78]. While physical activity is generally considered beneficial for strengthening the pelvic floor muscles (PFM), excessive stretching and straining of these muscles can have the opposite effect [51]. Recent studies have suggested a link between UI and high-impact physical activities, as the increased intra-abdominal pressure generated during such sports may surpass the intra-urethral pressure, leading to UI [45]. Additionally, an imbalance in abdominal force can alter the physiological urethrovesical angle, contributing to UI, particularly SUI, in high-impact athletes [86]. Interestingly, most athletes report experiencing leakage during training rather than during competitions (95.2% vs. 51.2%, respectively), likely due to elevated catecholamine levels during competition, which stimulate urethral alpha receptors and help maintain urethral closure.

Syeda and Pandit [84] conducted a systematic review to examine the prevalence of urinary incontinence (UI) in nulliparous female athletes and the effectiveness of physical therapy interventions. The review focused on studies investigating UI prevalence in athletes, particularly those involved in high-impact sports, and the role of physical therapy in managing the condition. The authors found a significant prevalence of UI among nulliparous athletes engaged in high-impact activities. Physical therapy interventions, primarily pelvic floor muscle training (PFMT) combined with education about pelvic anatomy, were identified as common approaches for preventing and managing UI in this population.

Goldstick and Constantini's [38] review highlighted the significant prevalence of urinary incontinence among physically active women and female athletes. High-impact sports and eating disorders were identified as major risk factors. While the exact mechanisms remain complex, pelvic floor muscle training emerged as a cornerstone treatment. However, there is a clear need for more tailored treatment protocols specifically designed for athletes. The study underscores the importance of raising awareness among athletes and their support teams to address this often-underreported issue and facilitate timely intervention.

A study investigated the prevalence and risk factors of urinary incontinence (UI) in competitive female weightlifters. The study found that approximately 31.9% of participants experienced UI within 3 months of the survey. Parity and age were significantly correlated with UI severity. While the squat was the most common exercise triggering UI, the study did not find a significant correlation between UI and years of resistance training, weightlifting experience, BMI, or competition total. Interestingly, some self-care strategies employed by weightlifters, such as training while dehydrated, may actually hinder performance and exacerbate UI.

24.1.3 Factors of Pelvic Health and Athletic Performance: An Integrated Perspective

The menstrual cycle and hormonal fluctuations significantly impact pelvic health and athletic performance. Hormones like estrogen influence connective tissue integrity and neuromuscular function, potentially affecting injury risk during specific cycle phases [66]. Pregnancy and postpartum periods further compound these changes, introducing muscle and ligament laxity that may predispose athletes to pelvic floor dysfunction. Addressing these challenges requires a multidisciplinary approach involving physiotherapists, sports medicine specialists, and coaches [76]. Preventative and rehabilitative strategies, such as pelvic floor muscle training (PFMT), biofeedback, and core stabilization exercises, have proven effective in managing and preventing pelvic floor dysfunction among athletes [77, 78]. Bladder training programs designed to meet the unique physiological needs of female athletes are essential for optimizing performance and minimizing injury risks [81].

Emerging imaging and biomechanical technologies, such as real-time ultrasound and magnetic resonance imaging (MRI), offer advanced insights into pelvic floor dynamics during athletic activities. These tools provide valuable data for developing intervention programs tailored specifically for female athletes [20, 24]. Future research should prioritize exploring the long-term impact of high-impact sports on pelvic health and evaluating the effectiveness of these specialized programs. Pelvic health is a critical aspect of women's health in sports, influencing performance, injury prevention, and overall well-being. Incorporating evidence-based practices and fostering interdisciplinary collaboration can address the unique needs of female athletes. Continued research and open discussions are vital to breaking the stigma around pelvic health issues and empowering women to achieve their athletic potential without compromise [21].

24.2 Pelvic Floor Muscle Architecture

The macroscopic arrangement of skeletal muscle, referred to as muscle architecture, is the organization of muscle fibers relative to the axis of force production. This architecture plays a crucial role in determining muscle function and adapts rapidly to loading. While sarcomere structure and fiber type distribution are often highlighted to explain muscle function and adaptation, the arrangement of muscle fibers is equally significant. Despite minor differences in fiber sizes across muscles, architectural variations primarily dictate force generation capacity [34, 56].

24.2.1 Factors Basic Architectural Definitions

Muscle fiber length and orientation are key parameters in functional classification. Fibers aligned parallel to the axis of force production are termed longitudinal or parallel fibers. These fibers do not span the entire muscle length but allow for greater excursion and faster contraction. The ratio of fiber length to muscle length ranges between 0.2 and 0.6, enabling fibers to stretch up to 60% of the muscle length. In contrast, unipennate muscles have fibers oriented at single angles (0° to 30°) relative to the force axis, enhancing force generation. Multipennate muscles feature fibers at multiple angles to the axis, further diversifying functionality [34, 56, 90].

Key parameters in architectural analysis include:

- Muscle Length (Lm): Distance between the most proximal and distal fibers.
- Fiber Length (Lf): Length of individual muscle fibers.
- Pennation Angle (PA): Angle of fiber orientation relative to the force axis. This angle changes

during contraction, increasing with muscle strengthening and decreasing with stretching.

- Physiological Cross-Sectional Area (PCA): Sum of the cross-sectional areas of all fibers, directly proportional to maximum tension but influenced by pennation angle. Large PCA with short fibers optimizes force generation, while small PCA with long fibers maximizes power [57].

Sarcomere length influences force production, with optimal lengths for maximum tension at approximately 2.6 μm. Stretching fibers to 3.65 μm eliminates actin-myosin overlap, halting force production. Conversely, shortening fibers reduces sarcomere length, increasing force production until overlap saturation occurs at 2.2 μm [58].

24.2.2 Mechanical Properties of the Muscle

The length-tension relationship, which describes skeletal muscle's mechanical properties, has two components:

- Active Length-Tension: Defined by actin-myosin overlap. Maximum tension occurs at optimal overlap, while too much or too little overlap reduces force.
- Passive Length-Tension: Involves elastic elements within the sarcomere that stretch and generate force as length increases.

Understanding the sarcomere-tension relationship is critical for designing effective treatment strategies, such as tendon transfers and stretching protocols. For instance, altering sarcomere length impacts movement and rehabilitation outcomes [57, 58].

24.2.3 Pelvic Floor Muscle (PFM) Architecture and Functional Insights

The architecture of pelvic floor muscles (PFM), including the urethral sphincter and perineal body, remains poorly understood due to limited accessibility and a reliance on dissection-based models. Although dissection provides clinical insights, its irreversible nature and potential for artifacts present challenges. Cross-sectional anatomical studies have emerged as ethical and reproducible alternatives for understanding PFM architecture [94]. Pelvic floor dysfunctions (PFD), such as prolapse and incontinence, significantly impact the quality of life and present social and economic burdens. Risk factors for PFD include vaginal childbirth, aging, obesity, and menopause [53, 91]. Understanding the architecture of PFMs is critical for evaluating and improving these dysfunctions, as changes in muscle architecture directly affect functional capacity [26]. Limited studies have investigated pelvic floor muscle (PFM) architecture in living humans, with most research relying on cadaveric data. These studies indicate that PFM muscles generally have smaller physiological cross-sectional areas compared to other pelvic muscles. The pubovisceral muscle within the levator ani complex, characterized by its long fibers, facilitates functions such as defecation and maintaining pelvic floor tension under increased abdominal pressure. Conversely, the coccygeus muscle, with shorter fibers and a larger physiological cross-sectional area, acts as a stabilizer for the coccyx, playing a crucial role in pelvic floor function. Sarcomere lengths in PFM muscles are shorter than the optimal 2.7 μm for human skeletal muscles, enhancing their resistance to intra-abdominal pressure [82].

A cadaveric study examining the coccygeus (C), iliococcygeus (IC), and pubovisceral (PV) muscles normalized fiber length to mitigate fixation-induced variability. The study found significant differences in fiber lengths among the muscles ($C = 5.29 \pm 0.32$ cm, IC = 7.55 ± 0.46 cm, PV = 10.45 ± 0.67 cm, $p < 0.001$), while physiological cross-sectional area values ($C = 0.71 \pm 0.06$ cm^2, IC = 0.63 ± 0.04 cm^2, PV = 0.59 ± 0.05 cm^2, $p = 0.21$) and sarcomere lengths ($C = 2.05 \pm 0.02$ μm, IC = 2.02 ± 0.02 μm, PV = 2.07 ± 0.01 μm, $p = 0.15$) did not show significant differences. These findings suggest that the pubovisceral muscle is capable of greater movement compared to other PFM components. Table 24.1 summarizes these architectural mea-

Table 24.1 Architectural features of the hip muscles [74]

Muscle	Muscle fiber length (cm)	Sarcomere length (μm)	PCA (cm^2)
Obturator internus	8.77 ± 0.34	2.57 ± 0.03	3.76 ± 0.28
Gluteus maximus	15.69 ± 2.57	2.63 ± 1.57	33.4 ± 8.8
Pectineus	10.38 ± 0.53	2.72 ± 0.05	2.27 ± 0.17
Piriformis	8.37 ± 0.51	2.47 ± 0.03	2.17 ± 0.15
Superior gemellus	4.85 ± 0.32	2.85 ± 0.09	0.68 ± 0.12
Inferior gemellus	5.64 ± 0.25	2.45 ± 0.03	1.02 ± 0.11
Gluteus minimus	10.30 ± 0.77	2.79 ± 0.06	8.29 ± 0.51

PCA Physiological cross-sectional area, Values are expressed as mean ± standard deviation

surements [32, 82, 93]. Magnetic resonance imaging and electromyography findings reveal functional links between pelvic floor muscles and hip muscles, such as the gluteus maximus and levator ani. Synergistic contractions of the hip adductor and gluteal muscles enhance pelvic floor stability. Additionally, the obturator internus contributes to levator ani function via the obturator fascia, supporting the pelvic viscera and distributing mechanical loads during PFM contractions [69, 74, 85].

24.2.4 Effects of Vaginal Delivery and Aging on Pelvic Floor Architecture

A study examining the muscle architecture of the coccygeus, iliococcygeus, and pubovisceralis muscles in 23 young and 23 elderly cadavers, both with and without vaginal delivery, revealed notable differences. Vaginal delivery significantly increased muscle fiber length in the coccygeus (38% in younger and 30% in older groups) and iliococcygeus (31% in both age groups). Conversely, the pubovis-ceral muscle's fiber length remained unchanged regardless of delivery status or age. While the physiological cross-sectional area showed minor reductions in younger vaginally delivered specimens compared to non-delivered individuals, these changes were not statistically significant. Additionally, vaginal delivery had no measurable impact on the physiological cross-sectional area in older groups [2].

In nulliparous cadavers, aging did not alter muscle fiber length, but the sarcomere length of the coccygeus muscle was significantly shorter in older individuals (2.46 μm) compared to younger ones (2.75 μm). This reduction in sarcomere length likely decreases the muscle's capacity for active force production, as the optimal sarcomere length for human skeletal muscle is 2.7 μm. Changes in muscle mass between young and old specimens were minimal and showed no significant statistical differences [2].

Knowledge about pelvic floor muscle architecture is limited. There is a strong need to develop rehabilitation approaches based on pelvic floor muscle architecture. Research involving different architecture-based rehabilitation methods in the treatment of pelvic floor muscle-related problems, such as urinary incontinence, constipation, and pelvic pain, should be designed.

24.3 Common Pelvic Health Issues in Female Athletes

Female athletes frequently encounter pelvic health issues that can significantly impact their athletic performance, quality of life, and long-term health. These issues are often associated with high-impact sports and the physiological demands placed on the pelvic region. Below is an in-depth discussion of common pelvic health problems experienced by female athletes, including stress urinary incontinence, pelvic girdle pain, and pelvic organ prolapse [21].

24.3.1 Stress Urinary Incontinence (SUI)

Pelvic floor dysfunction (PFD) refers to a range of signs, symptoms, and conditions impacting the pelvic floor [42]. Urinary incontinence (UI), which is the most prevalent form of PFD among women, is described as the 'involuntary leakage of urine' and is a frequent issue across women of all ages. The primary types of UI are stress urinary incontinence (SUI) and urgency urinary incontinence (UUI). According to the International Urogynecological Association (IUGA) and the International Continence Society (ICS), SUI is defined as the 'involuntary loss of urine during physical activity or exertion, such as during sports, or when sneezing or coughing,' while UUI is characterized by the 'involuntary loss of urine accompanied by a sudden, strong need to urinate.' Additional symptoms of PFD include anorectal dysfunction (ARD), sexual dysfunction (SD), pelvic organ prolapse (POP), and pelvic pain [13, 42]. Discussing PFD symptoms, including continence issues, can be uncomfortable for many women, and incontinence has been shown to adversely affect the quality of life [21].

Stress urinary incontinence is one of the most prevalent pelvic health issues among female athletes. Defined as the involuntary leakage of urine during physical activity, SUI is often triggered by increased intra-abdominal pressure, which challenges the strength and coordination of the pelvic floor muscles [62]. Research by Nygaard et al. (2015) [70] revealed that up to 70% of female athletes participating in high-impact sports, such as gymnastics, running, and volleyball, experience SUI. Despite its prevalence, many athletes do not seek medical advice due to stigma or a lack of awareness.

Factors contributing to SUI include repetitive impact forces, insufficient pelvic floor muscle training, and hormonal changes, particularly during pregnancy and postpartum periods. Studies emphasize the importance of tailored pelvic floor muscle training (PFMT) to address this condition effectively, as PFMT has been shown to enhance muscle strength, endurance, and coordination [77, 78].

Recent studies have also highlighted the role of biomechanics in exacerbating or mitigating SUI symptoms. For example, improper landing mechanics during jumps or poor running gait patterns can increase the load on the pelvic floor. Interventions focusing on movement reeducation and posture correction have shown promising results in reducing symptom severity [62, 80] (…). Furthermore, advancements in wearable sensor technology have allowed for real-time feedback on pelvic floor engagement, empowering athletes to take a proactive approach to managing their symptoms.

In a study investigating the awareness levels of female athletes regarding pelvic floor dysfunction in 2024, a total of 255 female athletes completed an anonymous online survey exploring their knowledge of urinary incontinence (UI), pelvic organ prolapse (POP), anal incontinence (AI), and sexual dysfunction (SexD), alongside their PFD symptoms and gender-stereotyped beliefs related to sports. Additional factors, such as educational level and sports characteristics (training volume, experience, and athletic modality), were also examined. The results revealed low knowledge levels about POP (52.5%), AI (64.0%), and SexD (40%), although knowledge about UI was relatively higher (70.8%). The prevalence of PFD symptoms was notable, with 63.5% reporting dyspareunia, 51.8% experiencing urine leakage, 42.4% reporting pelvic pain, 17.3% having AI, and 9.0% experiencing POP. However, no significant association was found between symptomatology and knowledge levels. Interestingly, lower knowledge about UI and SexD was linked to stronger gender stereotypes and a higher likelihood of rejecting professional healthcare. These findings indicate that female athletes in Spain have a limited understanding of PFD, particularly of sexual dysfunction, despite the high prevalence of symptoms such as dyspareunia and urinary leakage. This underscores the urgent need for targeted educational interventions to improve awareness of all PFD types, especially those related to sexual health. Given the influence of gender stereotypes, incorporating a gender perspective into these educational programs is essential to ensure their effectiveness [14].

24.3.2 Pelvic Organ Prolapse (POP)

Pelvic organ prolapse (POP) occurs when pelvic organs, including the bladder, uterus, or rectum, descend into or beyond the vaginal canal due to weakened pelvic floor support structures [52]. This condition is particularly relevant for female athletes engaged in high-impact sports such as weightlifting, gymnastics, or volleyball, where repetitive jumping, heavy lifting, or sustained high intra-abdominal pressure is common. Research highlights an increased risk of POP in these populations due to the significant strain placed on the pelvic floor during these activities [22, 96]. The primary symptoms of POP are a sensation of pelvic heaviness or pressure, urinary or bowel dysfunction, and discomfort during physical activity. These symptoms can compromise athletic performance and overall quality of life if left untreated [12]. Early intervention is essential, with preventative strategies including pelvic floor muscle training (PFMT) to enhance strength and support, education on proper breathing and lifting techniques, and biomechanical assessments to optimize movement patterns and minimize excessive pelvic strain [77, 78].

In cases of advanced POP, treatment options may extend to the use of pessary devices to provide structural support or surgical interventions for more permanent solutions. However, these interventions should be complemented by long-term rehabilitation programs focusing on restoring pelvic floor function and preventing recurrence [47]. Emerging studies also suggest the potential benefits of real-time ultrasound and biofeedback mechanisms to monitor and enhance pelvic floor engagement during training and rehabilitation [33].

24.3.3 Pelvic Pain and Dysfunction

Pelvic pain and dysfunction are complex issues affecting many athletes, particularly females engaged in high-impact and endurance sports. These conditions encompass chronic pelvic pain (CPP), myofascial dysfunction, and nerve-related pain syndromes, which collectively impair athletic performance, daily activities, and mental well-being [60].

CPP, defined as pain persisting for over 6 months in the pelvic region, often arises from repetitive microtrauma, muscle overuse, or conditions such as endometriosis or pelvic inflammatory disease [48]. A systematic review by Culleton-Quinn et al. [21] reported that up to 25% of female athletes experience CPP, with a higher prevalence in endurance sports like long-distance running and cycling [21]. Effective CPP management requires a multidisciplinary approach, incorporating physiotherapists, pain specialists, and psychologists. Interventions such as trigger point release, myofascial therapy, and transcutaneous electrical nerve stimulation (TENS) have shown efficacy in symptom relief [8]. Advances in neuroimaging have provided insights into central sensitization mechanisms, offering potential for targeted therapies. Hormonal factors also influence CPP, as fluctuations in estrogen and progesterone levels may heighten pain sensitivity. Addressing hormonal imbalances through medical or lifestyle changes has been shown to alleviate symptoms in hormone-sensitive CPP cases [15].

Myofascial dysfunction, stemming from overuse or poor biomechanics, is another major contributor to pelvic pain in athletes. Tightness or trigger points in muscles like the iliopsoas, obturator internus, and levator ani can result in referred pain and restricted mobility [37]. Srinivasan et al. [88] highlighted the importance of addressing fascial restrictions to optimize pelvic and core functionality [88]. Fascial health is crucial for athletic performance, as restricted fascia can reduce movement efficiency and increase injury risk. Therapeutic techniques such as instrument-assisted soft tissue mobilization (IASTM) and fascial stretching enhance pelvic mobility and alleviate pain. Incorporating foam rolling and self-myofascial release tools into training regimens provides long-term benefits in maintaining fascial flexibility and reducing dysfunction [65].

Nerve-related pain syndromes, such as pudendal neuralgia, are increasingly recognized contributors to pelvic dysfunction in athletes. These syndromes often result from nerve entrapment or irritation due to prolonged sitting (e.g., cycling) or repetitive hip flexion (e.g., sprinting) [79]. Symptoms typically include sharp, burning sensations or numbness in the perineal region. Advanced diagnostic tools, including magnetic resonance neurography and high-resolution ultrasound, have revolutionized the diagnosis and management of nerve-related pelvic pain [75, 79]. Current treatment strategies involve a combination of physical therapy, nerve blocks, and nerve glide exercises. Emerging approaches such as sacral nerve stimulation offer promising options for managing chronic nerve pain in athletes [31].

Campbell et al. [16] conducted a cross-sectional survey to investigate the prevalence of pelvic floor dysfunction (PFD), including urinary incontinence (UI), anal incontinence (AI), and pelvic organ prolapse (POP), in women engaging in recreational exercise. Despite a high prevalence of PFD across all participants, the study found no significant association between recreational exercise at or above UK health guidelines and PFD symptoms after adjusting for confounders. While some increased reporting of AI was observed in women exercising more than 10 h per week, the overall findings suggest that recreational exercise, as defined in the study, does not significantly increase the risk of PFD. However, the study highlights the high prevalence of PFD in the general female population and the low rate of seeking professional help among women experiencing these symptoms.

24.4 Impact of Different Sports on Pelvic Health

24.4.1 High-Impact Sports

High-impact sports such as gymnastics, basketball, and volleyball place considerable strain on the pelvic floor due to repetitive jumping and landing [49]. A study by Skaug et al. [82] found that gymnasts and volleyball players were at a higher risk of stress urinary incontinence and pelvic organ prolapse. The high intra-abdominal pressures generated during these activities can compromise pelvic floor integrity over time [82].

Preventative measures include educating athletes on proper landing techniques, incorporating plyometric exercises to enhance neuromuscular control, and emphasizing pelvic floor muscle training (PFMT) in strength and conditioning programs [21]. Additionally, real-time feedback systems, such as wearable sensors, have been used to monitor pelvic floor engagement during high-impact activities, enabling personalized interventions [59].

24.4.2 Endurance Sports

Endurance sports such as running and cycling present unique challenges to pelvic health due to the repetitive and prolonged nature of these activities. Among long-distance runners, pelvic girdle pain (PGP) and stress urinary incontinence (SUI) are frequently reported conditions. These issues stem from repetitive impact forces exerted on the pelvic floor during running, coupled with muscular fatigue and biomechanical alterations over time. High training loads and inadequate recovery periods exacerbate these problems by weakening pelvic floor structures and diminishing neuromuscular coordination [10, 11].

In contrast, cyclists often experience pudendal neuralgia and saddle-related pain syndromes due to prolonged pressure on the perineal region. Compression of the pudendal nerve, particularly in the area where it traverses the Alcock canal, can lead to numbness, pain, or dysfunction in the perineal and genital regions. Improper bike saddle design and prolonged seated positions are key contributors to these symptoms, which are collectively known as saddle-related neuropathies [4].

Recent advancements in biomechanical analysis have driven the development of targeted interventions to address these challenges. For runners, gait retraining programs focus on modifying stride length, cadence, and landing mechanics to reduce impact forces transmitted to the pelvic floor [36]. Studies have shown that increasing cadence can significantly decrease peak impact forces and reduce pelvic floor strain, thereby mitigating the risk of SUI and PGP [1, 40]. In cycling, the optimization of saddle design has been a pivotal focus. Pressure mapping technology has facilitated the development of ergonomic saddles that distribute weight more evenly and reduce perineal pressure. Saddles with cut-out designs, for example, have demonstrated significant benefits in alleviating pudendal nerve compression and improving overall comfort during long rides [61, 87].

Both sports benefit from core stability programs tailored to the unique demands of endurance athletes. Core strengthening exercises enhance pelvic support by improving the coordination and endurance of the deep stabilizing muscles, including the transverse abdominis, multifidus, and pelvic floor muscles. Evidence suggests that core-focused rehabilitation programs not only alleviate pelvic girdle pain but also improve running economy and cycling efficiency [44, 63]. Understanding the specific pelvic health challenges faced by endurance athletes enables the implementation of evidence-based interventions. Integrating biomechanical retraining, ergonomic equipment, and targeted strengthening programs into training regimens can significantly reduce the prevalence and severity of pelvic health issues. Further research is warranted to explore the long-term effects of these interventions and to develop sport-specific guidelines for injury prevention.

24.4.3 Weightlifting and Strength Training

Weightlifting and strength training involve heavy lifting and bracing techniques that generate significant intra-abdominal pressure (IAP) to stabilize the core and support the spine [9]. While essential for lifting performance, these mechanics pose specific pelvic health risks, particularly for female athletes. Two major concerns are pelvic organ prolapse (POP) and diastasis recti abdominis (DRA) [55]. POP occurs when pelvic organs, such as the bladder, uterus, or rectum, descend due to the weakening of the pelvic floor, a condition exacerbated by repetitive heavy lifting. DRA, defined as the separation of the rectus abdominis muscles along the linea alba, compromises core stability and increases the risk of injury during lifting. Research shows these conditions are more likely to occur with inadequate breathing techniques or incorrect bracing methods during strength exercises [26, 83, 89].

Breath control and proper lifting mechanics are critical in reducing these risks. Techniques such as diaphragmatic breathing and controlled exhalation during exertion help modulate IAP and protect the pelvic floor from excessive strain [26, 83, 89]. Hagins et al. [41] demonstrated that structured breath training significantly reduces IAP peaks during maximal lifting, lowering the risk of POP and DRA [41]. Furthermore, engaging the transverse abdominis muscle and maintaining a neutral spine during lifts reduces pelvic floor strain. The integration of intra-abdominal pressure monitoring devices into training routines is a promising advancement, offering real-time feedback that enables athletes and coaches to adjust techniques dynamically [25, 26].

Physiotherapists increasingly collaborate with strength coaches to develop comprehensive training programs that prioritize pelvic health while maintaining performance outcomes. These interdisciplinary approaches often include tailored pelvic floor muscle training programs to enhance muscle coordination and endurance, biomechanical assessments to identify compensatory patterns that increase pelvic floor stress, and progressive load management strategies to allow safe adaptation of pelvic and abdominal structures to training demands. Pelvic floor muscle training is particularly effective not only in preventing POP and DRA but also in enhancing overall athletic performance [29].

In summary, while weightlifting and strength training offer substantial benefits for health and athletic performance, they present pelvic health challenges for female athletes. Evidence-based interventions, including breath training, proper lifting mechanics, and intra-abdominal pressure monitoring, are essential to minimizing the risks of POP and DRA. Collaborative efforts between physiotherapists and strength coaches ensure training programs remain both effective and safe. Further research into the long-term effects of these interventions will be instrumental in refining sport-specific guidelines for pelvic health preservation.

24.4.4 Aquatic Sports

Aquatic sports, including swimming and synchronized swimming, are generally associated with a lower risk of pelvic health issues compared to high-impact or endurance sports due to the buoyant nature of water, which reduces joint loading and impact forces [65]. However, these disciplines are not without challenges. Athletes often perform repetitive motions and maintain prolonged hyperextension of the lumbar spine, which can lead to pelvic girdle pain (PGP) and myofascial dysfunction. These issues arise primarily due to the high demands on core stability and pelvic alignment during aquatic maneuvers, as well as the repetitive use of specific muscle groups, particularly in freestyle, butterfly, and synchronized routines [28, 43].

Pelvic girdle pain in aquatic athletes is often linked to muscle imbalances and poor postural alignment, which can be exacerbated by the continuous hyperextension required for streamlined positions and undulating movements [92]. Myofascial dysfunction, particularly in the iliopsoas and pelvic floor muscles, can result from repetitive activation patterns and insufficient recovery periods. Synchronized swimmers, for example, are at heightened risk due to prolonged inverted positions and the high degree of lumbar spine extension required for artistic elements [88].

Innovative interventions have been developed to address these biomechanical stresses and enhance pelvic health in aquatic athletes. Cross-training programs that incorporate land-based stability exercises have been shown to improve core and pelvic floor muscle function. These programs often include exercises such as planks, bridges, and resistance-based stability drills targeting the transverse abdominis, multifidus, and pelvic floor muscles. Evidence suggests that integrating these exercises into training regimens not only reduces PGP but also enhances swimming performance by improving stroke efficiency and stability [50, 64].

Underwater video analysis has also emerged as a valuable tool in refining techniques and reducing biomechanical stress. By providing real-time visual feedback, this technology allows coaches and athletes to identify and correct inefficient movement patterns that contribute to pelvic and lumbar strain. For instance, optimizing hip rotation and minimizing excessive lumbar hyperextension during strokes can significantly decrease the risk of myofascial dysfunction and improve overall biomechanical efficiency [6, 95].

The importance of adequate recovery and individualized training plans cannot be overstated. Ensuring sufficient rest and incorporating active recovery techniques, such as aquatic therapy and foam rolling, can help alleviate myofascial tension and prevent overuse injuries. Collaborative approaches involving physiotherapists, coaches, and sports scientists are essential for creating comprehensive strategies that balance performance demands with pelvic health preservation [7, 19].

In conclusion, while aquatic sports present lower overall risks to pelvic health compared to high-impact activities, the repetitive and specific demands of swimming and synchronized swimming require targeted interventions to mitigate pelvic girdle pain and myofascial dysfunction. Cross-training programs, underwater video analysis, and collaborative care models provide evidence-based solutions for optimizing both pelvic health and athletic performance. Future research should continue to explore the long-term effects of these interventions to inform training practices and improve outcomes for aquatic athletes.

24.5 Impact on Performance and Quality of Life

Stress urinary incontinence (SUI) has been found to discourage women from participating in sports and fitness activities, potentially posing a barrier to lifelong engagement in health and fitness pursuits. While urinary incontinence does not directly cause significant morbidity or mortality, it can contribute to physical inactivity. A sedentary lifestyle, in turn, is an independent risk factor for numerous diseases and conditions, including hypertension, coronary heart disease, type 2 diabetes, obesity, colon and breast cancer, osteoporosis, depression, and anxiety [10, 11].

Research indicates a higher prevalence of urinary incontinence (UI), particularly stress urinary incontinence (SUI), among young, nulliparous female athletes, with volleyball players and long-distance runners being notably affected. Nulliparous athletes engaging in high-impact activities have been observed to exhibit an increased cross-sectional area of the levator ani muscle (LAM) and greater puborectalis muscle width. SUI often goes unreported and undiagnosed due to a lack of knowledge and awareness, which can significantly impact the personal and social lives of these young women. Pelvic floor muscle (PFM) training is recognized as the primary treatment option for nulliparous athletes. However, it remains uncertain whether the high-impact nature of sports leads to UI by causing PFM fatigue or structural damage. Further studies are necessary to clarify this relationship [46].

PF symptoms significantly impacted women's participation, leading to limitations in the type, intensity, and frequency of exercise. Women reported experiencing negative emotions such as anger, fear, and isolation and employed meticulous coping strategies to manage symptoms, often impacting their social and mental well-being. The study highlights the need for strategies to address PF symptoms in women athletes, including improved screening, management, and the promotion of supportive and inclusive sporting environments to encourage continued participation [22]. In another study, the same author declared, "For 1 in 2 women, UI symptoms negatively affect exercise participation. Half of women with UI reported either stopping or modifying exercise due to their symptoms. Limited data on pelvic organ prolapse also demonstrated adverse exercise effect." The expression was said as a conclusion.

24.6 Prevention and Management of Pelvic Health Issues

In a study that compiled treatment approaches for pelvic floor dysfunction seen in female athletes, the most commonly used approach is pelvic floor muscle training. This is followed by biofeedback, other applications, lifestyle interventions, electrical stimulation, education, vaginal cones, bladder training, vaginal tampons, manual therapy, and pad and pessary applications [37].

It is plausible that targeted PFM strengthening exercises could help prevent stress urinary incontinence (SUI) and pelvic organ prolapse. Such exercises might enhance PFM volume and elevate the levator plate to a higher, more cranial position within the pelvis. Furthermore, if the pelvic floor attains a certain degree of stiffness, it is likely that the muscles will be able to resist the increased abdominal pressures that arise during physical activities [5, 39].

The elite athletes have the same condition, and one would therefore assume that they would respond to the same treatments as other women. There are methodological problems in assessing bladder and urethral function during physical activity before and after treatment [10, 11].

24.6.1 Effects of Exercise on the Pelvic Floor

There are two contrasting views regarding the pelvic floor in elite female athletes:

1. They have strong pelvic floor muscles (PFM).
2. They may overload, stretch, and weaken these muscles.

Hypothesis One: Female Athletes Have Strong Pelvic Floor Muscles

The reasoning behind this hypothesis is that any physical activity increasing abdominal pressure prompts a simultaneous or anticipatory contraction of the PFM, effectively training these muscles. This assumption suggests that general physical activity could help prevent and manage stress urinary incontinence (SUI). However, many women experience urine leakage during physical activity, particularly during high-impact exercises, which indicates that sports do not typically involve voluntary PFM contractions. Additionally, many women fail to demonstrate effective simultaneous or pre-contraction of the PFM during increased abdominal pressure. In nulliparous women, this may be attributed to factors such as genetically weak connective tissue, the lower and more caudal position of the PFM within the pelvis, a lower total number of muscle fibers (especially fast-twitch fibers), or untrained pelvic floor muscles in those who experience leakage.

Hypothesis Two: Female Athletes May Overload, Stretch, and Weaken the Pelvic Floor

Heavy lifting and intense physical exertion are recognized as risk factors for developing pelvic organ prolapse and stress urinary incontinence (SUI). Nichols and Milley proposed that repeated increases in abdominal pressure, caused by strenuous manual labor or chronic coughing, could lead to chronic damage of the cardinal and uterosacral ligaments, pelvic floor muscles (PFM), and the connective tissues of the perineum [10, 11].

In a study investigating the use of pelvic floor muscle training in elite volleyball players and its effect on stress urinary incontinence, the experimental group underwent a 4-month pelvic floor muscle training program, structured into three phases: awareness and stabilization, strength training, and power development. Meanwhile, the control group did not receive any intervention during the same timeframe. Data were collected at the start and end of the study for both groups. Maximum voluntary contractions were measured using a perineometer, urine loss was assessed through a pad test, and quality of life was evaluated using the King's Health Questionnaire. No significant differences were observed in the baseline sociodemographic and anthropometric characteristics between the groups. When comparing outcomes, the experimental group demonstrated enhanced maximum voluntary pelvic contractions ($p < 0.001$) and reduced urine loss ($p = 0.025$), highlighting significant differences between groups in changes from the initial to the final phases. The percentage of urine loss in the experimental group decreased from 71.4% to 42.9%, suggesting that the 16-week training program could benefit athletes experiencing stress urinary incontinence [77, 78].

According to the results of a review, pelvic floor muscle training (PFMT) led to a notable improvement in urinary incontinence (UI) symptoms, evidenced by a reduction in both the frequency ($n = 3$) and the severity ($n = 5$) of UI. Pelvic floor muscle function was evaluated in three studies, with two reporting improvements in maximal contraction strength and one noting increased vaginal resting pressure, all favoring PFMT. However, the two studies that examined the quality of life (QoL) outcomes found no significant differences following the PFMT intervention [35].

In another study, Bo and Nygaard published a review investigating whether physical activity is good or bad for the female pelvic floor. **Hypothesis 1** suggests that strengthening the pelvic floor muscles (PFM) and reducing the size of the levator hiatus through exercise can lower the risk of urinary incontinence, anal incontinence, and pelvic organ prolapse, though it may negatively impact the ease and safety of childbirth. **Hypothesis 2** proposes that overloading and stretching the PFM during exercise might increase the risk of these disorders but could facilitate labor and childbirth by reducing resistance during delivery. The key findings of this review support elements of both hypotheses. Women who exercise tend to have similar or greater PFM strength and larger levator ani muscles compared to non-exercisers, yet this does not seem to correlate with an increased risk of obstructed labor or childbirth complications. Moreover, pregnant women who engage in specific PFM training are not at a heightened risk of outcomes associated with obstructed labor. Mild-to-moderate physical activity, such as walking, appears to reduce the risk of urinary incontinence. However, female athletes are approximately three times more likely to experience urinary incontinence compared to non-athletes. While some evidence suggests that strenuous exercise may contribute to or exacerbate pelvic organ prolapse, the findings are inconsistent. Intra-abdominal pressure and PFM strength vary significantly depending on the type of activity and the individual, making the thresholds for beneficial or harmful effects on the pelvic floor highly variable from person to person. This review underscores several critical knowledge gaps that must be addressed to fully understand how both strenuous and non-strenuous physical activities affect pelvic floor health.

Stress urinary incontinence (SUI) is a prevalent issue among young female athletes, yet its underlying mechanisms remain poorly understood due to limited knowledge of pelvic floor support dynamics and the constraints of conventional diagnostic tools. Advanced computational modeling provides a powerful approach to investigating these dynamics during high-impact activities. A pelvic model constructed using high-resolution MRI scans of a healthy nulliparous young female demonstrates the behavior of the pelvic floor during athletic tasks. Simulations of a jump-landing process, incorporating realistic boundary conditions from experimental data, reveal significant differences in pelvic floor deformations compared to those observed during a Valsalva maneuver, commonly used in clinical settings. Alterations in levator ani muscle stiffness, simulating varying levels of muscle strength or weakness, have only a minimal impact on urethral mobility. These findings emphasize the need for clinical assessments to account for the distinct deformation patterns observed during athletic activities rather than relying solely on static maneuvers like the Valsalva. Furthermore, the evidence suggests that intrinsic sphincteric closure dysfunction may play a more critical role in SUI among young female athletes than urethral hypermobility. These insights offer valuable implications for refining diagnostic approaches, identifying risk factors, and optimizing treatment strategies for this population [25].

The study [86] revealed that physiotherapy interventions were generally more successful in improving continence for elite athletes, former athletes, and pregnant women engaging in regular aerobic activity, compared to non-athletic controls. Notably, the effectiveness of physiotherapy varied depending on the sport, with gymnastics, basketball, and some others showing less improvement. The authors conclude that PFD is associated with UI in high-performance athletes, and physiotherapy offers a valuable, non-invasive treatment option for this population [86].

24.6.2 Return-to-Sports

Okui et al. [72] conducted a study to identify predictive factors for a successful return-to-sports in elite female athletes (EFAs) experiencing postpartum stress urinary incontinence (SUI), using machine learning for analysis. The study included 153 EFAs and assessed factors such as pelvic floor muscle training (PFMT) frequency, treatment methods, 1-h pad test results at 3 months, and return-to-sports rates after 1 year. Key predictors included serum total testosterone levels, PFMT frequency, 1-HourPadtest outcomes, and combined vaginal erbium-doped yttrium–aluminum–garnet laser (VEL) and urethral laser (UEL) treatments. The findings highlighted the critical role of frequent PFMT, while those with suboptimal pad test results benefited from laser therapies, underscoring a multifactorial approach to enhancing sports resumption in EFAs with severe SUI.

A study [67] highlights key factors influencing postpartum women's ability to return to running and manage running-related stress urinary incontinence (SUI). Women who ran during pregnancy, maintained higher activity levels, and experienced less fear of movement or vaginal heaviness were more likely to resume running sooner. Returning to pre-pregnancy running levels was easier for younger women, those with shorter postpartum recovery periods, and those with multiple children. However, women with a history of running-related SUI before or during pregnancy were at higher risk of experiencing it postpartum, while cesarean delivery appeared to reduce this risk. These findings emphasize the importance of personalized support from healthcare providers to address physical and psychological barriers early, ensuring a safer and more successful return to running.

Elite female athletes (EFAs) with severe postpartum stress urinary incontinence (SUI) encounter distinct challenges when attempting to resume competitive sports. While various treatment options exist, pelvic floor muscle training (PFMT) has demonstrated efficacy among this population. However, research on the factors predicting successful sports return in EFAs with severe SUI, even after PFMT interventions, remains scarce. Despite limited data on the effectiveness of PFMT for EFAs, reviewing the available literature is essential. Other treatment modalities include vaginal and urethral erbium-doped yttrium–aluminum–garnet (Fotona) laser therapies and surgical approaches such as mid-urethral sling (MUS) surgery. Clustering-based analysis has proven effective in categorizing EFAs with SUI into subgroups, uncovering group-specific treatment outcomes. This method identified critical predictors of successful sports return and symptom relief, emphasizing the importance of tailored treatment strategies.

Future studies should aim to validate these findings in larger cohorts and incorporate advanced machine learning techniques to enhance personalized medicine approaches for managing SUI in EFAs. To improve the clinical application, subsequent research should focus on developing practical decision-making frameworks and tools to integrate these insights into routine clinical workflows [73].

24.7 Conclusion

Pelvic floor health in female athletes represents a complex interplay of anatomy, biomechanics, hormonal influences, and functional demands. The cumulative evidence presented across these sections highlights the unique challenges faced by this population, where high-impact sports, hormonal fluctuations, and insufficient rehabilitation strategies can lead to a spectrum of pelvic floor dysfunctions, including urinary incontinence, pelvic organ prolapse, and pain syndromes. Despite being highly trained, many female athletes remain underserved in terms of pelvic floor assessment, education, and individualized interventions.

A detailed understanding of pelvic floor muscle (PFM) architecture and function—encompassing fiber orientation, sarcomere length, muscle-tendon dynamics, and synergistic actions with surrounding musculature—reveals the sophistication and adaptability of this region. The PFMs are not isolated structures but integral components of a dynamic musculoskeletal system, closely linked to the hip, trunk, and breathing muscles. These relationships are especially important in high-demand activities where core stability, intra-abdominal pressure regulation, and load transfer must be finely coordinated.

Furthermore, structural and mechanical properties of the PFMs are influenced by age, hormonal milieu, and reproductive history, all of which must be considered in both preventive and rehabilitative strategies. Cadaveric and imaging-based studies provide valuable insights, yet future research must focus on real-time, functional assessments in living athletes to better translate anatomical knowledge into clinical applications.

In conclusion, optimizing pelvic health in female athletes requires an interdisciplinary and proactive approach—one that integrates sports science, rehabilitation, and pelvic health expertise. Only by bridging the gap between biomechanical understanding and practical intervention can we support the performance, health, and long-term well-being of female athletes at every stage of their careers.

References

1. Adams D, Pozzi F, Willy RW, et al. Altering cadence or vertical oscillation during running: effects on running-related injury factors. Int J Sports Phys Ther. 2018;13(4):633.
2. Alperin M, Cook M, Tuttle LJ, et al. Impact of vaginal parity and aging on the architectural design of pelvic floor muscles. Am J Obstet Gynecol. 2016;215(3):312.e1–9. https://doi.org/10.1016/j.ajog.2016.02.033.
3. Alves JO, Da LST BS, et al. Urinary incontinence in physically active young women: prevalence and related factors. Int J Sports Med. 2017;38(12):937–41.
4. Andersen KV, Bovim G. Impotence and nerve entrapment in long-distance amateur cyclists.

Acta Neurol Scand. 1997;95(4):233–40. https://doi.org/10.1111/j.1600-0404.1997.tb00104.x.
5. Ashton-Miller JA, Howard D, DeLancey JO, et al. The functional anatomy of the female pelvic floor and stress continence control system. Scand J Urol Nephrol. 2001;Suppl (207):1–7. discussion 106-25.
6. Barbosa TM, Barbosa AC, Simbaña Escobar D, et al. The role of the biomechanics analyst in swimming training and competition analysis. Sports Biomech. 2023;22(12):1734–51. https://doi.org/10.1080/14763141.2021.1960417.
7. Becker BE. Aquatic therapy: scientific foundations and clinical rehabilitation applications. PM&R. 2009;1(9):859–72. https://doi.org/10.1016/j.pmrj.2009.05.017.
8. Berghmans B. Physiotherapy for pelvic pain and female sexual dysfunction: an untapped resource. Int Urogynecol J. 2018;29(5):631–8. https://doi.org/10.1007/s00192-017-3536-8.
9. Blazek D, Stastny P, Maszczyk A, et al. Systematic review of intra-abdominal and intrathoracic pressures initiated by the Valsalva maneuver during high-intensity resistance exercises. Biol Sport. 2019;36(4):373–86. https://doi.org/10.5114/biolsport.2019.88759.
10. Bø K. Urinary incontinence, pelvic floor dysfunction, exercise and sport. Sports Med. 2004a;34(7):451–64.
11. Bø K. Pelvic floor muscle training is effective in treatment of female stress urinary incontinence, but how does it work? Int Urogynecol J Pelvic Floor Dysfunct. 2004b;15(2):76–84. https://doi.org/10.1007/s00192-004-1125-0.
12. Bø K, Anglès-Acedo S, Batra A, et al. Strenuous physical activity, exercise, and pelvic organ prolapse: a narrative scoping review. Int Urogynecol J. 2023;34(6):1153–64. https://doi.org/10.1007/s00192-023-05450-3.
13. Bo K, Frawley HC, Haylen BT, et al. An international Urogynecological association (IUGA)/international continence society (ICS) joint report on the terminology for the conservative and nonpharmacological management of female pelvic floor dysfunction. Neurourol Urodyn. 2017;36(2):221–44.
14. Bosch-Donate E, Vico-Moreno E, Fernández-Domínguez JC, et al. Symptomatology and knowledge regarding pelvic floor dysfunctions and influence of gender stereotypes in female athletes. Sci Rep. 2024;14(1):11052.
15. Brawn J, Morotti M, Zondervan KT, et al. Central changes associated with chronic pelvic pain and endometriosis. Hum Reprod Update. 2014;20(5):737–47. https://doi.org/10.1093/humupd/dmu025.
16. Campbell KG, Batt ME, Drummond A. Prevalence of pelvic floor dysfunction in recreational athletes: a cross-sectional survey. Int Urogynecol J. 2023;34(10):2429–37.
17. Carvalhais A, Natal Jorge R, et al. Performing high-level sport is strongly associated with urinary incontinence in elite athletes: a comparative study of 372 elite female athletes and 372 controls. Br J Sports Med. 2018;52(24):1586–90.
18. Caylet N, Fabbro-Peray P, Marès P, et al. Prevalence and occurrence of stress urinary incontinence in elite women athletes. Can J Urol. 2006;13(4):3174–9.
19. Cheatham SW, Kolber MJ, Cain M, et al. The effects of self-myofascial release using a foam roll or roller massager on joint range of motion, muscle recovery, and performance: a systematic review. Int J Sports Phys Ther. 2015;10(6):827.
20. Constantinou CE. Dynamics of female pelvic floor function using uro-dynamics, ultrasound, and magnetic resonance imaging (MRI). Eur J Obstet Gynecol Reprod Biol. 2009;144(Suppl 1):S159–65. https://doi.org/10.1016/j.ejogrb.2009.02.021.
21. Culleton-Quinn E, Bø K, Fleming N, et al. Elite female athletes' experiences of symptoms of pelvic floor dysfunction: a systematic review. Int Urogynecol J. 2022;33(10):2681–711. https://doi.org/10.1007/s00192-022-05302-6.
22. Dakic JG, Hay-Smith J, Lin KY, et al. Experience of playing sport or exercising for women with pelvic floor symptoms: a qualitative study. Sports Med Open. 2023;9:25. https://doi.org/10.1186/s40798-023-00565-9.
23. da Silva PF, Haupenthal A, Da Roza TH, et al. Urine loss during a volleyball competition: comparison between amateur and professional athletes. PM R. 2021;13(10):1122–6.
24. De Marzi L, Baumfeld Y, Wei Q, Shobeiri SA. Review of emerging technologies in pelvic floor ultrasonography. Open J Obstet Gynecol. 2022;12(5):375–85. https://doi.org/10.4236/ojog.2022.125034.
25. Dias N, Peng Y, Khavari R, et al. Pelvic floor dynamics during high-impact athletic activities: a computational modeling study. Clin Biomech (Bristol). 2017;41:20–7. https://doi.org/10.1016/j.clinbiomech.2016.11.003.
26. Dietze-Hermosa M, Hitchcock R, Nygaard IE, et al. Intra-abdominal pressure and pelvic floor health: should we be thinking about this relationship differently? Female Pelvic Med Reconstr Surg. 2020;26(7):409–14. https://doi.org/10.1097/SPV.0000000000000799.
27. Dominguez-Antuña E, Diz JC, Suárez-Iglesias D, et al. Prevalence of urinary incontinence in female CrossFit athletes: a systematic review with meta-analysis. Int Urogynecol J. 2023;34(3):621–34.
28. Dornowski M, Makar P, Sawicki P, et al. Effects of low- vs high-volume swimming training on pelvic floor muscle activity in women. Biol Sport. 2019;36(1):95–9. https://doi.org/10.5114/biolsport.2018.78909.
29. Dumoulin C, Hay-Smith J, Habée-Séguin GM, et al. Pelvic floor muscle training versus no treatment, or inactive control treatments, for urinary incontinence in women: a short version Cochrane systematic review with meta-

analysis. Neurourol Urodyn. 2015;34(4):300–8. https://doi.org/10.1002/nau.22700.
30. Easley DC, Abramowitch SD, Moalli PA. Female pelvic floor biomechanics: bridging the gap. Curr Opin Urol. 2017;27(3):262–7. https://doi.org/10.1097/MOU.0000000000000380.
31. Evancho A, Tyler WJ, McGregor K. A review of combined neuro-modulation and physical therapy interventions for enhanced neurorehabilitation. Front Hum Neurosci. 2023;17:1151218. https://doi.org/10.3389/fnhum.2023.1151218.
32. Felder A, Ward SR, Lieber RL. Sarcomere length measurement permits high-resolution normalization of muscle fibre length in architectural studies. J Exp Biol. 2005;208(Pt 17):3275–9. https://doi.org/10.1242/jeb.01763.
33. Franks Z, Krause HG. Pessary management for pelvic organ prolapse: a review of clinical practice and Australian medical device regulations. Aust N Z Continence J. 2023;29(3):67–73.
34. Frontera WR, Ochala J. Skeletal muscle: a brief review of structure and function. Calcif Tissue Int. 2015;96(3):183–95. https://doi.org/10.1007/s00223-014-9915-y.
35. Fukuda FS, Arbieto ERM, Da Roza T, et al. Pelvic floor muscle training in women practicing high-impact sports: a systematic review. Int J Sports Med. 2023;44(6):397–405.
36. Gaudette LW, Bradach MM, de Souza Junior JR, et al. Clinical application of gait retraining in the injured runner. J Clin Med. 2022;11(21):6497. https://doi.org/10.3390/jcm11216497.
37. Giagio S, Innocenti T, Pillastrini P, et al. What is known from the existing literature about the available interventions for pelvic floor dysfunction among female athletes? A scoping review. Neurourol Urodyn. 2022;41(2):573–84.
38. Goldstick O, Constantini N. Urinary incontinence in physically active women and female athletes. Br J Sports Med. 2014;48(4):296–8.
39. Haderer JM, Pannu HK, Genadry R, et al. Controversies in female urethral anatomy and their significance for understanding urinary continence: observations and literature review. Int Urogynecol J Pelvic Floor Dysfunct. 2002;13(4):236–52.
40. Hafer JF, Brown AM, deMille P, et al. The effect of a cadence retraining protocol on running biomechanics and efficiency: a pilot study. J Sports Sci. 2015;33(7):724–31. https://doi.org/10.1080/02640414.2014.962573.
41. Hagins M, Pietrek M, Sheikhzadeh A, et al. The effects of breath control on intra-abdominal pressure during lifting tasks. Spine (Phila Pa 1976). 2004;29(4):464–9. https://doi.org/10.1097/01.brs.0000092368.90019.d8.
42. Haylen BT, de Ridder D, Freeman RM, et al. International Urogynecological Association; International Continence Society. An International Urogynecological Association (IUGA)/International Continence Society (ICS) joint report on the terminology for female pelvic floor dysfunction. Neurourol Urodyn. 2010;29(1):4–20.
43. Hsu C, Krabak B, Cunningham B, et al. Swimming anatomy and lower back injuries in competitive swimmers: a narrative review. Sports Health. 2024;16(6):971–81. https://doi.org/10.1177/19417381231225213.
44. Hung KC, Chung HW, Yu CC, et al. Effects of 8-week core training on core endurance and running economy. PLoS One. 2019;14(3):e0213158. https://doi.org/10.1371/journal.pone.0213158.
45. Jiang K, Novi JM, Darnell S, et al. Exercise and urinary incontinence in women. Obstet Gynecol Surv. 2004;59:717–21.
46. Joseph C, Srivastava K, Ochuba O, et al. Stress urinary incontinence among young nulliparous female athletes. Cureus. 2021;13(9):e17986.
47. Jones KA, Harmanli O. Pessary use in pelvic organ prolapse and urinary incontinence. Rev Obstet Gynecol. 2010;3(1):3–9.
48. Juganavar A, Joshi KS. Chronic pelvic pain: a comprehensive review. Cureus. 2022;14(10):e30691. https://doi.org/10.7759/cureus.30691.
49. Karmakar D, Dwyer PL. High-impact exercise may cause pelvic floor dysfunction: FOR: scale, strengthen, protect! BJOG. 2018;125(5):614. https://doi.org/10.1111/1471-0528.15025.
50. Khiyami A, Nuhmani S, Joseph R, et al. Efficacy of core training in swimming performance and neuromuscular parameters of young swimmers: a randomized control trial. J Clin Med. 2022;11(11):3198. https://doi.org/10.3390/jcm11113198.
51. Khowailed IA, Pinjuv-Turney J, Lu C, et al. Stress incontinence during different high-impact exercises in women: a pilot survey. Int J Environ Res Public Health. 2020;17(22):8372.
52. Koroknai E, Rátonyi D, Pákozdy K, et al. Correlation between the female pelvic floor biomechanical parameters and the severity of stress urinary incontinence. BMC Urol. 2023;23(1):198. https://doi.org/10.1186/s12894-023-01375-7.
53. Lawrence JM, Lukacz ES, Nager CW, et al. Prevalence and co-occurrence of pelvic floor disorders in community-dwelling women. Obstet Gynecol. 2008;111(3):678–85. https://doi.org/10.1097/AOG.0b013e3181660c1b.
54. Leitner M, Moser H, Eichelberger P, et al. Evaluation of pelvic floor muscle activity during running in the continent and incontinent women: an exploratory study. Neurourol Urodyn. 2017;36(6):1570–6.
55. Leopold M, Santiago K, Cheng J, et al. Efficacy of a core strengthening program for diastasis rectus abdominis in postpartum women: a prospective observational study. J Women's Pelvic Health Phys Ther. 2021;45(4):147–63.
56. Lieber RL, Fridén J. Functional and clinical significance of skeletal muscle architecture. Muscle Nerve. 2000;23(11):1647–66. https://doi.org/10.

1002/1097-4598(200011)23:11<1647::aid-mus1>3.-0.co;2-m.
57. Lieber RL, Ward SR. Skeletal muscle design to meet functional demands. Philos Trans R Soc Lond Ser B Biol Sci. 2011;366(1570):1466–76. https://doi.org/10.1098/rstb.2010.0316.
58. Lieber RL, Roberts TJ, Blemker SS, et al. Skeletal muscle mechanics, energetics and plasticity. J Neuroeng Rehabil. 2017;14(1):108. https://doi.org/10.1186/s12984-017-0318-y.
59. Ling DI, Cepeda NA, Marom N, et al. Injury prevention programmes with plyometric and strengthening exercises improve on-field performance: a systematic review. J ISAKOS. 2020;5(1):48–59.
60. Louis-Charles K, Biggie K, Wolfinbarger A, et al. Pelvic floor dysfunction in the female athlete. Curr Sports Med Rep. 2019;18(2):49–52. https://doi.org/10.1249/JSR.0000000000000575.
61. Lowe BD, Schrader SM, Breitenstein MJ. Effect of bicycle saddle designs on the pressure to the perineum of the bicyclist. Med Sci Sports Exerc. 2004;36(6):1055–62. https://doi.org/10.1249/01.mss.0000128248.40501.73.
62. Mahoney K, Heidel RE, Olewinski L. Prevalence and normalization of stress urinary incontinence in female strength athletes. J Strength Cond Res. 2023;37(9):1877–81. https://doi.org/10.1519/JSC.0000000000004461.
63. Mamipour H, Farazmehr S, Negahban H, et al. Effect of core stabilization exercises on pain, functional disability, and quality of life in pregnant women with lumbar and pelvic girdle pain: a randomized controlled trial. J Manip Physiol Ther. 2023;46(1):27–36. https://doi.org/10.1016/j.jmpt.2023.05.005.
64. Marani IN, Subarkah A, Octrialin V. The effectiveness of core stability exercises on increasing core muscle strength for junior swimming athletes. Int J Hum Mov Sports Sci. 2020;8(1):22–8.
65. Martínez-Aranda LM, Sanz-Matesanz M, García-Mantilla ED, et al. Effects of self-myofascial release on athletes' physical performance: a systematic review. J Funct Morphol Kinesiol. 2024;9(1):20. https://doi.org/10.3390/jfmk9010020.
66. Martínez-Fortuny N, Alonso-Calvete A, Da Cuña-Carrera I, Abalo-Núñez R. Menstrual cycle and sport injuries: a systematic review. Int J Environ Res Public Health. 2023;20(4):3264. https://doi.org/10.3390/ijerph20043264.
67. Moore IS, James ML, Brockwell E, et al. Multidisciplinary, biopsychosocial factors contributing to return to running and running related stress urinary incontinence in postpartum women. Br J Sports Med. 2021;55(22):1286–92.
68. Moser H, Leitner M, Eichelberger P, et al. Pelvic floor muscle displacement during jumps in continent and incontinent women: an exploratory study. Neurourol Urodyn. 2019;38(8):2374–82.
69. Muro S, Nimura A, Ibara T, et al. Anatomical basis for contribution of hip joint motion by the obturator internus to defaecation/urinary functions by the levator ani via the obturator fascia. J Anat. 2023;242(4):657–65. https://doi.org/10.1111/joa.13810.
70. Nygaard I, Barber MD, Burgio KL, et al. Prevalence of symptomatic pelvic floor disorders in US women. JAMA. 2008;300(11):1311–6. https://doi.org/10.1001/jama.300.11.1311.
71. Nygaard I, DeLancey JO, Arnsdorf L, et al. Exercise and incontinence. Obstet Gynecol. 1990;75(5):848–51.
72. Okui N, Erel T, Okui MA. Analysis of predictive factors for return to sports in female athletes with stress urinary incontinence. Cureus. 2023;15(8):e44364.
73. Okui N, Okui M. Unsupervised clustering analysis of treatment strategies for elite female athletes with severe stress urinary incontinence: focusing on competition return and SUI improvement. Int Urol Nephrol. 2024; https://doi.org/10.1007/s11255-024-04337-6.
74. Parvaresh KC, Chang C, Patel A, et al. Architecture of the short external rotator muscles of the hip. BMC Musculoskelet Disord. 2019;20(1):611. https://doi.org/10.1186/s12891-019-2995-0.
75. Possover M, Forman A. Neuropelveological assessment of neuro-pathic pelvic pain. Gynecol Surg. 2014;11:139–44. https://doi.org/10.1007/s10397-014-0838-4.
76. Romeikienė KE, Bartkevičienė D. Pelvic-floor dysfunction prevention in prepartum and postpartum periods. Medicina (Kaunas). 2021;57(4):387. https://doi.org/10.3390/medicina57040387.
77. Pires TF, Pires PM, Moreira MH, et al. Pelvic floor muscle training in female athletes: a randomized controlled pilot study. Int J Sports Med. 2020a;41(4):264–70. https://doi.org/10.1055/a-1073-7977.
78. Pires TF, Pires PM, Moreira MH, et al. Prevalence of urinary incontinence in high-impact sport athletes: a systematic review and meta-analysis. J Hum Kinet. 2020b;73:279–88.
79. Ploteau S, Labat JJ, Riant T, et al. New concepts on functional chronic pelvic and perineal pain: pathophysiology and multidisciplinary management. Discov Med. 2015;19(104):185–92.
80. Rátonyi D, Koroknai E, Pákozdy K, et al. The impact of short-term pelvic floor muscle training on the biomechanical parameters of the pelvic floor among patients with stress urinary incontinence: a pilot study. Eur J Obstet Gynecol Reprod Biol. 2024;302:283–7. https://doi.org/10.1016/j.ejogrb.2024.09.037.
81. Selman R, Early K, Battles B, et al. Maximizing recovery in the postpar-tum period: a timeline for rehabilitation from pregnancy through return to sport. Int J Sports Phys Ther. 2022;17(6):1170–83. https://doi.org/10.26603/001c.37863.

82. Skaug KL, Engh ME, Frawley H, et al. Urinary and anal incontinence among female gymnasts and cheerleaders bother and associated factors. Int Urogynecol J. 2022;33(8):1267–76. https://doi.org/10.1007/s00192-021-04856-6.
83. Skoura A, Billis E, Papanikolaou DT, et al. Diastasis recti abdominis rehabilitation in the postpartum period: a scoping review of current clinical practice. Int Urogynecol J. 2024;35(3):491–520. https://doi.org/10.1007/s00192-024-05727-1.
84. Syeda F, Pandit U. Urinary incontinence in female athletes: a systematic review on prevalence and physical therapy approaches. Cureus. 16. 2024;16(7):e64544.
85. Soljanik I, Janssen U, May F, et al. Functional interactions between the fossa ischioanalis, levator ani and gluteus maximus muscles of the female pelvic floor: a prospective study in nulliparous women. Arch Gynecol Obstet. 2012;286(4):931–8. https://doi.org/10.1007/s00404-012-2377-4.
86. Sorrigueta-Hernández A, Padilla-Fernandez BY, Marquez-Sanchez MT, et al. Benefits of physiotherapy on urinary incontinence in high-performance female athletes. Meta-analysis. J Clin Med. 2020;9:3240.
87. Spears IR, Cummins NK, Brenchley Z, et al. The effect of saddle design on stresses in the perineum during cycling. Med Sci Sports Exerc. 2003;35(9):1620–5. https://doi.org/10.1249/01.MSS.0000084559.35162.73.
88. Srinivasan AK, Kaye JD, Moldwin R. Myofascial dysfunction associated with chronic pelvic floor pain: management strategies. Curr Pain Headache Rep. 2007;11(5):359–64. https://doi.org/10.1007/s11916-007-0218-0.
89. Talasz H, Kremser C, Talasz HJ, et al. Breathing, (S)training and the pelvic floor—a basic concept. Healthcare (Basel). 2022;10(6):1035. https://doi.org/10.3390/healthcare10061035.
90. Tirrell TF, Cook MS, Carr JA, et al. Human skeletal muscle biochemical diversity. J Exp Biol. 2012;215(15):2551–9. https://doi.org/10.1242/jeb.066704.
91. Tuttle LJ, Nguyen OT, Cook MS, et al. Architectural design of the pelvic floor is consistent with muscle functional subspecialization. Int Urogynecol J. 2014;25(2):205–12. https://doi.org/10.1007/s00192-013-2189-5.
92. Wanivenhaus F, Fox AJ, Chaudhury S, et al. Epidemiology of injuries and prevention strategies in competitive swimmers. Sports Health. 2012;4(3):246–51. https://doi.org/10.1177/1941738112442132.
93. Ward SR, Eng CM, Smallwood LH, Lieber RL. Are current measurements of lower extremity muscle architecture accurate? Clin Orthop Relat Res. 2009;467(4):1074–82. https://doi.org/10.1007/s11999-008-0594-8.
94. Wu Y, Dabhoiwala NF, Hagoort J, et al. Architectural differences in the anterior and middle compartments of the pelvic floor of young-adult and postmenopausal females. J Anat. 2017;230(5):651–63. https://doi.org/10.1111/joa.12598.
95. Veiga S, Pla R, Qiu X, et al. Effects of extended underwater sections on the physiological and biomechanical parameters of competitive swimmers. Front Physiol. 2022;13:815766.
96. Vergeldt TF, Weemhoff M, IntHout J, et al. Risk factors for pelvic organ prolapse and its recurrence: a systematic review. Int Urogynecol J. 2015;26(11):1559–73. https://doi.org/10.1007/s00192-015-2674-4.

Sleep Disorders in Pelvic and Women's Health

25

Özge Özkutlu and Özgü Inal Özün

25.1 Introduction

25.1.1 Sleep Physiology

Sleep and wake states are regulated by neural networks and circadian mechanisms, with sleep initiation and maintenance requiring the suppression of arousal systems, and adenosine acting as a sleep switch [8, 18]. The suprachiasmatic nucleus (SCN), located in the anterior hypothalamus, acts as the central coordinator of the body's circadian rhythms. It regulates a complex, hierarchically organized system of biological clocks distributed throughout the body. This master clock synchronizes with the environmental light–dark cycle through signals received by specialized photoreceptors and neural pathways. The regulation of these rhythms is driven by circadian clock genes, which form the molecular foundation of the system. These genes are expressed not only within the SCN but also in other brain regions and peripheral tissues. Together, they ensure the precise timing and coordination of physiological and behavioral processes. The coordination of this system is essential for maintaining optimal physical function as well as physical and mental health [116].

Sleep consists of two primary stages: rapid eye movement (REM) sleep, known for its heightened brain activity and the occurrence of vivid dreams, and non-rapid eye movement (NREM) sleep, which is characterized by lower levels of neuronal activity and the presence of non-visual thoughts [88]. NREM sleep is further categorized into three stages: N1, N2, and N3. Transitioning from wakefulness to light sleep involves 5 min of stage N1 sleep, marked by slow brain waves, decreased body temperature, muscle relaxation, and slow eye movements, and being easily jarred awake. The N2 stage of sleep, lasting 10–25 min, is characterized by a slower heart rate and breathing compared with awareness. During this phase of sleep, it is possible to observe the occurrence of sleep spindles and K complexes. Following N2, N3, also known as deep sleep, or slow-wave sleep, begins. Deep sleep is marked by slow brain waves called delta waves, regular breathing, reduced blood pressure, and reduced brain responsiveness to external stimuli. This period promotes body renewal and repair, with decreased blood flow to the brain along with increased levels of immune system activators, suggesting that deep sleep may aid in infection defense [8, 18, 34]. REM sleep, a complex neural state involving muscle paralysis, rapid eye movements, and an activated cerebral cortex, is a paradoxical state [11]. REM sleep,

Ö. Özkutlu (✉) · Ö. I. Özün
Department of Neurologic Physiotherapy and Rehabilitation,Gülhane Faculty of Physiotherapy and Rehabilitation, University of Health Sciences, Ankara, Türkiye
e-mail: ozge.coban@sbu.edu.tr; ozgu.inal@sbu.edu.tr

T. Akbayrak, E. Üzelpasaci (eds.), *Physiotherapy and Rehabilitation in Pelvic and Women's Health-Related Problems*, https://doi.org/10.1007/978-3-032-28741-0_25

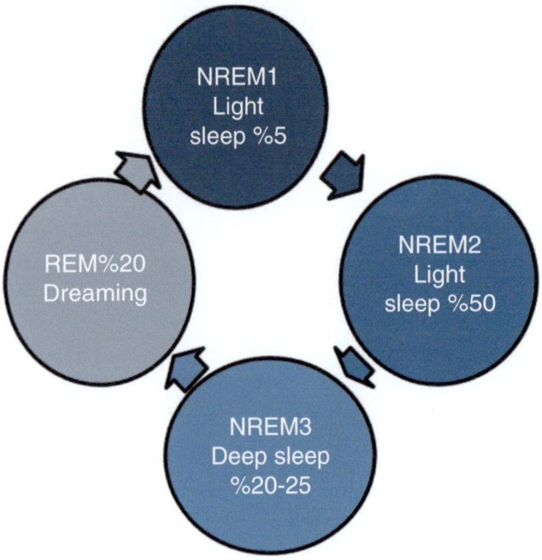

Fig. 25.1 Cycle of sleep*REM* rapid eye movement, *NREM* non-rapid eye movements

which accounts for 20% of normal sleep, is crucial for memory consolidation and dreaming. REM sleep is characterized by rapid heart and respiratory rates, (which become less regular), and longer REM cycles as the night progresses [8, 18]. A normal sleeper transitions between different sleep stages at night, alternating between REM and NREM sleep, in a predictable pattern [34] (Fig. 25.1).

Optimal sleep architecture involves 4–5 sleep cycles, each 90 min long, including light, deep sleep, and REM sleep, each playing a unique role in brain function and body repair [8].

Impaired sleep quality and quantity have several harmful effects on the metabolic, cardiovascular (CV), immune, and endocrine systems [8]. Sleep restriction causes alterations in metabolism and hormone regulation. It results in reduced glucose tolerance and lower insulin sensitivity. Additionally, it leads to elevated cortisol levels in the evening, as well as increased ghrelin and decreased leptin levels. These hormonal changes contribute to heightened hunger and appetite [79]. Sleep deprivation is associated with hypertension, coronary heart disease, and diabetes mellitus, as well as increased sympathetic nervous system activity. The U-shaped relationship indicates that both insufficient and excessive sleep are linked to higher disease risk, while moderate sleep duration is associated with a lower risk [94]. Nocturnal arousal is more strongly associated with long-term cardiovascular disease and all-cause mortality in women [125]. Sleep disruption, including insomnia and obstructive sleep apnea (OSA), leads to excessive neuronal activity and oxidative stress, contributing to neuronal dysfunction and cognitive impairment, ultimately leading to neurocognitive disorders [42]. In addition, sleep plays a crucial role in learning, memory, and cognitive processing. Sleep strengthens both declarative and nondeclarative memories, improves resistance to interference and aids in gaining insight, making connections, and integrating information [32].

Methods for sleep assessment are categorized into two main groups based on the need for medical devices. Assessment methods requiring medical devices include polysomnography, multiple sleep latency tests, maintenance of wakefulness tests, continuous positive airway pressure titration (CPAP) tests, and home sleep tests. Nonmedical device-based assessment methods consist of questionnaires, sleep diaries, and wearable devices. Wearable devices are further classified into those that make physical contact with the user, those that do not, and sound-based devices. The effectiveness of these devices in evaluating sleep can be ranked as follows: questionnaires < sleep diaries < non-contact devices < contact devices < polysomnography [53].

The increased public awareness of sleep disorders has led to more requests for sleep studies and referrals to specialists. Understanding technical and clinical information is important. Sleep latency (SL) is a crucial parameter in sleep studies. It indicates the duration between turning off the lights and falling asleep. Total sleep time (TST) is the sleep time, including onset from offset, and is divided into stages like Stage N1, Stage N2, Stage N3, and REM sleep, all in minutes. Sleep efficiency (SE) is an important parameter that measures the percentage of total bedtime spent in sleep. SE is calculated by dividing the sum of all sleep phases by total bedtime and then multiplying the result by 100. Wake after sleep onset (WASO) is a parameter that measures wakefulness after a defined sleep onset, excluding pre-sleep wakefulness, and is a better indicator of sleep fragmentation [127].

25.2 Sex Hormones and Sleep

A significant biological distinction between the sexes, particularly during the reproductive years, is the variation in the concentrations of sex hormones, including estrogen and progesterone.

25.2.1 Estrogen

Inconsistent results regarding the association between estrogen and sleep have been reported [50]. In premenopausal women, a significant positive relationship was found between SE and estrogen [80]; likewise, a negative relationship was found between estradiol and arousals [31]. Estradiol levels were not associated with sleep in perimenopausal women [31]. In a study examining perceived sleep quality in women with severe premenstrual syndrome (PMS), estradiol levels were associated with a lower percentage of REM sleep and a higher percentage of WASO in the control group, whereas no significant relationship was found with the percentage of either WASO or REM sleep in women with PMS. All-night NREM delta power was found to be correlated with estradiol level only in the control group [7].

25.2.2 Progesterone

Data show increased daytime growth hormone (GH) and prolactin (PRL) secretions in the luteal phase in cycling young women, suggesting that endogenous progesterone modulates pituitary hormone secretion, stimulating GH and PRL release and enhancing the inhibitory action of sleep on thyroid-stimulating hormone secretion and preventing sleep disorders [20]. In addition to endogenous progesterone's effects on sleep, progesterone administration itself can affect sleep. A study on eight postmenopausal women without sleep complaints found that progesterone administration significantly improved sleep quality, reducing WASO by 53% and increasing slow-wave sleep duration by nearly 50%. Progesterone also increases growth hormone and reduces TSH levels, suggesting its ability to regulate sleep in age-related disturbances [21]. However, in contrast to this, a study also showed that progesterone metabolite levels were associated with increased trouble sleeping in perimenopausal women [68]. Progesterone affects REM sleep during the luteal phase, resulting in shorter REM latency. However, no significant difference was found in sleep onset or REM sleep percentage [76]. Subjective research also supports the claim that progesterone promotes sleep, since women reported lower-quality sleep when progesterone levels decrease [50].

25.2.3 Gonadotropins

The hypothalamic–pituitary–ovarian (HPA) axis and sleep–wake regulatory systems interact in premenopausal and perimenopausal women without sleep complaints. Follicle-stimulating hormone (FSH) was positively associated with WASO, number of wakefulness events, and awakenings in perimenopausal women without sleep complaints, independent of age, body mass index, and hot flashes, while it also correlated with WASO and light NREM sleep I in premenopausal women [31]. FSH levels are associated with increased sleeping trouble in premenopausal women [68]. There have been conflicting reports on the association between LH levels and sleep, with one study finding no relationship [144], while another found a substantial correlation between SE and LH among women using hormonal contraceptives [47].

25.3 The Reproductive and Endocrine Life Stages of Sleep in Women

Female reproductive hormones have been implicated in women's sleep disturbances across different stages of reproductive aging [50].

25.3.1 Sleep and Menstrual Cycle

In premenopausal women, sleep is affected by the menstrual cycle. Women in the mid/late follicular phase had higher SE and reduced sleep onset latency (SOL) than during the menstrual and luteal phases [55]. Similarly, women reported decreased quality of sleep during their luteal phases [16]. Women with severe PMS reported worse subjective sleep quality when symptomatic in the late luteal phase compared with the follicular phase [7]. Sleep disturbances are often self-reported during the premenstrual and menstrual phases, particularly among women with PMS, irregular cycles, or dysmenorrhea. However, objective sleep assessments in young women without menstrual complaints generally show no significant variation across the cycle, although perimenstrual sleep disruptions may become evident during the late reproductive years. Notably, sleep spindle activity on electroencephalograms exhibits a significant menstrual cycle-related change, with higher activity during the luteal phase compared to the follicular phase, likely influenced by progesterone and its metabolites. This relationship is bidirectional: while reproductive hormone fluctuations can impact sleep, whereas sleep disturbances or altered sleep patterns can, in turn, influence reproductive function [2].

25.3.2 Sleep During Pregnancy and the Postnatal Period

Women experience significant changes in their physiology, social circumstances, and psychological well-being during the perinatal and postpartum periods, all of which impact the quality of their sleep. At every stage of pregnancy, women need good-quality sleep. For optimal health-related quality of life (QoL) and positive obstetric outcomes, it is crucial to increase both the quantity and quality of sleep throughout pregnancy [123].

Women who are pregnant or have recently given birth frequently experience sleep issues, such as disturbed or poor-quality sleep. Clinically significant insomnia symptoms are experienced by 14–76% of pregnant women and by 87.5% of postpartum women [67, 91]. Although all types of sleep disorders occur in pregnant women, insomnia, sleep disturbance, and poor sleep quality are the most common. The main sleep concerns in the early stages of pregnancy are increased exhaustion and numbness. However, by the third trimester, falling and staying asleep becomes especially difficult due to the physical obstacles of pregnancy, including increased urination, bodily discomfort or pain, and breathing difficulties brought on by increased pressure on the lungs [27].

Sleep disturbances and sleep quality in perinatal women have been associated with advanced gestational age, fluid retention, anemia, discomfort (such as awkwardness in sleep positions), body pain, and mood disorders (such as symptoms of depression) [151]. Compared with other periods during pregnancy and reproductive age, postpartum women generally sleep worse and less during the first few days after birth [100]. Although the birth of a child is a happy event, it is a stressful process, especially for the mother. Compared to the third trimester of pregnancy, postpartum women have lower SE due to short sleep–wake cycles and hormonal fluctuations. Due to these changes, women are particularly susceptible to sleep problems in the first few months after birth [108].

The sleep quality of postpartum mothers is affected by physical changes, postpartum stress, the demands of the newborn (e.g., feeding and care at night), bed-sharing with the infant, and family/social support. Multiparous women generally sleep less effectively than nulliparous women from pre-pregnancy to 3 months postpartum [77]. Additionally, cesarean procedures were linked to worse sleep quality and more frequent overnight awakenings than vaginal deliveries [75]. A higher risk of gestational diabetes during pregnancy is associated with short sleep duration [158].

Inadequate sleep can have detrimental effects on a person's physical and mental health. For example, inadequate sleep during pregnancy can increase the risk of depression and suicidal thoughts during pregnancy and the postpartum period, as well as the likelihood of preterm birth and prolonged labor. Poor sleep quality increases the risk of postpartum depression and increases the likelihood of preterm birth and cesarean section [22, 143].

In pregnancy-related situations, non-pharmacological approaches to sleep-related problems are often preferred. Individuals are encouraged to avoid triggers such as caffeine use and strenuous activities and to use massage and exercise-related approaches. Pregnancy is an excellent time to begin exercise, as it is a time when increased motivation and physical activity are required to start or maintain a healthy lifestyle [98]. Exercise has been shown to reduce anxiety and insomnia, and improve sleep quality. As a standard, healthy pregnant women should do at least 150 min of moderate-intensity aerobic exercise per week [3].

Progressive muscle relaxation, imagery training, meditation, biofeedback, hypnosis, and other non-pharmacological relaxation therapy techniques can also be very useful for promoting sleep [129]. Because they ease muscle tension, relaxation techniques are crucial. They entail the deliberate contraction and relaxation of all the body's major muscle groups. The goal is to assist people in examining their complete bodies, identifying any tensions, controlling their muscles, and releasing tension as quickly as possible. Relaxation techniques help pregnant women sleep more comfortably and with greater quality by easing muscle tension [74].

25.3.3 Sleep and Menopause

Premenopause (having at least one monthly period in the previous 12 months), perimenopause (having changes in menstrual flow and frequency for 12 months), and postmenopause (having no menstruation for ≥12 months) are the three categories of menopause status [1]. Perimenopause, another name for the menopausal transition, usually starts between the ages of 45 and 55. It may, however, begin earlier or later than this range. A woman's body experiences hormonal changes during the perimenopause, which cause her menstrual cycles to stop and her ability to conceive to end. Over the course of this shift, which may take years, women may encounter a variety of symptoms, such as mood changes, sleep difficulties, and hot flashes.

Sleep and menopause influence almost one-third of women's lives worldwide, and they both have a significant impact on health. The prevalence of these sleep disturbances is roughly 42% in premenopausal age groups, 47% in perimenopausal age groups, and 60% in postmenopausal age groups. Sleep disturbances during menopause are caused by several accelerating and persisting variables, such as mood disorders, menopausal symptoms, and hormonal changes. Sleeping for less than 7 h per night can increase mortality, cardiovascular disease, mood disorders, and obesity in postmenopausal women. Sleep disorders are frequently associated with depression and anxiety. Age, marital status, history of hypertension, body mass index, and other factors all play a part in postmenopausal women's declining sleep quality [10, 107].

A lot of women who experience menopause symptoms turn to complementary and alternative medicine choices such as herbal remedies and mind-body therapies. It is important to adopt a healthy lifestyle and incorporate behaviors such as exercise (such as yoga) into the lifestyle to reduce the intensity of menopause symptoms [4]. When waking up from sleep, a yoga routine can increase alpha activity and decrease autonomic arousal. Insomnia is one of the "domino effects" that can result from menopause symptoms. However, yoga may improve sleep quality. As a form of meditation, yoga helps strengthen the body, calm and heal the soul, and focus the mind. The stretching exercises used in yoga aim to improve joint flexibility and muscle strength; this activity can also increase blood flow. Women going through menopause experience significant physical changes; yoga helps to reduce tension by increasing flexibility and promoting mental and physical relaxation, which can help improve the quality of sleep for women going through menopause. Long-term yoga practice is often beneficial for postmenopausal and perimenopausal women to improve the quality of sleep [23].

Menopause symptoms can be effectively managed with physiotherapy without having a negative impact on a person's health. By increasing levels of hormones such as serotonin and brain-derived neurotrophic factor (BDNF) in the blood, sleep quality can be improved, and depression can be reduced [134, 138]. A safe, non-invasive, non-pharmacological method of treating sadness and poor sleep after menopause is physiotherapy. Perimenopausal, menopausal, and postmenopausal women may experience less depression and insomnia if they engage in aerobic exercise, stretching, strengthening, warm-up and cool-down exercises, yoga, walking, reflexology, and massage [81]. Exercise may increase metabolic rate, serotonin release, or core temperature in ways that improve sleep quality. Exercise is considered a thermogenic stimulus to improve sleep because the anterior hypothalamus regulates sleep in response to temperature increases. Pro-inflammatory cytokines are associated with fragmentation and disruption of sleep, and exercise may decrease resting plasma concentrations [51]. Additionally, exercise can increase anti-inflammatory cytokines, which can improve sleep quality. Exercise can also initiate the body's sleep cycle, which is controlled by the peripheral clock. Melatonin production and release are regulated by the circadian clock, which lowers body temperature and controls sleep. Exercise promotes the release of GH and growth hormone-releasing hormone, both of which improve sleep quality [60].

Stretching exercises before bedtime improve sleep quality and reduce sleep latency, which helps relieve symptoms of menopause and depression. In addition, the acute effect of stretching promotes better sleep by increasing parasympathetic neuroactivity and decreasing sympathetic nerve activity. Stretching exercises performed daily for 28 days may have long-term benefits on the autonomic nervous system [81]. In menopausal women, manual therapy practices also improve mental health and relieve menopausal symptoms such as depression and insomnia [89].

Physical activity is beneficial in reducing blood insulin levels, exercise systolic/diastolic blood pressure, psychiatric symptoms, metabolic syndrome, and breast cancer risk, and improving sleep and QoL in postmenopausal women [5, 13]. It is recommended that women receive comprehensive information about physical exercise before entering menopause. Menopausal symptoms, changes in quality of life, and their functions in preventing these should be well understood by physiotherapists. Creating a "menopause school" paradigm for lifestyle adjustments in this regard will also provide a significant advantage [70].

25.3.4 Sleep and Infertility

Infertility and sleep difficulties are common public health concerns worldwide in modern culture. Infertility is a disease of the male or female reproductive system defined by the failure to achieve a pregnancy after 12 months or more of regular unprotected sexual intercourse. Infertility has a multitude of causes, and research suggests that sleep disorders may also be a contributing factor to it. A person's mental health, brain function, metabolism, and hormone levels can all be affected by sleep quality, which can ultimately affect reproductive function and lead to infertility [6]. There are three possible mechanisms by which sleep disorders may lead to infertility [66]. First, endometrial receptivity may be reduced, and secretion of reproductive hormones and melatonin may be altered directly or indirectly through HPA axis activation. By interfering with critical times such as regular menstrual bleeding or effective ovulation, implantation, and placental growth and development, these changes may reduce fertility. Second, sleep disorders themselves may inhibit fertility by suppressing or increasing reproductive hormones and inflammatory reactions. Third, circadian dysrhythmia, which is associated with altered reproductive hormone secretion and adverse reproductive outcomes, may affect fertility.

Various sex hormones secreted along with the body's circadian rhythm control female reproductive function. The synthesis, release, and metabolism of these hormones, which are physiologically necessary for reproduction, depend on a regular circadian cycle to get enough sleep [72]. At the same time, hormones in the body have a close relationship with sleep. Lack of sleep can affect a person's fertility, as it can cause the body to produce more stress hormones and lower levels of estrogen, testosterone, and other reproductive hormones. Moreover, sleep patterns produce general characteristics that support the physiological processes necessary for hormone synthesis for reproduction [72].

Reproduction and sleep are related. Sleep disorders can affect the CV, immunologic, and neuroendocrine systems, leading to reproductive endocrine system disorders and increasing the risk of abnormal HPA axis outcomes, including amenorrhea, pregnancy loss, infertility, and failed embryo implantation [9, 148]. Sleep disorders are linked to decreased ovarian reserve, and sleep is crucial for the diurnal fluctuation of several neuroendocrine hormones that affect ovulation [140].

For women, infertility is a life crisis due to its high cost and emotionally exhausting nature. In addition to being a gynecological problem, it is a biopsychosocial health problem. Infertility often has significant psychological effects and is often associated with poorer QoL [45]. The outcome of infertility treatment is also affected by stress. Stress-related problems occur two to three times more frequently during treatment. Sleep habits also change in individuals who experience stress and anxiety.

Female fertility depends on the hormone PRL, which changes before sleep onset and reaches its peak at night. PRL is reduced in those who suffer from sleep deprivation and is prevented by short-term awakenings. Sleep disorders affect the ability of the HPA glands to function, which can lead to oxidative stress and the development of insulin resistance.

Stress can affect fertility at critical times for effective ovulation, implantation, and placental growth and development, or regular menstrual bleeding [44]. Reducing stress will both support infertility treatment and reduce sleep problems, which are a risk factor for infertility. Therefore, it is important to correctly implement physiotherapy interventions for parameters such as stress and anxiety.

Osteopathic manipulative therapy (OMT) is beneficial for various diseases such as melancholy, stress, and back pain. The sympathetic and parasympathetic nervous systems come into balance after osteopathic manipulative therapy sessions. The procedure involving OMT can improve general health and greatly increase the quality of life. Improving well-being is especially important in the treatment of infertility [137].

Relaxation and meditation increase mental clarity and help individuals overcome the challenges associated with infertility treatment. Yoga can help all women with infertility issues and is particularly effective in reducing stress levels in women with infertility issues. One of the main factors contributing to infertility is stress, which disrupts women's menstrual cycles and delays ovulation. Regular yoga practice can help reduce stress [64]. Additionally, regular yoga practice improves sleep quality. In addition to improving overall well-being, yoga also increases sleep duration, efficiency, and quality [48].

25.4 Sleep and Female Athlete

Optimal preparation and adequate performance between training and competition are essential for success in elite sports. Athletes typically sleep less than 7 h per night, despite recommendations of ≥7 h to support optimal health and cognitive function among adults [30]. Compared to male athletes, female athletes who train and perform late at night often exhibit higher levels of sleep disturbances [86]. High levels of anxiety have been observed in female athletes, which is thought to increase pre-sleep hyperarousal (increased psychological and physiological tension) and result in a reduced sense of restorative sleep [120].

The importance of sleep for the performance and recovery of highly skilled athletes is increasingly recognized. However, elite athletes often face situational challenges such as competition schedules and travel demand. Additionally, factors such as increased body temperature after exercise, increased muscle tension and soreness after training and competition, exposure to light and noise, and increased psychological stress contribute to poorer sleep quality in elite athletes compared to the general population [99].

Examples of typical situations that may affect sleep cycles in team sports are:

- Performing at night (such as after 8 p.m.)
- Long-term travel
- Busy schedule (such as playing three games in 7 days)
- Competition stress
- Pain after training and competition

Attention, concentration, perceptual function, language, memory, executive and intellectual function, and other sleep parameters (sleep architecture and efficiency) are interconnected [95]. In many sports, but especially in team sports, it is essential to have adequate cognitive function. Therefore, sleep deprivation can negatively affect the athlete's performance by impairing cognitive function [49].

Sleep deprivation can aggravate or trigger pain, and the discomfort felt can disrupt sleep by causing awakenings during sleep. Pain or sleep deprivation can then start a cycle in which these two problems reinforce or sustain each other [73]. Training, competition, and/or injuries can cause pain in athletes [78]. Therefore, it is important for athletes to benefit greatly from appropriate pain management and adequate sleep in terms of pain and sleep.

There is also a bidirectional relationship between sleep and immunity. Sleep deprivation can have deleterious effects on immune function, and immune responses feed back into sleep architecture [12]. Sleep deprivation can disrupt endocrine and physiological circadian rhythms, which can impair immune responses and increase disease risk [149]. Short sleep durations can reduce immune function, and the resulting decreased immunity can have a negative impact on athletic performance.

Practicing behaviors that promote sleep and avoiding behaviors that interfere with sleep is called sleep hygiene [49]. Educating people about sleep hygiene involves providing them with guidance on lifestyle and behavioral choices and environmental factors such as temperature, light, and noise that affect sleep. It is important to teach athletes ways to optimize their sleep quantity and quality through instruction on sleep and sleep hygiene practices [71].

25.5 Sleep Disorders in Women

Sleep disorders are classified into seven major categories according to the International Classification of Sleep Disorders (ICSD) [119].

25.5.1 Insomnia

Insomnia is a sleep disorder characterized by difficulties in falling asleep or staying asleep, which leads to impaired daytime functioning and reduced QoL. The condition includes three primary aspects: difficulty initiating or maintaining sleep despite adequate opportunity and environment for rest, and experiencing daytime consequences such as fatigue, concentration issues, mood changes, and cognitive impairment. In diagnosing chronic insomnia, these symptoms must persist for at least 3 months and occur at least three times per week [119]. The prevalence of insomnia increases with age for both genders. In a large sample of approximately 5000 individuals aged over 65 years, 70% reported experiencing at least one symptom of insomnia. Difficulty in maintaining sleep was the most reported symptom in both genders. Women reported experiencing more insomnia symptoms than men. Loud snoring was found to be highly associated with difficulty maintaining sleep, with a high body mass index increasing the risk of difficulty initiating sleep in men alone [56].

The meta-analysis, which included 13 articles, revealed a significantly higher prevalence of insomnia in women than in men [154]. The increased risk of insomnia in women might be attributable to various factors, including sex differences, hormonal variations, mood disorders, environmental factors, socioeconomic vulnerability, and psychosocial stressors [106]. Insomnia is an expected symptom of many medical and psychiatric conditions [119]. The prevalence and comorbidity of anxiety disorders are significantly different between women and men, with research showing a greater impact on women. When examining factors related to gender and sex differences in anxiety, masculinity may act as a protective factor against the development of anxiety, whereas femininity may serve as a risk factor. The potential influence of brain structures, genetic factors, and fluctuations in sex hormones was identified as a reason for the higher prevalence of anxiety in women. Regarding comorbidity, findings indicate that women are more likely to develop other internalizing disorders (e.g., depression), whereas men are more likely to develop externalizing disorders (e.g., substance abuse) [37]. A meta-analysis found that women are twice as likely to experience depression as men, partly because of their tendency to ruminate more [59]. Rumination involves repetitive, prolonged, and recurrent negative thinking about oneself, feelings, personal concerns, and upsetting experiences [150]. Women experience higher worry around bedtime than men, possibly due to life stress resulting from work demands and gendered expectations [128]. Worry and rumination predict nighttime sleep in older adults, with better sleep predicting less worry the next morning and more sleep buffering worry overnight [157]. In addition, there are some specific types of depression-related disorders, such as postpartum depression and premenstrual dysphoric disorder, that women experience during periods when hormonal processes change.

Insomnia is highly prevalent in the last trimester of pregnancy. Pregnant women often neglect sleep disorders, which can cause mental and physical issues and can also affect the fetus [117]. Both objective nighttime sleep of less than 6 h and self-reported poor sleep quality in healthy third-trimester pregnant women were associated with significant risks of clinical depression [145]. The presence of other sleep disorders can cause or worsen insomnia symptoms.

Insomnia is one of the most frequent symptoms of menopause [109]. The etiology of insomnia during menopause can be attributed to reproductive hormonal changes, vasomotor symptoms, mood disorders, circadian rhythm modifications, and decreased secretion of melatonin [57]. Insomnia in postmenopausal women was found to be associated with vasomotor and depressive symptoms. In addition, mood symptoms affect sleep independently of vasomotor symptoms [155].

In recent years, numerous systematic reviews have been conducted to explore the effects of exercise in individuals with insomnia. According to the results of a recent umbrella review that combines multiple systematic reviews and/or meta-analyses, the available evidence suggests that different exercise modalities have varied effects on insomnia [141]. Table 25.1 summarizes these results.

Regular moderate-intensity aerobic exercise is particularly recommended for the treatment and prevention of sleep disorders because it can increase total sleep duration and enhance slow-wave sleep. Exercising before bedtime does not necessarily disturb the sleep of individuals with good sleep quality. The beneficial effects of exercise on sleep are attributed to multiple pathways,

Table 25.1 Effects of different exercise types on insomnia

Exercise type	Effects of insomnia
Moderate-intensity aerobic exercise	Reduced wakefulness after sleep onset and improved sleep efficiency (objectively measured) Reduced sleep onset latency
Moderate-intensity aerobic exercise + Light-intensity strength exercises	Reduced wakefulness after sleep onset and improved sleep efficiency (objectively measured) Improved sleep efficiency (subjectively measured) Reduced ISI and PSQI scores
Mind-body exercise	Reduced wakefulness after sleep onset and improved sleep efficiency (objectively and subjectively measured) Reduced latency of sleep onset and increases total sleep time (subjectively measured) Reduced ISI and PSQI scores
Low-intensity strength exercise	Improved sleep efficiency Reduced ISI and PSQI scores
Moderate-intensity strength exercise	ImproveD sleep efficiency Reduced ISI and PSQI scores

ISI Insomnia Severity Index, *PSQI* Pittsburgh Sleep Quality Index

including the regulation of circadian rhythm through melatonin, mood improvement via increased BDNF, and reduced inflammation by lowering prostaglandin E2 and tumor necrosis factor-alpha levels. Exercise can also affect body core temperature, boost growth factor levels, decrease insulin resistance, and modulate vagal nerve activity [25].

25.5.2 Sleep-Related Breathing Disorders

Sleep-related breathing disorders are defined by abnormal respiratory patterns during sleep, with OSA being the most common form [119].

25.5.2.1 Obstructive Sleep Apnea

The diagnosis of OSA is based on the presence of specific signs and symptoms. These can include sleepiness, fatigue, insomnia, snoring, subjective nocturnal respiratory disturbances, or observed episodes of apnea. Additionally, it is important to consider any associated medical or psychiatric conditions. A diagnosis is confirmed through polysomnography, where five or more predominantly obstructive respiratory events are observed per hour of sleep. These events typically include episodes of apnea or hypopnea, which reflect reduced or blocked airflow. The combination of clinical symptoms and polysomnographic findings is essential for a definitive diagnosis. Therefore, both subjective reports and objective data are required for accurate assessment [119]. OSA is more common in men than in women [41]. Men have greater upper airway collapsibility than women due to longer airway length, larger soft tissue volume on the lateral pharyngeal walls, and fluid displacement during recumbency, which contributes to upper airway narrowing, despite similar pharyngeal cross-sectional areas [61, 85, 135]. Although OSA is more common in men across all age groups, the prevalence of OSA increases with age in both sexes [38]. The sex difference narrows in older individuals (>50 years) because of an increase in OSA prevalence in women during the postmenopausal period [121]. Women with OSA often report atypical symptoms, such as insomnia, depression/mood disturbance, morning headache, and fatigue, but less commonly report snoring, witnessed apnea, and excessive daytime sleepiness [41]. The association between OSA and several adverse outcomes may be more pronounced in women [121]. While the presence of OSA in women has been found to be associated with a high risk of heart failure, this association is not observed in men. The same study's 13-year follow-up indicates a greater occurrence of mortality in women [115]. Polysomnographic studies reveal differences between genders. It was found that women experienced more severe desaturations after 30–45 s of obstructive apneas, whereas their desaturation areas after hypopneas (with related hypopnea event durations ⩽ of 30 s) are smaller. This suggests that longer obstructive apneas may be more detrimental to females than males [69]. Women typically exhibit lower apnea-hypopnea index (AHI) scores compared to men. Their apneic episodes are generally shorter in duration. Women also have a smaller proportion of positional OSA. In women, apneas predominantly occur during REM sleep, with a lower frequency of respiratory disturbances observed during NREM sleep [40, 41, 102]. Females with OSA experience a higher frequency of hypopneas and fewer desaturation events per hour, more daytime functioning, and QoL impairment compared to men [36, 121, 153].

Significant differences in symptoms, diagnosis, and OSA outcomes have been reported. Understanding these gender differences can enhance awareness and diagnosis of OSA in women and develop therapeutic options that consider the unique physiology and presentation of OSA in women, potentially improving patient outcomes [152]. Further studies are needed on potential sex-specific differences in responsiveness to OSA treatment because female patients with OSA are more likely to be underdiagnosed, resulting in inadequate treatment [121]. The most common treatment options are lifestyle modification, continuous positive airway pressure therapy, mandibular advancement devices, and surgery [35]. The treatment options for OSAS, their

Table 25.2 Treatment options for obstructive sleep apnea: characteristics, effects, and gender-specific considerations

Treatment options	The characteristics or effects of the treatment	Gender-specific considerations
Weight loss	Weight loss in overweight/obese adults, induced by behavioral means, significantly reduced AHI [65], whereas weight loss induced by medication or surgery also improved AHI proportionately [83]	There is a notable gender difference in bariatric surgery, with women accounting for 80% of those undergoing the procedure, even though the prevalence of obesity is similar in both sexes [126]. After surgery, 77.5% of men and 90.0% of women with obstructive sleep apnea ceased using CPAP therapy [62]
Oral appliance	Oral appliances are recommended by qualified dentists for treating OSA, especially for patients who cannot tolerate CPAP or who prefer alternative therapies [112]	Individual characteristics like lower BMI and female sex can predict positive responses to mandibular advancement device treatment [24] A mandibular advancement device for OSA reduces nocturnal blood pressure in women but not in men [114]
Positive airway pressure	The four primary guidelines for PAP therapy are as follows: (1) utilizing PAP to manage excessive daytime sleepiness, (2) initiating therapy with either home-based APAP or in-lab CPAP titration, (3) maintaining PAP treatment for OSA with either CPAP or APAP, and (4) implementing educational strategies to assist adults with OSA in starting PAP therapy [103]	Female gender was significantly correlated with increased CPAP use [130] CPAP use in pregnancy is well tolerated with good adherence and may be linked to lower blood pressure, reduced risk of preeclampsia, increased birth weight, and decreased risk of preterm birth [101] CPAP treatment significantly reduced diastolic blood pressure and preeclampsia incidence in women with mild-to-moderate OSA and high-risk pregnancy [139]

(continued)

Table 25.2 (continued)

Treatment options	The characteristics or effects of the treatment	Gender-specific considerations
Exercise	Exercise reduces OSA severity without BMI changes, and aerobic exercise combined with resistance training had a better effect on AHI reduction compared to AE alone. Moreover, exercise enhances cardiopulmonary fitness, sleep quality, and excessive daytime sleepiness [105] The oropharyngeal exercise program did not significantly change the BMI but did significantly reduce the neck circumference. It improved daytime sleepiness, witnessed apnea, and snoring intensity. It significantly improved sleep indices such as minimum oxygen saturation, duration of Sao2 < 90%, sleep efficiency, arousal index, and total sleep time N3 stage [147]	A significant negative correlation was found between OSA severity as measured by AHI and peak VO_2 in women but not in men [28]
Upper airway surgery	The following five categories cover the primary surgical options for sleep-disordered breathing: nasal surgery, oropharyngeal surgery, tongue surgery, craniofacial surgery, and tracheostomy [19]	Most studies about surgery outcomes are male-dominated, with little data on gender's role in surgical decision-making or outcomes, including effective procedures in carefully selected patients like maxillomandibular advancement and multilevel airway surgery ([156]; [41]; [133])
Neurostimulation	Hypoglossal nerve stimulation can be considered a second-line option for certain patients when first-line treatments are ineffective [52]	The majority of participants in existing studies were male, and the potential influence of gender as a predictor of treatment response has yet to be explored ([132]; [41])
Treatment alternatives		
Hormone replacement treatment	Hormonal replacement therapy alone cannot alleviate sleep-related breathing disorders in midlife women, as there is no evidence that hormonal changes during menopause explain the increase in sleep-disordered breathing [82]	Despite the increased prevalence of sleep-related breathing disorders in women during menopausal transition, menopause's role as an independent risk factor has been weak or absent, according to various studies [82]

OSA obstructive sleep apnea, *BMI* body mass index, *AHI* apnea–hypopnea index, VO_2 volume or amount of oxygen your body consumes, *PAP* positive airway pressure, *APAP* auto-adjusting positive airway pressure, *CPAP* continuous positive airway pressure, *AE* aerobic exercise

effects, and specific gender considerations are listed in Table 25.2.

Snoring, a symptom of OSA, tends to increase during pregnancy and is linked to greater sleepiness, a higher BMI at the beginning of pregnancy, and a higher occurrence of edema [118].

25.5.3 Central Disorders of Hypersomnolence

The most characteristic condition among central disorders of hypersomnolence is narcolepsy, which is characterized by excessive daytime sleepiness that persists even with adequate nocturnal sleep duration and quality, and other associated symptoms [63]. Gender differences in human narcolepsy have not been thoroughly evaluated, but female mice exhibit an earlier onset of cataplexy during active hypocretin cell loss and doubling of cataplexy during the estrous phases of the cycle [122]. The treatment of hypersomnia in pregnancy is limited because of concerns about teratogenicity. Patients with narcolepsy have similar pregnancy outcomes but have higher incidences of impaired glucose metabolism and anemia. Possible treatments include discontinuing medications, using the lowest effective doses, and considering non-pharmacologic options like sleep hygiene and scheduled naps [39].

25.5.4 Circadian Rhythm Sleep–Wake Disorders

Plasma estradiol, progesterone, LH, FSH, sex hormone-binding globulin (SHBG), melatonin, and core body temperature exhibit significant 24-h rhythms under standard sleep–wake conditions during the follicular phase, whereas only FSH and SHBG are rhythmic during the luteal phase [111]. There are certain differences in the context of circadian rhythms between men and women [84]. The effect of age on chronotype changes was observed across genders. The data showed that women were more morning-oriented until 30 years old, with no significant differences between 30 and 45 years, and later, more evening-oriented than men [33]. Social jetlag was found to be lower in women and older participants, with some evidence suggesting a diminishing sex difference in older age [146]. Women were found to have a significantly higher melatonin amplitude and lower temperature amplitude than men [17].

Extrinsic misalignment, like jet lag during trans meridian travel, occurs when external factors misalign with the body's internal circadian rhythms. Intrinsic circadian rhythm sleep-wake disorders involve a mismatch between the individual's internal clock and preferred sleep-wake timing, leading to sleep difficulties and daytime dysfunction [104]. Common treatments for these disorders include sleep hygiene education, time therapy, light therapy, melatonin, and hypnotic drug therapy [136]. Melatonin production suppression triggered by exposure to bright light after the onset of melatonin production is not influenced differently by sex [96, 97].

25.5.5 Parasomnia

Parasomnias are abnormal events related to sleep entry, during, or arousal. They are categorized into NREM-related, REM-related parasomnias, and others. Gender differences are not observed in NREM-related parasomnias, except for sleep-related eating disorder, which is more frequently reported in women. The lifetime prevalence of NREM-related parasomnias is estimated to reach up to 40%, though their occurrence declines significantly with advancing age. In contrast, REM-related parasomnias exhibit considerable variability in prevalence, with gender differences depending on the specific disorder; for instance, REM sleep behavior disorder is less common in women, whereas isolated sleep paralysis shows similar prevalence across genders [131].

25.5.6 Sleep-Related Movement Disorders

Several movement disorders can manifest during nocturnal rest, leading to disruptions in sleep. These disturbances are often characterized by involuntary, repetitive, and typically stereotypical movements that lack purposeful intent [90]. This section focuses on restless legs syndrome and periodic limb movement disorder, which are the most common sleep-related movement disorders.

25.5.6.1 Restless Leg Syndrome

The diagnosis of restless legs syndrome (RLS) is based on several key criteria. Patients must experience an urge to move their legs, often accompanied by uncomfortable sensations. These symptoms primarily occur during periods of rest or inactivity. The discomfort is typically alleviated, either partially or completely, by movement, as long as the movement continues. Additionally, the symptoms are most prominent in the evening or at night [119]. RLS is a common disorder in the general adult population, with a higher prevalence in women [14]. Pregnant women were found to be at higher risk of RLS, with increased parity being a predisposing factor [124]. Symptoms typically subside shortly after parturition, but some patients may experience further symptoms postpartum [46]. Paradoxically, menopause increases the prevalence and severity of symptoms. This study suggests that symptoms may be triggered by changes in estrogen levels rather than absolute levels, indicating a complex role for reproductive hormones [124]. Present understanding suggests that a strong family history, low serum iron and ferritin levels, and high estrogen levels during pregnancy might play important roles [46]. Iron and estrogen play a role in dopamine and glutamate transmission, potentially explaining pregnant women's susceptibility to RLS [124]. Pregnancy-related RLS treatment can be challenging due to risks to both mother and fetus, but severe cases may necessitate treatment [46]. Non-pharmacological approaches, along with dietary supplementation, may be initially administered to pregnant women with RLS. Considering that aerobic and stretching exercises can effectively reduce symptom severity in the primary RLS group, exercise practices may be preferred during pregnancy [29]. Various drugs are also available for RLS treatment. In general, all medications should be avoided, but if the symptoms are severe, this safety approach must be considered. Supplemental oral iron should be provided to all pregnant women, and intravenous iron therapy may be beneficial for those with RLS [46].

25.5.6.2 Periodic Limp Movement Disorder

Periodic limb movement disorder is diagnosed when the frequency of limb movement exceeds 15/h in adults and 5/h in children, accompanied by sleep disturbance or functional impairment [119]. RLS is often accompanied by periodic limb movements. The occurrence of periodic limb movements increases with age in both sexes; however, it tends to plateau at an earlier age in women. The periodicity of movements rises to around 35 in men, whereas in women, it continues to increase until around the age of 45–50. After this age, it remains at a higher level than in men for an additional decade [93]. A previous study demonstrated that women show greater acute responsiveness to dopamine agonists (pramipexole and ropinirole) for periodic limb movements in RLS compared to men. This finding suggests a need for a more tailored, sex-specific approach to treating RLS associated with PLMS, as dopamine agonists may lead to better outcomes in women than in men [92].

25.5.6.3 Sleep-Related Leg Cramps

Sleep-related leg cramps are probably the most frequent sleep disorder. They are easy to diagnose but difficult to treat [15]. Nocturnal leg cramps are commonly observed and are associated with reduced sleep quality. Diuretic and long-acting beta-agonist therapy may predispose individuals to cramps. The effectiveness of prophylactic stretching exercises is controversial. Cramp frequency has been shown to be reduced by quinine, although with modest benefits and potential risks and side effects [110].

25.6 Sleep Hygiene

All individuals, including women, should prioritize sleep hygiene, regardless of the diagnosis of a specific sleep disorder. The standard sleep hygiene training recommendations can be summarized as follows:

- Consuming caffeine near bedtime can interfere with sleep, with its disruptive effects increasing in proportion to the amount consumed. Individuals with caffeine sensitivity may be particularly affected by these adverse impacts on sleep [54].
- Nicotine use, or smoking, disrupts sleep. In the early stages of smoking cessation, arousal may temporarily increase [54].
- Acute alcohol consumption before sleep reduces SOL and increases arousal during the

second half of the night. The effects of alcohol on sleep exhibit a dose-response relationship. Individuals who quit alcohol may experience sleep problems during the acute phase. Although there is a modest improvement in sleep in the long term, sleep problems can persist in abstinent users [54].

- Regular or acute exercise provides modest improvement, regardless of the presence of sleep complaints [54]. Exercise, regardless of the time, enhances NREM sleep without significantly affecting other aspects of sleep quality. The current evidence does not support the claim that late-night exercise disrupts sleep because exercise enhances NREM sleep without significantly affecting other sleep quality aspects [43, 54].
- Two different methods can be recommended for restful sleep: journaling and mindful and meditative walking. Journaling is a personal, unfiltered expression in which you write freely without structure or rules, focusing on thoughts, feelings, memories, and dreams. It is a journey of self-discovery that can be undertaken daily, without judgment, allowing one to process emotions and gain insights [58].
- Relaxation and breathing exercises can help you fall asleep. Some examples include diaphragmatic breathing exercises such as the 4-7-8 breathing technique (inhale deeply through your nose for 4 s, hold for 7 s, and then exhale through your mouth for 8 s, making a gentle sound as if blowing out a candle), visualization exercises such as body scan, Yoga Nidra, progressive relaxation exercise, and non-sleep deep rest [113].
- The sleep environment must be sleep-friendly to ensure a high-quality sleep experience. Nocturnal noise can increase arousals, and even if individuals seem to adapt to the noise, arousal recorded via EEG during sleep may persist. Strategies to reduce noise can improve sleep [54] . It is essential to sleep in completely dark environments to optimize sleep hygiene. Sleeping with lights on can lead to shallow sleep, frequent arousals, and persistent disruptions in brain oscillations that are critical for maintaining sleep depth and stability [26]. Some evidence suggests that a cooler sleep environment promotes deeper sleep [142]. Therefore, creating a dark, cool, and quiet sleep environment is recommended [8].
- In healthy young individuals, a midday nap, which can facilitate cognitive and emotional health, is beneficial. Frequent napping is linked to negative health outcomes in older adults. Therefore, it is important to be cautious about the frequency of napping in this population. Encouraging a structured sleep routine and minimizing daytime naps can help maintain overall health and support better nighttime sleep quality [87].

25.7 Conclusion

This exploration of the fundamental characteristics of sleep, changes during specific periods in women, and sleep disorders provides valuable insights into an essential aspect of women's health. Sleep, with its biological, psychological, and social dimensions, can significantly vary across different stages of a woman's life. In this context, there are countless ways to explore the impact of sleep on women. Future research in this field will contribute to developing more targeted and effective approaches, including physiotherapy, to improve women's sleep health.

References

1. Agarwal AK, Kiron N, Gupta R, Sengar A, Gupta P. A study of assessment menopausal symptoms and coping strategies among middle age women of North Central India. Int J Commun Med Public Health. 2018;5(10):4470–7. https://doi.org/10.18203/2394-6040.ijcmph20180001.
2. Alzueta E, Baker FC. The menstrual cycle and sleep. Sleep Med Clin. 2023;18(4):399–413. https://doi.org/10.1016/j.jsmc.2023.06.003.
3. American College of Obstetricians and Gynecologists (ACOG). Committee opinion no. 650. Obstet Gynecol. 2015;126(6):e135–42.
4. Amrutha V, Miranda JP. A study to assess the effectiveness of yoga therapy on menopausal symptoms among women in a selected area at Mangaluru. Indian J Pub Health Res Dev. 2019;10(11)

5. Anderson D, Seib C, Rasmussen L. Can physical activity prevent physical and cognitive decline in postmenopausal women?: A systematic review of the literature. Maturitas. 2014;79(1):14–33. https://doi.org/10.1016/j.maturitas.2014.06.010.
6. Auger N, Healy-Profitós J, Wei SQ. In the arms of Morpheus: meta-analysis of sleep and fertility. Fertil Steril. 2021;115(3):596–8. https://doi.org/10.1016/j.fertnstert.2020.12.030.
7. Baker FC, Sassoon SA, Kahan T, Palaniappan L, Nicholas CL, Trinder J, Colrain IM. Perceived poor sleep quality in the absence of polysomnographic sleep disturbance in women with severe premenstrual syndrome. J Sleep Res. 2012;21(5):535–45. https://doi.org/10.1111/j.1365-2869.2012.01007.x.
8. Baranwal N, Yu PK, Siegel NS. Sleep physiology, pathophysiology, and sleep hygiene. Prog Cardiovasc Dis. 2023;77:59–69. https://doi.org/10.1016/j.pcad.2023.02.005.
9. Besedovsky L, Lange T, Haack M. The sleep-immune crosstalk in health and disease. Physiol Rev. 2019; https://doi.org/10.1152/physrev.00010.2018.
10. Bezerra AG, Andersen ML, Pires GN, Tufik S, Hachul H. The effects of hormonal contraceptive use on sleep in women: a systematic review and meta-analysis. J Sleep Res. 2023;32(3):e13757. https://doi.org/10.1111/jsr.13757.
11. Blumberg MS, Lesku JA, Libourel P-A, Schmidt MH, Rattenborg NC. What is REM sleep? Curr Biol. 2020;30(1):R38–49. https://doi.org/10.1016/j.cub.2019.11.045.
12. Bollinger T, Bollinger A, Oster H, Solbach W. Sleep, immunity, and circadian clocks: a mechanistic model. Gerontology. 2010;56(6):574–80. https://doi.org/10.1159/000281827.
13. Bonaiuti D, Shea B, Iovine R, Negrini S, Robinson V, Kemper HC, et al. Exercise for preventing and treating osteoporosis in postmenopausal women. Cochrane Database Syst Rev. 2002;3:CD000333. https://doi.org/10.1002/14651858.cd000333.
14. Broström A, Alimoradi Z, Lind J, Ulander M, Lundin F, Pakpour A. Worldwide estimation of restless legs syndrome: a systematic review and meta-analysis of prevalence in the general adult population. J Sleep Res. 2023;32(3):e13783. https://doi.org/10.1111/jsr.13783.
15. Brown TM. Sleep-related leg cramps a review and suggestions for future research. Sleep Med Clin. 2015;10(3):385. https://doi.org/10.1016/j.jsmc.2015.05.002.
16. Brown SG, Morrison LA, Calibuso MJ, Christiansen TM. The menstrual cycle and sexual behavior: relationship to eating, exercise, sleep, and health patterns. Women Health. 2008;48(4):429–44. https://doi.org/10.1080/03630240802575179.
17. Cain SW, Dennison CF, Zeitzer JM, Guzik AM, Khalsa SB, Santhi N, Schoen MW, Czeisler CA, Duffy JF. Sex differences in phase angle of entrainment and melatonin amplitude in humans. J Biol Rhythm. 2010;25(4):288–96. https://doi.org/10.1177/0748730410374943.
18. Carley DW, Farabi SS. Physiology of sleep. Diabetes Spectr. 2016;29(1):5–9. https://doi.org/10.2337/diaspect.29.1.5.
19. Carvalho B, Hsia J, Capasso R. Surgical therapy of obstructive sleep apnea: a review. Neurotherapeutics. 2012;9(4):710–6. https://doi.org/10.1007/s13311-012-0141-x.
20. Caufriez A, Leproult R, L'Hermite-Balériaux M, Moreno-Reyes R, Copinschi G. A potential role of endogenous progesterone in modulation of GH, prolactin and thyrotrophin secretion during normal menstrual cycle. Clin Endocrinol. 2009;71(4):535–42. https://doi.org/10.1111/j.1365-2265.2009.03539.x.
21. Caufriez A, Leproult R, L'Hermite-Balériaux M, Kerkhofs M, Copinschi G. Progesterone prevents sleep disturbances and modulates GH, TSH, and melatonin secretion in postmenopausal women. J Clin Endocrinol Metabol. 2011;96(4):E614–23. https://doi.org/10.1210/jc.2010-2558.
22. Chang JJ, Pien GW, Duntley SP, Macones GA. Sleep deprivation during pregnancy and maternal and fetal outcomes: is there a relationship? Sleep Med Rev. 2010;14(2):107–14. https://doi.org/10.1016/j.smrv.2009.05.001.
23. Chen KM, Chen MH, Chao HC, Hung HM, Lin HS, Li CH. Sleep quality, depression state, and health status of older adults after silver yoga exercises: cluster randomized trial. Int J Nurs Stud. 2009;46(2):154–63.
24. Chen H, Eckert DJ, van der Stelt PF, Guo J, Ge S, Emami E, Almeida FR, Huynh NT. Phenotypes of responders to mandibular advancement device therapy in obstructive sleep apnea patients: a systematic review and meta-analysis. Sleep Med Rev. 2020;49:101229. https://doi.org/10.1016/j.smrv.2019.101229.
25. Chennaoui M, Arnal PJ, Sauvet F, Léger D. Sleep and exercise: a reciprocal issue? Sleep Med Rev. 2015;20:59–72. https://doi.org/10.1016/j.smrv.2014.06.008.
26. Cho JR, Joo EY, Koo DL, Hong SB. Let there be no light: the effect of bedside light on sleep quality and background electroencephalographic rhythms. Sleep Med. 2013;14(12):1422–5. https://doi.org/10.1016/j.sleep.2013.09.007.
27. Christian LM, Carroll JE, Teti DM, Hall MH. Maternal sleep in pregnancy and postpartum part I: mental, physical, and interpersonal consequences. Curr Psychiatry Rep. 2019;21:1–8. https://doi.org/10.1007/s11920-019-0999-y.
28. Cintra F, Poyares D, Rizzi CF, Risso TT, Skomro R, Montuori E, Mello-Fujita L, de Paola A, Tufik S. Cardiorespiratory response to exercise in men and women with obstructive sleep apnea. Sleep Med. 2009;10(3):368–73. https://doi.org/10.1016/j.sleep.2008.04.006.
29. Çoban Ö, Ün Yıldırım N, Yaşa ME, Sonkaya AR. Effects of different exercise programs

on symptoms, sleep, and quality of life in patients with primary restless legs syndrome. Mov Disord Clin Pract. 2023;10(9):1349–59. https://doi.org/10.1002/mdc3.13833.
30. Consensus Conference Panel, Watson NF, Badr MS, Belenky G, Bliwise DL, Buxton OM, et al. Recommended amount of sleep for a healthy adult: a joint consensus statement of the American Academy of Sleep Medicine and Sleep Research Society. J Clin Sleep Med. 2015;11(6):591–2. do
31. de Zambotti M, Colrain IM, Baker FC. Interaction between reproductive hormones and physiological sleep in women. J Clin Endocrinol Metab. 2015;100(4):1426–33. https://doi.org/10.1210/jc.2014-3892.
32. Deak MC, Stickgold R. Sleep and cognition. Wiley Interdiscip Rev Cogn Sci. 2010;1(4):491–500. https://doi.org/10.1002/wcs.52.
33. Duarte LL, Menna-Barreto L, Miguel MA, Louzada F, Araújo J, Alam M, Areas R, Pedrazzoli M. Chronotype ontogeny related to gender. Braz J Med Biol Res. 2014;47(4):316–20. https://doi.org/10.1590/1414-431x20143001.
34. Epstein LJ. Improving sleep: a guide to a good night's rest. Harvard Health Publications; 2010.
35. Epstein LJ, Kristo D, Strollo PJ Jr, Friedman N, Malhotra A, Patil SP, Ramar K, Rogers R, Schwab RJ, Weaver EM, Weinstein MD. Clinical guideline for the evaluation, management and long-term care of obstructive sleep apnea in adults. J Clin Sleep Med. 2009;5(3):263–76.
36. Fabozzi A, Pasqualotto F, Laguardia M, Natuzzi PF, Capone R, Steffanina A, Pellegrino D, Olmati F, Antonaglia C, Palange P. Gender differences in obstructive sleep apnea syndrome: a pilot study. Sleep Breath. 2024;28(4):1645–50. https://doi.org/10.1007/s11325-024-03052-x.
37. Farhane-Medina NZ, Luque B, Tabernero C, Castillo-Mayén R. Factors associated with gender and sex differences in anxiety prevalence and comorbidity: a systematic review. Sci Prog. 2022;105(4):00368504221135469. https://doi.org/10.1177/00368504221135469.
38. Fietze I, Laharnar N, Obst A, Ewert R, Felix SB, Garcia C, Gläser S, Glos M, Schmidt CO, Stubbe B, Völzke H, Zimmermann S, Penzel T. Prevalence and association analysis of obstructive sleep apnea with gender and age differences – results of SHIP-trend. J Sleep Res. 2019;28(5):e12770. https://doi.org/10.1111/jsr.12770.
39. Freedom T, Rasameesoraj T. Management of hypersomnia in pregnancy. In: Sleep disorders in women, Current clinical neurology. Cham: Humana; 2020. p. 295–310.
40. Gabbay IE, Lavie P. Age- and gender-related characteristics of obstructive sleep apnea. Sleep Breath. 2012;16(2):453–60. https://doi.org/10.1007/s11325-011-0523-z.
41. Geer JH, Hilbert J. Gender issues in obstructive sleep Apnea. Yale J Biol Med. 2021;94(3):487–96.
42. Gilley RR. The role of sleep in cognitive function: the value of a good night's rest. Clin EEG Neurosci. 2022;54(1):12–20. https://doi.org/10.1177/15500594221090067.
43. Goldberg M, Pairot de Fontenay B, Blache Y, Debarnot U. Effects of morning and evening physical exercise on subjective and objective sleep quality: an ecological study. J Sleep Res. 2024;33(1):e13996. https://doi.org/10.1111/jsr.13996.
44. Gordon CM. Functional hypothalamic amenorrhea. N Engl J Med. 2010;363(4):365–71. https://doi.org/10.1056/NEJMcp0912024.
45. Greil AL. Infertility and psychological distress: a critical review of the literature. Soc Sci Med. 1997;45(11):1679–704. https://doi.org/10.1016/S0277-9536(97)00102-0.
46. Gupta R, Dhyani M, Kendzerska T, Pandi-Perumal SR, BaHammam AS, Srivanitchapoom P, Pandey S, Hallett M. Restless legs syndrome and pregnancy: prevalence, possible pathophysiological mechanisms and treatment. Acta Neurol Scand. 2016;133(5):320–9. https://doi.org/10.1111/ane.12520.
47. Hachul H, Andersen ML, Bittencourt L, Santos-Silva R, Tufik S. A population-based survey on the influence of the menstrual cycle and the use of hormonal contraceptives on sleep patterns in São Paulo, Brazil. Int J Gynaecol Obstet. 2013;120(2):137–40. https://doi.org/10.1016/j.ijgo.2012.08.020.
48. Halpern J, Cohen M, Kennedy G, Reece J, Cahan C, Baharav A. Yoga for improving sleep quality and quality of life for older adults. Altern Ther Health Med. 2014;20(3):37–46.
49. Halson SL. Sleep in elite athletes and nutritional interventions to enhance sleep. Sports Med. 2014;44(Suppl 1):13–23.
50. Haufe A, Leeners B. Sleep disturbances across a woman's lifespan: what is the role of reproductive hormones? J Endocr Soc. 2023;7(5) https://doi.org/10.1210/jendso/bvad036.
51. Herrero Babiloni A, Baril AA, Charlebois-Plante C, Jodoin M, Sanchez E, De Baets L, et al. The putative role of neuroinflammation in the interaction between traumatic brain injuries, sleep, pain and other neuropsychiatric outcomes: a state-of-the-art review. J Clin Med. 2023;12(5):1793.
52. Hsieh Y-H, Schell AE, Yeh E, Strohl MP, Curado TF, Strohl KP. Neurostimulation in the management of obstructive sleep Apnea. Curr Sleep Med Rep. 2022;8(4):168–79.
53. Ibáñez V, Silva J, Cauli O. A survey on sleep assessment methods. PeerJ. 2018;6:e4849. https://doi.org/10.7717/peerj.4849.
54. Irish LA, Kline CE, Gunn HE, Buysse DJ, Hall MH. The role of sleep hygiene in promoting public health: a review of empirical evidence. Sleep Med Rev. 2015;22:23–36. https://doi.org/10.1016/j.smrv.2014.10.001.
55. Ishikura IA, Moysés-Oliveira M, Fernandes GL, Hachul H, Tufik S, Andersen ML. How do phases of the menstrual cycle affect sleep?

A polysomnographic study of the EPISONO database. Sleep Breath. 2024;28(3):1399–407. https://doi.org/10.1007/s11325-024-02996-4.
56. Jaussent I, Dauvilliers Y, Ancelin M-L, Dartigues J-F, Tavernier B, Touchon J, Ritchie K, Besset A. Insomnia symptoms in older adults: associated factors and gender differences. Am J Geriatr Psychiatry. 2011;19(1):88–97. https://doi.org/10.1097/JGP.0b013e3181e049b6.
57. Jeon G-H. Insomnia in postmenopausal women: how to approach and treat it? J Clin Med. 2024;13(2):428.
58. Johnson D. A good night's sleep: three strategies to rest, relax and restore energy. J Interprofessional Educ Pract. 2023;30:100591. https://doi.org/10.1016/j.xjep.2022.100591.
59. Johnson DP, Whisman MA. Gender differences in rumination: a meta-analysis. Personal Individ Differ. 2013;55(4):367–74. https://doi.org/10.1016/j.paid.2013.03.019.
60. Karandikar-Agashe G, Agrawal R. Comparative study of the effect of resistance exercises versus aerobic exercises in postmenopausal women suffering from insomnia. J Mid-life Health. 2020;11(1):2–5. https://doi.org/10.4103/jmh.JMH_35_19.
61. Kasai T, Motwani SS, Elias RM, Gabriel JM, Taranto Montemurro L, Yanagisawa N, Spiller N, Paul N, Bradley TD. Influence of rostral fluid shift on upper airway size and mucosal water content. J Clin Sleep Med. 2014;10(10):1069–74. https://doi.org/10.5664/jcsm.4102.
62. Kennedy-Dalby A, Adam S, Ammori BJ, Syed AA. Weight loss and metabolic outcomes of bariatric surgery in men versus women – a matched comparative observational cohort study. Eur J Intern Med. 2014;25(10):922–5. https://doi.org/10.1016/j.ejim.2014.10.020.
63. Khan Z, Trotti LM. Central disorders of hypersomnolence. Chest. 2015;148(1):262–73. https://doi.org/10.1378/chest.14-1304.
64. Kirca N, Pasinlioglu T. The effect of yoga on stress level in infertile women. Perspect Psychiatr Care. 2019;55(2):319–27.
65. Kline CE, Burke LE, Sereika SM, Imes CC, Rockette-Wagner B, Mendez DD, Strollo PJ, Zheng Y, Rathbun SL, Chasens ER. Bidirectional relationships between weight change and sleep apnea in a behavioral weight loss intervention. Mayo Clin Proc. 2018;93(9):1290–8. https://doi.org/10.1016/j.mayocp.2018.04.026.
66. Kloss JD, Perlis M, Zamzow JA, Culnan EJ, Gracia CR. Sleep, sleep disturbance, and fertility in women. Sleep Med Rev. 2015;22:78–87. https://doi.org/10.1016/j.smrv.2014.10.005.
67. Ko SH, Chen CH, Wang HH, Su YT. Postpartum women's sleep quality and its predictors in Taiwan. J Nurs Scholarsh. 2014;46(2):74–81. https://doi.org/10.1111/jnu.12053.
68. Kravitz HM, Janssen I, Santoro N, Bromberger JT, Schocken M, Everson-Rose SA, Karavolos K, Powell LH. Relationship of day-to-day reproductive hormone levels to sleep in midlife women. Arch Intern Med. 2005;165(20):2370–6. https://doi.org/10.1001/archinte.165.20.2370.
69. Kulkas A, Duce B, Leppänen T, Hukins C, Töyräs J. Gender differences in severity of desaturation events following hypopnea and obstructive apnea events in adults during sleep. Physiol Meas. 2017;38(8):1490–502. https://doi.org/10.1088/1361-6579/aa7b6f.
70. Kurbonboyev A, Kaygisiz BB. The effect of preventive physiotherapy training on physical activity level and functional capacity in postmenopausal women. Medicina Sportiva J Rom Sports Med Soc. 2019;15(1):3021–9.
71. Lastella M, Roach GD, Halson SL, Sargent C. Sleep/wake behaviours of elite athletes from individual and team sports. Eur J Sport Sci. 2015;15(2):94–100. https://doi.org/10.1080/17461391.2014.932016.
72. Lateef OM, Akintubosun MO. Sleep and reproductive health. J Circadian Rhythms. 2020;18 https://doi.org/10.5334/jcr.190.
73. Lautenbacher S, Kundermann B, Krieg JC. Sleep deprivation and pain perception. Sleep Med Rev. 2006;10(5):357–69. https://doi.org/10.1016/j.smrv.2005.08.001.
74. Lee KA. Sleep promotion in the childbearing family 16. In: Sleep disorders and sleep promotion in nursing practice. Springer; 2011. p. 261.
75. Lee SY, Lee KA. Early postpartum sleep and fatigue for mothers after cesarean delivery compared with vaginal delivery: an exploratory study. J Perinat Neonatal Nurs. 2007;21(2):109–13. https://doi.org/10.1097/01.JPN.0000270627.73993.b0.
76. Lee KA, Shaver JF, Giblin EC, Woods NF. Sleep patterns related to menstrual cycle phase and premenstrual affective symptoms. Sleep. 1990;13(5):403–9.
77. Lee KA, Zaffke ME, Mcenany G. Parity and sleep patterns during and after pregnancy. Obstet Gynecol. 2000;95(1):14–8. https://doi.org/10.1016/S0029-7844(99)00486-X.
78. Leeder J, Glaister M, Pizzoferro K, Dawson J, Pedlar C. Sleep duration and quality in elite athletes measured using wristwatch actigraphy. J Sports Sci. 2012;30(6):541–5. https://doi.org/10.1080/02640414.2012.660188.
79. Leproult R, Van Cauter E. Role of sleep and sleep loss in hormonal release and metabolism. Endocr Dev. 2010;17:11–21. https://doi.org/10.1159/000262524.
80. Li DX, Romans S, De Souza MJ, Murray B, Einstein G. Actigraphic and self-reported sleep quality in women: associations with ovarian hormones and mood. Sleep Med. 2015;16(10):1217–24. https://doi.org/10.1016/j.sleep.2015.06.009.
81. Lialy HE, Mohamed MA, AbdAllatif LA, Khalid M, Elhelbawy A. Effects of different physiotherapy modalities on insomnia and depression in perimenopausal, menopausal, and post-menopausal women: a systematic review. BMC Womens Health. 2023;23(1):363.

82. Lindberg E, Bonsignore MR, Polo-Kantola P. Role of menopause and hormone replacement therapy in sleep-disordered breathing. Sleep Med Rev. 2020;49:101225. https://doi.org/10.1016/j.smrv.2019.101225.
83. Locke BW, Gomez-Lumbreras A, Tan CJ, Nonthasawadsri T, Veettil SK, Patikorn C, Chaiyakunapruk N. The association of weight loss from anti-obesity medications or bariatric surgery and apnea-hypopnea index in obstructive sleep apnea. Obes Rev. 2024;25(4):e13697. https://doi.org/10.1111/obr.13697.
84. Lok R, Qian J, Chellappa SL. Sex differences in sleep, circadian rhythms, and metabolism: implications for precision medicine. Sleep Med Rev. 2024;75:101926. https://doi.org/10.1016/j.smrv.2024.101926.
85. Malhotra A, Huang Y, Fogel RB, Pillar G, Edwards JK, Kikinis R, Loring SH, White DP. The male predisposition to pharyngeal collapse: importance of airway length. Am J Respir Crit Care Med. 2002;166(10):1388–95. https://doi.org/10.1164/rccm.2112072.
86. Mallampalli MP, Carter CL. Exploring sex and gender differences in sleep health: a society for women's health research report. J Women's Health. 2014;23(7):553–62. https://doi.org/10.1089/jwh.2014.4816.
87. Mantua J, Spencer RMC. Exploring the nap paradox: are mid-day sleep bouts a friend or foe? Sleep Med. 2017;37:88–97. https://doi.org/10.1016/j.sleep.2017.01.019.
88. McCarley RW. Neurobiology of REM and NREM sleep. Sleep Med. 2007;8(4):302–30. https://doi.org/10.1016/j.sleep.2007.03.005.
89. Mehrnoush V, Darsareh F, Roozbeh N, Ziraeie A. Efficacy of the complementary and alternative therapies for the management of psychological symptoms of menopause: a systematic review of randomized controlled trials. J Menopausal Med. 2021;27(3):115. https://doi.org/10.6118/jmm.21022.
90. Merlino G, Gigli GL. Sleep-related movement disorders. Neurol Sci. 2012;33(3):491–513. https://doi.org/10.1007/s10072-011-0905-9.
91. Mindell JA, Cook RA, Nikolovski J. Sleep patterns and sleep disturbances across pregnancy. Sleep Med. 2015;16(4):483–8. https://doi.org/10.1016/j.sleep.2014.12.006.
92. Mogavero MP, Antelmi E, Lanza G, Marelli S, Castelnuovo A, Tinazzi M, DelRosso LM, Silvestri R, Ferri R, Ferini Strambi L. Sex-based disparities in dopamine agonist response in patients with restless legs syndrome. J Sleep Res. 2024a:e14311. https://doi.org/10.1111/jsr.14311.
93. Mogavero MP, Lanza G, DelRosso LM, Lanuzza B, Bruni O, Ferini Strambi L, Ferri R. Exploring sex differences in periodic leg movements during sleep across the lifespan of patients with restless legs syndrome. Sleep Med. 2024b;122:253–7. https://doi.org/10.1016/j.sleep.2024.08.023.
94. Nagai M, Hoshide S, Kario K. Sleep duration as a risk factor for cardiovascular disease- a review of the recent literature. Curr Cardiol Rev. 2010;6(1):54–61. https://doi.org/10.2174/157340310790231635.
95. Nami MT, Sadeghniaat K. Understanding the interplay between neurobiochemistry of sleep-wake systems and cognition. Webmed Central Brain. 2011;2(10):1–10.
96. Nathan PJ, Burrows GD, Norman TR. The effect of dim light on suppression of nocturnal melatonin in healthy women and men. J Neural Transm (Vienna). 1997;104(6–7):643–8. https://doi.org/10.1007/bf01291882.
97. Nathan PJ, Wyndham EL, Burrows GD, Norman TR. The effect of gender on the melatonin suppression by light: a dose response relationship. J Neural Transm. 2000;107(3):271–9. https://doi.org/10.1007/s007020050022.
98. Nawaz H, Adams ML, Katz DL. Physician – patient interactions regarding diet, exercise, and smoking. Prev Med. 2000;31(6):652–7. https://doi.org/10.1006/pmed.2000.0760.
99. Nédélec M, Halson S, Abaidia A, Ahmaidi S, Dupont G. Stress, sleep and recovery in elite soccer: a critical review of the literature. Sports Med. 2015;45:1387–400.
100. Nishihara K, Horiuchi S, Eto H, Uchida S. Comparisons of sleep patterns between mothers in post-partum from 9 to 12 weeks and non-pregnant women. Psychiatry Clin Neurosci. 2001;55(3):227–8. https://doi.org/10.1046/j.1440-1819.2001.00835.x.
101. Nugent R, Wee A, Kearney L, de Costa C. The effectiveness of continuous positive airway pressure for treating obstructive sleep apnoea in pregnancy: a systematic review. Aust N Z J Obstet Gynaecol. 2023;63(3):290–300. https://doi.org/10.1111/ajo.13654.
102. O'Connor C, Thornley KS, Hanly PJ. Gender differences in the polysomnographic features of obstructive sleep apnea. Am J Respir Crit Care Med. 2000;161(5):1465–72. https://doi.org/10.1164/ajrccm.161.5.9904121.
103. Patil SP, Ayappa IA, Caples SM, Kimoff RJ, Patel SR, Harrod CG. Treatment of adult obstructive sleep Apnea with positive airway pressure: an American Academy of sleep medicine clinical practice guideline. J Clin Sleep Med. 2019;15(2):335–43. https://doi.org/10.5664/jcsm.7640.
104. Pavlova M. Circadian rhythm sleep-wake disorders. Continuum (Minneapolis, Minn). 2017;23(4 Sleep Neurology):1051–63. https://doi.org/10.1212/con.0000000000000499.
105. Peng J, Yuan Y, Zhao Y, Ren H. Effects of exercise on patients with obstructive sleep apnea: a systematic review and meta-analysis. Int J Environ Res Public Health. 2022;19(17) https://doi.org/10.3390/ijerph191710845.
106. Pengo MF, Won CH, Bourjeily G. Sleep in women across the life span. Chest. 2018;154(1):196–206. https://doi.org/10.1016/j.chest.2018.04.005.

107. Pérez-López FR, Chedraui P, Gilbert JJ, Pérez-Roncero G. Cardiovascular risk in menopausal women and prevalent related co-morbid conditions: facing the post-women's health initiative era. Fertil Steril. 2009;92(4):1171–86. https://doi.org/10.1016/j.fertnstert.2009.06.032.
108. Posmontier B. Sleep quality in women with and without postpartum depression. J Obstet Gynecol Neonatal Nurs. 2008;37(6):722–37. https://doi.org/10.1111/j.1552-6909.2008.00298.x.
109. Proserpio P, Marra S, Campana C, Agostoni EC, Palagini L, Nobili L, Nappi RE. Insomnia and menopause: a narrative review on mechanisms and treatments. Climacteric. 2020;23(6):539–49. https://doi.org/10.1080/13697137.2020.1799973.
110. Rabbitt L, Mulkerrin EC, O'Keeffe ST. A review of nocturnal leg cramps in older people. Age Ageing. 2016;45(6):776–82. https://doi.org/10.1093/ageing/afw139.
111. Rahman SA, Grant LK, Gooley JJ, Rajaratnam SMW, Czeisler CA, Lockley SW. Endogenous circadian regulation of female reproductive hormones. J Clin Endocrinol Metab. 2019;104(12):6049–59. https://doi.org/10.1210/jc.2019-00803.
112. Ramar K, Dort LC, Katz SG, Lettieri CJ, Harrod CG, Thomas SM, Chervin RD. Clinical practice guideline for the treatment of obstructive sleep Apnea and snoring with oral appliance therapy: an update for 2015. J Clin Sleep Med. 2015;11(7):773–827. https://doi.org/10.5664/jcsm.4858.
113. Rehman RNA. Relaxation exercises to help fall asleep. 2024. https://www.sleepfoundation.org/sleep-hygiene/relaxation-exercises-to-help-fall-asleep. Accessed 14 Nov 2024.
114. Rietz H, Franklin KA, Carlberg B, Sahlin C, Marklund M. Nocturnal blood pressure is reduced by a mandibular advancement device for sleep Apnea in women: findings from secondary analyses of a randomized trial. J Am Heart Assoc. 2018;7(13) https://doi.org/10.1161/jaha.118.008642.
115. Roca GQ, Redline S, Claggett B, Bello N, Ballantyne CM, Solomon SD, Shah AM. Sex-Specific Association of Sleep Apnea Severity with subclinical myocardial injury, ventricular hypertrophy, and heart failure risk in a community-dwelling cohort: the atherosclerosis risk in communities-sleep heart health study. Circulation. 2015;132(14):1329–37. https://doi.org/10.1161/circulationaha.115.016985.
116. Rosenwasser AM, Turek FW. Neurobiology of circadian rhythm regulation. Sleep Med Clin. 2015;10(4):403–12. https://doi.org/10.1016/j.jsmc.2015.08.003.
117. Salari N, Darvishi N, Khaledi-Paveh B, Vaisi-Raygani A, Jalali R, Daneshkhah A, Bartina Y, Mohammadi M. A systematic review and meta-analysis of prevalence of insomnia in the third trimester of pregnancy. BMC Pregnancy Childbirth. 2021;21(1):284. https://doi.org/10.1186/s12884-021-03755-z.
118. Sarberg M, Svanborg E, Wiréhn A-B, Josefsson A. Snoring during pregnancy and its relation to sleepiness and pregnancy outcome – a prospective study. BMC Pregnancy Childbirth. 2014;14(1):15. https://doi.org/10.1186/1471-2393-14-15.
119. Sateia MJ. International classification of sleep disorders-third edition: highlights and modifications. Chest. 2014;146(5):1387–94. https://doi.org/10.1378/chest.14-0970.
120. Schaal K, Tafflet M, Nassif H, Thibault V, Pichard C, Alcotte M, et al. Psychological balance in high level athletes: gender-based differences and sport-specific patterns. PLoS One. 2011;6(5):e19007. https://doi.org/10.1371/journal.pone.0019007.
121. Schiza SE, Bouloukaki I. Does gender matter: sex-specific aspects of symptoms, outcome, and therapy of obstructive sleep apnea. Curr Opin Pulm Med. 2020;26(6):642–9. https://doi.org/10.1097/mcp.0000000000000728.
122. Schmidt MH, Bassetti CLA. Gender differences in narcolepsy: what are recent findings telling us? Sleep. 2022;45(12) https://doi.org/10.1093/sleep/zsac126.
123. Sedov ID, Cameron EE, Madigan S, Tomfohr-Madsen LM. Sleep quality during pregnancy: a meta-analysis. Sleep Med Rev. 2018;38:168–76. https://doi.org/10.1016/j.smrv.2017.06.005.
124. Seeman MV. Why are women prone to restless legs syndrome? Int J Environ Res Public Health. 2020;17(1) https://doi.org/10.3390/ijerph17010368.
125. Shahrbabaki SS, Linz D, Hartmann S, Redline S, Baumert M. Sleep arousal burden is associated with long-term all-cause and cardiovascular mortality in 8001 community-dwelling older men and women. Eur Heart J. 2021;42(21):2088–99. https://doi.org/10.1093/eurheartj/ehab151.
126. Sherif A, Krista H, Luise IMP. Gender disparities in weight loss surgery. Mini-invasive Surg. 2020;4:21. https://doi.org/10.20517/2574-1225.2019.57.
127. Shrivastava D, Jung S, Saadat M, Sirohi R, Crewson K. How to interpret the results of a sleep study. J Community Hosp Intern Med Perspect. 2014;4(5):24983. https://doi.org/10.3402/jchimp.v4.24983.
128. Sidani S, Guruge S, Fox M, Collins L. Gender differences in perpetuating factors, experience and management of chronic insomnia. J Gend Stud. 2019;28(4):402–13. https://doi.org/10.1080/09589236.2018.1491394.
129. Siebern AT, Suh S, Nowakowski S. Non-pharmacological treatment of insomnia. Neurotherapeutics. 2012;9(4):717–27. https://doi.org/10.1007/s13311-012-0142-9.
130. Sin DD, Mayers I, Man GC, Pawluk L. Long-term compliance rates to continuous positive airway pressure in obstructive sleep apnea: a population-based study. Chest. 2002;121(2):430–5. https://doi.org/10.1378/chest.121.2.430.
131. Stahl SM, Bodkin C. Parasomnias in women. In: A clinical casebook of sleep disorders in women. Springer; 2023. p. 129–35.
132. Strollo PJ Jr, Soose RJ, Maurer JT, de Vries N, Cornelius J, Froymovich O, Hanson RD, Padhya

TA, Steward DL, Gillespie MB, Woodson BT, Van de Heyning PH, Goetting MG, Vanderveken OM, Feldman N, Knaack L, Strohl KP. Upper-airway stimulation for obstructive sleep apnea. N Engl J Med. 2014;370(2):139–49. https://doi.org/10.1056/NEJMoa1308659.
133. Stuck BA, Ravesloot MJL, Eschenhagen T, de Vet HCW, Sommer JU. Uvulopalatopharyngoplasty with or without tonsillectomy in the treatment of adult obstructive sleep apnea – a systematic review. Sleep Med. 2018;50:152–65. https://doi.org/10.1016/j.sleep.2018.05.004.
134. Stuenkel CA, Davis SR, Gompel A, Lumsden MA, Murad MH, Pinkerton JV, Santen RJ. Treatment of symptoms of the menopause: an endocrine society clinical practice guideline. J Clin Endocrinol Metabol. 2015;100(11):3975–4011. https://doi.org/10.1210/jc.2015-2236.
135. Su MC, Chiu KL, Ruttanaumpawan P, Shiota S, Yumino D, Redolfi S, Haight JS, Yau B, Lam J, Bradley TD. Difference in upper airway collapsibility during wakefulness between men and women in response to lower-body positive pressure. Clin Sci (Lond). 2009;116(9):713–20. https://doi.org/10.1042/cs20080321.
136. Sun SY, Chen GH. Treatment of circadian rhythm sleep-wake disorders. Curr Neuropharmacol. 2022;20(6):1022–34. https://doi.org/10.2174/1570159x19666210907122933.
137. Szafarowska M, Rosiński M, Segiet-Święcicka A, Jędrzejczyk S, Jerzak M, Jerzak M. Effect of physiotherapy on infertility treatment in polycystic ovary syndrome patients. Menopause Rev. 2024;23(1) https://doi.org/10.5114/pm.2024.136439.
138. Takahashi M, Lim PJ, Tsubosaka M, Kim HK, Miyashita M, Suzuki K, Tan EL, Shibata S. Effects of increased daily physical activity on mental health and depression biomarkers in postmenopausal women. J Phys Ther Sci. 2019;31(4):408–13. https://doi.org/10.1589/jpts.31.408.
139. Tantrakul V, Ingsathit A, Liamsombut S, Rattanasiri S, Kittivoravitkul P, Imsom-Somboon N, Lertpongpiroon S, Jantarasaengaram S, Somchit W, Suwansathit W, Pengjam J, Siriyotha S, Panburana P, Guilleminault C, Preutthipan A, Attia J, Thakkinstian A. Treatment of obstructive sleep apnea in high risk pregnancy: a multicenter randomized controlled trial. Respir Res. 2023;24(1):171. https://doi.org/10.1186/s12931-023-02445-y.
140. Thurston L, Abbara A, Dhillo WS. Investigation and management of subfertility. J Clin Pathol. 2019;72(9):579–87. https://doi.org/10.1136/jclinpath-2018-205579.
141. Tian C, Wei Y, Xu M, Liu J, Tong B, Ning J, Wang Y, Wang Y, Estill J, Ge L. The effects of exercise on insomnia disorders: an umbrella review and network meta-analysis. Sleep Med. 2024;115:66–75. https://doi.org/10.1016/j.sleep.2024.02.002.
142. Togo F, Aizawa S, Arai J-i, Yoshikawa S, Ishiwata T, Shephard RJ, Aoyagi Y. Influence on human sleep patterns of lowering and delaying the minimum core body temperature by slow changes in the thermal environment. Sleep. 2007;30(6):797–802. https://doi.org/10.1093/sleep/30.6.797.
143. Tomfohr LM, Buliga E, Letourneau NL, Campbell TS, Giesbrecht GF. Trajectories of sleep quality and associations with mood during the perinatal period. Sleep. 2015;38(8):1237–45. https://doi.org/10.5665/sleep.4900.
144. Touzet S, Rabilloud M, Boehringer H, Barranco E, Ecochard R. Relationship between sleep and secretion of gonadotropin and ovarian hormones in women with normal cycles. Fertil Steril. 2002;77(4):738–44. https://doi.org/10.1016/s0015-0282(01)03254-x.
145. Tsai SY, Lin JW, Wu WW, Lee CN, Lee PL. Sleep disturbances and symptoms of depression and daytime sleepiness in pregnant women. Birth (Berkeley, Calif). 2016;43(2):176–83. https://doi.org/10.1111/birt.12215.
146. Ujma PP, Horváth CG, Bódizs R. Daily rhythms, light exposure and social jetlag correlate with demographic characteristics and health in a nationally representative survey. Sci Rep. 2023;13(1):12287. https://doi.org/10.1038/s41598-023-39011-x.
147. Verma RK, Johnson JJ, Goyal M, Banumathy N, Goswami U, Panda NK. Oropharyngeal exercises in the treatment of obstructive sleep apnoea: our experience. Sleep Breath. 2016;20(4):1193–201. https://doi.org/10.1007/s11325-016-1332-1.
148. Vgontzas AN, Bixler EO, Lin HM, Prolo P, Mastorakos G, Vela-Bueno A, et al. Chronic insomnia is associated with nyctohemeral activation of the hypothalamic-pituitary-adrenal axis: clinical implications. J Clin Endocrinol Metabol. 2001;86(8):3787–94. https://doi.org/10.1210/jcem.86.8.7778.
149. Walsh NP, Gleeson M, Shephard RJ, Gleeson M, Woods JA, Bishop NC, et al. Position statement part one: immune function and exercise. Exerc Immunol Rev. 2011;17
150. Watkins ER. Constructive and unconstructive repetitive thought. Psychol Bull. 2008;134(2):163–206. https://doi.org/10.1037/0033-2909.134.2.163.
151. Wen SY, Ko YL, Jou HJ, Chien LY. Sleep quality at 3 months postpartum considering maternal age: a comparative study. Women Birth. 2018;31(6):e367–73. https://doi.org/10.1016/j.wombi.2018.02.004.
152. Wimms A, Woehrle H, Ketheeswaran S, Ramanan D, Armitstead J. Obstructive sleep Apnea in women: specific issues and interventions. Biomed Res Int. 2016;2016:1764837. https://doi.org/10.1155/2016/1764837.
153. Ye L, Pien GW, Ratcliffe SJ, Weaver TE. Gender differences in obstructive sleep apnea and treatment response to continuous positive airway pressure. J Clin Sleep Med. 2009;5(6):512–8.
154. Zeng LN, Zong QQ, Yang Y, Zhang L, Xiang YF, Ng CH, Chen LG, Xiang YT. Gender difference in the prevalence of insomnia: a meta-analysis of observational studies. Front Psych. 2020;11:577429. https://doi.org/10.3389/fpsyt.2020.577429.

155. Zervas IM, Lambrinoudaki I, Spyropoulou AC, Koundi KL, Voussoura E, Tzavara C, Verdeli H, Aravantinos L, Creatsa M, Paparrigopoulos T. Additive effect of depressed mood and vasomotor symptoms on postmenopausal insomnia. Menopause. 2009;16(4)
156. Zhou N, Ho J-PTF, Huang Z, Spijker R, de Vries N, Aarab G, Lobbezoo F, Ravesloot MJL, de Lange J. Maxillomandibular advancement versus multilevel surgery for treatment of obstructive sleep apnea: a systematic review and meta-analysis. Sleep Med Rev. 2021;57:101471. https://doi.org/10.1016/j.smrv.2021.101471.
157. Zhou Z, Birditt KS, Leger KA, Fingerman KL. Daily worry, rumination, and sleep in late life. J Psychosom Res. 2024;179:111622. https://doi.org/10.1016/j.jpsychores.2024.111622.
158. Zhu B, Bronas UG, Carley DW, Lee K, Steffen A, Kapella MC, Izci-Balserak B. Relationships between objective sleep parameters and inflammatory biomarkers in pregnancy. Ann N Y Acad Sci. 2020;1473(1):62–73. https://doi.org/10.1111/nyas.14375.

26 Pelvic and Women's Health in People with Disabilities

Nuriye Özengin and Necmiye Ün Yıldırım

26.1 Introduction

Pelvic health and women's health in individuals with disabilities is a comprehensive issue that needs to be addressed in terms of medical, social, and psychological dimensions. These individuals experience processes such as sexual development, changes specific to puberty, and expectations regarding reproductive health and menopause, just like their non-disabled peers. However, different conditions that lead to disability can significantly affect the needs and difficulties individuals may face related to pelvic health. Therefore, understanding the unique dynamics of pelvic health and women's health in individuals with disabilities, developing appropriate screening and assessment methods, and providing accessible health services are becoming a critical necessity [1–3].

Pelvic health problems are not limited to physical discomfort but can also directly affect an individual's quality of life, psychosocial well-being, and general health. Difficulties in accessing reproductive health services, lack of knowledge about sexual health, and inadequate approaches by health professionals toward individuals with disabilities can cause these individuals to not benefit sufficiently from health services. Women with disabilities, in particular, face various inequalities in reproductive health, pregnancy management, and menopause due to prejudices in society and structural deficiencies in health services [1, 4, 5].

This book chapter aims to shed light on important issues in this area by presenting the current knowledge on pelvic health and women's health in disabled individuals. Starting from the definition and prevalence of disability, it will be discussed how life cycle processes such as puberty, pregnancy, and menopause are shaped in disabled individuals. In addition, pelvic health problems commonly seen in these individuals and inequalities experienced by disabled individuals in accessing health services will be discussed. Clinical assessment, physiotherapy, and rehabilitation treatment methods are examined in detail in other chapters of the book, so they are not mentioned in this chapter.

N. Özengin (✉)
Department of Physiotherapy and Rehabilitation, Faculty of Health Sciences, Bolu Abant İzzet Baysal University, Bolu, Türkiye
e-mail: ozengin_n@ibu.edu.tr

N. Ü. Yıldırım
Gülhane Faculty of Physiotherapy and Rehabilitation, University of Health Sciences, Ankara, Türkiye
e-mail: necmiyeun.yildirim@sbu.edu.tr

T. Akbayrak, E. Üzelpasaci (eds.), *Physiotherapy and Rehabilitation in Pelvic and Women's Health-Related Problems*, https://doi.org/10.1007/978-3-032-28741-0_26

26.2 The Importance of Pelvic Health and Women's Health in Disabled Individuals

Individuals with disabilities experience the same sexual development, pubertal changes, anxieties, and reproductive desires as their typically developing counterparts. The conditions that lead to disabilities can arise from many different causes. Some are the result of genetic changes or congenital anomalies (e.g., Down syndrome), some are acquired during the neonatal or perinatal period (e.g., cerebral palsy), and some are acquired through traumatic injuries (e.g., spinal cord injury), chronic diseases (e.g., amputation due to diabetes), or unknown causes (e.g., multiple sclerosis) [6]. Individuals with disabilities may be more prone to pelvic health problems or feel the effects of these problems more intensely due to the nature of their disabilities. Therefore, it is of great importance to understand the special health needs of individuals with disabilities, to conduct appropriate screening and assessments, and to provide accessible treatment and support services. This is a critical step in improving their health and well-being, and enhancing their quality of life [1, 3, 7].

26.3 Definition, Epidemiology, and Prevalence of Disability

There are different definitions of the concept of disability, and this has played an important role in shaping research and public health understanding in the field. The lack of a single definition of disability also results in the absence of a valid incidence or prevalence of disability [6]. The World Health Organization divides the term "disability" into three areas: deviations from the norm in society, activity, and participation. The first area includes losses in body structure or function. The activity area is defined as a person's ability to perform a task. The third area is participation or involvement in life situations. Whether a person is disabled or not is partly due to contextual factors. Contextual factors include the roles imposed by society rather than looking at the individual and their own strengths [3].

Disability epidemiology is a relatively new field of science that systematically examines the patterns, distribution, determinants, and consequences of disabilities in specific populations. This field can support improved health status for individuals with disabilities by quantifying the prevalence of disability, identifying factors that reduce the quality of life of individuals with disabilities, and designing interventions to address these factors [6].

In epidemiology, surveillance data and special studies are used to assess the health of a population, identify risk factors for health problems, and evaluate whether interventions to improve health and well-being are effective [6].

Disability is a major public health problem worldwide, and its prevalence varies by age, gender, socioeconomic status, and geographic location. The prevalence of disability is defined as the number of people with a disability in each population at a given time. The incidence of disability (the number of new cases occurring in each population during a given time period) can be difficult to determine [6]. The prevalence of disability among adults worldwide is estimated at approximately 14%. This rate is higher in low- and middle-income countries and more common among women and older people [8, 9]. In Türkiye, the prevalence of disability varies among different groups and regions. In a study conducted in the Southeastern Anatolia Region of Türkiye, the prevalence of disability was determined as 13.8% [10].

26.4 Hormonal Changes and Reproductive Health in Disabled Individuals

Puberty

Puberty is a difficult time for all adolescents but especially for those with disabilities. Life itself is challenging for a youth with a disability. The onset of puberty or menstruation can disrupt the delicate balance of a youth's life. Adolescence typically occurs in predictable, sequential stages. These stages include preadolescence, early adolescence (ages 11–14), middle adolescence (ages 15–17), and late adolescence (ages 18–25), and each stage involves unique physical and psychological changes [3]. It is important to address both the disabled person and their caregivers at these stages. The disabled person should be given the opportunity to speak privately and confidentially with the health professional at the appropriate time. This is important to support the needs for privacy and independence during adolescence [1].

In general, puberty and menarche, and monthly menstrual cycles are the same in adolescents with disabilities as in those without disabilities. The typical progression of puberty in females is the onset of breast development, which occurs at an average age of 10 years in Caucasian females and 8–9 years in African-American females, followed by pubic hair development, a growth spurt, and finally menarche. On physical examination, breast development and pubic hair development can be staged according to the Sexual Maturity Rating [3].

There are several conditions associated with early puberty. In general, children with neurodevelopmental disabilities are 20 times more likely to experience early pubertal changes than their typically developing peers. The reason for this is not fully understood, but it is thought to be related to neurological changes involving the pathways that lead to pubertal development. It has been shown that sexual maturation generally occurs earlier in women with spina bifida. The frequency of precocious puberty (<12 years of age) in this group is 12% to 16%, while this rate is reported to be 0.6% in their non-disabled peers. It is thought that this difference may be because most studies associate a history of hydrocephalus with precocious puberty in girls with spina bifida. However, it is stated in the literature that there are insufficient studies examining precocious puberty in women with spina bifida without hydrocephalus [11]. The mean age of menarche in women with spina bifida ranges from 10.9 to 11.4 years, while the mean age in women without spina bifida is 12.7 years. Other disorders associated with precocious puberty include obesity, intellectual disability, Williams syndrome, meningomyelocele, and neurofibromatosis [3].

The literature indicates that the average age of menarche in women with intellectual disabilities is similar to that of women in the general population. Most of them appear to have regular menstrual cycles [12].

People with cerebral palsy tend to enter puberty earlier and complete puberty later than their typically developing peers. The average age of menarche in white women with cerebral palsy is 14. One hypothesis for why children with developmental disabilities enter or end puberty later is that they often have difficulty swallowing and gastrointestinal motility disorders that may affect their nutritional status. There is a known link between poor nutritional status and delayed puberty [3].

Adolescence is a difficult period even for typically developing individuals, and the difficulties that individuals with disabilities may face may be greater. It is stated that as young women with physical disabilities reach adolescence, they become increasingly aware of how different their bodies are from the bodies of their peers. Society's prejudices about disability can also have negative effects on self-esteem and sexual identity development during this period [13]. It is recommended that health professionals make some modifications (such as visual materials or drawings) in their relationships and communication with disabled individuals [1]. Parents should also be advised to encourage their children to maximize their independence in the areas of self-care and social skills and to avoid the tendency to "infantilize" their children [3].

In women with spinal cord injuries, hormonal imbalances in the months following the injury can disrupt menstrual cycles. Ninety percent of women return to their menstrual cycles within a year of the injury, an average of 5 months [14]. Increases in prolactin and/or follicle-stimulating hormone (FSH) levels may be seen as a neurochemical response to spinal cord injury [15].

In most women with intellectual disability, gonadal endocrine function is generally supported to be within normal limits. However, psychotropic medications may affect a number of hormonal and metabolic functions. Hyperprolactinemia is a common finding associated with neuroleptic drug use. Long-term anti-epileptic drug therapy has been associated with primary gonadal dysfunction and an increased risk of polycystic ovary syndrome [12]. Hypothyroidism is more common in individuals with Down syndrome and may cause amenorrhea or abnormal uterine bleeding [1].

Pregnancy

Historically, women with disabilities have been discouraged from pregnancy based on beliefs that pregnancy could be life-threatening, that pregnancy could worsen the disability, or that the disability was incompatible with motherhood. Research has shown that women with disabilities naturally desire to parent [13, 16, 17]. Some disabled women have expressed their desire to have children to prove whether they can give birth to a "normal child" [5].

Literature has shown that women with disabilities have difficulty finding healthcare professionals and hospitals experienced in pregnancy and birth management for women with disabilities. Women may "settle" for less experienced healthcare professionals [16]. When women with disabilities shared their experiences of pregnancy and birth, they stated that some health professionals constantly focused on their disabilities and did not sufficiently consider "normal health" issues [5].

In the literature, when pregnancy characteristics were compared between physically disabled women and the non-disabled control group, it was reported that disabled women had more premature births, low birth weight, and pregnancy complications [18]. These increased complications highlight the need for women with disabilities to have access to comprehensive reproductive health services, including pre-pregnancy, prenatal, and postnatal care. The care of women with disabilities is best managed by an interdisciplinary team of primary care professionals, obstetricians, anesthesiologists, neurologists, psychiatrists, physiotherapists, and occupational therapists [3, 16].

Women with disabilities may experience bladder spasms, infections, urinary incontinence, and related problems with catheter use. Constipation and back pain are common problems during pregnancy [9, 11]. Skin problems may increase during pregnancy due to possible decreased mobility. Decreased lung volume due to the expanding uterus may cause breathing difficulties and an increased risk of pneumonia. The risk of autonomic dysreflexia also increases during pregnancy, as does the risk of blood clots [16]. Women with neurological disabilities may be more likely to experience pelvic floor problems such as urinary and fecal incontinence during and after pregnancy. Pregnant women with neurological disabilities should have their pelvic floor health closely monitored and be offered appropriate supportive care [19]. Women with disabilities may encounter some problems not only during pregnancy but also during birth. The birth positions and pushing mechanics of women with physical disabilities may differ, and this may affect the risk of perineal trauma. The birth team must be sensitive to the special needs and limitations of the disabled woman and adopt appropriate approaches [20]. The management of pregnancy and birth processes of women with disabilities should be planned and carried out with a multidisciplinary approach, considering the type and severity of the disability, accompanying health problems, and individual needs. In this process, it is of great importance that women with disabilities feel comfortable and safe and have access to the necessary support services.

Menopause

Menopause is the natural end of menstrual bleeding and fertility. It typically occurs when women are in their forties or fifties. Complications of menopause are caused by decreasing estrogen levels and include an increased risk of cardiovascular disease, osteoporosis, urinary incontinence, decreased skin integrity, decreased sexual function, and weight gain [3]. For women with disabilities, menopause can worsen existing health problems. For example, postmenopausal changes such as accelerated bone loss and increased risk of heart disease pose greater risks for people with mobility impairments [21, 22].

As women with disabilities live longer, healthier lives, the risk of complications during and after menopause increases. For example, women with poor mobility may be at increased risk of osteoporosis and weight gain. If sexual dysfunction is already present, vaginal dryness or decreased sensation may worsen it. Reduced skin integrity may increase the risk of decubitus ulcers [3].

It is reported in the literature that menopause tends to occur earlier in women with learning disabilities, especially those with Down syndrome. It has been shown that women with Down syndrome enter menopause at an earlier age compared to other women with mental disabilities, suggesting a connection with the acceleration of the aging process [12, 23–25]. Menopause can also be a turning point in the progression of diseases such as multiple sclerosis; some studies show worsening disability after menopause [26, 27]. Menopausal symptoms such as fatigue, cognitive, mood, and bladder disorders often overlap with multiple sclerosis (MS) symptoms, making management difficult and potentially worsening quality of life [28, 29].

Andropause

Andropause, commonly referred to as male menopause, is a condition characterized by a gradual decline in testosterone levels in aging men, typically over the age of 50. This decline can lead to a variety of symptoms and has been linked to a variety of health conditions. Low testosterone levels are associated with a higher risk of multiple sclerosis in men, potentially affecting immune response and neuroprotective mechanisms. Because testosterone has protective effects that decline with age, the decline in testosterone during andropause may contribute to the onset and progression of MS in men. Epidemiological studies suggest that men have a later onset of MS compared to women, potentially because of the protective effects of testosterone that decline with age. This later onset in men may be related to the gradual decline in testosterone levels during andropause and may influence the progression and severity of MS [30].

26.5 Common Pelvic Health Issues in People with Disabilities

- **Lower Urinary Tract Symptoms**

People with disabilities are significantly more likely to experience urinary incontinence than those without disabilities. Literature has shown that people with disabilities are three times more likely to experience urinary incontinence, highlighting the need for targeted interventions in this group [31].

A systematic review of Lower Urinary Tract Symptoms (LUTS) in children and young adults with cerebral palsy reported that urinary incontinence was common in this population. The prevalence of total urinary incontinence in individuals with cerebral palsy was 55.5%, the prevalence of daytime incontinence was 46%, and the prevalence of enuresis was 38.5%. Other lower urinary tract symptoms seen in individuals with cerebral palsy include urgency, frequency, and nocturia. It has been reported that the condition known as neurogenic detrusor overactivity, characterized by involuntary bladder contractions, negatively affects incontinence and reduces bladder capacity [32].

LUTS in individuals with multiple sclerosis range from 63.95% to 87.6%. Common symptoms include urinary frequency (73.45%), urgency (63.87%), and detrusor overactivity (42.9%). The severity of multiple sclerosis is associated with the likelihood of experiencing Urgency Urinary Incontinence (UUI), and the likelihood of UUI increases as the disease becomes more severe [33–35].

Urinary incontinence is a common problem affecting both men and women with spinal cord injury. Studies show that approximately half of women with spinal cord injury experience urinary incontinence, and 27% experience it daily.

In the larger population of individuals with spinal cord injury, 43% report incontinence at rates ranging from less than once a week to daily. This condition has been associated with decreased quality of life, reduced mobility, and being unmarried or not living together [36, 37].

- **Sexual Dysfunctions**

Sexual well-being includes not only physical function but also environmental, social, interpersonal, and personal factors [4]. Sexual dysfunction is a significant problem affecting both physical and psychological health among people with disabilities. Despite its impact on quality of life, this problem is often underdiagnosed and undertreated. Sexual dysfunction is common among people with disabilities, and studies report high rates [38]. In patients with multiple sclerosis (MS), 40% to 80% of women and 50% to 90% of men report sexual complaints, and these complaints are often underdiagnosed [39].

A variety of factors contribute to sexual dysfunction in populations with disabilities. Age, gender, and type of disability are important determinants, with younger individuals and men generally reporting higher levels of dysfunction [40]. Sexual dysfunction in Parkinson's disease occurs independently of disease severity and motor disability, indicating a complex interaction of neurological and hormonal factors [41]. Also, high self-esteem and self-efficacy are very important, as they can reduce sexual dysfunction [40].

It is stated that conditions such as sexual experiences of physically disabled women and lower urinary tract problems may also affect sexual function [5, 32]. The literature indicates that sexual dysfunction may be more common in disabled women and that sexual response may be affected by disability [4, 11]. Men with disabilities experience higher rates of difficulties with sexual function than men without disabilities. Common problems include premature ejaculation, sexual desire instability, and general sexual dissatisfaction [42].

It is noted that there is little information about the effects of spina bifida on women's sexual response. It is also reported that there is no data on the incidence of sexual dysfunction in women with spina bifida. Therefore, careful sexual history is recommended when treating women with spina bifida [11].

It is stated that women with physical disabilities experience more sexual dysfunction, are typically less sexually active, and have less sexual intercourse than women without disabilities. In addition, the literature emphasizes that the sexual well-being of women with physical disabilities is not limited to physical function alone but also includes personal factors [4].

After a spinal cord injury, women may experience decreased desire for sexual activity due to urinary incontinence, pain, and spasticity. The rate of reaching orgasm in these women is significantly reduced, but vaginal lubrication and blood flow are usually preserved [43].

Individuals with intellectual disabilities face a significant prevalence of sexual dysfunction, compounded by factors such as a lack of sexual education and high rates of sexual abuse. Approximately 35% of adults with intellectual disabilities have experienced sexual victimization, which can further exacerbate sexual dysfunction [44–46].

- **Colorectal Dysfunctions**

Individuals with disabilities frequently experience bowel problems such as constipation and bowel dysfunction. These problems are common and are often related to the severity of the disability and associated comorbidities.

Chronic constipation affects a significant proportion of individuals with intellectual disabilities, with prevalence rates ranging from 25% to 69% in different studies [47–49]. This condition is associated with significant morbidity and may contribute to early mortality [49, 50]. The impact of constipation goes beyond physical discomfort to affect psychological and emotional well-being and is linked to anxiety and behavioral difficulties [51]. Risk factors for constipation include the severity of disability, reduced mobility, the use of medications (antipsychotic, anticholinergic, and antiseizure drugs), low physical activity, poor eating habits, and inadequate fluid intake [48, 52, 53].

Bowel dysfunction, including constipation and fecal incontinence, affects a significant proportion of MS patients. Studies indicate a prevalence of bowel dysfunction in 68% of MS patients, with 43% having constipation and 51% having fecal incontinence. The severity of bowel problems is related to the level of disability, disease duration, and genitourinary symptoms [54, 55].

Adults with cerebral palsy and spina bifida also experience high rates of bowel problems, with 49.2% of individuals with spina bifida reporting fecal incontinence. These conditions often occur with other comorbidities, such as pain and fatigue, which can further exacerbate bowel problems [56].

26.6 Health Inequalities and Access Challenges Faced by People with Disabilities

There are a number of obstacles to providing access to care for people with disabilities. These obstacles include physical access barriers, lack of knowledge and training of health professionals, lack of attitude and respect, difficulties in communication and providing information, financial and logistical barriers, inadequate appointment times, and inequalities in access to sexual and reproductive health [2, 57, 58]. Barriers to treating individuals with disabilities may include a lack of time for the healthcare professional, as there may be other medical, physical, and functional needs that need to be addressed during the examination. Other barriers include difficulty navigating narrow office corridors, waiting rooms, or small exam rooms with a wheelchair or special equipment. The healthcare professional may lack knowledge or be unable to communicate a concern to the patient. In addition, myths and misinformation about individuals with disabilities exist among healthcare professionals [2, 3, 59]. A significant problem that disabled individuals face when receiving healthcare is the attitudes and lack of respect of healthcare professionals. Brace et al.'s study showed that disabled women reported more negative experiences of healthcare professionals not respecting them as individuals [17].

26.7 Conclusion

As a result, the overall health and well-being of individuals, whether they have a disability, is fundamental to their physical, mental, and social well-being. Individuals with disabilities may experience additional health challenges due to their disability, which may impact their access to and utilization of health services. Addressing pelvic and women's health in individuals with disabilities requires a comprehensive, multidisciplinary approach that considers the unique challenges faced by this population. The hormonal changes and special conditions of puberty, pregnancy, and menopause, examined in this chapter provide a holistic view of the health of individuals with disabilities. The high prevalence of pelvic health problems among individuals with disabilities, such as common lower urinary tract symptoms, sexual dysfunction, and anorectal dysfunction, clearly demonstrates the need for special attention and interventions in this area.

Health inequalities and access difficulties constitute significant barriers to accessing quality health services for people with disabilities. Physical access problems, lack of knowledge and training of health professionals, negative attitudes, communication difficulties, financial and logistical barriers, and inadequate appointment times significantly limit the equal access of people with disabilities to health services. Improving access to specialized care, raising awareness of the role of physiotherapy, and developing targeted outcome measures are fundamental steps toward reducing health inequalities and improving quality of life.

Special attention needs to be paid to pelvic and women's health in people with disabilities. This means not only ensuring physical accessibility but also ensuring that health professionals adopt a disability-sensitive approach, provide adequate information and training, and address the specific health needs of people with disabilities in a holistic manner. It is vital that continued efforts are made to improve the health and well-being of people with disabilities, support their participation in their own health decisions, and reduce stigma.

References

1. Abells D, Kirkham YA, Ornstein MP. Review of gynecologic and reproductive care for women with developmental disabilities. Curr Opin Obstet Gynecol. 2016;28(5):350–8.
2. Sonalkar S, Chavez V, McClusky J, Hunter TA, Mollen CJ. Gynecologic care for women with physical disabilities: a qualitative study of patients and providers. Womens Health Issues. 2020;30(2):136–41.
3. Stockburger S, Omar HA. Women with disabilities: reproductive care and women's health. Int J Child Health Hum Dev. 2015;4(8):429–47.
4. Nery-Hurwit MB, Kalpakjian CZ, Kreschmer JM, Quint EH, Ernst S. Development of a conceptual framework of sexual well-being for women with physical disability. Womens Health Issues. 2022;32(4):376–87.
5. Kalpakjian CZ, Kreschmer JM, Slavin MD, Kisala PA, Quint EH, Chiaravalloti ND, et al. Reproductive health in women with physical disability: a conceptual framework for the development of new patient-reported outcome measures. J Women's Health. 2020;29(11):1427–36.
6. Drum CE, Krahn GL, Bersani H, editors. Disability and public health. Washington, DC: American Public Health Association; 2009. p. 1–212.
7. Fletcher S, Nosek MA, Rizk DEE. Mobility impairments and pelvic health disorders in women: the need for innovative treatment and research. Int Urogynecol J Pelvic Floor Dysfunct. 2014;25:1003–4.
8. Mitra S, Sambamoorthi U. Disability prevalence among adults: estimates for 54 countries and progress toward a global estimate. Disabil Rehabil. 2014;36(11):940–7.
9. Mont D. Measuring disability prevalence. 2007.
10. Arca M, Saka G. The prevalence of disability and contributory factors in Turkey's Southeastern Anatolia region. J Public Health (Bangkok). 2022;30(3):545–51.
11. Jackson AB, Mott PK. Reproductive health care for women with spina bifida. Sci World J. 2007;7:1875–83.
12. Walsh PN, Heller T, Schupf N, Van Schrojenstein Lantman-de Valk H, Saxena S. Healthy ageing – adults with intellectual disabilities: women's health and related issues. J Appl Res Intellect Disabil. 2001;14(3):195–217.
13. Piotrowski K, Snell L. Health needs of women with disabilities across the lifespan. J Obstet Gynecol Neonatal Nurs. 2007;36:79–87.
14. Schopp LH, Sanford TC, Hagglund KJ, Gay JW, Coatney MA. Removing service barriers for women with physical disabilities: promoting accessibility in the gynecologic care setting. J Midwifery Womens Health. 2002;47(2):74–9.
15. Dillaway H, Cross K, Lysack C, Schwartz J. Normal and natural, or burdensome and terrible? Women with spinal cord injuries discuss ambivalence about menstruation. Sex Roles. 2013;68(1–2):107–20.
16. Huff MB. Disabled women and reproductive healthcare in the USA. In: Adults with childhood illnesses: considerations for practice; 2011. p. 231.
17. Brace M, Copel L, McKeever A, Smeltzer SC. Reproductive health care inequities by disability status: experiences with providers and barriers to care. Res Nurs Health. 2025:1–11.
18. Morton C, Le JT, Shahbandar L, Hammond C, Murphy EA, Kirschner KL. Pregnancy outcomes of women with physical disabilities: a matched cohort study. PM R. 2013;5(2):90–8.
19. Gianfranco L, Donatella G, Stefania M, editors. Suprapontine lesions and neurogenic pelvic dysfunctions assessment, treatment and rehabilitation. Springer; 2020. p. 1–114.
20. Sultan AH, Thakar R, Lewicky-Gaupp C. Pelvic floor, perineal, and anal sphincter trauma during childbirth diagnosis, management and prevention. 2nd ed; 2024. p. 1–416.
21. Vandenakker CB, Glass DD. Menopause and aging with disability. Phys Med Rehabil Clin N Am. 2001;1(12)
22. Welner S, Simon J, Menopause BW. Maximizing health in menopausal women with disabilities. Menopause. 2002;3(9)
23. Martin DM, Cassidy G, Ahmad F, Martin MS. Women with learning disabilities and the menopause. J Learn Disabil. 2001;5(2):121–32.
24. Schupf N, Zigman W, Kapell D. Early menopause in women with Down's syndrome. J Intellect Disabil Res. 1997;41(3):264–7.
25. Carr J, Hollins S. Menopause in women with learning disabilities. J Intellect Disabil Res. 1995;39(2):137–9.
26. Midaglia L, Otero S, Baró F, Montalban X, Tintoré M. Menopause and multiple sclerosis: influence on prognosis and role of disease-modifying drugs and hormonal replacement therapy. Mult Scler J. 2022;28(2):173–82.
27. Baroncini D, Annovazzi P, De Rossi N, Mallucci G, Clerici V, Tonietti S, et al. Impact of natural menopause on multiple sclerosis: a multicentre study. J Neurol Neurosurg Psychiatry. 2019;11(90):1201–6.
28. Bove R, Okai A, Houtchens M, Elias-Hamp B, Lugaresi A, Hellwig K, et al. Effects of menopause in women with multiple sclerosis: an evidence-based review. Front Neurol. 2021:12.
29. Lorefice L, Nicola D'alterio M, Firinu D, Fenu G, Cocco E. Impact of menopause in patients with multi-

ple sclerosis: current perspectives. J Women's Health. 2023;15:103–9.

30. Ysrraelit MC, Correale J. Impact of andropause on multiple sclerosis. Front Neurol. 2021;12
31. Wilbur J, Morrison C, Bambery L, Tanguay J, Baker S, Sheppard P, et al. "I'm scared to talk about it": exploring experiences of incontinence for people with and without disabilities in Vanuatu, using mixed methods. Lancet Reg Health West Pac. 2021;21(14)
32. Samijn B, Van Laecke E, Renson C, Hoebeke P, Plasschaert F, Vande Walle J, et al. Lower urinary tract symptoms and urodynamic findings in children and adults with cerebral palsy: a systematic review. Neurourol Urodyn. 2017;36(3):541–9.
33. Nazari F, Shaygannejad V, Sichani MM, Mansourian M, Hajhashemi V. The prevalence of lower urinary tract symptoms based on individual and clinical parameters in patients with multiple sclerosis. BMC Neurol. 2020;20(1)
34. Al Dandan HB, Mngt A, Coote S, Mcclurg D. Prevalence of lower urinary tract symptoms in people with multiple sclerosis: a systematic review and meta-analysis. Int J MS Care. 2020;22(2):91–9.
35. Khalaf K, Globe D, Armstrong E, Malone D, Coyne K. Prevalence of lower urinary tract symptoms among patients with multiple sclerosis. J Urol. 2012;187(4S)
36. Hansen R, Biering-Sørensen F, Cord JK. Urinary incontinence in spinal cord injured individuals 10–45 years after injury. Spinal Cord. 2010;48:27–33.
37. Sekido N, Igawa Y, Kakizaki H, Kitta T, Sengoku A, Takahashi S, et al. Clinical guidelines for the diagnosis and treatment of lower urinary tract dysfunction in patients with spinal cord injury. Int J Urol. 2020;27(4):276–88.
38. Aslan E, Yılmaz B, Acar Z. Reproductive health, sexual function and satisfaction levels in women with physical, hearing, and visual disabilities. Sex Disabil. 2021;39(3):595–608.
39. Calabrò R, De Luca R, Conti-Nibali V, Reitano S, Leo A, Bramanti P. Sexual function in young individuals with multiple sclerosis: does disability matter? Int J Neurosci. 2013;
40. Oladele O, Adejumo A, Agberotimi S, Ojedokun S. Influence of psycho-demographic factors on sexual dysfunction among people living with disabilities. Int Neuropsychiatr Dis J. 2023;20(4):64–70.
41. Mousli A, Zouari R, Lahmer A, et al. Sexual dysfunction and motor disability in Parkinson's disease: any link? Eur Psychiatry. 2023;66(S1):S1095.
42. Bollier A, King T, Shakespeare T, Hocking J, Kavanagh A. Sexual functioning in men with and without disabilities: findings from a representative sample of Australian men. J Sex Med. 2019;11:1749–57.
43. Özengin N, Çankaya H. Nörolojik Hastalıklarda Pelvik Taban Disfonksiyonunda Fizyoterapi ve Rehabilitasyon. In: Türkan A, Serap Ö, Ceren G, editors. Multidisipliner Bakış Temeli ile Pelvik Sağlıkta Fizyoterapi ve Rehabilitasyon. 1st ed. Hedef Yayıncılık; 2023.
44. Tomsa R, Gutu S, Cojocaru D, Gutiérrez-Bermejo B, Flores N, Jenaro C. Prevalence of sexual abuse in adults with intellectual disability: systematic review and meta-analysis. Int J Environ Res Public Health. 2021;18(4)
45. Codina M, Pereda N. Characteristics and prevalence of lifetime sexual victimization among a sample of men and women with intellectual disabilities. J Interpers Violence. 2021;37(15–16):NP14117–39.
46. Spytska L. Understanding sexual dysfunctions in individuals with intellectual disabilities from a psychological perspective. J Intellect Disabil Diagn Treat. 2024;12:22–31.
47. Böhmer C, Taminiau J, Klinkenberg-Knol E, Meuwissen S. The prevalence of constipation in institutionalized people with intellectual disability. J Intellect Disabil Res. 2001;45(3):212–8.
48. Laugharne R, Wilcock M, Rees J, Wainwright D, Newton N, Sterritt J, et al. Clinical characteristics of people with intellectual disability admitted to hospital with constipation: identifying possible specific high-risk factors. J Intellect Disabil Res. 2024;68(3):277–84.
49. Laugharne R, Sawhney I, Perera B, Wainwright D, Bassett P, Caffrey B, et al. Chronic constipation in people with intellectual disabilities in the community: cross-sectional study. BJPsych Open. 2024;10(2):e55.
50. Roberts C, Ding J, Bishara D, Riaz S, Hospital B, Rory Sheehan D, et al. Constipation prevalence and risk from prescribed medications in people with intellectual disability: findings from an English mortality programme. J Intellect Disabil. 2024:1–17.
51. Kelly AM. Constipation in community-dwelling adults with intellectual disability. Br J Community Nurs. 2019;24(8):392–6.
52. Robertson J, Baines S, Emerson E, Hatton C. Constipation management in people with intellectual disability: a systematic review. J Appl Res Intellect Disabil. 2018;31(5):709–24.
53. Maslen C, Hodge R, Tie K, Laugharne R, Lamb K, Shankar R. Constipation in autistic people and people with learning disabilities. Br J Gen Pract. 2022;720(72):348–51.
54. Alvino B, Arianna F, Assunta B, Antonio C, Emanuele A, Giorgia M, et al. Prevalence and predictors of bowel dysfunction in a large multiple sclerosis outpatient population: an Italian multicenter study. J Neurol. 2021;269(3):1610–7.
55. Hinds J, Eidelman B, Wald A. Prevalence of bowel dysfunction in multiple sclerosis: a population survey. Gastroenterology. 1990;98(6):1538–42.
56. Sattoe JNT, Hilberink SR. Impairments and comorbidities in adults with cerebral palsy and spina bifida: a meta-analysis. Front Neurol. 2023:14.
57. Haregewoine Gebreselassie E, Dereje Wale D, Kassahun Tarekegn T, Worku Molla M, Adamu Gebremedhin R, Abera Tumdedo B, et al. Assessment of challenges of disabled women towards accessing medical health care services in Addis Ababa

Ethiopia; a qualitative study-2022Gc. Am J Gyne Obst. 2024:251.
58. Joseph M, Saravanabavan S, Jeff N. Physicians' perceptions of barriers to equal access to reproductive health promotion for women with mobility impairment. Can J Disabil Stud. 2018;7(1):62–100.
59. Lehman CA. APN knowledge, self-efficacy, and practices in providing women's healthcare services to women with disabilities. Rehabil Nurs. 2009;34(5):186–94.

Pelvic Health in Children

27

Seda Yakıt Yeşilyurt and Büşra İnal

27.1 Introduction

In children, age-related differences and developmental maturity are critical factors to consider when making informed decisions about optimal clinical interventions. It is essential to recognize that children undergo rapid changes in their physical and cognitive functions and abilities. Furthermore, cognitive abilities and motor performance are interconnected, working together to enhance functional outcomes in children [1]. On the other hand, the evidence-based data on pelvic floor development, biomechanics, and the musculoskeletal system in children are extremely limited.

The pelvic floor is a key component of the musculoskeletal system, playing an essential role in maintaining continence, supporting pelvic organs, and facilitating various reproductive and excretory functions [2]. Proper motor development during childhood is fundamental for the optimal functioning of the pelvic floor muscles, establishing the foundation for lifelong pelvic health. Conversely, disruptions in normal motor development may contribute to pelvic floor dysfunctions later in life, such as incontinence, pelvic organ prolapse, and sexual dysfunction. While the clinical presentation of pelvic floor disorders varies between adults and children, the underlying pathophysiological mechanisms often share common roots. During childhood, the development of the pelvic floor is closely tied to the overall motor maturation of the individual, encompassing gross and fine motor skills development, muscle strength, and coordination [1].

As motor development progresses, the pelvic floor undergoes a parallel process of maturation, with its muscles and connective tissues gradually gaining strength, tone, and flexibility [3]. The pelvic floor's ability to effectively contract, relax, and coordinate with other muscle groups is essential for maintaining continence, supporting pelvic organs, and facilitating activities such as bowel movements [4]. Normal motor development refers to the sequential acquisition of muscular control and coordination from infancy through adulthood. Early in development, infants first gain control over head movements, followed by trunk stability and later fine motor skills. This progression establishes the foundational muscle strength and coordination necessary for various bodily functions, including those involving the pelvic floor.

Motor development in children follows a predictable sequence, progressing from head to toe (cephalocaudal) and from the center of the body

S. Yakıt Yeşilyurt (✉)
Department of Physiotherapy and Rehabilitation, Faculty of Health Sciences, Izmir University of Economics, Izmir, Türkiye
e-mail: seda.yesilyurt@izmirekonomi.edu.tr

B. İnal
Department of Physiotherapy and Rehabilitation, Faculty of Health Sciences, Bolu Abant Izzet Baysal University, Bolu, Türkiye

T. Akbayrak, E. Üzelpasaci (eds.), *Physiotherapy and Rehabilitation in Pelvic and Women's Health-Related Problems*, https://doi.org/10.1007/978-3-032-28741-0_27

outward (proximodistal) [5]. This orderly development highlights the interconnected nature of motor skills and pelvic floor function throughout childhood.

27.2 Normal Motor Development

The subcortical level of motor control within the central nervous system (CNS) emerges and predominantly matures during the first year of life. The maturation of the second level of the subcortical CNS is associated with the initiation of postural-locomotor functions. After the neonatal period, basic trunk stabilization develops, which is a prerequisite for any phasic movement and for the locomotor function of the extremities [6]. Before movements of an extremity, head, or neck can occur, the core must provide support against the gravitational field [7].

Subsequently, the cortical level of motor control gradually becomes active. Cortical control plays a crucial role in shaping the individual qualities and characteristics of movement, enabling isolated segmental movements and relaxation [6]. Forward activation of the neck flexors and extensors is a vital mechanism for the stability of extremity movements and the integration of the visual and vestibular systems. This mechanism ensures both cervical spine stabilization and protection [8].

A complex synergy between the diaphragm, pelvic floor, abdominal wall, and spinal extensors is required to stabilize the lower thoracic and lumbar spine. This involves coordinated concentric activity of the diaphragm and pelvic floor, followed by eccentric activation of all sections of the abdominal wall. This synergy increases intra-abdominal pressure (IAP), stabilizing the lower thoracic spine from the front. Ideally, this activity is balanced with that of the spinal extensors [9–12]. This stabilizing synergy develops during the first 4–5 months of life.

After the neonatal period, infants begin raising their legs while lying on their backs and lifting their heads while on their stomachs. A balance between all stabilizers is required for effective postural activity. By 3 months of age, infants can lift their legs and shift their weight to the upper gluteal muscles while maintaining an upright spine [13]. At this stage, the chest and pelvis align in a neutral position, with their axes parallel. This alignment supports balanced postural function.

In musculoskeletal development, functional neonatal immaturity corresponds with anatomical immaturity. For instance, spinal curves are not yet well-defined, the chest remains barrel-shaped (the anteroposterior diameter is longer than the width, unlike in adults), the tibial plateau is inclined, and the foot arch has yet to form. Postnatal anatomical maturation depends on muscle function controlled by the CNS, alongside genetic, hormonal, metabolic, and immunological factors [6].

In newborns, the diaphragm functions primarily as a respiratory muscle [14]. However, after the neonatal period, it also becomes a critical stabilizer [12]. Proportional activity among all stabilizers is essential for maintaining balance. If one component (a muscle or part of a muscle) is weak, compensatory activity from another muscle can create an imbalance in the global stabilization chain. Without early intervention, these imbalances can persist throughout life, contributing to various motor dysfunctions [6, 15, 16]. During motor development, the presence of symmetry has a unique value for the success of more complex and detailed movements. Three months of age is critically important for achieving symmetrical movement, especially in the lower extremities. Stabilization of the upper part of the trunk and the cranium leads to movement in the pelvic area. The longitudinal axis of the body (the spine) is correctly curved in all planes, which is of great importance for subsequent developmental stages, including the ability to turn, crawl, and walk. In accordance with the cranio-caudal development theory, the pelvis is the final element to achieve the optimal position [17].

Therefore, assessing motor development from the neonatal period can serve as a valuable pediatric screening tool to identify potential dysfunctions early [13, 18].

27.2.1 Pelvic Floor Muscle Function in Children

There is very little information on the function of the pelvic floor muscles (PFM) in children. The newborn pelvis is funnel-shaped and has no postural function, and when the baby cries or is held upright, pressure is transmitted directly to the visceral organs, causing the organs to move toward the pelvic cavity and resulting in the PFM contracting to counteract this pressure. As the child begins to stand and walk, the diaphragm contracts more. The sudden contraction of the diaphragm directs pressure toward the anterior abdominal wall, and this pressure is then directed downward and posteriorly toward the sacrum, resulting in sacral concavity during adolescence. This fully protects the pelvic floor from visceral impingement [1, 19].

In the initial stages of life, there is a lack of postural synergy between the intrinsic back muscles and the abdominal muscles. As the intrinsic back muscles exert control, the spine assumes a straightened position. The chest is stabilized by the pulling action of the ribs and abdominal muscles. The ribs have steeper angles than in the neonatal period. The straightening of the spine and the stabilization efficiency of the abdominal muscles change the anchoring point of the diaphragm's joints, bringing the diaphragm into a horizontal position. This is a specific adaptation to upright posture in humans. The increased IAP and the pulling action of the abdominal and gluteal muscles enable the pelvic floor to perform its postural function [19].

The existing literature on the relationship between posture and PFM dysfunction in children is limited. Inal et al. [20] reported that children with primary monosymptomatic nocturnal enuresis exhibited altered postural alignment, as well as static and dynamic postural instability, when compared to same-aged controls. Similarly, differences in abdominal and spinal musculoskeletal function were observed in children with slow-transit constipation when compared with the control group [21].

In 2008, Delancey et al. [22] developed the Pelvic Floor Model and described a graphical tool that integrates pelvic floor function related to pelvic floor disorders in three stages. The first stage was the "development of functional reserve" during the individual's growth. According to this model, a child who develops this reserve will be less prone to pelvic floor dysfunction in adulthood. However, in some individuals, this reserve is depleted, and a threshold is crossed where symptoms begin to manifest. When and how this occurs will depend on the amount of reserve gained during initial development, the rate of decline, the extent to which lifestyle stresses the pelvic floor, and the effects of any triggering events. There are normal variations in the initial growth and development of all body parts. Variation in height is perhaps the most familiar. Like height, pelvic floor development is influenced by factors including genetic code, nutrition, and environment. An individual who develops excellent pelvic floor function may lead their life without experiencing any pelvic floor disorder symptoms, even in the face of injurious or lifestyle events, as long as they have sufficient functional reserve. However, an individual with less robust growth and development may become symptomatic throughout their life, even due to normal age-related decline [22]. Both internal and external factors are likely to affect PFM function. For example, children who experience difficulty during defecation are prone to stool retention, failure of the PFM to relax during defecation, and the risk of functional constipation. Therefore, developing such a model for children would be beneficial [1]. In the female sexual dysfunction study, it was stated that "primary pelvic floor hyperactivity in children and adolescents is one of the most neglected predisposing factors for later dyspareunia and vulvar vestibulitis" [23].

In children with bladder and/or bowel dysfunction, there is a high prevalence of movement problems, which indicate muscle dysfunction, alongside considerable rates of core muscle stability and motor skill challenges [24]. A study involving children with cerebral palsy showed that the degree of motor dysfunction was associated with increased urinary symptoms and urodynamic findings [17]. Consequently, it appears that there is an opportunity to learn from adult studies, and further investigation is needed to determine whether pelvic floor dysfunction is a contributing factor in pediatric incontinence. Evaluating muscle dysfunction is essential for prescribing an effective muscle training program.

27.3 Bladder and Bowel Dysfunctions in Pediatrics

27.3.1 Pediatric Bladder Dysfunctions

Toilet training is an important step in a child's development. The age at which toilet training is acquired and the beliefs about toilet training differ across cultures. Most children usually acquire the physiological, cognitive, and emotional development necessary for toilet training between 18 and 30 months. In Turkey, toilet training starts at an average age of 22–28 months, whereas it has been reported that toilet training starts between 24 and 36 months in the United States. In Asian and African countries, toilet training starts in the first month and can be completed by 12 months of age [25–28]. There are some signs that indicate that children are ready for toilet training, and parents should read these signs for proper toilet training. Signs that indicate a child's readiness for toilet training include being able to walk to the toilet or to walk back from the toilet, being able to take off their clothes, a change in facial expression when they go to the toilet, being uncomfortable when their diaper is dirty, and asking for a change [26]. Especially in the last 50 years, there have been significant global changes, such as the delayed initiation of toilet training. The main reasons for this are disposable diapers and working parents [28]. It is known that pelvic floor dysfunction may develop in children due to some errors in toilet training. Many studies have shown that late toilet training causes pelvic floor dysfunction. Li et al. reported that toilet training starting after 24 months caused lower urinary tract dysfunction, and Barone et al. reported that toilet training given after 32 months caused urge incontinence [29–32]. Hodges et al. showed a relationship between dysfunctional voiding in children with early toilet training (before 24 months) and constipation in children with late toilet training (after 36 months) [33].

The minimum age for inclusion is 4 years for lower urinary tract dysfunction and 5 years for bowel dysfunction. According to the latest standardization paper by the International Child Continence Society (ICCS) published in 2016, the term bladder and bowel dysfunction is used as an umbrella term to cover both lower urinary tract and bowel dysfunctions due to the close relationship between the bladder and bowel [34]. Pediatric bladder dysfunctions are shown in Table 27.1.

Table 27.1 Pediatric bladder dysfunctions

Terminology [34]	Definition
Urinary incontinence	Urinary incontinence is involuntary leakage of urine. Pediatric urinary incontinence is divided into two types: Intermittent and continuous. Continuous urinary incontinence means continuous urine leakage day and night and is usually associated with congenital malformations (ectopic ureter, ex-trophic variables, etc.), functional loss of the external urethral sphincter (external sphincterotomy, etc.), or iatrogenic causes (vesicovaginal fistula, etc.). Intermittent urinary incontinence is leakage of different amounts of urine. When intermittent urinary incontinence occurs during the daytime, it is called daytime urinary incontinence, and when it occurs during sleep, it is called nocturnal enuresis. If a child has both daytime urinary incontinence and urinary incontinence during sleep, it is called daytime incontinence and nocturnal enuresis

(continued)

Table 27.1 (continued)

Terminology [34]	Definition
Increased or decreased voiding frequency	Voiding frequency is variable and is influenced by diuresis and fluid intake rather than bladder capacity. A voiding frequency of 8 or more than 8 voids per day is defined as increased voiding frequency, whereas 3 or less than 3 voids per day is defined as decreased voiding frequency. Voiding frequency cannot be fully understood without a voiding frequency/volume chart or voiding diary
Urgency	Urgency is a sudden and unexpected feeling of urgency, a compulsion to urinate. Urgency symptom is often a sign of an overactive bladder
Nocturia	Nocturia is the complaint of waking up at night to urinate and is common among school children. Nocturia is not indicative of lower urinary tract dysfunction or a pathologic condition. Unlike nocturnal enuresis, nocturia does not result in incontinence
Overactive bladder	Overactive bladder is characterized by frequent urination and nocturia (with or without urinary incontinence), usually in the absence of urinary urgency, urinary tract infection, or other specific pathologies. Children with overactive bladder usually have detrusor overactivity, although this term can only be used with cystometric evaluation. Urgency urinary incontinence is a complaint of involuntary urine leakage with urgency and is present in many children with overactive bladder
Voiding postponement	Children who habitually delay voiding by using holding maneuvers may suffer from this condition. The clinical history of this behavior is often accompanied by a decrease in micturition frequency, a feeling of urgency, and possible incontinence due to a full bladder. Some children simultaneously restrict their fluid intake to reduce incontinence. These children also often have behavioral disorders such as oppositional defiant disorder and psychological comorbidities
Underactive bladder	This clinical term is used for children who need to increase intra-abdominal pressure to initiate, maintain, and complete voiding. Children may have low voiding frequencies but urinate frequently due to inadequate urine evacuation, and bladder refill may be very rapid. These children often present with an intermittent voiding curve on uroflowmetry evaluation, and urodynamic evaluation reveals detrusor underactivity
Dysfunctional voiding	Children with dysfunctional voiding have the habit of contracting the urethral sphincter or pelvic floor during voiding, and when EMG activity is evaluated simultaneously with uroflowmetry, they produce a staccato-shaped voiding curve and sometimes an intermittent voiding curve
Giggle incontinence	Giggle urinary incontinence is a rare condition. It is urinary incontinence that occurs immediately after or during laughter. Bladder function is normal when the person is not laughing

27.3.1.1 Other Symptoms

Hesitancy

Hesitancy denotes difficulty in initiating voiding when the child is ready to void.

Straining

Straining means the child complains of needing to make an intense effort to increase intra-abdominal pressure (e.g., Valsalva) in order to initiate and maintain voiding [34].

Weak Stream

This term describes an observed stream or uroflow that is weak [34].

Intermittency

Intermittency implies micturition that is not continuous but rather has several discrete stop-and-start [34].

Dysuria

Dysuria is the complaint of burning or discomfort during micturition. The timing of dysuria may be noted during voiding. Dysuria at the start of voiding suggests a urethral source of pain, whereas dysuria at the completion of voiding suggests a bladder [34].

Holding Maneuvers
These are observable strategies used to postpone voiding or suppress urgency that may be associated with bladder overactivity. The child may or may not be fully aware of the purpose of these maneuvers, but they are usually obvious to caregivers. Common behaviors include standing on tiptoes, forcefully crossing the legs, grabbing or pushing on the genitals or abdomen, and placing pressure on the perineum (e.g., squatting with the heel pressed into the perineum or sitting on the edge of a chair) [34].

Feeling of Incomplete Emptying
This refers to the complaint that the bladder does not feel empty after voiding and may result in the need to return to the toilet to void again [34].

Urinary Retention
This refers to the sensation of an inability to void despite persistent effort in the presence of a fully distended bladder. Duration of time is particularly beneficial in characterizing the retention [34].

Post-Micturition Dribble
This term is used when the child describes involuntary leakage of urine immediately after voiding has finished. This symptom may be associated with vaginal reflux in girls or syringocoele in boys (see below). Spraying (splitting) of the urinary stream. This refers to the complaint that urine passes as a spray or a split rather than a single, discrete stream. It usually implies a mechanical obstruction at or just below the meatus (e.g., meatal stenosis) [34].

27.3.2 Pediatric Bowel Dysfunctions

See Table 27.2.

Table 27.2 Pediatric bowel dysfunctions

Terminology (Rome IV) [35]	Definition
Organic constipation	Organic constipation is very rare and is caused by Hirschsprung's disease, hypothyroidism, hypercalcemia, spina bifida, anorectal malformations, and some medications [36]
Functional constipation	Functional constipation is defined as the occurrence of 2 or more of the Rome IV criteria for functional constipation for children and adolescents at least 1 time per week for at least 1 month and no other underlying medical condition [35]
	Rome IV diagnostic criteria for child functional constipation [35][a]
	1. 2 or fewer defecations per week (at least in a 4-year-old child)
	2. Fecal incontinence at least once a week
	3. History of retentive posturing or excessive volitional stool retention
	4. History of painful or hard bowel movements
	5. Presence of a large fecal mass in the rectum
	6. History of large diameter stools that can obstruct the toilet
Organic fecal incontinence	Fecal incontinence is defined as the involuntary leakage of liquid feces or the complete loss of solid feces. Organic FI is generally defined as associated with structural or physiologic abnormalities in the gastrointestinal tract or the nervous system that controls continence mechanisms. Organic FI is less common than functional FI
Functional FI	Functional FI is defined according to Rome IV criteria and has two types: retentive FI (associated with constipation) and non-retentive FI (FNRFI)
Functional retentive FI	Functional retentive FI resulted from constipation. Long-term constipation and dilated rectum may cause fecal incontinence
Functional non-retentive FI	Rome IV diagnostic criteria for child non-retentive fecal incontinence[b]
	1. Defecation into places inappropriate to the sociocultural context
	2. No evidence of fecal retention
	3. After appropriate medical evaluation, the fecal incontinence cannot be explained by another medical condition

(continued)

Table 27.2 (continued)

Terminology (Rome IV) [35]	Definition
Irritable bowel syndrome	Rome IV diagnostic criteria child IBS[c]
	1. Abdominal pain >4 days per month associated with one or more of the following:
	(a) Related defecation
	(b) Change in frequency of stool
	(c) Change in form (shape) of stool
	2. In children with constipation, the pain does not resolve with resolution of the constipation (children in whom the pain resolves have functional constipation, not irritable bowel syndrome)
	3. After appropriate evaluation, the symptoms cannot be fully explained by another medical condition
Hirschsprung's disease	Hirschsprung's disease is a congenital malformation of the enteric nervous system characterized by the absence of ganglia in the distal part of the intestine. In this disease, the anal canal is always affected, and the rectum and sigmoid colon are often involved
Functional abdominal pain disorders (FAPD)	Functional abdominal pain disorders (FAPD) are among the most common types of chronic pain disorders in children. FAPD defined in the Rome IV criteria includes functional dyspepsia, IBS, abdominal migraine, and functional abdominal pain not otherwise specified

FI fecal incontinence, *FNRFI* functional non-retentive fecal incontinence, *IBS* irritable bowel syndrome, *FAPD* functional abdominal pain disorders

[a]2 or more of these criteria must occur at least 1 time per week for at least 1 month, and there must be no other underlying medical condition

[b]A child older than 4 years should have these symptoms for at least 1 month

[c]These symptoms must be present for at least 2 months

27.4 Evaluation in Pediatric Pelvic Floor Dysfunction

27.4.1 Differences in Assessing the Pelvic Floor in Children and Adults

Pelvic floor muscle training is a mainstay of treatment for both pediatric and adult pelvic floor dysfunction. According to the literature, there is a lack of studies investigating the pediatric pelvic floor compared with the adult pelvic floor literature [37–39]. Also, the existing pediatric pelvic floor studies are not homogeneous in terms of design.

There are some important points that researchers and clinicians should pay attention to regarding the assessment of the pediatric pelvic floor. Firstly, children are not young adults and should not be assessed as adults. Secondly, when deciding on the appropriate pelvic floor assessment for the child, not only parents but also children should be consulted and informed well. Thirdly, invasive methods should be avoided in pelvic floor evaluation as much as possible in order not to cause possible trauma in children [1]. Lastly, even though we do not have enough information about how pelvic floor muscles mature during childhood, to decrease possible failure, researchers may assess similar age groups, such as 7 years and below, 7 to 11 years, and 12 years and above [1].

Pediatric patients are less likely to experience conditions such as pelvic organ prolapse or stress urinary incontinence, which are more common in adults, particularly in women after childbirth or due to aging. These conditions are often related to the weakening or damage to the PFMs and connective tissue [40, 41].

In clinical practice, the treatment and assessment of pelvic floor disorders need to be age-appropriate, taking into account the anatomical and functional maturity of the pelvic floor in pediatric patients compared with adults. These differences underscore the importance of specialized approaches in diagnosing and treating pelvic floor issues across different age groups. For a comprehensive understanding, it is beneficial to consult detailed literature on anatomical and clinical pelvic floor anatomy and development.

In this part of the chapter, the focus will be on differences in pelvic floor assessment between children and adults from the perspective of pedi-

Table 27.3 Comparison of pelvic floor assessment methods between children and adults

Pelvic floor assessment methods	Invasive/ noninvasive	Direct/ indirect	Children	Adults	Position	Why do we use this method?
Visual observation	Noninvasive	Indirect	√	√	Lithotomy or left lateral lying position	Perineal and perianal skin assessment (scar, lesion color changes), anal gaping, keyhole deformity, and reflexes (anal reflex, bulbospongiousus and bulbocavernosus reflex, sacral reflex) [39]
Digital rectal examination (DRE)	Invasive	Indirect	√	√	Left lateral lying position	Presence of anal fissure and blood, stool, and pain. Ability of contraction and relaxation of PFM and anal sphincter [42, 43]
Digital vaginal examination	Invasive	Indirect	X	√	Lithotomy position	Presence of scar and pain. Ability of contraction and relaxation of PFM [39]
EMG		Direct [44]				
Perineal surface EMG	Noninvasive	Direct	√	√	Lithotomy position Left lateral lying position	Ability of contraction and relaxation of PFM. Duration of fast or slow contraction. Reaction time, baseline muscle activity [39, 45]
Perianal surface EMG	Noninvasive	Direct	√	√	Lithotomy position Left lateral lying position Defecation posture on commode	Ability of contraction and relaxation of PFM. Duration of fast or slow contraction. Reaction time, baseline muscle activity [39, 45]

(continued)

Table 27.3 (continued)

Pelvic floor assessment methods	Invasive/ noninvasive	Direct/ indirect	Children	Adults	Position	Why do we use this method?
Intervaginal EMG probe	Invasive	Direct	X	√	Lithotomy position	Ability of contraction and relaxation of PFM. Duration of fast or slow contraction. Reaction time, baseline muscle activity [46]
Interanal EMG probe	Invasive	Direct	X	√	Left lateral lying position	Ability of contraction and relaxation of PFM. Duration of fast or slow contraction. Reaction time, baseline muscle activity [39, 45]
Ultrasound (US)		Indirect [44]				
Transabdominal US	Noninvasive	Indirect	√	√	Supine position	Primarily used to assess the lifting aspect of a PFM contraction by observation of movement of the bladder base as a marker for PFM activity during voluntary PFM contraction [1]
Transperineal US	Noninvasive	Indirect	√	√	Lithotomy position	Assesses pelvic floor muscle contractility and relaxation by anorectal angle and/ or bladder neck and proximal urethra [1, 47]
Endovaginal ultrasound	Invasive	Indirect	X	√	Lithotomy position	Assesses bladder neck, urethra, and PFM [39]
Endoanal ultrasound	Invasive	Indirect	X	√	Left lateral lying position	Assesses anal sphincter and puborectalis muscle contractility and check sphincter defects [48]
Manometer/ perineometer	Invasive	Direct				

(continued)

Table 27.3 (continued)

Pelvic floor assessment methods	Invasive/ noninvasive	Direct/ indirect	Children	Adults	Position	Why do we use this method?
Anal pressure probe	Invasive	Direct	X	√	Left lateral lying position	Assesses anal sphincter muscle contractility and anorectal complex [39]
Vaginal probe	Invasive	Direct	X	√	Lithotomy position	Assesses levator ani and PFM contractility [39]
Uroflowmetry	Noninvasive	Indirect	√	√	Voiding position [49]	Gives information about voiding dysfunction and pelvic floor activity during voiding and also assesses urine flow, volume, and rate [50]
Urodynamic	Invasive	Direct	√	√	Comfortably seated and/or standing [49]	Evaluates bladder physiology such as detrusor function, bladder capacity and volume, bladder sensation, compliance, and urethral function [51]
Anorectal manometry	Noninvasive	Direct	√	√	Left lateral lying position	Assesses the following parameters: maximum rest pressure, high-pressure zone, anal sphincter and puborectalis muscles contractility and relaxation ability, duration of squeeze, straining ability, rectal sensation, and rectal reflexes [52, 53]
MRI	Noninvasive	Indirect [44]	√	√	Supine position	Provides any information about spinal nerves and malfunctions and abnormality of bladder and bowel-related structures [54]
Balloon expulsion test	Noninvasive	Direct	√	√	Defecation posture on commode	Gives information about the presence of dyssynergic defecation [55]

PFM pelvic floor muscle, *DRE* digital rectal examination, *EMG* electromyography, *US* ultrasound, *MRI* magnetic resonance imaging atric pelvic floor assessment literature (Table 27.3).

27.4.2 History

The most important part of the evaluation of pelvic floor dysfunction is history-taking. Therefore, history taking should be very thorough, specific, and at the same time not boring so as not to distract the child. As described above, even if the child has only bladder or bowel complaints, other organ-related symptoms should also be evaluated.

It is essential to consider the following factors when assessing pelvic dysfunction: when (day or night), where (school/public place and/or home), the frequency (once a week or daily), and the amount (mild or severe). Additionally, the voiding and defecation posture, the frequency of defecation, and the presence of any associated symptoms must be taken into account. It is essential to ascertain the following information: the age at which toilet training commenced, the efficiency of defecation, the presence of any behavioral traits that may indicate a tendency to delay defecation, the density of stool, and the presence of rectal, anal, or other pain during the act of defecation. In the event that fecal incontinence is present, it is essential to ascertain the quantity of soiling in the underwear, the frequency and severity of the fecal incontinence, the duration of the fecal incontinence (such as before/after noon, evening, or after school), and the activity performed at the time of the incontinence [56, 57].

27.4.3 Bladder and Bowel Diary

A bladder and bowel diary should be kept for objective recording and documentation of bladder and bowel function. A 7-night bladder diary (incontinence frequencies and nocturnal voiding volume measurements) should be kept to evaluate nocturnal enuresis. A 2-day bladder diary (daytime voiding frequencies and volumes) should be recorded to evaluate lower urinary tract dysfunction [57].

Bowel history should be recorded with a 7–14-day bowel diary. The bowel diary assesses the frequency of defecation and fecal incontinence, the shape and intensity of the stool, whether the defecation is spontaneous or effortful, whether there is any straining, bleeding, or pain during defecation, and whether the patient ignores the feeling of urgent defecation. The Bristol Stool Scale is used in combination with a bowel diary to classify stool [57].

27.4.4 Pelvic Floor Assessment in Children

27.4.4.1 Digital Rectal Examination

During digital rectal examination, anal position, presence of FI, skin irritation, eczema, anal fissures, hemorrhoids, and the possibility of sexual abuse are examined by inspection and palpation. Although digital rectal examination is generally not preferred in children, if an evaluation is to be performed, it should be explained in detail to the child and parents why this evaluation will be performed, what will be evaluated, in which position, and where the evaluation will be performed. The evaluation position is the left lateral position with knees bent, and the child should be covered with a sheet, and privacy should be ensured. In addition, the fifth finger can be used in the assessment according to the age of the child or the thickness of the assessor's finger. During the examination, the perianal, perineal, and sacral regions can be observed for congenital defects, sacral dimple/hair/tumor. Anal sphincter muscle tone, contraction, and relaxation ability can be evaluated. The presence of intra-rectal mass (feces, tumor, etc.) and blood can be evaluated [43].

27.4.4.2 Uroflowmetry

Uroflowmetry is a simple and noninvasive test. Therefore, it is accepted as the first diagnostic tool used to evaluate lower urinary tract function in children. Uroflow studies evaluate the rate, volume, duration, and pattern of voiding. The child must be toilet-trained to perform uroflow studies. In addition, since the curve changes when the voided volume is less than 50% of the expected bladder capacity for age, it is important that the voided volume is sufficient and that multiple curves are obtained to improve the accuracy, reliability, and interpretation of the test.

Uroflowmetry can be performed by evaluation of the perineal muscles with or without EMG. The advantage of performing EMG and uroflowmetry tests together is that they evaluate the synergy or dyssynergy between the bladder and pelvic floor [49, 50].

27.4.4.3 Urodynamic Evaluation

Urodynamic studies are frequently used in the evaluation of infants and children with neurogenic or non-neurogenic bladder dysfunction or lower urinary tract dysfunction. Urodynamics in infants, children, and adolescents requires some adaptations to produce meaningful results and to accurately assess the lower urinary tract to enable evidence-based treatment. In pediatric cases, specific adaptations to staff training, the environment, and child and parental support should be made so that the entire examination is child-friendly [49].

27.4.4.4 Anorectal Manometry

Anorectal manometry provides objective information about the neuromuscular function of the rectum and anal sphincter complex. With this measurement, anorectal physiology data such as the presence of recto-anal inhibitory reflex, resting pressure, compression pressure, rectal sensation, and recto-anal coordination are evaluated [53].

27.4.4.5 Ultrasound

Ultrasound (US) is a very important assessment tool for evaluating lower urinary tract and bowel function in children. It can be performed before voiding with a full bladder and after voiding. Pre-voiding images also contribute to the overall assessment of the bladder wall, lower urethral dilatation, and bladder neck appearance. Bladder ultrasound can also show whether the bladder is full enough for normal voiding [58].

- *Post-Void Residual*: Residual urine can be demonstrated by evaluation of the bladder after voiding. To be reliable, a post-void ultrasound should be performed within 5 min after voiding. Post-void residual values are highly variable in neurologically normal children. Two measurements are recommended for post-void residual [34, 58]
- *Bladder Wall Thickness*: A thickened bladder wall will cause long-lasting problems like storing and emptying urine. Bladder wall thickness depends on the degree of bladder filling and is likely to be associated with lower urinary tract dysfunction [34]
- *Rectal Diameter*: Rectal diameter is significantly enlarged in constipated children and can also be used as a predictor of constipation [59]

27.4.5 Physical Assessment

The physical assessment includes general, abdominal, perineal, perianal, posture, balance, and sensory integration. However, the assessment of the perineal and perianal area is described in the pelvic floor assessment section and will not be described in this section. The general physical assessment should first obtain information about the child's body composition by measuring the child's height and weight (Fig. 27.1). Growth parameters should also be considered as part of the general physical assessment. The child's muscle strength and deep tendon reflexes should be evaluated. As a result of the evaluation, the presence of abnormal muscle strength or reflex response may indicate cerebral or spinal abnormalities [56, 60].

The child's abdomen can be examined manually. This assessment detects the presence of gas or feces. Fecal matter is usually found in the sigmoid colon in the lower left quadrant of the abdomen. The presence of an abdominal fecal mass may be associated with both constipation and fecal incontinence [54, 61, 62].

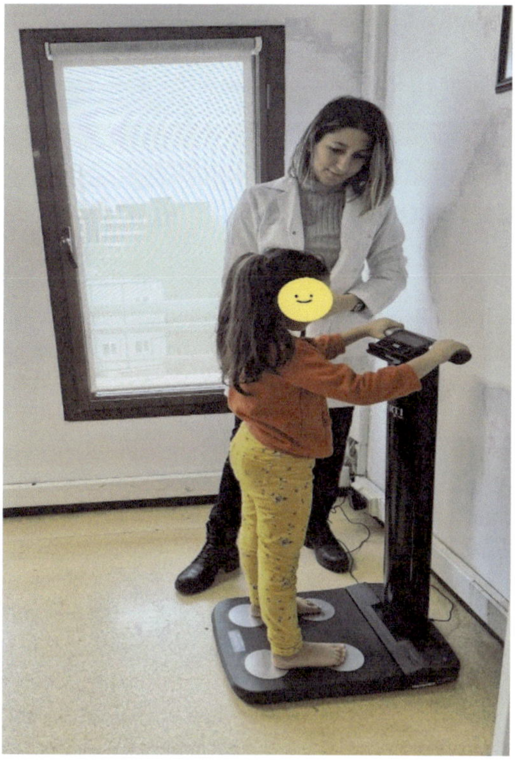

Fig. 27.1 Bioelectrical impedance measurement

It has been shown that the posture of children with nocturnal enuresis is impaired compared to healthy children [20, 63] (Fig. 27.2). In children with constipation, it is predicted that joint hypermobility, trunk muscle imbalances, and posture disorders may be present [21, 64]. Besides, the child's posture should be evaluated for signs of sacral dysraphism, such as scoliosis, the presence of sacral dimples or hair in the lumbosacral area, and deviation of the gluteal cleft.

There are studies showing that the balance of children with nocturnal enuresis is negatively affected [20, 63]. According to the Dutch pelvic physiotherapy protocol, it is reported that in the presence of constipation, it should be treated with balance exercises (Fig. 27.3) [65].

27.4.6 Sensory Integration

Sensory integration is the processing, integration, and organization of sensory information from the body and the environment. Sensory processing disorder is a term that includes difficulties in pro-

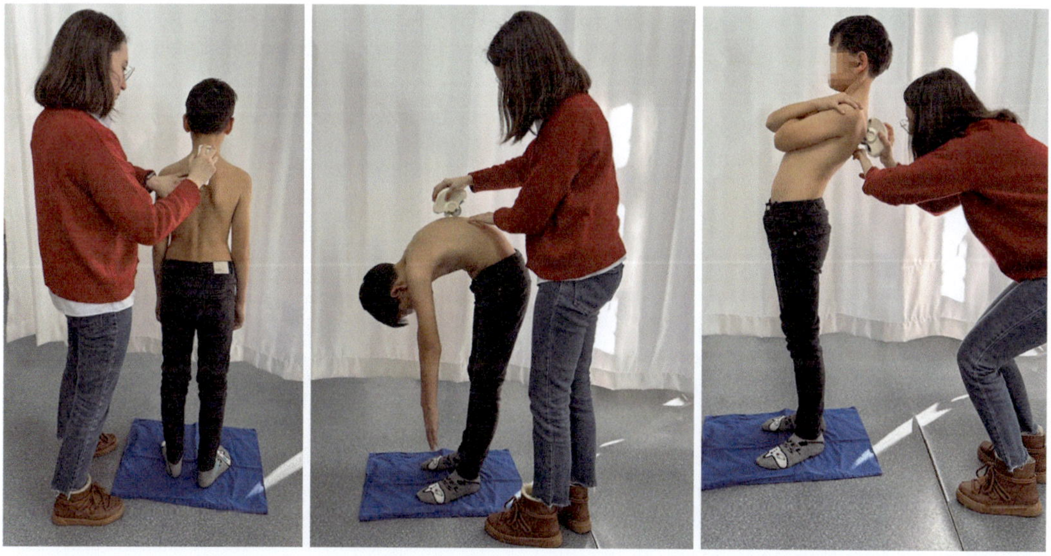

Fig. 27.2 Posture evaluation using the Spinal Mouse Device

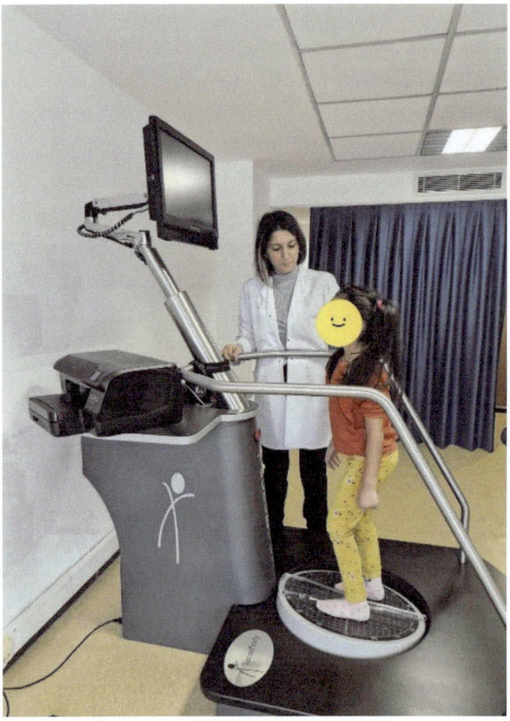

Fig. 27.3 Dynamic balance evaluation

cessing and using sensory information for the regulation of physiological, motor, affective, and/or attentional responses that interfere with the organization of behavior and participation in activities of daily living [66].

Children with bowel problems often have atypical bowel habits that lead to bowel dysfunction. Pilot studies suggest that problems with sensory reactivity (the process of modulation of neural activity in response to sensory stimulation) and perception (the ability to detect and interpret sensory stimulation) might be related to atypical bowel patterns. In recent years, new studies have been conducted on sensory integration, especially in children with bowel problems. In recent years, new studies have been conducted on sensory integration, especially in children with bowel problems. The following tests can be used in the evaluation of these children [67–69]. The following tests can be used in the evaluation of these children: Sensory Integration and Praxis Tests, Sensory Processing Measure, and Sensory Integration Inventory-Revised [70].

27.4.7 Questionnaires

Quality of life scales assess the physical, mental, and social well-being of the individual, with the understanding that the individual is situated within a dynamic interaction with the environment. Health-related quality of life (HRQOL) is defined as the patient's perception of the effects of a disease and its treatment. HRQOL measures can be divided into two categories: general and condition-specific. General condition-specific HRQOL measures can be used in both healthy and sick individuals, thus providing the opportunity to make comparisons. Quality of life scales that are used in pediatric pelvic floor dysfunction is shown in Table 27.4.

Symptom severity questionnaires are used to assess the presence and severity of symptoms. There are a few symptom scales used in the presence of pediatric bladder and bowel dysfunction. Symptom scales used in the presence of pediatric pelvic floor dysfunction are shown in Table 27.5.

Table 27.4 Pediatric pelvic floor dysfunction-specific quality of life questionnaires

Condition	Name of Questionnaire
Urinary incontinence	Pediatric Incontinence Related Quality of Life [71]
Nocturnal enuresis	Pediatric Enuresis Module to Assess Quality of Life [72]
Functional constipation	Pediatric Functional Constipation Questionnaire-Parent Report [73]
FI in anorectal malformations and Hirschsprung's disease	Questionnaire for the Assessment of Quality of Life Related to Fecal Continence in Children and Adolescents [74]

Table 27.5 Pediatric pelvic floor dysfunction-specific symptom severity questionnaires

Condition	Name of Questionnaire
Non-neurogenic LUT	Vancouver Non-Neorogenic Lower Urinary Tract Dysfunction/ Dysfunctional Elimination Syndrome Questionnaire [75]
Lower urinary tract dysfunctions	Dysfunctional Voiding and Incontinence Scoring System [76]
Bladder and bowel dysfunction	Child Bladder And Bowel Dysfunction Questionnaire (CBBDQ) [77]
FI in anorectal malformations and Hirschsprung's disease	Fecal Incontinence Index [74]
Urinary incontinence	Incontinence Symptom Index-Pediatric [78]
Daytime UI and enuresis	Wetting and Functional Voiding Disorder Score [79]

LUT lower urinary tract, *FI* fecal incontinence, *UI* urinary incontinence

27.5 Treatment of Bladder and Bowel Dysfunction in Children

Bladder and/or bowel dysfunction in children may occur independently or simultaneously. When both bladder and bowel dysfunctions coexist, it is recommended that treatment priorities follow a specific sequence: addressing fecal incontinence or constipation first, followed by daytime urinary incontinence, and finally nocturnal enuresis [38, 80].

The involvement of both the child and their family in the treatment process is crucial. The child must be willing to participate in the treatment, and parents should be actively involved in decision-making. Before initiating treatment, parents should receive education to avoid punitive behaviors, foster the child's awareness of their condition, and provide consistent encouragement and support [81].

Table 27.6 Response to treatment according to ICCS

Percentage reduction in symptoms	Definition
<50%	No response to treatment
50–99%	Partial response to treatment
100%	Full response to treatment

The ICCS rates treatment efficacy and success based on the reduction of symptoms rather than classifying them as "responders" and "non-responders." If the percentage reduction in symptoms after treatment in children is below 50%, it is classified as "no response to treatment", between 50 and 99% as "partial response to treatment", and 100% as "full response to treatment" (Table 27.6) [57]. The literature suggests different treatment protocols for bladder and bowel dysfunctions and colorectal-anal problems [54, 56, 60, 82–85].

27.5.1 Urotherapy

Urotherapy is one of the most used treatment methods for children with bladder and bowel dysfunction. The term "urotherapy" was first defined by the ICCS (International Children's Continence Society) as the "non-surgical and non-pharmacological treatment of lower urinary tract dysfunction (LUTD)." More recently, it has been described as "a conservative therapy and treatment method that rehabilitates lower urinary tract dysfunction." The primary aim of urotherapy is to normalize bladder and bowel function and to prevent potential functional disorders through repeated training. The secondary aim is to improve the quality of life for the child and their parents/caregivers, enhance the ability to cope with symptoms, and increase self-efficacy [38, 80, 82].

Urotherapy is mainly used for daytime urinary incontinence. However, the 2020 ICCS paper reported that urotherapy is not only used for daytime urinary incontinence but also for nocturnal enuresis, functional constipation, and fecal incontinence. Urotherapy is divided into two types: standard urotherapy and specific urotherapy. Standard urotherapy is the first treatment option for many functional disorders, while specific urotherapy is used for the treatment of particular lower urinary tract dysfunctions [38, 80, 82].

27.5.1.1 Standard Urotherapy

(a) *Patient and Parents' Education*

Education, along with explanations and recommendations, plays a crucial role in the treatment of children with bladder and bowel dysfunction. Explanations should be tailored to the child's age using tools like models, presentations, and brochures (Fig. 27.4). Effective education is vital for successful treatment. The goal of this information session is to educate both the child and their parents about the anatomy, function, and physiology of the bladder and bowel; how urination and defecation occur; the PFMs and their function; and the relationship between the bladder and bowel.

Besides, physiotherapists should focus on avoiding behaviors such as delaying urination and defecation, prevalence, symptoms, and the prognosis of dysfunction. It can be explained that FI and UI occur involuntarily and are often linked to social issues like shame and discomfort [54, 60].

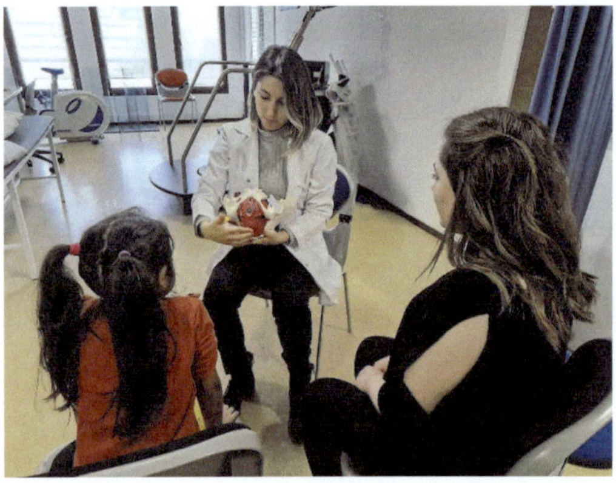

Fig. 27.4 Patient and parents' education

(b) *Toilet Program/Education*

Correct toilet posture and relaxation of the pelvic floor muscles are essential for effective urination and defecation. In the appropriate toilet posture, the hips should be positioned at approximately a 90° angle, with the knees higher than the hips, and a footstool placed under the feet to ensure full contact with the footstool (Fig. 27.5).

The therapist can act as a role model by demonstrating the correct way to sit on the toilet. Additionally, a timed voiding method can be employed to encourage children to use the toilet at regular intervals [38, 86]. A timer watch or a chart can help to remind the child to take time to go to the toilet, thereby increasing compliance. Timed voiding can lead to positive results because the child does not wet as often, and it gives the child a feeling of self-control [87].

Inadequate toilet training can lead to the development of constipation and fecal incontinence (FI). If a child receives insufficient training, this may result in painful defecation, causing the child to voluntarily withhold stool, which in turn can lead to constipation and eventually FI. Therefore, proper toilet training is a cornerstone of treatment [56]. Toilet training should involve going to the bathroom 15–30 min after

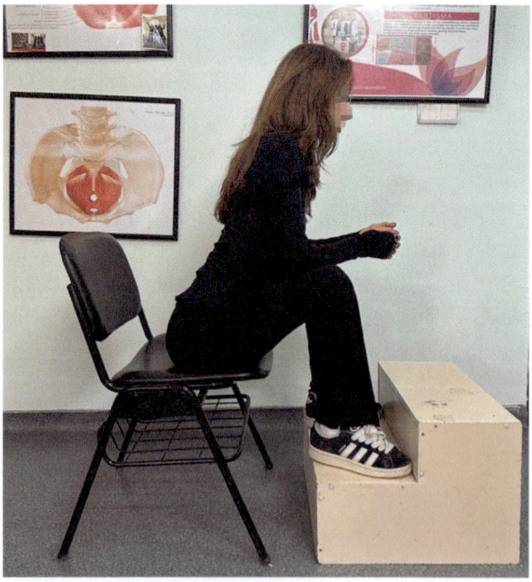

Fig. 27.5 Correct toilet posture

main meals (to take advantage of the gastrocolic reflex) and sitting on the toilet for about 5 min [38, 56, 60, 88].

(c) *Dietary Changes*

Some foods and drinks have been reported to affect bladder function [89, 90]. Foods and beverages such as caffeine, carbonated drinks, and artificial sweeteners can lead to urgency and frequency or stimulate diuresis. Various types of drinks and foods, including coffee, tea, soda, alcoholic beverages, citrus fruits, fruit juices, artificial sweeteners, and spicy peppers, may exacerbate symptoms in patients with painful bladder syndrome/interstitial cystitis (BPS/IC) [91]. The BPS/IC Diet Special Committee has published a list of "bladder-friendly foods" to help identify and avoid foods that may trigger symptoms or compromise the effectiveness of treatment. The guidelines recommend avoiding known bladder irritants such as coffee and citrus products [89].

In terms of dietary changes for children with colorectal problems, there are conflicting views in the literature. According to some studies, children with constipation and functional retentive fecal incontinence benefit from consuming high-fiber foods, while other studies show no significant changes. The ESPGHAN and NASPGHAN guidelines do not recommend fiber supplements for children with constipation [92]. Additionally, high-fiber food consumption is not recommended for children with functional retentive FIF [60]. It has also been shown that the use of probiotics in pediatric constipation and FIF is ineffective and lacks sufficient evidence [93, 94]. Therefore, it is important to refer children to nutrition and dietetic specialists for proper dietary management.

(d) *Recording* Symptoms

During the treatment, recording stool and/or bladder diary helps to get objective information about children's symptoms, such as the frequency of urination, defecation, and incontinence. Besides, it gives feedback to children, gaining control over their bodies, and provides motivation to children and parents. Further, a reward system using a diary including a star chart, dry/wet night in nocturnal enuresis treatment is a common behavioral therapy. The child is rewarded with a positive reinforcer for a dry night or waking up for urination, and it provides motivation for both children and parents [60, 87].

27.5.1.2 Specific Urotherapy

In the management of children diagnosed with bladder and bowel dysfunction, various specific urotherapy approaches are utilized, including pelvic floor muscle training, electrotherapy, breathing exercises, different exercise modalities, manual therapy techniques, and sensory integration interventions.

27.5.1.2.1 Physiotherapy and Rehabilitation

(a) *Pelvic Floor Muscle Training*

In children, very little is known about pelvic floor muscle training. Teaching the difference between PFM contraction and relaxation to enhance PFM awareness is used to facilitate defecation and urination. The aim of Pelvic Floor Muscle Training (PFMT) is to ensure that the child internalizes the difference between PFM contraction and relaxation and has sufficient awareness to apply it correctly. The method of teaching PFM awareness may vary depending on many factors, such as the child's age, sensorimotor awareness, and cognitive ability. PFM contraction and relaxation can be taught by EMG-biofeedback, anorectal manometry, transabdominal, or transperineal US [38, 56, 60, 83, 88, 92, 95–97].

Pelvic Floor Muscle Training with Biofeedback

Biofeedback (BF) is a noninvasive behavioral therapy, and it gives information back to the body using visual or verbal feedback. BF treatment was initiated in the late 1970s, and interest in treating children with voiding dysfunction has increased over time [98]. BF is generally considered a method different from PFMT; however, BF is an assistive therapy to PFMT. BF provides information to patients about muscle function and helps correct taught contractions, or enhances their performance, and increases patient motivation and performance during training [23].

In the treatment of pediatric pelvic floor dysfunctions, basically, there are two primary mechanisms by which PFMT with BF therapy:

The first is providing real-time flow rates using uroflowmetry/anorectal manometers and a visual display.

The second involves feedback on the activity of the pelvic floor and abdominal muscles through visual or auditory cues.

Electromyography-BF

BF, especially with animated computer games, has become a preferred option due to its positive results in treating conditions such as Dysfunctional Voiding (DV), vesicoureteral reflux, and constipation [99]. The goal of BF treatment is to teach neurologically healthy children proper urination/defecation habits and help them gain control over urination/defecation function [100, 101].

BF combined with PFMT in children is usually done via EMG-BF with electrodes placed on the perineum. Proper guidance, motivation of both the child and the parents, and the rapport between the therapist and the patient are crucial for success [99]. EMG-BF is frequently used in clinical practice in pediatric pelvic floor units to provide visual feedback during PFM contraction, but they show both elevation and straining of PFM activity as increased values [102].

Transperineal and/or Transabdominal US-BF

Many physiotherapists adopt US imaging as a way of providing personalized rehabilitation. Three clinical categories for the use of US have been identified: for rehabilitation purposes, diagnostic purposes, and interventional US [103]. In the literature, the most common use of US by physiotherapists falls within real-time US imaging, which is used in various musculoskeletal problems, including sports medicine, orthopedics, respiratory health, and pelvic health. In the context of pelvic health, real-time US imaging is used to understand [104], predict [105], and manage urinary incontinence [103]. Additionally, it has been reported that US biofeedback may be helpful in PFMT training and effective in different populations [106].

In evaluating the morphology of the pelvic floor muscles using transperineal and transabdominal imaging approaches, US imaging is utilized to measure PFM contraction and determine the effect of increased IAP on the bladder [104]. Transabdominal US of the bladder and pelvic floor was first used by White to investigate women with stress urinary incontinence [107]. The transabdominal approach (in both sagittal and transverse planes) is a relatively noninvasive method that provides clinicians with new insights into certain components of PFM function and serves as a biofeedback source during PFMT. Transabdominal US is primarily used to evaluate the cranial movement of the pelvic floor by observing the movement of the bladder base as an indicator of PFM activity during voluntary PFM contraction. The technique has also been used to assess the amount of movement of the bladder base during various functional maneuvers that increase IAP, such as the Valsalva maneuver and lower limb functions [104]. Good intra-rater and inter-rater reliability (ICC, 0.81–0.88) has been reported for measuring bladder base displacement during PFM contraction (in both transverse and sagittal views) [108]. The transabdominal US method is relatively easier to learn compared to the transperineal approach, with simpler measurements and image interpretation, and placement of the transducer does not restrict lower limb movement. Providing PFMT with transabdominal BF is particularly important in specific populations where internal examination is not desired, such as children, adolescents, males, victims of sexual abuse, and certain ethnic groups, because transabdominal US is completely noninvasive (there is no need for the patient to undress). Due to its noninvasive nature, errors associated with low patient compliance and increased parental/patient anxiety seen with more invasive traditional methods can be minimized. Thus, this technique provides an alternative BF source for individuals who do not wish to undergo internal examination while learning PFM exercises [104]. Most studies on PFMT using US have been conducted with adults, and its use in pediatric pelvic health will guide future research [99].

(b) *Diaphragmatic Breathing*

The first and most important phase of PFMT is teaching diaphragmatic exercises. During inspiration, the diaphragm contracts and increases the volume of the thoracic cavity [109]. Additionally, the diaphragm contributes to core stabilization and postural control during voluntary limb movements [110, 111]. The stability of the spine, shoulder, and pelvic girdle is regulated by a central feedback mechanism prior to performing a postural task, independently of the diaphragm's respiratory activity [110].

The relationship between the PFMs and the diaphragm and their role in regulating IAP [112, 113] has been demonstrated by many studies [114–117]. Increased IAP periods occur during both inspiration and expiration. During inspiration, the diaphragm moves caudally with concentric contraction, causing the abdominal organs to displace downward, leading to an increase in IAP due to the simultaneous reflex coactivation of the transverse abdominis (TA) and PFM [112]. The flattening of the diaphragm dome leads to changes in the volume and shape of the thoracic cavity, causing cylindrical expansion of the thoracic wall in all directions. This requires the synchronized eccentric activity of all the muscles that make up the thoracic and abdominal walls [112]. With the eccentric activity of these muscles, the expansion of the thoracic, abdominal, and pelvic cavities is achieved [118]. During expiration, the diaphragm contracts eccentrically, arching upwards into the thoracic cavity. During forced expiration, the concentric contraction of the abdominal muscles reduces the volume of the abdominal cavity, increases IAP, and facilitates the upward displacement of the diaphragm. Additionally, during forced expiration, the PFMs, together with the anterolateral muscles, function like bellows, directing the increased IAP toward the diaphragm. It has been reported in the literature that the PFM contributes to the increase in IAP during breathing and forced expiratory maneuvers and responds to sudden increases in IAP through a precontraction reflex [11, 23, 114, 119–122].

Studies have reported that an abnormal breathing pattern may develop in patients with pelvic floor dysfunction [102, 122]. Additionally, restricted diaphragm movement can impair the coordination between the diaphragm, TA muscle, and PFMs during functional movement [9, 11, 123]. Along with PFMT, both breathing coordination and control of IAP should be applied in a combined manner. The superficial and deep abdominal muscles, diaphragm, and PFM form a muscular unit that promotes regular defecation and peristalsis. Exercises that stimulate and relax the abdominal muscles indirectly affect the pelvic floor. When these exercises are performed in conjunction with diaphragmatic breathing, they can lead to the contraction of the intestinal and rectal muscles, contributing to improvements in children with colorectal-anal problems (Fig. 27.6). The stimulation of colonic movements through diaphragmatic breathing has mechanical effects such as improved coordination of muscles, progression of feces, and increased abdominal muscle tone. Additionally, parasympathetic nervous system stimulation increases motility, while sympathetic nervous system stimulation reduces anxiety and increases endogenous serotonin levels [124].

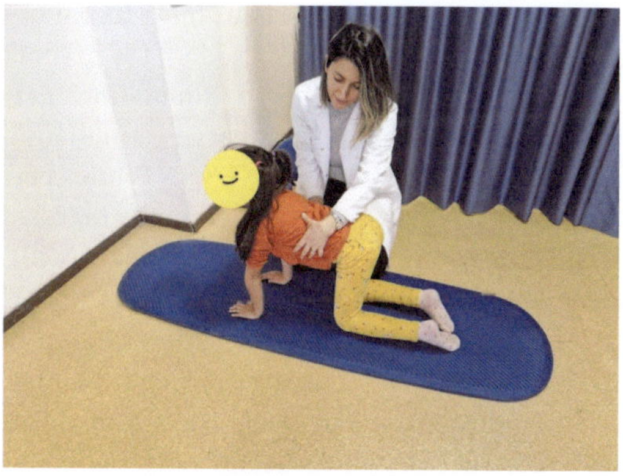

Fig. 27.6 Diaphragm exercises in the quadripedal position

(c) *Electrotherapy*

Electrotherapy has been used for the treatment of LUTD in both adults and children in recent years [125, 126]. Electrical currents that stimulate nerves or muscles are used for purposes such as pain relief, improving blood flow, relieving muscle spasms, promoting wound healing, muscle training, and strengthening [127, 128].

On the other hand, electrical currents can also affect sensory, motor, glandular, and secretory functions. Some chemical changes have been reported after electrical stimulation therapy, such as increased beta-adrenergic activity, decreased cholinergic activity, and changes in the availability of neurotransmitters (dopamine, serotonin, vasopressin, and nitric oxide) [129]. Electrical currents can reduce detrusor pressure and increase bladder capacity or compliance [45, 130–132]. Additionally, significant improvements were observed in two-thirds of children with slow-transit constipation treated with transcutaneous Electrical Stimulation (ES) applied to the abdominal region, including an increase in defecation frequency, reduction in fecal incontinence, and abdominal pain. It was also reported that in one-third of the children who improved, the clinical symptoms continued to improve for more than 2 years [133].

Neurostimulation or neuromodulation is a term that refers to the modulation of neuronal activity through electrical stimulation applied to nerve fibers. Sacral neuromodulation (SNM), developed by Tanagho, Schmidt, and Orvis in 1989, has become a successful third-line treatment option for overactive bladder [134]. There are two types of tibial nerve stimulation: percutaneous transcutaneous nerve stimulation (TNS) and transcutaneous TNS. While percutaneous TNS involves a minimally invasive procedure (a needle inserted near the nerve), transcutaneous TNS is a noninvasive procedure. The tibial nerve, which originates from the fourth and fifth lumbar nerves and the first, second, and third sacral nerves, is stimulated by TNS. In contrast to sacral nerve stimulation (SNS), TNS is less expensive and has no adverse effects [135, 136].

SNM has been used for various other disease processes, including interstitial cystitis, pelvic pain syndrome, and fecal incontinence. Although it has only been approved for adults, it has been used in pediatric patients since the early 2000s. Even 5-year-old children with both neurogenic and non-neurogenic bladder dysfunction and bowel-bladder dysfunction have benefited from SNM implantation [137]. Acutely, SNM regulates sensorimotor learning. Chronic SNM improves awareness of bladder emptying, the sensation of bladder filling, and urgency. The mechanism of action of neurostimulation on chronic constipation and fecal incontinence remains unclear. There are many different neurostimulation techniques [138]. Transcutaneous electrical nerve stimulation is a noninvasive and painless technique. Surface electrodes can be applied to the third sacral foramen, posterior tibial nerve, or invasively as percutaneous electrical nerve stimulation using needle electrodes in the same areas. Additionally, neurostimulation can be applied invasively by surgically placing electrodes in the sacral foramen [38]. The posterior tibial nerve consists of branches from the fourth and fifth lumbar and the first, second, and third sacral nerves. Stimulation of the nerve fibers at the level of the ankle inhibits the preganglionic neurons of the relevant branches. As a result, there is regulation in the afferent rectal sensory perception and the function of the rectal striated muscle. Clinically, this results in an increase in maximum resting and squeezing pressures [139]. A systematic review conducted in 2019 noted that there were few studies on transcutaneous and percutaneous electrical nerve stimulation in children with fecal incontinence and constipation. Despite the limited studies, it has been reported that neurostimulation increases the frequency of defecation and reduces abdominal pain. Additionally, it was observed that noninvasive techniques have no complications [138, 140].

Interferential (IF) electrical stimulation, which is a medium-frequency current, painlessly penetrates deep tissues with low skin resistance and has been used for over 20 years to strengthen the pelvic floor in patients with overactive bladder, urinary incontinence, and women [141].

Recently, the use of IF in the treatment of slow-transit constipation in children has also been reported [142]. IF currents are produced by the intersection of two different medium-frequency currents at 4000 Hz applied to the body using four surface electrodes. This creates an amplitude-modulated current in deep tissues such as the bladder or pelvic floor [143].

The possible mechanism of action of IF stimulation involves the activation of local sensory and motor nerves in the skin, spinal nerves (sensory and motor T9-L2), sympathetic and parasympathetic nerves leading to the intestines, enteric neurons, pacemaker cells (Cajal's interstitial cells), or smooth muscle cells in the intestinal wall [142]. It has been reported that IF current is an effective and safe option for managing overactive bladder and urinary incontinence issues in children [144]. In the literature, IF stimulation has been used to treat chronic treatment-resistant constipation and soiling in children [142]. It has been indicated that IF stimulation, in conjunction with diaphragmatic exercises, is effective in children with chronic constipation and bowel-bladder dysfunction [145].

(d) *Exercise*

The positive effects of physical activity on children have long been recognized. It has been reported that physical activity contributes to a reduction in the risk of obesity and depression in children, improvement in lung function, reduction in asthma symptoms, enhancement of mental health, and maintenance of glycemic control [146]. Physical inactivity can lead to pelvic floor dysfunctions and urinary incontinence, while individuals with dysfunction may also restrict their physical activity [147, 148]. Therefore, although urinary incontinence itself may not cause significant morbidity or mortality, it can lead to physical inactivity [149].

A sedentary lifestyle is also an independent risk factor for various diseases and conditions, such as high blood pressure, coronary heart disease, type 2 diabetes mellitus, obesity, colon and breast cancer, osteoporosis, depression, and anxiety [150]. Further, Inal et al. [20] showed that children with nocturnal enuresis had abnormal posture and balance compared with their healthy peers. Therefore, determining the level of physical activity in children with urinary incontinence and making the necessary recommendations will also be important for potential pediatric or adolescent comorbidities in the future. Physical activity has also been shown to be beneficial for colonic motility and to reduce the development of constipation in children [38, 151]. Muddasani et al. [83] reported that exercise training, combined with manual techniques and PFMT, reduced the frequency of fecal incontinence in children with pelvic floor dyssynergia. Brands et al. reported [152] that yoga training reduced abdominal pain and pain frequency in children with irritable bowel syndrome. In another study, it was reported that the addition of game-based core stabilization exercises to the biofeedback program applied to children aged 6–13 years with non-neuropathic bladder dysfunction was superior to the biofeedback program alone or game-based core exercises alone in improving uroflowmetry results and symptoms [153]. In a study, children with dysfunctional voiding were given PFMT together with behavioral therapy. It was reported that PFMT integrated with functional exercises and a Swiss ball decreased the frequency of urinary incontinence, PVR, and severity of constipation in children with DV and was a safe and effective therapeutic method [154]. A review of the literature indicates that there are very few studies involving exercise training in the treatment of pediatric colorectal problems. Therefore, there is a need for randomized controlled trials in the pediatric population (Figs. 27.7 and 27.8).

(e) *Manual Therapy*

Classical massage is a manual technique applied to the surfaces of soft tissues such as skin, fascia, muscles, and ligaments. The general aim of classical massage is to increase circulation, promote relaxation, and reduce muscle tension. Additionally, classical massage induces sedative effects by increasing parasympathetic activity [155]. The goal of abdominal classical

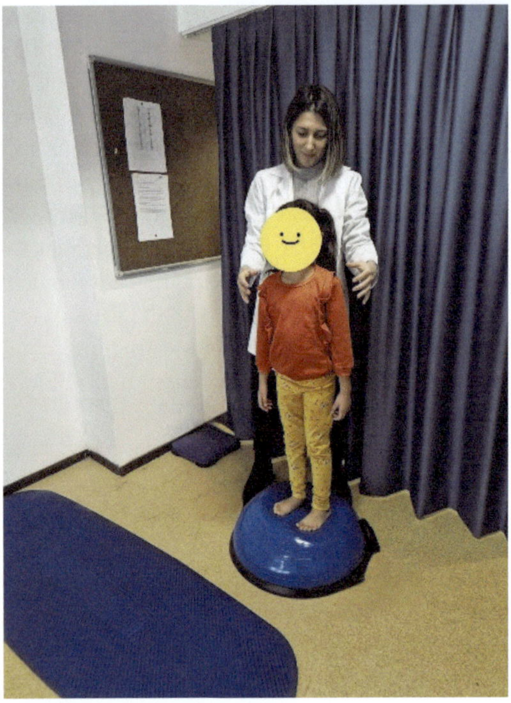

Fig. 27.7 Balance training-1

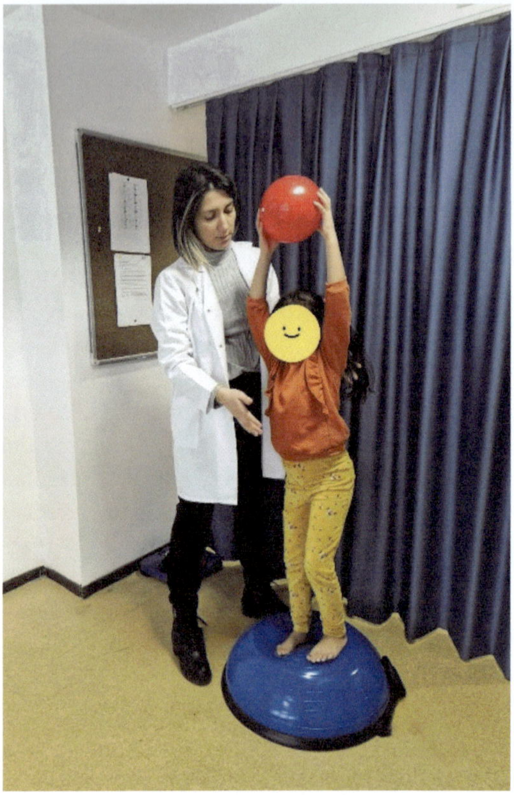

Fig. 27.8 Balance training-2

massage is to enhance colonic and rectal motility. The physiotherapist should perform the massage with slow circular movements from the ascending colon toward the sigmoid colon. In a study conducted by Silva et al. [124], children with constipation who received isometric abdominal muscle contractions, diaphragmatic breathing exercises, and classical abdominal massage for 6 weeks showed greater improvement in constipation compared to the group using only medication.

Connective tissue massage is a reflex therapy that stimulates the autonomic nerve endings in the skin through pulling forces applied to the connective tissue. The mechanism of action of connective tissue massage is thought to establish a balance between the sympathetic and parasympathetic divisions of the autonomic nervous system via segmental or suprasegmental cutaneo-visceral reflexes [155]. Orhan et al. [156] divided children with cerebral palsy and constipation into three groups: the first group received connective tissue massage to the sacral, lumbar, lower thoracic, scapular, and inter-scapular areas; the second group underwent kinesiotaping to the sacrum and lower abdominal area; and the third group served as the control group. At the end of this study, it was shown that the groups receiving connective tissue massage and kinesiotaping had a greater reduction in constipation complaints.

(f) *Sensory Integration*

The sensory profile is a neurological process that organizes the sensations coming from a person's body and the environment, enabling effective use of the body within the environment. "Sensory processing" (SP) is a broad term that refers to the ability of the CNS to interpret sensory information [157]. Jean Ayres compared sensory processing disorder to a neurological "traffic jam" that prevents certain areas of the brain from receiving the information needed to correctly interpret sensory data [158].

Interruptions in sensory processing and changes in neurological thresholds to sensory inputs can lead to hypersensitivity or hyposensitivity [159]. Individuals with sensory hypersensitivity exhibit a behavioral pattern characterized by a tendency to be overwhelmed by various external factors [160].

According to Dunn's sensory processing framework, children display behaviors in four sensory processing models: sensitivity (increased awareness of sensory stimuli); avoidance (actively withdrawing from sensory stimuli); seeking (intense interest in sensory stimuli); and registration (insufficient or delayed response to sensory stimuli). Sensory processing differences manifest across systems (e.g., tactile, auditory) and reflect a community of behaviors that mirror underlying neurological thresholds and self-regulation strategies [161]. Previous research has linked sensory sensitivity to toileting difficulties [161–163]. For instance, it has been shown that children with chronic constipation possess underlying sensory characteristics (patterns of sensory processing) that contribute to their difficulties with toilet behavior [164]. When the findings are combined, they provide a rationale for how sensory profiles contribute to the development of chronic constipation: children with low sensitivity may not realize they need to have a bowel movement, while children with high sensitivity may avoid the toilet, resulting in higher levels of fecal retention [164]. When examining specific sensory modalities that may be predictive of chronic constipation, two factors emerged: oral processing and attention. Oral processing presented as the most significant factor in predicting toileting behavior overresponsiveness. More recently, research has suggested a bidirectional association between fussy eating and functional constipation was reported in preschool children [165]. These findings point to a vicious cycle in which a child's gastrointestinal problems and problematic eating behavior mutually affect each other, and it may be that there are underlying factors that contribute to the cooccurrence of such behaviors. The second modality that emerged as a predictor of toilet behavior was attention. However, this finding was less robust and was only associated with low sensitivity in toilet behavior (not hypersensitivity). Children who experienced more difficulties with attention tended to exhibit more characteristics of low sensitivity in toilet behavior (e.g., not feeling the urge to defecate, not noticing bowel movements). Attention difficulties have been previously identified as significantly higher in children with "soiling difficulties." However, attention has been studied from a psychological perspective rather than in terms of sensory processing. As a modality, attention skills are multifaceted and can vary depending on the sensory system (vision, hearing, touch, taste, smell) [166]. For instance, children who are highly attentive to visual inputs may be less attentive to auditory inputs. In addition to the five basic senses, attention can also affect lesser-known senses like proprioception (body awareness), vestibular input (movement), and interoception (the ability to register, understand, and feel sensations within the body) [167].

Children with incontinence problems appear different from those without. Common symptoms mentioned in the literature include urinary urgency, abnormal posture, bedwetting at night, and fecal incontinence [168]. These children tend to exhibit higher rates of behavioral or psychological problems such as anxiety, attention deficit/hyperactivity disorder (ADHD), oppositional defiant behavior, or conduct disorders compared to their continent peers [169]. Children with monosymptomatic nocturnal enuresis also display higher rates of behavioral issues, such as conduct disorders [169]. Enuretic children also seem to be at greater risk for behavioral or emotional problems [170].

The literature indicates a relationship between toilet skill issues and sensory processing dysfunctions, and it has been noted that sensory integration therapy provides benefits for toilet skill issues in addition to the benefits mentioned in the literature [171]. In the 1970s, Jean Ayres introduced the term "sensory integration therapy" (SIT). Information processing is the integration of the senses. The brain must selectively enhance, inhibit, compare, and associate sensory information in a fluid, continuously changing, or integrated manner. The SIT approach supports a child's normal development by enhancing their ability to receive and process sensory data [172].

It is a theory and neurological procedure that enables a person to organize and produce structured action by analyzing, incorporating, and using the spatial-temporal components from the environment. It suggests that for children to learn, they must be able to interpret sensory input from their surroundings, internalize these impulses throughout the CNS, and use this information to produce organized behavior [173]. The integration of the neuromuscular system is essential for maintaining balance and adequate elimination function (Fig. 27.9). It is hypothesized that difficulties in processing and integrating sensory information may be a contributing factor to the development of some problematic behaviors in children [174]. Sensory overresponsivity is also documented to be associated with certain gastrointestinal dysfunctions [175]. Findings indicated that children with any type of gastrointestinal problem, including chronic constipation, had higher levels of sensory overresponsivity than children without such problems. Using logistic regression analyses, researchers found that sensory overresponsivity significantly contributed to the prediction of constipation, abdominal pain, nausea, and bloating [175].

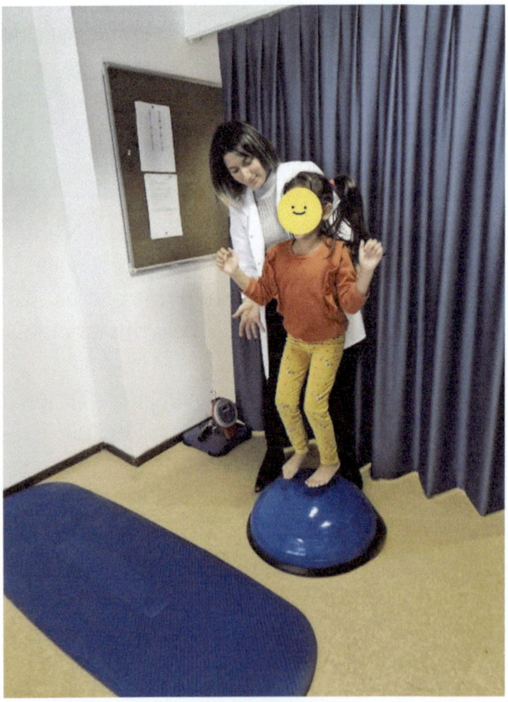

Fig. 27.9 Sensory integration exercise example

Children often exhibit sensory disorders, negative or avoidant behaviors, reduced body awareness, poor nutrition, insufficient fluid intake, and additional disorders such as nonfunctioning or hypertonic PFMs. Due to the multifactorial nature of the condition, some children may not respond to standard medical treatment alone and may benefit from non-pharmacological therapies in the treatment of functional constipation and fecal incontinence. Pelvic physiotherapy specifically targets the muscular chains of the PFM and sensory integration [11, 21]. According to the Dutch Pelvic Physiotherapy Protocol, pelvic physiotherapy consists of education and patient-centered instruction, similar to standard medical care, as well as specific physiotherapy interventions. Specific physiotherapy interventions include (i) balance and stability training to maintain effective toilet posture, (ii) locomotor exercises to learn proper abdominal breathing and effective contraction and relaxation of muscles, all prerequisites for normal defecation, (iii) sensory integration training to achieve body awareness, the sensation of a full bowel, and the urge to defecate, and (iv) a musculoskeletal approach involving awareness, relaxation, and proper functioning of the abdominal and PFM. Rectal balloon training and EMG-BF are used only in cases of dysfunctional PFMs [95].

(g) *Dynamic Neuromuscular Stabilization Training*

Dynamic neuromuscular stabilization (DNS) is a manual and rehabilitative approach developed by Professor Pavel Kolar, aimed at optimizing the movement system based on the scientific principles of developmental kinesiology [176]. Today, DNS is successfully used in the rehabilitation of various neurological, musculoskeletal, pediatric, and sports injury cases [177–180]. Great emphasis is placed on the correct activation of the diaphragm, breathing patterns, and core stability before any purposeful movement [181]. Around 6 months of age, abdominal breathing is coordinated with chest breathing, and the diaphragm fully performs its dual function as both a respiratory and postural stabilization muscle. This foundation of developmental kinesiology, on which DNS is based, uses the theory that every human has a genetically predetermined motor development model, and as the central nervous system matures from the early stages of life, this kinesiological development continues to take place. From the DNS perspective, a lack of motor development in infancy can lead to neuromuscular disorders that will manifest as biomechanical deficiencies later in life. The result of this assumption is that the movement correction process must begin with the correction of neuromuscular disorders. The primary reason for DNS's effectiveness may be due to the practitioner's ability to absorb the chest during breathing, resulting in the diaphragm's eccentric contraction and downward descent, which increases IAP. Additionally, DNS utilizes the subconscious and synkinetic activation of the deep core muscles (diaphragm, TA, multifidus, and pelvic floor) responsible for optimal IAP and associated spinal stability, along with the global muscles. The coactivation (timing, synergy) between the diaphragm, abdominal muscles (particularly the TA), and pelvic floor is crucial during urination and defecation. A deficiency in coactivation can result in paradoxical contraction of the pelvic floor during defecation and urination [182].

It has been shown that DNS activates the anterior cingulate cortex, which may be related to subcortical processing, learning, and memory, as well as core stabilization and respiratory control. DNS exercises modulate core muscle activation and the learning process by activating both cortical areas and the subcortical cerebellum-basal ganglia-thalamus-cingulate cortex network. Therefore, it is suggested that DNS exercises can be applied for subcortical motor relearning in patients with hemiplegia and cerebral palsy, whose cortical network is impaired but whose subcortical network is relatively preserved [181]. Imaging studies provide evidence that the prefrontal cortex and other supraspinal regions (periaqueductal gray matter, insula, thalamus, hypothalamus, anterior cingulate cortex) are metabolically active during bladder filling and emptying. It is assumed that these processes are similar in children. Given their greater capacity for neuroplasticity, it is possible that children can change more easily than adults. According to current understanding, the pontine micturition center is active during both the storage and emptying phases. It is actively inhibited during storage and is also activated by input from the periaqueductal gray matter [54]. Therefore, we hypothesize that IAP directed to the pelvic cavity through DNS exercises, which contributes to stabilization, may also have a controlled effect on the bladder, facilitating complete bladder emptying (Fig. 27.10).

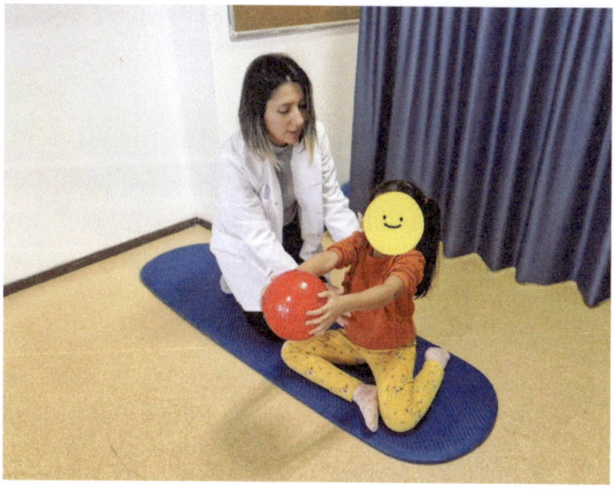

Fig. 27.10 Stabilization exercise in sitting position according to the principles of DNS

(h) *Therapeutic Motor Control Interventions*

The aim of motor control interventions in childhood Bladder and Bowel Dysfunction (BBD) is to support toilet training by practicing a stabilized and relaxed posture on the toilet and adequate straining to defecate, to increase awareness of abdominal sensations as the urge to urinate or defecate, to increase awareness of the muscles (abdominal and PFM) to avoid DV or dyssynergic defecation, to achieve continence, and to prevent constipation and urinary tract infections. Varying methods, techniques, and materials (appropriate for the age and complaints) can be used [86].

Therapeutic motor control interventions include the following:

1. Motor control exercises and functional training (training the body for the normal activities performed in daily life), such as core stability and balance training, to maintain an adequate posture on the toilet.
2. Sensory processing techniques, such as filtering, organizing, and integrating sensory information to become aware of the urge to urinate and defecate.
3. Relaxation and breathing exercises can be used to learn to relax, to teach adequate abdominal breathing and straining while defecating, which are all prerequisites for a normal micturition and defecation, and to stay continent.
4. Pelvic floor and abdominal muscle training (awareness, relaxation, and functional training).

27.5.1.2.2 Clean Intermittent Catheterization

Children with an underactive bladder can have such an over-distended bladder that spontaneously urinating without straining is no longer possible. When these children do not have sufficient results with conservative treatment, they will benefit from catheterization. Children aged 6 years and older can learn how to self-catheterize well. This is recommended because self-catheterization is more acceptable and makes the child less dependent. Support in this process is very important to let the treatment integrate well into daily life. Level of evidence: Clean intermittent catheterization is recommended for children with significant PVR and urinary retention. It shows effectiveness, but Randomized Controlled Trials (RCTs) in neurologically normal children are lacking [80].

27.5.1.2.3 Alarm Therapy

Alarm therapy has been used to treat pediatric nocturnal enuresis for decades. The alarm device consists of a moisture detector connected to a sound system that triggers a warning signal when urine is detected. Alarm therapy is considered the first-line treatment for enuresis, with long-term improvement rates nearing 50% [183]. Numerous studies have demonstrated that alarm therapy is highly effective in terms of achieving dryness, providing a better treatment response, and having a lower recurrence rate compared to other treatment methods [183–185].

Alarm therapy requires collaboration between parents and children with appropriate training programs, which enhances compliance and success rates [185]. It has been shown that alarm therapy has a better response rate in proactive parents compared to desmopressin [186]. However, families and children undergoing alarm therapy have been reported to require more support from healthcare professionals to adhere to the treatment compared to those receiving desmopressin therapy [187].

The goal of alarm therapy is to wake the child to urinate before they wet the bed or to prevent them from emptying their bladder during sleep. However, waking up to urinate is not the only effect of alarm therapy; it has also been found that using alarm therapy in children increases bladder capacity throughout the night [188].

If alarm therapy is decided upon, the treatment duration should be 2–3 months or until the child remains dry for 14 consecutive nights. However, the most effective duration of alarm intervention is expected to be continuous therapy for 16–20 weeks. Due to the potential for sleep deprivation from repeated alarms, a single alarm per night is sufficient. Despite its high effectiveness, selecting alarm therapy is critical, as it is not easy to find the right families for this option and to provide them with comprehensive information. Frustration and withdrawal between parents and children are common [189]. After 10–12 weeks of treatment, success rates have been observed to range between 50% and 80%, with recurrence occurring in 12–30% of cases within the first 6 months following treatment. However, in cases of recurrence, a second course of alarm therapy may yield a good response [80].

27.5.2 Alternative Methods (Acupuncture, Kinesiotaping)

Many studies have reported that kinesiotaping (KT) is an effective method for increasing blood and lymph flow in local and peripheral areas, enhancing proprioceptive sensation, increasing muscle strength, alleviating pain, and improving joint range of motion [190, 191]. It has been indicated that KT can be used as an effective complementary physiotherapy approach in children with urinary incontinence [192].

It is believed that acupuncture therapy has developed over thousands of years in China. Acupuncture aims to restore internal homeostasis through the stimulation of specific acupuncture points using techniques such as laser acupuncture, acupressure, and electroacupuncture [193]. It has been applied in various pelvic floor disorders (PFDs) such as overactive bladder, fecal incontinence, hypoactive sexual desire disorder, and chronic pelvic pain, with reports of its effectiveness [194].

There are very few studies on the application of acupuncture for PFDs in children. The application of acupuncture in children has been shown to be safe when performed by trained practitioners. Common minor side effects and rare serious injuries have also been reported in pediatric acupuncture [195]. Electroacupuncture treatment has been shown to reduce residual urine volume in pediatric patients experiencing chronic urinary retention after lumbar sacral surgery [196]. It has been suggested that laser acupuncture could be considered a noninvasive, painless, and alternative treatment for children with functional chronic constipation [197].

27.5.3 Treatment of Accompanying Psychological Disorders

Counseling is an active process that involves both parents and the child. It means providing support and guidance in resolving personal, social, and psychological challenges. Treatment includes methods such as cognitive-behavioral therapy, family therapy, and psychodynamic therapy [60].

27.5.4 Pharmacological Treatment

Antimuscarinics, alpha-blockers, desmopressin, and laxatives are used as pharmacological treatments for bladder and bowel dysfunction in children. Antimuscarinics have remained the mainstay of treatment in children with Overactive Bladder (OAB) and Urinary Incontinence (UI) when standard urotherapy and neuromodulation are unable to help the child achieve continence and/or normal elimination habits. This is commonly the case when children present with extreme urgency and severe incontinence. Urotherapy should be continued during pharmacotherapy [82].

The use of α-adrenergic antagonists in children with non-neurogenic bladder dysfunction is still considered "off-label." Theoretically, α-blockers facilitate bladder emptying by blocking α-adrenergic receptors at the bladder neck, reducing bladder outlet resistance associated with high voiding pressure, thus avoiding obstruction-related detrusor overactivity [82].

Desmopressin is a synthetic analogue of the natural antidiuretic hormone arginine vasopressin. Over the years, it has been clinically used to manage nocturnal polyuria in children with enuresis. Lee et al. evaluated the efficacy of desmopressin monotherapy versus desmopressin combined with oxybutynin (anticholinergic) and versus imipramine (tricyclic antidepressant) monotherapy in children with enuresis (5–15 years). The authors concluded that the efficacy of combination therapy was higher in comparison with both monotherapies [198]. Laxatives are frequently used in children with constipation and functional retention fecal incontinence (FI). In chronic constipation, osmotic laxatives are recommended as a first-line treatment because they help with soft stool formation and facilitate the passage of bowel movements by improving intestinal motility. However, although laxatives can reduce fecal leakage into underwear by emptying the rectum, their use is not recommended. While the use of laxatives is suggested in cases of constipation and functional retention fecal incontinence, it is not recommended in cases of non-retentive fecal incontinence. This is because laxatives cause softer stools, which can lead to fecal incontinence in this group of children [60, 92, 199].

27.6 Conclusion

Bladder and bowel dysfunctions can lead to significant difficulties in children's daily life activities and social relationships. Conditions such as constipation, fecal incontinence, and nocturnal enuresis, in particular, can place a serious psychosocial burden on both children and their families. The evaluation and treatment processes related to the pediatric pelvic floor should be customized according to the developmental needs of children. Additionally, urological and anorectal problems experienced during childhood can pave the way for serious health problems in later life if not addressed early. Conditions such as constipation, fecal incontinence, and nocturnal enuresis can negatively affect the development of PFMs, leading to chronic issues in adulthood such as pelvic organ prolapse, stress urinary incontinence, and sexual dysfunction. Therefore, investments in pelvic floor health during childhood are of great importance in preventing pelvic floor disorders in later life. For the effective management of pelvic floor dysfunctions, physiotherapists should specialize in pediatric pelvic floor health and develop holistic and individualized treatment plans by considering the psychological, social, and physical development of the child.

References

1. Chase J, Schrale L. Childhood incontinence and pelvic floor muscle function: can we learn from adult research? J Pediatr Urol. 2017;13(1):94–101.
2. Martínez-Gómez M, Corona-Quintanilla DL, Cruz-Gómez Y, Zempoalteca R, Rodríguez-Antolín J, Castelán F. The role of pelvic and perineal muscles in reproductive and excretory functions. In: Applications of EMG in clinical and sports medicine; 2012.
3. Eickmeyer SM. Anatomy and physiology of the pelvic floor. Phys Med Rehabil Clin N Am. 2017;28(3):455–60.
4. Wallace SL, Miller LD, Mishra K. Pelvic floor physical therapy in the treatment of pelvic floor dysfunction in women. Curr Opin Obstet Gynecol. 2019;31(6):485–93.
5. Gerber RJ, Wilks T, Erdie-Lalena C. Developmental milestones: motor development. Pediatr Rev. 2010;31(7):267–76. quiz 77.
6. Kobesova A, Kolar P. Developmental kinesiology: three levels of motor control in the assessment and treatment of the motor system. J Bodyw Mov Ther. 2014;18(1):23–33.
7. Hodges P. Lumbopelvic stability: a functional model of the biomechanics and motor control. In: Therapeutic exercise for lumbopelvic stabilization; 2004. p. 13–28.
8. Falla D, Rainoldi A, Merletti R, Jull G. Spatio-temporal evaluation of neck muscle activation during postural perturbations in healthy subjects. J Electromyogr Kinesiol. 2004;14(4):463–74.
9. Hodges PW, Gandevia SC. Changes in intra-abdominal pressure during postural and respiratory activation of the human diaphragm. J Appl Physiol. 2000;89:967.
10. Hodges PW, Eriksson AM, Shirley D, Gandevia SC. Intra-abdominal pressure increases stiffness of the lumbar spine. J Biomech. 2005;38(9):1873–80.
11. Hodges PW, Sapsford R, Pengel LH. Postural and respiratory functions of the pelvic floor muscles. Neurourol Urodyn. 2007;26(3):362–71.
12. Kolář P, Neuwirth J, Šanda J, Suchanek V, Svata Z, Volejnik J, et al. Analysis of diaphragm movement during tidal breathing and during its activation while breath holding using MRI synchronized with spirometry. Physiol Res 2009;58(3).
13. Adde L, Rygg M, Lossius K, Oberg GK, Støen R. General movement assessment: predicting cerebral palsy in clinical practise. Early Hum Dev. 2007;83(1):13–8.
14. Mantilla CB, Fahim MA, Brandenburg JE, Sieck GC. Functional development of respiratory muscles. In: Fetal and neonatal physiology, 2-Volume Set. Elsevier; 2017. p. 692–705. e3.
15. Kolar P, Kobesova A. 2. A. 2.Postural–locomotion function in the diagnosis and treatment of movement disorders. Clin Chiropractic. 2010;13(1):58–68.
16. Kolar P, Sulc J, Kyncl M, Sanda J, Cakrt O, Andel R, et al. Postural function of the diaphragm in persons with and without chronic low back pain. J Orthop Sports Phys Ther. 2012;42(4):352–62.
17. Bross S, Honeck P, Kwon ST, Badawi JK, Trojan L, Alken P. Correlation between motor function and lower urinary tract dysfunction in patients with infantile cerebral palsy. Neurourol Urodyn. 2007;26(2):222–7.
18. Burger M, Louw QA. The predictive validity of general movements--a systematic review. Eur J Paediatr Neurol. 2009;13(5):408–20.
19. Sharma K, Yadav A. Dynamic neuromuscular stabilization-a narrative. Int J Health Sci Res. 2020;10(9):221–31.

20. Inal B, Ozengin N, Bakar Y, Ankaralı H, Ozturk Y. Examination of posture and balance in children with primary monosymptomatic nocturnal enuresis. J Pediatr Rehabil Med. 2023;16(3):529–37.
21. Chase JW, Stillman BC, Gibb SM, Clarke MC, Robertson VJ, Catto-Smith AG, et al. Trunk strength and mobility changes in children with slow transit constipation. J Gastroenterol Hepatol. 2009;24(12):1876–84.
22. Delancey JO, Kane Low L, Miller JM, Patel DA, Tumbarello JA. Graphic integration of causal factors of pelvic floor disorders: an integrated life span model. Am J Obstet Gynecol. 2008;199(6):610.e1–5.
23. Bo K, Berghmans B, Morkved S, Kampen MV. Evidence-based physical therapy for the pelvic floor bridging science and clinical practice 2014.
24. van Engelenburg-van Lonkhuyzen ML, Bols EM, Benninga MA, Verwijs WA, de Bie RA. Bladder and bowel dysfunctions in 1748 children referred to pelvic physiotherapy: clinical characteristics and locomotor problems in primary, secondary, and tertiary healthcare settings. Eur J Pediatr. 2017;176(2):207–16.
25. Tarhan H, Çakmak Ö, Akarken İ, Ekin RG, Ün S, Uzelli D, et al. Toilet training age and influencing factors: a multicenter study. Turk J Pediatr. 2015;57(2):172–6.
26. Baird DC, Bybel M, Kowalski AW. Toilet training: common questions and answers. Am Fam Physician. 2019;100(8):468–74.
27. Koc I, Camurdan AD, Beyazova U, Ilhan MN, Sahin F. Toilet training in Turkey: the factors that affect timing and duration in different sociocultural groups. Child Care Health Dev. 2008;34(4):475–81.
28. de Carvalho Mrad FC, da Silva ME, Moreira Lima E, Bessa AL, de Bessa JJ, Netto JMB, et al. Toilet training methods in children with normal neuropsychomotor development: a systematic review. J Pediatr Urol. 2021;17(5):635–43.
29. Hellström AL, Sillén U. Early potty training advantageous in bladder dysfunction. Decreases the risk of urinary infection. Lakartidningen. 2001;98(28–29):3216–9.
30. Li X, Wen JG, Xie H, Wu XD, Shen T, Yang XQ, et al. Delayed in toilet training association with pediatric lower urinary tract dysfunction: a systematic review and meta-analysis. J Pediatr Urol. 2020;16(3):352.e1–.e8.
31. Barone JG, Jasutkar N, Schneider D. Later toilet training is associated with urge incontinence in children. J Pediatr Urol. 2009;5(6):458–61.
32. Bakker E, Wyndaele JJ. Changes in the toilet training of children during the last 60 years: the cause of an increase in lower urinary tract dysfunction? BJU Int. 2000;86(3):248–52.
33. Hodges SJ, Richards KA, Gorbachinsky I, Krane LS. The association of age of toilet training and dysfunctional voiding. Res Rep Urol. 2014;6:127–30.
34. Austin PF, Bauer SB, Bower W, Chase J, Franco I, Hoebeke P, et al. The standardization of terminology of lower urinary tract function in children and adolescents: update report from the standardization committee of the International Children's Continence Society. Neurourol Urodyn. 2016;35(4):471–81.
35. Hyams JS, Di Lorenzo C, Saps M, Shulman RJ, Staiano A, van Tilburg M. Functional disorders: children and adolescents. Gastroenterology. 2016;150(6):1456–1468.e2.
36. Mulhem E, Khondoker F, Kandiah S. Constipation in children and adolescents: evaluation and treatment. Am Fam Physician. 2022;105(5):469–78.
37. Bø K, Mørkved S, Frawley H, Sherburn M. Evidence for benefit of transversus abdominis training alone or in combination with pelvic floor muscle training to treat female urinary incontinence: a systematic review. Neurourol Urodyn. 2009;28(5):368–73.
38. Nieuwhof-Leppink AJ, Hussong J, Chase J, Larsson J, Renson C, Hoebeke P, et al. Definitions, indications and practice of urotherapy in children and adolescents: – a standardization document of the International Children's Continence Society (ICCS). J Pediatr Urol. 2021;17(2):172–81.
39. Frawley H, Shelly B, Morin M, Bernard S, Bø K, Digesu GA, et al. An International Continence Society (ICS) report on the terminology for pelvic floor muscle assessment. Neurourol Urodyn. 2021;40(5):1217–60.
40. Rentea RM, St Peter SD. Pediatric rectal prolapse. Clin Colon Rectal Surg. 2018;31(2):108–16.
41. Raju R, Linder BJ. Evaluation and management of pelvic organ prolapse. Mayo Clin Proc. 2021;96(12):3122–9.
42. Rao SSC. Digital rectal examination: an invaluable clinical tool. Gastro Hep Adv. 2024;3(5):592–3.
43. Orenstein SR, Wald A. Pediatric rectal exam: why, when, and how. Curr Gastroenterol Rep. 2016;18(1):4.
44. Worman RS, Stafford RE, Cowley D, Prudencio CB, Hodges PW. Evidence for increased tone or overactivity of pelvic floor muscles in pelvic health conditions: a systematic review. Am J Obstet Gynecol. 2023;228(6):657–74.e91.
45. Sollini ML, Capitanucci ML, Foti C, Nocentini U, Castelli E, Mosiello G. Home pelvic floor exercises in children with non-neurogenic lower urinary tract symptoms: is fitball an alternative to classic exercises? Neurourol Urodyn. 2023;42(1):146–52.
46. Oleksy Ł, Wojciechowska M, Mika A, Antos E, Bylina D, Kielnar R, et al. Normative values for Glazer protocol in the evaluation of pelvic floor muscle bioelectrical activity. Medicine (Baltimore). 2020;99(5):e19060.
47. Nieuwhof-Leppink AJ, van Geen FJ, van de Putte EM, Schoenmakers M, de Jong T, Schappin R. Pelvic floor rehabilitation in children with functional LUTD: does it improve outcome? J Pediatr Urol. 2019;15(5):530.e1–.e8.

48. Rao SS. Pathophysiology of adult fecal incontinence. Gastroenterology. 2004;126(1 Suppl 1):S14–22.
49. Rosier P, Schaefer W, Lose G, Goldman HB, Guralnick M, Eustice S, et al. International Continence Society Good Urodynamic Practices and terms 2016: urodynamics, uroflowmetry, cystometry, and pressure-flow study. Neurourol Urodyn. 2017;36(5):1243–60.
50. Wen JG, Djurhuus JC, Rosier P, Bauer SB. ICS educational module: pressure flow study in children. Neurourol Urodyn. 2018;37(8):2311–4.
51. de Jong TP, Klijn AJ. Urodynamic studies in pediatric urology. Nat Rev Urol. 2009;6(11):585–94.
52. Lee TH, Bharucha AE. How to perform and interpret a high-resolution anorectal manometry test. J Neurogastroenterol Motil. 2016;22(1):46–59.
53. Frye J, SSC R. Anorectal manometry: when, how to perform and interpret, and is it useful? Am J Gastroenterol. 2024;119(8):1449–55.
54. Franco I, Austin P, Bauer S, von Gontard A, Homsy Y. Pediatric incontinence: evaluation and clinical management. Wiley; 2015.
55. Rao SS, Patcharatrakul T. Diagnosis and treatment of dyssynergic defecation. J Neurogastroenterol Motil. 2016;22(3):423–35.
56. Rajindrajith S, Devanarayana NM, Benninga MA. Review article: faecal incontinence in children: epidemiology, pathophysiology, clinical evaluation and management. Aliment Pharmacol Ther. 2013;37(1):37–48.
57. Chase J, Bower W, Gibb S, Schaeffer A, von Gontard A. Diagnostic scores, questionnaires, quality of life, and outcome measures in pediatric continence: a review of available tools from the International Children's Continence Society. J Pediatr Urol. 2018;14(2):98–107.
58. Hoebeke P, Bower W, Combs A, De Jong T, Yang S. Diagnostic evaluation of children with daytime incontinence. J Urol. 2010;183(2):699–703.
59. Joensson IM, Siggaard C, Rittig S, Hagstroem S, Djurhuus JC. Transabdominal ultrasound of rectum as a diagnostic tool in childhood constipation. J Urol. 2008;179(5):1997–2002.
60. Koppen IJ, von Gontard A, Chase J, Cooper CS, Rittig CS, Bauer SB, et al. Management of functional nonretentive fecal incontinence in children: Recommendations from the International Children's Continence Society. J Pediatr Urol. 2016;12(1):56–64.
61. Burgers RE, Mugie SM, Chase J, Cooper CS, von Gontard A, Rittig CS, et al. Management of functional constipation in children with lower urinary tract symptoms: report from the Standardization Committee of the International Children's Continence Society. J Urol. 2013;190(1):29–36.
62. Nurko S, Zimmerman LA. Evaluation and treatment of constipation in children and adolescents. Am Fam Physician. 2014;90(2):82–90.
63. Pavione Rodrigues Pereira R, Nascimento Fagundes S, Surry Lebl A, Azevedo Soster L, Machado MG, Koch VH, et al. Children with nocturnal enuresis have posture and balance disorders. J Pediatr Urol. 2016;12(4):216.e1–6.
64. Adib N, Davies K, Grahame R, Woo P, Murray KJ. Joint hypermobility syndrome in childhood. A not so benign multisystem disorder? Rheumatology (Oxford). 2005;44(6):744–50.
65. van Engelenburg-van Lonkhuyzen ML, Bols EM, Benninga MA, Verwijs WA, Bluijssen NM, de Bie RA. The effect of pelvic physiotherapy on reduction of functional constipation in children: design of a multicentre randomised controlled trial. BMC Pediatr. 2013;13:112.
66. Lane SJ, Mailloux Z, Schoen S, Bundy A, May-Benson TA, Parham LD, et al. Neural foundations of ayres sensory integration(®). Brain Sci. 2019;9(7):153.
67. Beaudry-Bellefeuille I, Ramos-Polo E. Improving participation in toileting routines in a child with functional constipation: a case study using the integrated sensory toileting® approach. Occup Ther Health Care. 2024;39(3):685–96.
68. Beaudry-Bellefeuille I, Lane SJ, Lane AE. Sensory integration concerns in children with functional defecation disorders: a scoping review. Am J Occup Ther. 2019;73(3):7303205050p1-p13.
69. Beaudry-Bellefeuille I, Booth D, Lane SJ. Defecation-specific behavior in children with functional defecation issues: a systematic review. Perm J. 2017;21:17–047.
70. Camarata S, Miller LJ, Wallace MT. Evaluating sensory integration/sensory processing treatment: issues and analysis. Front Integr Neurosci. 2020;14:556660.
71. Bower WF, Sit FK, Bluyssen N, Wong EM, Yeung CK. PinQ: a valid, reliable and reproducible quality-of-life measure in children with bladder dysfunction. J Pediatr Urol. 2006;2(3):185–9.
72. Landgraf JM. Precision and sensitivity of the short-form pediatric enuresis module to assess quality of life (PEMQOL). J Pediatr Urol. 2007;3(2):109–17.
73. Gamarra ACQ, Carvalho MA, Machado NC. Pediatric functional constipation questionnaire-parent report (PedFCQuest-PR): development and validation. J Pediatr (Rio J). 2022;98(1):46–52.
74. Mathias AL, Tannuri AC, Ferreira MA, Santos MM, Tannuri U. [Validation of questionnaires to assess quality of life related to fecal incontinence in children with anorectal malformations and Hirschsprung's disease]. Rev Paul Pediatr. 2016;34(1):99–105.
75. Afshar K, Mirbagheri A, Scott H, MacNeily AE. Development of a symptom score for dysfunctional elimination syndrome. J Urol. 2009;182(4 Suppl):1939–43.

76. Farhat W, Bägli DJ, Capolicchio G, O'Reilly S, Merguerian PA, Khoury A, et al. The dysfunctional voiding scoring system: quantitative standardization of dysfunctional voiding symptoms in children. J Urol. 2000;164(3 Pt 2):1011–5.
77. van Engelenburg-van Lonkhuyzen ML, EMJ B, CHG B, Benninga MA, de Bie RA. Childhood bladder and bowel dysfunction questionnaire: development, feasibility, and aspects of validity and reliability. J Pediatr Gastroenterol Nutr. 2017;64(6):911–7.
78. Nelson CP, Park JM, Bloom DA, Wan J, Dunn RL, Wei JT. Incontinence symptom index-pediatric: development and initial validation of a urinary incontinence instrument for the older pediatric population. J Urol. 2007;178(4 Pt 2):1763–7. discussion 7
79. Akbal C, Genc Y, Burgu B, Ozden E, Tekgul S. Dysfunctional voiding and incontinence scoring system: quantitative evaluation of incontinence symptoms in pediatric population. J Urol. 2005;173(3):969–73.
80. Gontard AV, Kuwertz-Bröking E. The diagnosis and treatment of enuresis and functional daytime urinary incontinence. Dtsch Arztebl Int. 2019;116(16):279–85.
81. Bogaert G, Stein R, Undre S, RJM N, Quadackers J, t Hoen L, et al. Practical recommendations of the EAU-ESPU guidelines committee for monosymptomatic enuresis-Bedwetting. Neurourol Urodyn. 2020;39(2):489–97.
82. Chang SJ, Van Laecke E, Bauer SB, von Gontard A, Bagli D, Bower WF, et al. Treatment of daytime urinary incontinence: a standardization document from the International Children's Continence Society. Neurourol Urodyn. 2017;36(1):43–50.
83. Muddasani S, Moe A, Semmelrock C, Gilbert CL, Enemuo V, Chiou EH, et al. Physical therapy for fecal incontinence in children with pelvic floor dyssynergia. J Pediatr. 2017;190:74–8.
84. Paknejad MS, Motaharifard MS, Barimani S, Kabiri P, Karimi M. Traditional, complementary and alternative medicine in children constipation: a systematic review. Daru. 2019;27(2):811–26.
85. Hjalmas K, Arnold T, Bower W, Caione P, Chiozza LM, von Gontard A, et al. Nocturnal enuresis: an international evidence based management strategy. J Urol. 2004;171(6 Pt 2):2545–61.
86. van Engelenburg-van Lonkhuyzen ML, Bols E, Benninga M, Groen LA, Chase J, de Bie R. Physiotherapy interventions for functional bladder and bowel dysfunctions in neurologically normal and otherwise healthy children (Protocol). Cochrane Database Syst Rev. 2016(11):CD012434.
87. Hagstroem S, Rittig S, Kamperis K, Djurhuus JC. Timer watch assisted urotherapy in children: a randomized controlled trial. J Urol. 2010;184(4):1482–8.
88. Assis GM, Silva C, Martins G. Urotherapy in the treatment of children and adolescents with bladder and bowel dysfunction: a systematic review. J Pediatr (Rio J). 2019;95(6):628–41.
89. Lukacz ES, Sampselle C, Gray M, Macdiarmid S, Rosenberg M, Ellsworth P, et al. A healthy bladder: a consensus statement. Int J Clin Pract. 2011;65(10):1026–36.
90. Burgio KL, Newman DK, Rosenberg MT, Sampselle C. Impact of behaviour and lifestyle on bladder health. Int J Clin Pract. 2013;67(6):495–504.
91. Shorter B, Lesser M, Moldwin RM, Kushner L. Effect of comestibles on symptoms of interstitial cystitis. J Urol. 2007;178(1):145–52.
92. Tabbers MM, DiLorenzo C, Berger MY, Faure C, Langendam MW, Nurko S, et al. Evaluation and treatment of functional constipation in infants and children: evidence-based recommendations from ESPGHAN and NASPGHAN. J Pediatr Gastroenterol Nutr. 2014;58(2):258–74.
93. Gomes D, Morais MB. Gut microbiota and the use of probiotics in constipation in children and adolescents: systematic review. Rev Paul Pediatr. 2020;38:e2018123.
94. Wojtyniak K, Szajewska H. Systematic review: probiotics for functional constipation in children. Eur J Pediatr. 2017;176(9):1155–62.
95. van Engelenburg-van Lonkhuyzen ML, Bols EM, Benninga MA, Verwijs WA, de Bie RA. Effectiveness of pelvic physiotherapy in children with functional constipation compared with standard medical care. Gastroenterology. 2017;152(1):82–91.
96. Farahmand F, Abedi A, Esmaeili-Dooki MR, Jalilian R, Tabari SM. Pelvic floor muscle exercise for paediatric functional constipation. J Clin Diagn Res. 2015;9(6):Sc16–7.
97. van Summeren J, Holtman GA, Lisman-van Leeuwen Y, Louer L, van Ulsen-Rust AHC, Vermeulen KM, et al. Physiotherapy plus conventional treatment versus conventional treatment only in the treatment of functional constipation in children: design of a randomized controlled trial and cost-effectiveness study in primary care. BMC Pediatr. 2018;18(1):249.
98. Maizels M, King LR, Firlit CF. Urodynamic biofeedback: a new approach to treat vesical sphincter dyssynergia. J Urol. 1979;122(2):205–9.
99. Koenig JF, PH MK. Biofeedback therapy for dysfunctional voiding in children. Curr Urol Rep. 2011;12(2):144–52.
100. Kaye JD, Palmer LS. Animated biofeedback yields more rapid results than nonanimated biofeedback in the treatment of dysfunctional voiding in girls. J Urol. 2008;180(1):300–5.
101. Oktar T, Dönmez M, Özkuvancı Ü, Ander H, Ziylan O. Animated versus non-animated biofeedback therapy for dysfunctional voiding treatment: does it change the outcome? J Pediatr Surg. 2018;53(4):825–7.
102. Thompson JA, O'Sullivan PB, Briffa NK, Neumann P. Altered muscle activation patterns in symptom-

atic women during pelvic floor muscle contraction and Valsalva manouevre. Neurourol Urodyn. 2006;25(3):268–76.
103. Whittaker JL, Ellis R, Hodges PW, OS C, Hides J, Fernandez-Carnero S, et al. Imaging with ultrasound in physical therapy: what is the PT's scope of practice? A competency-based educational model and training recommendations. Br J Sports Med. 2019;53(23):1447–53.
104. Whittaker JL, Thompson JA, Teyhen DS, Hodges P. Rehabilitative ultrasound imaging of pelvic floor muscle function. J Orthop Sports Phys Ther. 2007;37(8):487–98.
105. Chen L, Luo D, Yu X, Jin M, Cai W. Predicting stress urinary incontinence during pregnancy: combination of pelvic floor ultrasound parameters and clinical factors. Acta Obstet Gynecol Scand. 2018;97(8):966–75.
106. Dietz HP, Wilson PD, Clarke B. The use of perineal ultrasound to quantify levator activity and teach pelvic floor muscle exercises. Int Urogynecol J Pelvic Floor Dysfunct. 2001;12(3):166–8. discussion 8–9
107. White RD, McQuown D, McCarthy TA, Ostergard DR. Real-time ultrasonography in the evaluation of urinary stress incontinence. Am J Obstet Gynecol. 1980;138(2):235–7.
108. Smith MD, Coppieters MW, Hodges PW. Postural activity of the pelvic floor muscles is delayed during rapid arm movements in women with stress urinary incontinence. Int Urogynecol J Pelvic Floor Dysfunct. 2007;18(8):901–11.
109. De Troyer A, Boriek AM. Mechanics of the respiratory muscles. Compr Physiol. 2011;1(3):1273–300.
110. Hodges PW, Gandevia SC. Activation of the human diaphragm during a repetitive postural task. J Physiol. 2000;522(Pt 1(Pt 1)):165–75.
111. Hodges PW, Butler JE, McKenzie DK, Gandevia SC. Contraction of the human diaphragm during rapid postural adjustments. J Physiol. 1997;505(Pt 2):539–48.
112. Emerich Gordon K, Reed O. The role of the pelvic floor in respiration: a multidisciplinary literature review. J Voice. 2020;34(2):243–9.
113. Tahan N, Rasouli O, Arab AM, Khademi K, Samani EN. Reliability of the ultrasound measurements of abdominal muscles activity when activated with and without pelvic floor muscles contraction. J Back Musculoskelet Rehabil. 2014;27(3):339–47.
114. Talasz H, Kofler M, Kalchschmid E, Pretterklieber M, Lechleitner M. Breathing with the pelvic floor? Correlation of pelvic floor muscle function and expiratory flows in healthy young nulliparous women. Int Urogynecol J. 2010;21(4):475–81.
115. Talasz H, Kremser C, Kofler M, Kalchschmid E, Lechleitner M, Rudisch A. Phase-locked parallel movement of diaphragm and pelvic floor during breathing and coughing-a dynamic MRI investigation in healthy females. Int Urogynecol J. 2011;22(1):61–8.
116. Talasz H, Kremser C, Kofler M, Kalchschmid E, Lechleitner M, Rudisch A. Proof of concept: differential effects of Valsalva and straining maneuvers on the pelvic floor. Eur J Obstet Gynecol Reprod Biol. 2012;164(2):227–33.
117. Neumann P, Gill V. Pelvic floor and abdominal muscle interaction: EMG activity and intra-abdominal pressure. Int Urogynecol J Pelvic Floor Dysfunct. 2002;13(2):125–32.
118. Talasz H, Kremser C, Talasz HJ, Kofler M, Rudisch A. Breathing, (S)Training and the pelvic floor-a basic concept. Healthcare (Basel). 2022;10(6):1035.
119. Sapsford RR, Hodges PW, Richardson CA, Cooper DH, Markwell SJ, Jull GA. Co-activation of the abdominal and pelvic floor muscles during voluntary exercises. Neurourol Urodyn. 2001;20(1):31–42.
120. Berghmans B, Seleme M. The '5 F's concept for pelvic floor muscle training: from finding the pelvic floor to functional use. J Womens Health Dev. 2020;3(2):131–4.
121. Bø K. Pelvic floor muscle training is effective in treatment of female stress urinary incontinence, but how does it work? Int Urogynecol J Pelvic Floor Dysfunct. 2004;15(2):76–84.
122. Sapsford R. Rehabilitation of pelvic floor muscles utilizing trunk stabilization. Man Ther. 2004;9(1):3–12.
123. Bradley H, Esformes J. Breathing pattern disorders and functional movement. Int J Sports Phys Ther. 2014;9(1):28–39.
124. Silva CA, Motta ME. The use of abdominal muscle training, breathing exercises and abdominal massage to treat paediatric chronic functional constipation. Colorectal Dis. 2013;15(5):e250–5.
125. Barroso U Jr, Tourinho R, Lordêlo P, Hoebeke P, Chase J. Electrical stimulation for lower urinary tract dysfunction in children: a systematic review of the literature. Neurourol Urodyn. 2011;30(8):1429–36.
126. Schreiner L, Santos TG, Souza AB, Nygaard CC, Silva Filho IG. Electrical stimulation for urinary incontinence in women: a systematic review. Int Braz J Urol. 2013;39(4):454–64.
127. Xu X, Zhang H, Yan Y, Wang J, Guo L. Effects of electrical stimulation on skin surface. Acta Mech Sin. 2021;37(12):1843–71.
128. Rahmati M, Gondin J, Malakoutinia F. Effects of neuromuscular electrical stimulation on quadriceps muscle strength and mass in healthy young and older adults: a scoping review. Phys Ther. 2021;101(9):pzab144.
129. Bower W, Yeung C. A review of non-invasive electro neuromodulation as an intervention for non-neurogenic bladder dysfunction in children. Neurourol Urodyn. 2004;23(1):63–7.
130. de Oliveira LF, de Oliveira DM, da Silva de Paula LI, de Figueiredo AA, de Bessa J Jr, de Sá CA, et al. Transcutaneous parasacral electrical neural stimulation in children with primary monosymptomatic

enuresis: a prospective randomized clinical trial. J Urol. 2013;190(4):1359–63.
131. Malm-Buatsi E, Nepple KG, Boyt MA, Austin JC, Cooper CS. Efficacy of transcutaneous electrical nerve stimulation in children with overactive bladder refractory to pharmacotherapy. Urology. 2007;70(5):980–3.
132. Sillén U, Arwidsson C, Doroszkiewicz M, Antonsson H, Jansson I, Stålklint M, et al. Effects of transcutaneous neuromodulation (TENS) on overactive bladder symptoms in children: a randomized controlled trial. J Pediatr Urol. 2014;10(6):1100–5.
133. Leong LC, Yik YI, Catto-Smith AG, Robertson VJ, Hutson JM, Southwell BR. Long-term effects of transabdominal electrical stimulation in treating children with slow-transit constipation. J Pediatr Surg. 2011;46(12):2309–12.
134. Tanagho EA, Schmidt RA, Orvis BR. Neural stimulation for control of voiding dysfunction: a preliminary report in 22 patients with serious neuropathic voiding disorders. J Urol. 1989;142(2 Pt 1):340–5.
135. Horrocks EJ, Thin N, Thaha MA, Taylor SJ, Norton C, Knowles CH. Systematic review of tibial nerve stimulation to treat faecal incontinence. Br J Surg. 2014;101(5):457–68.
136. Assmann SL, Keszthelyi D, Kleijnen J, Anastasiou F, Bradshaw E, Brannigan AE, et al. Guideline for the diagnosis and treatment of Faecal Incontinence-a UEG/ESCP/ESNM/ESPCG collaboration. United European Gastroenterol J. 2022;10(3):251–86.
137. Tong CMC, Kitchens DM. Neuromodulation for treatment of refractory non-neurogenic lower urinary tract symptoms in children: an overview. Curr Bladder Dysfunct Rep. 2023;18(1):59–63.
138. Iacona R, Ramage L, Malakounides G. Current state of neuromodulation for constipation and fecal incontinence in children: a systematic review. Eur J Pediatr Surg. 2019;29(6):495–503.
139. Abdelrahman EM, Abdel Ghafar MA, Selim AO, Ali OI, Balbaa MA. Biofeedback versus bilateral transcutaneous posterior tibial nerve stimulation in the treatment of functional non-retentive fecal incontinence in children: a randomized controlled trial. J Pediatr Surg. 2021;56(8):1349–55.
140. Mohamed A, Mahgoub MS, Elshafey MA. Efficacy of biofeedback and precautenous tibial nerve stimulation on functional faecal incontinence in children. Int J Ther Rehabil Res. 2016;5(4):215–23.
141. Southwell BR. Electro-neuromodulation for colonic disorders-review of meta-analyses, systematic reviews, and RCTs. Neuromodulation. 2020;23(8):1061–81.
142. Chase J, Robertson VJ, Southwell B, Hutson J, Gibb S. Pilot study using transcutaneous electrical stimulation (interferential current) to treat chronic treatment-resistant constipation and soiling in children. J Gastroenterol Hepatol. 2005;20(7):1054–61.
143. Goats G. Interferential current therapy. Br J Sports Med. 1990;24(2):87.
144. Sharifi-Rad L, Ladi-Seyedian SS, Kajbafzadeh AM. Interferential electrical stimulation efficacy in the management of lower urinary tract dysfunction in children: a review of the literature. Urol J. 2021;18(5):469–76.
145. Zivkovic VD, Stankovic I, Dimitrijevic L, Kocic M, Colovic H, Vlajkovic M, et al. Are interferential electrical stimulation and diaphragmatic breathing exercises beneficial in children with bladder and bowel dysfunction? Urology. 2017;102:207–12.
146. Dimitri P, Joshi K, Jones N. Moving more: physical activity and its positive effects on long term conditions in children and young people. Arch Dis Child. 2020;105(11):1035–40.
147. Nygaard IE, Shaw JM. Physical activity and the pelvic floor. Am J Obstet Gynecol. 2016;214(2):164–71.
148. Dakic JG, Cook J, Hay-Smith J, Lin KY, Frawley H. Pelvic floor disorders stop women exercising: a survey of 4556 symptomatic women. J Sci Med Sport. 2021;24(12):1211–7.
149. Wilkinson TJ, O'Mahoney LL, Highton P, Viana JL, Ribeiro HS, Lightfoot CJ, et al. Physical activity and the 'pediatric inactivity triad' in children living with chronic kidney disease: a narrative review. Ther Adv Chronic Dis. 2022;13:20406223221109971.
150. Bø K. Urinary incontinence, pelvic floor dysfunction, exercise and sport. Sports Med. 2004;34(7):451–64.
151. Seidenfaden S, Ormarsson OT, Lund SH, Bjornsson ES. Physical activity may decrease the likelihood of children developing constipation. Acta Paediatr. 2018;107(1):151–5.
152. Brands MM, Purperhart H, Deckers-Kocken JM. A pilot study of yoga treatment in children with functional abdominal pain and irritable bowel syndrome. Complement Ther Med. 2011;19(3):109–14.
153. Kilcik MH, Ozdemir F, Elmas AT. Effectiveness of game-based core exercise in children with non-neuropathic bladder dysfunction and comparison to biofeedback therapy. Low Urin Tract Symptoms. 2023;15(1):16–23.
154. Ladi Seyedian SS, Sharifi-Rad L, Ebadi M, Kajbafzadeh AM. Combined functional pelvic floor muscle exercises with Swiss ball and urotherapy for management of dysfunctional voiding in children: a randomized clinical trial. Eur J Pediatr. 2014;173(10):1347–53.
155. Akbayrak T, Özgül S, Orhan C. Fizyoterapi ve Rehabilitasyonda Klasik Masaj ve Konnektif Doku Masajı. Temel Fizyoterapi Rehabilitasyon. 2019.
156. Orhan C, Kaya Kara O, Kaya S, Akbayrak T, Kerem Gunel M, Baltaci G. The effects of connective tissue manipulation and Kinesio Taping on chronic constipation in children with cerebral palsy: a randomized controlled trial. Disabil Rehabil. 2018;40(1):10–20.
157. Dunn W. The sensations of everyday life: empirical, theoretical, and pragmatic considerations. Am J Occup Ther. 2001;55(6):608–20.
158. Fisher AG, Murray EA, Bundy AC. Sensory integration: theory and practice. Philadelphia: Davis Company; 1991.

159. Ermer J, Dunn W. The sensory profile: a discriminant analysis of children with and without disabilities. Am J Occup Ther. 1998;52(4):283–90.
160. Miller LJ, Anzalone ME, Lane SJ, Cermak SA, Osten ET. Concept evolution in sensory integration: a proposed nosology for diagnosis. The American Occupational Therapy Association, Inc.; 2007. p. 135–40.
161. Dunn W, Little L, Dean E, Robertson S, Evans B. The state of the science on sensory factors and their impact on daily life for children: a scoping review. OTJR (Thorofare N J). 2016;36(2 Suppl):3s–26s.
162. Beaudry-Bellefeuille I, Lane SJ, Ramos-Polo E. The toileting habit profile questionnaire: screening for sensory-based toileting difficulties in young children with constipation and retentive fecal incontinence. J Occup Ther Sch Early Interv. 2016;9(2):163–75.
163. Bellefeuille IB, Schaaf RC, Polo ER. Occupational therapy based on Ayres sensory integration in the treatment of retentive fecal incontinence in a 3-year-old boy. Am J Occup Ther. 2013;67(5):601–6.
164. Little LM, Benton K, Manuel-Rubio M, Saps M, Fishbein M. Contribution of sensory processing to chronic constipation in preschool children. J Pediatr. 2019;210:141–5.
165. Tharner A, Jansen PW, Kiefte-de Jong JC, Moll HA, Hofman A, Jaddoe VW, et al. Bidirectional associations between fussy eating and functional constipation in preschool children. J Pediatr. 2015;166(1):91–6. e1.
166. Leekam SR, Nieto C, Libby SJ, Wing L, Gould J. Describing the sensory abnormalities of children and adults with autism. J Autism Dev Disord. 2007;37:894–910.
167. Craig AD. How do you feel? Interoception: the sense of the physiological condition of the body. Nat Rev Neurosci. 2002;3(8):655–66.
168. Swithinbank L, Heron J, Von Gontard A, Abrams P. The natural history of daytime urinary incontinence in children: a large British cohort. Acta Paediatr. 2010;99(7):1031–6.
169. Franco I. Neuropsychiatric disorders and voiding problems in children. Curr Urol Rep. 2011;12(2):158–65.
170. von Gontard A, Heron J, Joinson C. Factors associated with low and high voiding frequency in children with diurnal urinary incontinence. BJU Int. 2010;105(3):396–401.
171. Koshy NM, Sugi S, Rajendran K. A study to identify prevalence and effectiveness of sensory integration on toilet skill problems among sensory processing disorder. Indian J Occup Ther. 2018;50(3):86–91.
172. Shamsoddini A, Hollisaz M. Effect of sensory integration therapy on gross motor function in children with cerebral palsy. Iran J Child Neurol. 2009;3(1):43–8.
173. Shamsoddini A. Comparison between the effect of neurodevelopmental treatment and sensory integration therapy on gross motor function in children with cerebral palsy. Iran J Child Neurol. 2010;4(1):31–8.
174. Dunn W. Supporting children to participate successfully in everyday life by using sensory processing knowledge. Infants Young Children. 2007;20(2):84–101.
175. Mazurek MO, Vasa RA, Kalb LG, Kanne SM, Rosenberg D, Keefer A, et al. Anxiety, sensory over-responsivity, and gastrointestinal problems in children with autism spectrum disorders. J Abnorm Child Psychol. 2013;41:165–76.
176. Frank C, Kobesova A, Kolar P. Dynamic neuromuscular stabilization & sports rehabilitation. Int J Sports Phys Ther. 2013;8(1):62.
177. Davidek P, Andel R, Kobesova A. Influence of dynamic neuromuscular stabilization approach on maximum kayak paddling force. J Hum Kinet. 2018;61:15–27.
178. Yoon HS, You JSH. Reflex-mediated dynamic neuromuscular stabilization in stroke patients: EMG processing and ultrasound imaging. Technol Health Care. 2017;25(S1):99–106.
179. Kim DH, An DH, Yoo WG. Effects of 4 weeks of dynamic neuromuscular stabilization training on balance and gait performance in an adolescent with spastic hemiparetic cerebral palsy. J Phys Ther Sci. 2017;29(10):1881–2.
180. Son MS, Jung DH, You JSH, Yi CH, Jeon HS, Cha YJ. Effects of dynamic neuromuscular stabilization on diaphragm movement, postural control, balance and gait performance in cerebral palsy. NeuroRehabilitation. 2017;41(4):739–46.
181. Kim DH, Lee JJ, You SJH. Best core stabilization exercise to facilitate subcortical neuroplasticity: A functional MRI neuroimaging study. Technol Health Care. 2018;26(3):401–7.
182. Kolar P, Kobesova A, Valouchova P, Bitnar P. Dynamic neuromuscular stabilization: developmental kinesiology: breathing stereotypes and postural-locomotion function. Recognizing and treating breathing disorders. 2014. p. 11–22.
183. Teles A, Lordêlo P. Alarm for the treatment of enuresis: review of treatment types and treatment efficacy. J Sleep Med Disord 2016;3(6):1066.
184. Keten T, Aslan Y, Balci M, Erkan A, Senel C, Oguz U, et al. Comparison of the efficacy of desmopressin fast-melting formulation and enuretic alarm in the treatment of monosymptomatic nocturnal enuresis. J Pediatr Urol. 2020;16(5):645.e1–.e7.
185. Peng CC, Yang SS, Austin PF, Chang SJ. Systematic review and meta-analysis of alarm versus desmopressin therapy for pediatric monosymptomatic enuresis. Sci Rep. 2018;8(1):16755.
186. Purnomo AF, Daryanto B, Nurhadi P. Monosymptomatic nocturnal enuresis treatment using alarm-therapy and desmopressin: a meta-analysis approach. Med Arch. 2021;75(6):431–5.
187. Perrin N, Sayer L, While A. The efficacy of alarm therapy versus desmopressin therapy in the treatment of primary mono-symptomatic nocturnal enuresis: a systematic review. Prim Health Care Res Dev. 2015;16(1):21–31.

188. Bayne AP, Skoog SJ. Nocturnal enuresis: an approach to assessment and treatment. Pediatr Rev. 2014;35(8):327–34. quiz 35
189. Alqannad EM, Alharbi AS, Almansour RA, Alghamdi MS. Alarm therapy in the treatment of enuresis in children: types and efficacy review. Cureus. 2021;13(8):e17358.
190. Yeşilyurt SY, Birinci T, Hantal SB. Function, pain and dynamic balance before and after kinesio taping in older women with knee osteoarthritis: a pilot study. Celal Bayar Üniversitesi Sağlık Bilimleri Enstitüsü Dergisi. 2022;9(2):283–9.
191. Lu Z, Li X, Chen R, Guo C. Kinesio taping improves pain and function in patients with knee osteoarthritis: a meta-analysis of randomized controlled trials. Int J Surg. 2018;59:27–35.
192. Krajczy M, Luniewski J, Bogacz K, Szczegielniak J. Evaluation of applying Kinesio taping in children with urinary incontinence. J Pediatr Urol. 2018;14(6):550.e1–.e6.
193. Yang C, Hao Z, Zhang LL, Guo Q. Efficacy and safety of acupuncture in children: an overview of systematic reviews. Pediatr Res. 2015;78(2):112–9.
194. Arnouk A, De E, Rehfuss A, Cappadocia C, Dickson S, Lian F. Physical, complementary, and alternative medicine in the treatment of pelvic floor disorders. Curr Urol Rep. 2017;18(6):47.
195. Adams D, Cheng F, Jou H, Aung S, Yasui Y, Vohra S. The safety of pediatric acupuncture: a systematic review. Pediatrics. 2011;128(6):e1575–87.
196. Yang M, Gao S, Yao H, He X, Fang J, Chen Y, et al. Effects of electroacupuncture on pediatric chronic urinary retention: a case-series study. Front Pediatr. 2023;11:1194651.
197. Abd El Azeem AM, Alsharnoubi J, Abd El-Rahman Mohamed M. Laser acupuncture improving functional chronic constipation in children: a randomized controlled trial. Lasers Med Sci. 2023;38(1):72.
198. Lee T, Suh HJ, Lee HJ, Lee JE. Comparison of effects of treatment of primary nocturnal enuresis with oxybutynin plus desmopressin, desmopressin alone or imipramine alone: a randomized controlled clinical trial. J Urol. 2005;174(3):1084–7.
199. Gordon M, MacDonald JK, Parker CE, Akobeng AK, Thomas AG. Osmotic and stimulant laxatives for the management of childhood constipation. Cochrane Database Syst Rev. 2016;2016(8):Cd009118.